Patient Treatment Adherence
Concepts, Interventions,
and Measurement

Patient Treatment Adherence Concepts, Interventions, and Measurement

Edited by

Hayden B. Bosworth
Eugene Z. Oddone
Morris Weinberger

Center for Health Services Research in Primary Care,
Durham Veterans Affairs Medical Center (VAMC)
Division of General Internal Medicine,
Duke University Medical Center
Department of Health Policy and Administration,
University of North Carolina at Chapel Hill

LEA LAWRENCE ERLBAUM ASSOCIATES, PUBLISHERS
2006   Mahwah, New Jersey   London

Lawrence Erlbaum Associates, Inc., Publishers
10 Industrial Avenue
Mahwah, New Jersey 07430
www.erlbaum.com

Cover design by Kathryn Houghtaling Lacey

Library of Congress Cataloging-in-Publication Data

Bosworth, Hayden B.
  Patient treatment adherence concepts, interventions, and measurement /
Hayden B. Bosworth, Eugene Z. Oddone, and Morris Weinberger.
      p.   cm.
  Includes bibliographical references and index.
  ISBN 0-8058-4833-9 (alk. paper)
  1. Patient compliance.   I. Oddone, Eugene Z.   II. Weinberger, Morris.   III. Title.

R727.43.B67   2005
615.5—dc22   2004062505
                                                                    CIP

Books published by Lawrence Erlbaum Associates are printed on acid-free paper,
and their bindings are chosen for strength and durability.

Printed in the United States of America
10 9 8 7 6 5 4 3 2 1

Contents

Preface

Although investigators have studied patient adherence since at least the late 1940s, the past 25 years has witnessed an explosion of adherence-related research in response to the growing burden of chronic diseases and the emphasis on patient self-management. Understanding the nature, causes, and consequences of nonadherence is critical to developing effective strategies to enhance adherence and, ultimately, improve patient outcomes. Thus, the goal of the book is to summarize the state of the adherence literature for a number of specific health behaviors and populations.

As described in this book, there exists a bewildering literature regarding the conceptualization, interventions, and measurement of treatment adherence, thereby creating inefficiencies and confusion among investigators. Thus, this book provides: (a) a conceptual definition of treatment adherence using multiple models, (b) a summary of existing literature regarding the impact of treatment nonadherence (e.g., costs, clinical outcomes, health-related quality of life), and (c) a review of patient factors related to treatment adherence for specific behaviors (i.e., diet, exercise, medication use), as well as across diseases and special populations (e.g., children, patient–physician interaction). Finally, we discuss important methodological issues related to treatment adherence, including community-based interventions, measurement and analytical issues, assessing cost-effectiveness, translation and dissemination of results into practice, and the use of new technological advances to improve treatment adherence.

Our primary audiences are researchers including health service researchers, health psychologists, social psychologists, and cognitive psychologists, as well as primary-care physicians, policymakers, and health managers responsible for quality improvement within a health organization. It is anticipated that the book could be used as a potential text for graduate courses on health behaviors, applied statistics, and public health as well as medical school programs on patient–physician interaction.

We have organized the book into four parts. Part I (chaps. 1 and 2) presents problems associated with treatment adherence and summarizes various theoretical models that have commonly been used to understand, predict, and/or improve adherences (e.g., health belief model, theory of planned behavior, and transtheoretical model). These models share an emphasis on patients' cognitive and social processes (e.g., beliefs, norms) and patients' resources (e.g., psychologic and social support). Part II addresses adherence with specific behaviors, including exercise, diet, smoking, rehabilitation, medication, and psychological therapies (chaps. 3–7). Understanding adherence to these behaviors is important because factors affecting adherence for each specific behavior are likely to be similar across chronic diseases and conditions. Each chapter begins by discussing the impact of treatment adherence for specific health behaviors (e.g., prevalence, costs, clinical outcomes, health-related quality of life). Part III (chaps. 8–12) is organized by special areas and populations, including depression, children, parent–provider communication, and provider guideline adherence. Chapters throughout this part highlight strategies that were both successful and unsuccessful in enhancing adherence. Each chapter provides a discussion on the clinical, research, and when appropriate, policy implications. The final part of the book (chaps. 13–17) discusses methodological issues related to treatment adherence including community-based models of interventions, analytical and methodological issues specifically related to nonadherence, assessing the cost-effectiveness of adherence interventions, translation and dissemination of results into practice, and the use of new technological advances to improve treatment adherence.

Introductory Remarks

As health care has transitioned from treating acute illness to treating chronic ailments, we have moved from curing disorders to controlling symptoms and improving quality of life. Sometimes, these regimens can be quite complex and difficult for patients to follow. Moreover, beyond therapeutic agents, improved health often requires modifying behaviors to encourage such changes as weight loss, cessation of smoking, and increasing exercise. Following complex medication regimens and modifying activities require complex and difficult behavioral changes by patients. Thus, patients must have a long-term commitment to complex regimens that emphasize patient self-management (1–3). Perhaps Mark Twain's astute comment best summarizes the problem: "Habit is habit, and not to be flung out the window, but coaxed downstairs a step at a time."

Though enhancing adherence is complex, the rationale for doing so is clear: Patients' outcomes will be maximized if health care providers make appropriate recommendations *and* patients have the requisite knowledge, motivation, skills, and resources to follow the recommendations. Viewed in this way, patient adherence to physicians' recommendations is the key mediator between medical practice and patient outcome. However, there are many places where this process may break down. Some individuals do not receive appropriate advice; others may follow the advice exactly, but not benefit from treatments; and others follow the advice incompletely, inconsistently, or not at all.

Adherence has been a major focus of researchers from various disciplines: A Medline search identified more than 10,000 papers related to nonadherence that were published during the last 10 years. The vast majority of these papers characterized factors associated with, and barriers to, adherence. However, relatively little progress has been made in demonstrating the effectiveness of pragmatic strategies to enhance adherence. Whereas randomized controlled trials have identified several strategies to help patients to follow their treatment regimens (4), many other interventions have been either ineffective or too labor-intensive and expensive to be pragmatic. In addition, there is a lot of "reinventing the wheel." That is, practitioners and scientists interested in resolving barriers to adherence often begin from scratch, rather than capitalize on the research of others. Once effective and pragmatic strategies have been identified, the challenge will be to get this information to providers, administrators, and policymakers in order to improve patients' health outcomes.

For the effective provision of care for chronic conditions, it is necessary to activate the patient and the patient's community of support (5). A continuous effort must be made to improve the provision of information to patients, but motivation, which drives sustainable good adherence, is one of the most difficult elements for the health care system to provide. Although health professionals have an important role in activating patients through promoting optimism, providing enthusiasm, and encouraging maintenance of health behaviors (6), the health systems and health care teams experience difficulties in sustaining these efforts. These difficulties have led to an increased interest in the role of community-based educational and/or self-management programs aimed at the creation and maintenance of healthy habits, including adherence to health recommendations.

Brief descriptions of each chapter follow:

• In chapter 1, Bosworth, Weinberger, and Oddone provide a general introduction to the issue of treatment adherence.

• In chapter 2, Bosworth and Voils present various theoretical models that have been used to understand, predict, and/or improve adherence.

• In chapter 3, Dominick and Morey focus on the initiation and maintenance of exercise. They summarize the vast literature on factors related to poor exercise adherence, and they describe various behavioral interventions that have demonstrated efficacy in enhancing physical-activity levels among communities and within structured programs.

• In chapter 4, Yancy and Boan review problems with assessing adherence to diet, the current media interest in low-carbohydrate versus low-fat diets, and interventions clinicians can easily implement to improve diet and reduce weight.

• In chapter 5, Bastian and colleagues discuss the importance of short- and long-term smoking cessation. The most successful interventions (cessation rates over 50%) incorporate multiple components (e.g., tailored print materials, telephone counseling, nicotine replacement therapy). They discuss the importance of capitalizing on "teachable moments" by targeting special populations (e.g., patients with a recent diagnosis of heart disease or cancer) using multicomponent interventions.

• Bosworth, in chapter 6, highlights important advances in medication adherence. Beyond describing potential factors related to medication adherence, this chapter reviews the relative strengths and weaknesses of alternative measures of medication adherence. Educational, behavioral, and multifaceted interventions are discussed.

• Zinn, in chapter 7, highlights developments in rehabilitation, a relatively unexplored area of adherence. Adding complexity to studies of adherence in rehabilitation are three considerations not generally found in chronic-disease management: (a) many conditions that require rehabilitation have both an acute and postacute or chronic phase that have different treatments, (b) the rehabilitation population includes a large proportion of patients with physical or cognitive impairments that are not readily accounted for in the normative-based theoretical models of adherence presented in chapter 2, and (c) many rehabilitation patients who require adaptive technology (e.g., wheelchairs, walkers) experience stigma not found in many other chronic diseases.

• In chapter 8, Cheng and Walter discuss unique issues related to maintaining treatment adherence among children such as need for independence among children and the need for practitioners to be aware of the additional dimension of complexity introduced by the interests of the parent or caregiver. Specific methods for enhancing treatment adherence for this group are provided.

• Chapter 9 addresses adherence issues related to depression. Specifically, the authors identify the independent effects of depression on adherence to medical treatments, mental-health treatments, and preventive care. This chapter is particularly important given that the increased number of problems and severity of depression is correlated with increased complexity of the treatment, increased risk of depression, and increased likelihood of treatment nonadherence.

• Chapter 10 addresses treatment adherence among individuals with severe mental illness, particular schizophrenia and posttraumatic stress disorder. The cost of nonadherence for these extremely disabling diseases is discussed, as are potential factors related to nonadherence. Notably, impaired thought processes and potential side effects of many prescribed medications pose significant challenges to patients and clinicians.

• Provider–patient communication has been identified as one of the most important factors for improving patient adherence. In chapter 11, Alexander and colleagues examine the underlining mechanisms that mediate how provider–patient communication affects treatment adherence. They discuss the unique communication challenges encountered when providers work with diverse patient populations, specifically covering issues related to cultural competency, health literacy, and working with elderly patients with complex treatment regimens. Then, they review interventions to improve provider–patient communication and patient adherence to treatment regimens. The chapter closes with a discussion of the limitations of existing research on provider–patient communication and treatment adherence and directions for future research.

• Weinberger and Salz (chap. 12) focus on physician adherence to clinical practice guidelines. The authors review the development of clinical practice guidelines; issues related to defining and measuring adherence to guidelines; strategies that have been successful or unsuccessful in increasing adherence to guidelines; and challenges for researchers and policymakers interested in evaluating and/or implementing innovative strategies to enhance adherence to guidelines.

• In chapter 13, Ammerman and Tajik present three frameworks that help improve treatment adherence at multiple levels of a continuum rather than solely at the individual level: (a) a socioecologic framework, which provides a multilevel model that describes the impact on behavior at various levels; (b) the RE-AIM model (7) on translating "proven" interventions to everyday settings; and (c) the importance of community-based participatory research, which allows researchers to reach a broader population more effectively and have a meaningful and sustainable impact on adherence at multiple levels over time.

• Van Houtven, Weinberger, and Carey (chap. 14) present a model to illustrate how researchers might consider the cost of nonadherence in their work. They review the economics literature on studies of nonadherence, as well as economic evaluation methods and health utility preference measures. The mechanics of adapting the cost-effectiveness calculation to incorporate nonadherence are discussed and a template of costs and effects that researchers should consider, including how these considerations influence the study design and interpretation, is presented. Finally, the authors discuss the implications of considering nonadherence costs in health policy.

• In chapter 15, Anstrom, Weinfurt, and Allen focus on the effects of nonadherence on the interpretations of clinical study findings. This has been the subject of much recent work in statistical methods. The intent in this chapter is to convey the key concepts using simple examples without focusing on computational and implementation issues.

• One possible reason for the lack of improvement in treatment adherence may be the ineffective dissemination of interventions. Chapter 16 addresses the issue that developing and disseminating evidence-based guidelines to improve treatment adherence is a complex system that exists in a dynamic equilibrium. Matchar and colleagues discuss the substantial efforts have been made to find tools that will improve adherence with guidelines, and many are creative solutions to specific barriers to practice improvement. They describe one approach to practice improvement that builds on the general principles of total quality management for process improvement and discuss their experience implementing this approach.

- Skinner and colleagues (chap. 17) describe new technologies and their influence on existing adherence interventions focuses on how tailoring technology has been used in adherence-promoting interventions. They present examples that illustrate various types of tailored interventions and summarize what can and cannot be concluded about the effectiveness of tailored adherence interventions.

REFERENCES

1. DiMatteo M, DiNicola, DD. *Achieving Patient Compliance*. Elmsford, NY: Pergamon Press Inc.; 1982.
2. DiMatteo MR. Enhancing patient adherence to medical recommendations. *JAMA*. 1994;271(1):79, 83.
3. Shumaker SA. *The Handbook of Health Behavior Change*. 2nd ed. New York: Springer; 1998.
4. Haynes RB, Montague P, Oliver T, et al. Interventions for helping patients to follow prescriptions for medications. *Cochrane Database Syst Rev*. 2000(2): CD000011.
5. McCann K. AIDS in the Nineties: from science to policy. Care in the community and by the community. *AIDS Care*. 1990;2(4):421–424.
6. Lo R. Correlates of expected success at adherence to health regimen of people with IDDM. *J Adv Nurs*. 1999;30(2):418–424.
7. Glasgow RE, Davis CL, Funnell MM, et al. Implementing practical interventions to support chronic illness self-management. *Jt Comm J Qual Saf*. 2003;29(11): 563–574.

Contributors

Stewart Alexander, PhD
Durham Veterans Affairs Medical
    Center

Andrew Allen, PhD
Duke University Medical Center

Alice Ammerman, PhD
University of North Carolina at
    Chapel Hill

Kevin Anstrom, PhD
Duke University Medical Center

Lori Bastian, MD, MPH
Durham Veterans Affairs Medical
    Center
Duke University Medical Center

Hayden B. Bosworth, PhD
Durham Veterans Affairs Medical
    Center
Duke University Medical Center

Jarol Boan, MD
Duke University Medical Center

Marian Butterfield, MD, MPH
Durham Veterans Affairs Medical
    Center
Duke University Medical Center

Patrick Calhoun, PhD
Durham Veterans Affairs Medical
    Center
Duke University Medical Center

Marci Campbell
University of North Carolina at
    Chapel Hill

Tim Carey, MD
University of North Carolina at
    Chapel Hill

Jennifer Cheng, MD
Duke University Medical Center

Kelli Dominick, PhD
Durham Veterans Affairs Medical
    Center
Duke University Medical Center

Laura Fish, MPH
Duke University Medical Center

Carol Golin, MD
University of North Carolina at
  Chapel Hill

Jodi Gonzalez, PhD
UT Health Science Center

Carolyn T. Kalinowski, MPH
University of North Carolina at
  Chapel Hill

Sarah Kobrin, PhD
Duke University Medical Center

David Matchar, MD
Center for Clinical Health Policy
  Research
Duke University Medical Center
Durham Veterans Affairs Medical
  Center

Colleen McBride, PhD
Branch Chief, Social and Behavioral
  Research Branch, National Institutes
  of Health

Stephanie Molner, MSW
Duke University Medical Center

Miriam Morey, PhD
Durham Veterans Affairs Medical
  Center
Duke University Medical Center

Eugene Oddone, MD, MHSc
Durham Veterans Affairs Medical
  Center
Duke University Medical Center

Meenal B. Patwardhan, MD, MHSA
Duke Center for Clinical Health
  Policy Research
Duke University Medical Center

Talya Salz
University of North Carolina at
  Chapel Hill

Greg Samsa, PhD
Duke Center for Clinical Health
  Policy Research
Duke University Medical Center

Celette Skinner, PhD
Duke University Medical Center

Betsy Sleath, PhD
University of North Carolina at
  Chapel Hill

Lisa A. Sutherland
School of Public Health
University of North Carolina at
  Chapel Hill

Mansoureh Tajik, PhD
University of North Carolina at
  Chapel Hill

Courtney Van Houtven, PhD
Durham Veterans Affairs Medical
  Center
Duke University Medical Center

Corrine Voils, PhD
Durham Veterans Affairs Medical
  Center
Duke University Medical Center

Emmanuel Chip Walter, MD
Duke University Medical Center

Morris Weinberger, PhD
Durham Veterans Affairs Medical
  Center
School of Public Health
University of North Carolina at
  Chapel Hill

Kevin Weinfurt, PhD
Duke University Medical Center

John Williams, MD
Durham Veterans Affairs Medical
  Center
Duke University Medical Center

William Yancy, MD
Durham Veterans Affairs Medical
  Center
Durham Veterans Affairs Medical

Sandra Zinn, PhD
Durham Veterans Affairs Medical
  Center
Duke University Medical Center

Part I

WHAT IS TREATMENT ADHERENCE?

Chapter 1

Introduction

Hayden B. Bosworth
Morris Weinberger
Eugene Z. Oddone

DEFINING TREATMENT NONADHERENCE

Treatment adherence has been examined from various scientific perspectives and it has an important influence on treatment effectiveness. There is confusion about the conceptual and operational definitions of treatment adherence. In part, this may be attributed to the multitude of terms that have often been used interchangeably to refer to this concept. For example, *compliance, cooperation, concordance, mutuality,* and *therapeutic alliance* have been used, and operational definitions of these terms vary widely across studies (1). Most definitions contain elements relating to patients' self-care responsibilities, their role in the treatment process, and their collaboration with health care providers.

Though providers have known about the problem of patient adherence since beginning of medicine, researchers have studied patient adherence since at least the late 1940s (2). As a response to the growing burden of chronic diseases and providers' increasing reliance on patient self-management, research in patient adherence has grown significantly over the last 30 years since Sackett (3); later Haynes (4) provided us with the most cited definition of compliance: "the extent to which a person's behavior [in terms of taking medication, following a diet, modifying habits, or attending clinics] coincides with medical or health advice" (4). Subsequent authors have objected to the term compliance because it implies subservience on the part of the patient. Thus, the terms adherence or concordance are generally more preferred (5). The term adherence is used through this book. Adherence connotes the patient's participation and engagement in maintaining a regimen she or he believes will be beneficial, strongly implying a therapeutic partnership with providers that is essential for the patients' successfully following the prescribed treatment regimen. Similar to the World Health Organization recommendation (6), it is also recognized that adherence to a regimen may reflect behavior ranging from seeking medical attention and filling prescriptions to obtaining immunizations and executing behavioral modifications that address self-management of disease (e.g., medications, smoking, diet, physical activity).

The lack of a generally accepted definition of treatment adherence makes it difficult to measure the concept. As a behavioral concept, treatment adherence involves complex actions, intentions, emotions, and phenomena that may not be directly observable. Therefore, self-reports have the advantage of revealing the patient's own assessment of treatment adherence. Outcome-oriented definitions (e.g., cure rate, serum level, clinical parameters) have the advantage of being "objective," but may not reflect adherence because of the complex processes required to achieve these outcomes. Process-oriented indicators make use of intermediate variables such as appointment keeping or pill counts to measure adherence (7). Other measurement issues include: (a) the degree of adherence (e.g., perfect adherence, partial adherence, complete nonadherence), (b) scale of measurement, that is, as a continuous ratio (percent adherence) versus categorical (e.g., good vs. poor adherence), and (c) combining indicators of adherence with multiple aspects of the regimen (e.g., index score vs. separate analyses). Measurement issues may also vary with the disease being studied. For example, to receive benefits for HIV/AIDS requires complete adherence, whereas patients with many other chronic diseases can miss some medication doses and still receive the benefits. Another issue involves differences between short- (e.g., antibiotics) and long-term (e.g., chronic medication, exercise, diet) behavioral regimens.

MAGNITUDE OF TREATMENT NONADHERENCE

Given these challenges to conceptualizing and measuring regimen adherence, it is not surprising that research reviews find wide ranges of adherence among patients, ranging from 0% to over 100% (overuse) with 50% adherence being an average (8–10). In a recent meta-analysis of 569 studies reporting adherence to medical treatment prescribed by a nonpsychiatrist physician, the average nonadherence rate was 24.8%. Adherence was highest in HIV disease, arthritis, gastrointestinal disorders, and cancers; it was lowest in pulmonary disease, diabetes, and sleep disorders (2). For behaviors involving lifestyle modifications (e.g., exercise, diet, smoking cessation), treatment adherence rates are distressingly poor (11, 12). Smoking cessation, exercise, and dietary modification can be extraordinarily difficult for patients to carry out and maintain successfully. Some medical practitioners are discouraged by their patients' failures to adhere and may be reluctant even to make preventive recommendations or provide reminders regarding the actions that may protect a patient's health. A 2003 Institute of Medicine report suggests that greater efforts to help people quit smoking, lose weight, and change other unhealthy behaviors could lead to a 29% decline in United States cancer rates by 2015; by decreasing risky health behaviors, the number of lung cancer cases could be cut in half and the number of colon cancers cut by a third (http://www.nap.edu/catalog/10263.html?onpi_newbooks_031403).

IMPACT OF MEDICAL REGIMEN NONADHERENCE

Nonadherence can result in tangible and intangible consequences, including suffering and death; diminished quality of life; and provider and patient frustration, anger, and hopelessness. Poor adherence can compromise the effectiveness of treatment and result in increased morbidity and health care costs. Nonadherence to medication regimens is estimated to result in 125,000 deaths in the United States per year (13). At least 10% of all hospitalizations and nearly one quarter of all nursing home admissions result from to patients' nonadherence with medications (14). More than one third of hospital admissions for heart failure results from nonadherence with dietary and medication regimens (15, 16). Small deviations from immunosuppressive therapy are associated with untoward outcomes, including organ rejections in transplant recipients. However, it is important to acknowledge that, in some cases, nonadherence may be beneficial if it prevents adverse drug reactions that might have occurred (17). Nonadherence may represent rational choice as patients attempt to maintain their personal identity to achieve their goals and preserve their quality of life (18–20).

Poor treatment adherence can have societal impacts as well. Nonadherence, for example, has a significant role in the reemergence of drug-resistant organisms (21) including tuberculosis (22). Nonadherence also contributes to waste of resources and the loss of health care dollars and productivity. It has been suggested that the offering of medical recommendations that are misunderstood or subsequently forgotten or ignored is a waste of scarce health care resources and suggests a systemic problem (2).

In research, nonadherence impacts the evaluation of the therapies. Because poor adherence to a treatment protocol can underestimate that intervention's effectiveness, either study power is reduced or additional subjects are required in order to attain a measurable effect, at increased study cost (23). Furthermore, nonadherence to experimental treatment may underestimate the incidence of side effects or result in an overestimation of the optimal dosage for therapeutic efficacy. The trial's internal validity may be threatened by differential adherence across experimental conditions (24). Though much research regarding adherence has been focused on the negative impact of nonadherence, it is important to acknowledge that adherence can also be detrimental. In one trial, for example, adherence to what turned out to be a detrimental medication resulted in increased arrhythmic mortality among the active medication group and expedited the termination of two of the active drugs (25).

KEY DETERMINANTS OF TREATMENT NONADHERENCE

In general, a multitude of studies examining determinants of treatment adherence demonstrate that there is no "stereotypical" nonadherer, and clinicians are unable to predict who is likely to adhere any better than chance. There are, however, four characteristics that do increase patients' risk of nonadherence. First, difficult social circumstances (e.g., marital discord, social isolation, family conflict and dysfunction) predict adherence difficulty, whereas increased levels of family support, cohesion, and organization are associated with better adherence (26). DiMatteo, for example, reported in a meta-analysis of 122 studies that treatment adherence is 1.74 times higher in patients from cohesive families and 1.52 times lower in patients from families in conflict (27). Second, access to care and financial barriers limit treatment adherence. For example, after controlling for various covariates, more-educated HIV-positive patients were found to be more likely to adhere to therapy; and similarly among diabetics, the less-educated were much more likely to switch treatment, which led to more health problems (28). In another study, it was reported that 2 million elderly beneficiaries did not adhere to drug treatment regimens due to cost. Lower income beneficiaries with high out-of-pocket drug spending appear especially vulnerable to nonadherence (29). Third, patients with psychiatric disorders including dementia (30, 31) and substance use problems (32–34) are less likely to adhere to medication regimens. Fourth, medical regimen nonadherence is less problematic when the recommended regimen is a short-term intervention for an acute problem, particularly one with a salient symptom such as pain. However, chronic illnesses, especially those that are asymptomatic, are associated with higher nonadherence. For example, after 5 years of statin treatment only 25% of patients maintained an adherence rate (proportion of days covered) of at least 80% (35) and within 6 months of statin initiation at least 25% of the patients discontinued therapy (36). This makes sense, because chronic disease is defined by a lifelong commitment to a regimen.

ASSESSING TREATMENT ADHERENCE IN CLINICAL PRACTICE

Because physician assessments of patients' adherence is often inaccurate, other measures of adherence are more difficult to implement in clinical practice. However, there are three simple techniques that can be used by providers to detect poor treatment adherence. First, providers can watch for patients who fail to attend appointments. Not only can these patients be dropping out of treatment, but they are also less likely to be following their prescribed regimens. Second, clinicians should watch for treatment responses. For patients whose conditions fail to respond to appropriate therapy, for example, nonadherence is one plausible explanation. Third, and most important, clinicians should ask patients about their nonadherence. When asked in a nonthreatening manner (e.g., "Many people have difficulty time exercising. During the past week, how much physical activity have you gotten?"), patients will often admit nonadherence. A meta-analysis has shown that simply asking the patient has a sensitivity of 55% with a specificity of 87% (37). Armed with this knowledge, physicians can elicit barriers to adherence and offer potential solutions. Notably, treatment adherence is not a unidimensional construct: Adherence to one component of a regimen is not necessarily related to other self-treatment behaviors (38). For example, medication recommendations are more likely to be followed, whereas such lifestyle changes as diet and exercise tend to be more problematic (39). Thus, physicians should ask about adherence to each aspect of a patient's regimen.

SUMMARY OF ADHERENCE INTERVENTIONS

Treatment adherence is a complex behavioral process determined by many interacting factors. These include attributes of the patient, the patient's environment (e.g., social support) the health care system (e.g., functioning of the health care team, availability of health care resources), and characteristics of the disease. Most research on adherence focuses on a health outcome and presumes that adherence to selected recommendations mediates or facilitates achievement of the desired outcome. Although studies have examined efforts to improve adherence, few are randomized controlled trials with adherence as the outcome (40, 41). The most promising strategies for improving treatment adherence involve patient education (42), contracts (43), self-monitoring (44), social support (45), telephone follow-up, and tailoring (46, 47); multicomponent strategies tend to be more effective in improving poor adherence (48). Managing risk factors by multidisciplinary teams within systems designed to modify health care delivery and respond to patient and provider needs have been more successful than physicians alone providing interventions in a traditional, minimally structured environment (49, 50).

Increasing the effectiveness of adherence interventions may have a far greater impact on health of the population than any improvements in specific medical treatments (51). There continues to be a tendency to focus on patient-related factors as the causes of problems with adherence to relative neglect of provider and health system–related determinants. In general, the ability of patients to follow treatment plans is frequently compromised by a number of barriers, which may include social and economic factors, the health care system, the characteristics of the disease, disease therapies, and patient-related factors. Thus, successful interventions must address these multiple factors if patients' adherence to therapies is to be improved. Because there is no single intervention strategy shown to be effective across all patients, conditions, and settings, interventions that target adherence must be tailored to the particular illness-related demands experienced by the patient. To accomplish this, health professionals need to be trained in assessing risk of nonadherence, factors that influence adherence, and delivering intervention to optimize adherence. Furthermore, improve adherence requires a continuous and dynamic process, and for effective provision of care, it is necessary that the patient, the family, and the community who support the individual all play an active role.

In summary, simplistic approaches to improve treatment adherence and subsequently improve the quality of life of people are not possible. What is required instead is a deliberative approach that starts with reviewing the way health professionals are trained and rewarded and addresses the many barriers patients and their families encounter as they strive to maintain optimal health. The following chapters discuss the prevalence and barriers to adherence for specific behaviors and populations, methods for improving adherence across various behaviors and populations, and ways to analyze and disseminate this information.

REFERENCES

1. Farmer KC. Methods for measuring and monitoring medication regimen adherence in clinical trials and clinical practice. *Clin Ther.* 1999;21(6):1074–1090.
2. DiMatteo MR. Variations in patients' adherence to medical recommendations: a quantitative review of 50 years of research. *Med Care.* 2004;42(3):200–209.

3. Sackett D. Preface. In: Sackett DL, Haynes RB, eds. *Compliance With Therapeutic Regimens.* Baltimore and London: Johns Hopkins University Press; 1976:xi–xiv.

4. Haynes R, Taylor DW, Sackett DL. *Compliance in Health Care.* Baltimore: Johns Hopkins University Press; 1978.

5. Mullen PD. Compliance becomes concordance. *BMJ.* 1997;314(7082):691–692.

6. World Health Organization. *Adherence to Long-Term Therapies: Evidence for Action.* Geneva: World Health Organization; 2003.

7. Urquhart J. Patient non-compliance with drug regimens: measurement, clinical correlates, economic impact. *Eur Heart J.* 1996;17(Suppl A):8–15.

8. Haynes RB, McKibbon KA, Kanani R. Systematic review of randomised trials of interventions to assist patients to follow prescriptions for medications. *Lancet.* 1996;348(9024):383–386.

9. Eraker S, Kirscht JP, Becker MH. Understanding and improving patient compliance. *Ann Intern Med.* 1984;100:258–268.

10. Rudd P. Clinicians and patients with hypertension: unsettled issues about compliance. *Am Heart J.* 1995;130(3 Pt 1):572–579.

11. Lawrence D, Graber JE, Mills SL, et al. Smoking cessation interventions in U.S. racial/ethnic minority populations: an assessment of the literature. *Prev Med.* 2003;36(2):204–216.

12. Fiore MC, Smith SS, Jorenby DE, Baker TB. The effectiveness of the nicotine patch for smoking cessation. A meta-analysis. *JAMA.* 1994;271(24):1940–1947.

13. Peterson AM, Takiya L, Finley R. Meta-analysis of trials of interventions to improve medication adherence. *Am J Health Syst Pharm.* 2003;60(7):657–665.

14. Berg JS, Dischler J, Wagner DJ, et al. Medication compliance: a healthcare problem. *Ann Pharmacother.* 1993;27(9 Suppl):S1–S24.

15. Vinson JM, Rich MW, Sperry JC, et al. Early readmission of elderly patients with congestive heart failure. *J Am Geriatr Soc.* 1990;38(12):1290–1295.

16. Ghali J, Kadakia S, Cooper R, Ferlinz J. Precipitating factors leading to decompensation of heart failure. *Arch Intern Med.* 1988;148:2013–2016.

17. Vik SA, Maxwell CJ, Hogan DB. Measurement, correlates, and health outcomes of medication adherence among seniors. *Ann Pharmacother.* 2004;38(2):303–312.

18. Trostle JA, Hauser WA, Susser IS. The logic of noncompliance: management of epilepsy from the patient's point of view. *Cult Med Psychiatry.* 1983;7(1):35–56.

19. Lynn J, DeGrazia D. An outcomes model of medical decision making. *Theor Med.* 1991;12(4):325–343.

20. Conrad P. The meaning of medications: another look at compliance. *Soc Sci Med.* 1985;20(1):29–37.

21. Gibbons A. Exploring new strategies to fight drug-resistant microbes. *Science.* 1992;257(5073):1036–1038.

22. Gourevitch MN, Wasserman W, Panero MS, Selwyn PA. Successful adherence to observed prophylaxis and treatment of tuberculosis among drug users in a methadone program. *J Addict Dis.* 1996;15(1):93–104.

23. Burke L, Dunbar-Jacob J. Adherence to medication, diet, and activity recommendations: from assessment to maintenance. *J Cardiovasc Nurs.* 1995;9:62–79.

24. Schron EB, Brooks MM, Gorkin L, et al. Relation of sociodemographic, clinical, and quality-of-life variables to adherence in the cardiac arrhythmia suppression trial. *J Cardiovasc Nurs.* 1996;32(2):1–6.

25. Obias-Manno D, Friedmann E, Brooks MM, et al. Adherence and arrhythmic mortality in the cardiac arrhythmia suppression trial (CAST). *Ann Epidemiol.* 1996;6(2):93–101.

26. Hauser ST, Jacobson AM, Lavori P, et al. Adherence among children and adolescents with insulin-dependent diabetes mellitus over a four-year longitudinal follow-up: II. Immediate and long-term linkages with the family milieu. *J Pediatr Psychol.* 1990;15(4):527–542.

27. DiMatteo MR. Social support and patient adherence to medical treatment: a meta-analysis. *Health Psychol.* 2004;23(2):207–218.

28. Goldman DP, Smith JP. Can patient self-management help explain the SES health gradient? *Proc Natl Acad Sci U S A.* 2002;99(16):10929–10934.

29. Mojtabai R, Olfson M. Medication costs, adherence, and health outcomes among Medicare beneficiaries. *Health Aff (Millwood).* 2003;22(4):220–229.

30. Nikolaus T, Kruse W, Bach M, et al. Elderly patients' problems with medication. An in-hospital and follow-up study. *Eur J Clin Pharmacol.* 1996;49(4):255–259.

31. Ruscin JM, Semla TP. Assessment of medication management skills in older outpatients. *Ann Pharmacother.* 1996;30(10):1083–1088.

32. Ferrando SJ, Wall TL, Batki SL, Sorensen JL. Psychiatric morbidity, illicit drug use and adherence to zidovudine (AZT) among injection drug users with HIV disease. *Am J Drug Alcohol Abuse.* 1996;22(4):475–487.

33. Pablos-Mendez A, Knirsch CA, Barr RG, et al. Nonadherence in tuberculosis treatment: predictors and consequences in New York City. *Am J Med.* 1997; 102(2):164–170.

34. Chesney MA, Ickovics JR, Chambers DB, et al. Self-reported adherence to antiretroviral medications among participants in HIV clinical trials: the AACTG adherence instruments. Patient Care Committee & Adherence Working Group of the Outcomes Committee of the Adult AIDS Clinical Trials Group (AACTG). *AIDS Care.* 2000;12(3):255–266.

35. Benner JS, Glynn RJ, Mogun H, et al. Long-term persistence in use of statin therapy in elderly patients. *JAMA.* 2002;288(4):455–461.

36. Jackevicius CA, Mamdani M, Tu JV. Adherence with statin therapy in elderly patients with and without acute coronary syndromes. *JAMA.* 2002;288(4):462–467.

37. Stephenson BJ, Rowe BH, Haynes RB, et al. Is this patient taking the treatment as prescribed? *JAMA.* 1993;269(21):2779–2781.

38. Johnson SB, Freund A, Silverstein J, et al. Adherence-health status relationships in childhood diabetes. *Health Psychol.* 1990;9(5):606–631.

39. Glasgow RE, McCaul KD, Schafer LC. Self-care behaviors and glycemic control in type I diabetes. *J Chronic Dis.* 1987;40(5):399–412.

40. Dunbar-Jacob J, Burkem LE, Pucyynski S, ed. *Clinical Assessment and Management of Adherence to Medical Regimens.* Washington, DC: American Psychological Association; 1995.

41. McDonald HP, Garg AX, Haynes RB. Interventions to enhance patient adherence to medication prescriptions: scientific review. *JAMA*. 2002;288(22): 2868–2879.
42. Morisky D. Five year blood pressure control and mortality following health education for hypertensive patients. *Am J Pub Health*. 1983;73:153–162.
43. Oldridge N, Jones NL. Improving patient compliance in cardiac rehabilitation: effects of written agreement and self-monitoring. *J Cardiopulmonary Rehab*. 1983; 3:257–262.
44. Baker R, Kirschenbaum DS. Self-monitoring may be necessary for successful weight control. *Behavior Therapy*. 1993;24:377–394.
45. Garay-Sevilla ME, Nava LE, Malacara JM, et al. Adherence to treatment and social support in patients with non-insulin dependent diabetes mellitus. *J Diabetes Complications*. 1995;9(2):81–86.
46. The Diabetes Prevention Program (DPP): description of lifestyle intervention. *Diabetes Care*. 2002;25(12):2165–2171.
47. Holzemer WL, Henry SB, Portillo CJ, Miramontes H. The Client Adherence Profiling-Intervention Tailoring (CAP-IT) intervention for enhancing adherence to HIV/AIDS medications: a pilot study. *J Assoc Nurses AIDS Care*. 2000;11(1):36–44.
48. Dunbar-Jacob JSS, Burke LE, Starz T, Rohay JH, Kwoh CK. Can poor adherence be improved? *Ann Behav Med*. 1995;1995:17.
49. DeBusk RF, Miller NH, Superko HR, et al. A case-management system for coronary risk factor modification after acute myocardial infarction. *Ann Intern Med*. 1994;120(9):721–729.
50. Peters AL, Davidson MB, Ossorio RC. Management of patients with diabetes by nurses with support of subspecialists. *HMO Pract*. 1995;9(1):8–13.
51. Haynes RB, McDonald H, Garg AX, Montague P. Interventions for helping patients to follow prescriptions for medications. *Cochrane Database Syst Rev*. 2002(2):CD000011.

Chapter 2

Theoretical Models to Understand Treatment Adherence

Hayden B. Bosworth
Corrine I. Voils

In this chapter, we review the models or theoretical approaches that have been used to describe and understand treatment adherence. Space constraints prevent us from reviewing every model, so we have selected those that have received the most attention and empirical support. For each, we describe the model, review empirical evidence for the model, and review applications to treatment adherence. We next discuss suggested strategies providers and researchers can use to encourage adherence based on the model's theoretical constructs. We conclude by discussing challenges with existing theories and models and suggest why and how the theories might be integrated to gain a better understanding of treatment adherence.

SOCIAL LEARNING (COGNITIVE) THEORY

Social learning theory (recently relabeled social cognitive theory) combines aspects of cognitive psychology and behavioral psychology. The theory suggests that behavior results from external stimuli and is explained in terms of rewards and punishment. According to social learning theory, behavior results from mental processes such as reasoning, decision making, and problem solving. Social learning theory also assumes that the majority of reinforcers of human behavior are social in nature (e.g., acceptance, smiles). As a result, theories that come out of the social learning tradition have been labeled social cognition theories (1). Although there are several theoretical models that can be applied to treatment adherence, most have their roots in social learning theory.

The social aspect of learning is evident from research suggesting that people can learn behaviors from watching others perform them—a process called observational learning. Observational learning may prove useful to increase treatment adherence to some behaviors such as exercise (e.g., by watching Richard Simmons on television), diet, and cancer screening (e.g., following Katie Couric undergoing a colonoscopy on national television), as these behaviors are highly recommended by health professionals and examples may be more readily available.

The cognitive aspect of learning is highlighted by research suggesting outcome expectancies (or response efficacy) influence behavior. Outcome expectancies, overlapping with parallel concepts in the theory of reasoned action and the health belief model, represent the expectancy that a positive outcome or consequence will occur as a function of the behavior. Two major competing views emerged from social learning theory to explain how this occurs: *locus of control* and *self-efficacy*. Locus of control refers to the belief that one has at one's disposal a response that can influence an event (2). Self-efficacy refers an individual's confidence in his or her ability to perform a given task (3). Thus, locus of control refers to one's perception of the availability of a response, whereas self-efficacy refers to one's confidence in the ability to effect that response.

Locus of Control

Rotter's Locus of Control Theory.   Rotter (4, 5) suggested that, when presented with the same information, different people learn very different things. Some individuals respond to reinforcement, as behavioral psychologists predict. That is, when people are rewarded for a behavior, they are more likely to repeat it in the future; when they are punished for a behavior, they are less likely to repeat it. Other individuals do not respond to reinforcement in that way. Indeed, they may convey the impression that they learned nothing at all because they often shift their expectancies in the direction opposite to the prior outcome; it is as though they believe chance determines behavior. The variable that represents these individual differences is termed locus of control. Locus of control has two dimensions: internal and external. People high in internal locus of control believe that reinforcement is contingent on one's behavior—for example, if one exercises, one will be rewarded with a slim figure and better health. In contrast, people high in external locus of control believe that reinforcement is contingent on outside forces such as luck, fate, or chance.

Wallston's Locus of Control Theory. Wallston and colleagues (6) expanded on Rotter's concept of locus of control to understand health-related behaviors. Like Rotter's theory, Wallston et al. suggested there are people who are high in internal locus of control who believe health rewards are contingent on healthy behavior. However, Wallston et al. also suggested that there are different ways to have an external control orientation. In their conceptualization, external locus of control refers to relying on powerful others, such as health care providers, as a source of reinforcement, whereas chance locus of control refers to relying on fate or chance for reinforcement (as in Rotter's concept of external locus of control).

Several studies have used locus of control to understand individual differences in the likelihood of engaging in healthy behaviors. Some research has suggested that individuals high in internal locus of control are more likely to be adherent to medical regimens (7). For example, such individuals are more likely to be nonsmokers (8), adhere to HIV medication (9) and hypertension medication (10), and are more successful at weight control (11). Other studies have found no relationship between locus of control and treatment adherence (12). Some have suggested this discrepancy may be resolved by examining locus of control in interactions with other variables (e.g., expectancies, social support, motivation) rather than as a main effect (7, 13). For example, adherence to depression medication was predicted by an interaction between locus of control and social support, such that increasing social support was associated with greater adherence among people high in internal locus of control (14).

Self-Efficacy

A second variation in the role of expectancies is based on Bandura's (15) concept of *self-efficacy*. Bandura suggested that just knowing what to do is not sufficient for one to behave; instead, one must also be confident that one is capable of performing the specific behavior. This belief is called self-efficacy (3). Self-efficacy is the product of both efficacy expectations (an individual's perception of his or her ability to achieve a specific level of performance) and outcome expectations (an individual's evaluation of the probable consequences of a specific behavior) (16). Hundreds of studies have shown that self-efficacy predicts the extent to which people are likely to engage in a behavior (17, 18). People who do not think they can stop smoking, for example, are more likely to relapse (19). Likewise, women who feel capable of performing breast self-examination are more likely to do so (20). Self-efficacy is also related to medication and exercise adherence (9, 21). However, it is important to emphasize that self-efficacy is behavior-specific. That is, someone may feel capable of performing one particular behavior, but not another.

Efficacy expectations are derived from four different sources: performance mastery, vicarious experience, social or verbal persuasion, and physiological states or cues experienced by the individual (22). Performance mastery refers to doing a task well. Vicarious experience refers to seeing another person model a behavior, often with the situational context and the consequences that follow. Persuasion, or trying to convince someone to do something, can occur socially (e.g., when norms support a behavior, such as not smoking) or verbally (e.g., by presenting information supporting one's position, such as evidence that smoking can cause lung cancer). Physiological states or cues refer to affect or arousal that one experiences in a situation; how one interprets the arousal influences one's beliefs. For example, experiencing a runner's high may lead one to think one is capable of increasing one's exercise routine.

The effect of performance mastery will be maximized when one believes that a positive outcome (e.g., weight loss) is the result of one's behavior (e.g., adhering to an exercise program). Additionally, performance mastery will be achieved most easily when learning or adopting a new behavior is broken down into manageable chunks. For example, patients will be more likely to adhere to an exercise program if they slowly increase their amount of physical activity each day. Although interventions designed to improve performance mastery generally are the most effective means of building patient self-efficacy, health care professionals also can develop strategies specific to the other sources of efficacy expectations (23). For example, verbal persuasion may be more successful if providers use past performance information, such as emphasizing past or recent weight loss. In addition, physiological arousal will influence self-efficacy to the extent that it is perceived as positive. For example, an increase in energy can help one feel capable of walking two miles, whereas nervousness may make one feel unable to give oneself a shot of insulin.

Strategies Using Social Learning Theory Concepts

There are several strategies providers and researchers can use to enhance self-efficacy. For example, providers can provide opportunities for the patient to master the necessary skills. This may be done by modeling the behavior or providing an example in order to facilitate learning the new behavior. For example, providers can teach their patients how to monitor their blood pressure or show a videotape of an individual engaging in the prescribed activity. Clinicians can also provide an opportunity for patients to rehearse the new behavior in front of them for feedback. For example, providers can have patients check their insulin after being shown how this is done. Previous experience with the health behavior change in question should also be addressed with patients. Providers can address previously failed attempts and explore individual and environmental factors that may have contributed to these unsuccessful attempts. Finally, verbal positive re-inforcement should be given when patients practice or perform the recom-mended behavior. Feelings of self-efficacy may give rise to greater internal locus of control, which in turn should be associated with greater adherence to a medical regimen.

CONTINUUM THEORIES

Several concepts that came out of the social learning tradition formed the basis for current models of health decision making. In general, these theo-ries can be grouped under two broad categories: continuum models, which include the theory of reasoned action/theory of planned behavior, protec-tion motivation theory, health belief model, self-regulatory model of illness; and stage models, which include the transtheoretical model and precau-tion adoption process model. Continuum models assume that all variables that influence behavior can be combined into a single equation that pre-dicts the likelihood of action. Furthermore, the way the variables combine to influence behavior is presumed to be the same for everyone.

Theory of Reasoned Action/Theory of Planned Behavior

The theory of reasoned action (24) was an attempt to resolve a debate in so-cial psychology concerning whether attitudes predict behavior. According to the theory, the strongest predictor of behavior is intention to perform that behavior. Intention, in turn, is determined by attitude toward a behav-ior (i.e., a person's overall evaluation of performing the behavior) and sub-jective norms (i.e., a person's perceptions of how others feel about the be-havior) (see Fig. 2.1). Determinants of attitudes toward a behavior include one's beliefs about the consequences of performing a behavior and one's evaluation of those possible consequences, whereas determinants of subjec-tive norms include perceived expectations of significant others and motiva-tion to meet those expectations.

The theory of reasoned action was later modified to explain behaviors that are not completely under volitional control; the revised theory was named the theory of planned behavior (25). The theory of planned behav-ior included a third determinant of intention, perceived behavioral control (i.e., the extent to which one believes one has control over performing the behavior, or the ease or difficulty of performing the behavior). Determi-nants of perceived behavioral control include beliefs about controllability

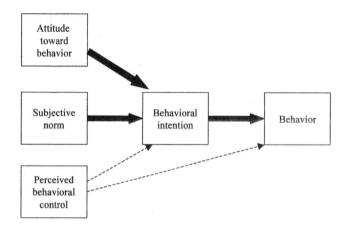

FIG. 2.1.   Theories of reasoned action (solid) and planned behavior.

and perceived power to perform the behavior. The theory of planned behavior stipulated that, whenever people's perceptions of control are accurate, perceived behavioral control would not only predict behavioral intention, but behavior as well (see Fig. 2.1). The concept of perceived
behavioral control is related to Bandura's (26) concept of self-efficacy (27).

In sum, the theory of reasoned action and theory of planned behavior
postulate that the more positive people's attitudes and subjective norms regarding behavior are, and the greater their perceived behavioral control,
the stronger people's intentions to perform the behavior will be. Similarly,
the stronger people's intentions, and the greater the perceived behavioral
control, the more likely it is that people will perform the behavior.

In general, theory of reasoned action and theory of planned behavior
concepts are good predictors of behavioral intentions; meta-analyses have
shown that theory of reasoned action and theory of planned behavior variables account for 40% to 50% of the explained variance for health behaviors (see ref. 28 for a review of meta-analyses). However, there are at least
three limitations of the theory of planned behavior. First, the theory has not
addressed potential changes in individuals' beliefs and attitudes over time.
Second, because the theory of planned behavior is primarily an account of
goal setting rather than goal pursuit (29), the model is less equipped to explain patterns of behavior change. Third, the theory does not account for
the discrepancy between intention to adhere and actual adherence; the latter may be a distinctly different process. For example, the relationship between intentions and behavior is less strong; in prospective studies, theory
of reasoned action and theory of planned behavior variables account for
only 20% to 40% of the variance in health behaviors (30–32). The relation-

ship appears to be attenuated by intentional abstainers—people who intend to perform a behavior but fail to do so.

Considerable research has been devoted to understanding why the intention–behavior relationship is so weak and how it might be strengthened. Several factors play a role, including behavior type, intention type, and cognitive and personality variables (33). Specific examples include past behavior (34, 35), certainty about intentions or attitudes (36), anticipated regret (37), and attitudinal versus normative control (38). These moderators function by strengthening one's intentions (39).

The intention–behavior relationship can also be strengthened by forming implementation intentions—specific intentions that denote when, where, and how a behavior is to be performed (40). People who form implementation intentions are more likely to perform a behavior than people who have general behavioral intentions for at least two reasons (41, 42). First, behavioral intentions are often accompanied by uncertainty (43, 44). For example, people may "intend to get screened for cancer" but lack details about how or when they will do so. Therefore, making a specific plan to carry out the behavior eliminates the uncertainty. Second, implementation intentions create memory traces that can be activated by environmental cues (40). For example, one may be reminded to take one's medication in the morning after seeing one's toothbrush if one normally takes one's medication after brushing one's teeth.

Applications to Treatment Adherence. The theories of reasoned action and planned behavior have been applied to understand several health-related behaviors, including addictive behaviors (e.g., smoking, alcohol, drugs), automobile-related behaviors (e.g., speeding, wearing seat belts), screening (cancer screening, breast self-exam), eating and exercise, HIV/AIDs behaviors (e.g., using condoms), and oral hygiene (for reviews, see refs. 32 and 45). Implementation intentions have also been used to increase treatment adherence, including breast self-examination (46), healthy eating (47), cervical cancer screening (34), and exercise (48).

The extent to which the theory of reasoned action and theory of planned behavior variables predict behavioral intentions appears to vary across treatment adherence behaviors (32). Attitudes are more predictive of intentions related to addictive behaviors, screening, and exercising than to eating; subjective norms are more predictive of intentions related to oral hygiene than to eating and exercising; and perceived behavioral control is more predictive of intentions related to oral hygiene and exercising than to eating and HIV/AIDS behaviors. The variables also vary in their ability to predict behaviors; perceived behavioral control is more predictive of addictive behaviors and screening behaviors than are intentions (32).

Strategies Using the Theory of Reasoned Action/Theory of Planned Behavior. Because patients must have a positive attitude toward the targeted behavior, providers might start by assessing patients' attitude toward treatment adherence. Negative attitudes could be changed through techniques of persuasion, including presenting a strong argument for the recommended behavior (e.g., increased life expectancy due to reducing risk of cardiovascular disease), providing knowledge that can serve as a basis for one's attitude, and alleviating fears. Social norms must also favor the recommended behavior. Providers could determine whether the patient thinks family members and friends endorse the behavior. They should highlight social pressure to engage in the behavior, if it exists, and provide examples of similar others who are currently engaging in the behavior. Often, patients with weight management problems are surrounded by people who do not believe the patient should lose weight (49). This creates a problem for the patient as he or she is often motivated to behave similarly to others (50). Providers should also provide social norms by adhering to the very behaviors that they recommend. It has been shown that patients are less confident about health advice given by obese than nonobese physicians (51). Perceived behavioral control can be increased using the strategies discussed previously for increasing self-efficacy. In addition, providers might try to address any perceived external constraints, such as cost and access to facilities. To increase the behavior intention and behavior relationship, specific examples of behaviors should be used when assessing behavioral intentions (52). Finally, providers should have patients form implementation intentions concerning the targeted behavior. For example, patients can decide that they will take their diuretics every morning after breakfast.

Protection Motivation Theory

Rogers's (53) protection motivation theory was originally designed to specify and operationalize the components of a fear appeal (i.e., a message that uses fear to persuade) that lead to attitude change and ultimately behavioral change. He later revised his theory into a more general theory of cognitive change (54), which has been used to understand decision making in relation to health threats. As in theory of reasoned action/theory of planned behavior, protection motivation theory stipulates that behavioral intentions, or what Rogers termed "protection motivation," is the best and most immediate protector of behavior. However, the models suggest different determinants of behavioral intentions. Whereas theory of planned behavior suggests that attitudes, social norms, and perceived behavioral control influence behavioral intentions, protection motivation theory suggests threat and coping appraisal influence them (see Fig. 2.2). Threat appraisal refers to the evaluation of the components of a fear appeal to determine

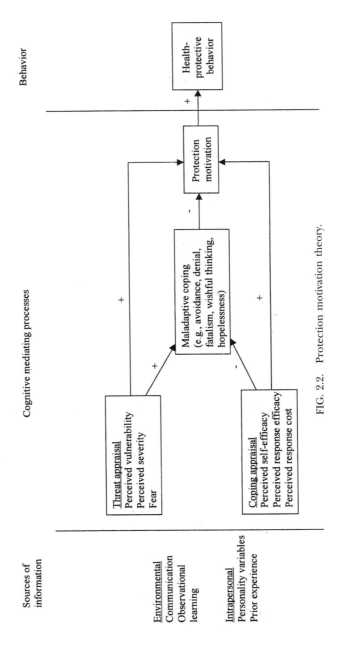

Sources of
information

Cognitive mediating processes

Behavior

Environmental
Communication
Observational
learning

Intrapersonal
Personality variables
Prior experience

Threat appraisal
Perceived vulnerability
Perceived severity
Fear

Coping appraisal
Perceived self-efficacy
Perceived response efficacy
Perceived response cost

Maladaptive coping
(e.g., avoidance, denial,
fatalism, wishful thinking,
hopelessness)

Protection
motivation

Health-
protective
behavior

+

+

−

+

−

+

FIG. 2.2.   Protection motivation theory.

how personally endangered one feels by the threat. It involves perceived vulnerability, or how susceptible one feels to a threat; perceived severity, or how serious one feels the threat is to one's life; and fear arousal evoked by the threat. One will be more likely to form intentions to adopt the recommended behavior if one believes one is susceptible to the threat, the threat is severe, and one is fearful of the threat. Coping appraisal refers to the evaluation of the recommended suggestion(s) for coping with the threat. Coping comprises self-efficacy, or how capable one feels of performing the recommended behaviors; response efficacy, or the belief about how effective a behavior will be in reducing a threat; and response costs, or beliefs about how costly the recommended response would be. One will be more likely to form intentions to adopt the recommended behavior if one is capable of performing that behavior, one believes a behavior will effectively reduce the threat, and the recommended response is not costly.

Protection motivation theory postulates that threat and coping appraisal are instigated by environmental (communication, observational learning) and intrapersonal (e.g., personality variables, prior experience) sources. It also postulates that threat and coping appraisal not only affect behavioral intentions, but also may lead to maladaptive coping responses (avoidance, denial, fatalism, wishful thinking, and hopelessness), which in turn may influence behavioral intentions. For example, through threat appraisal, one may determine that a threat is not personally relevant, which is associated with a denial coping response, which leads to low intentions to adopt the recommended behavior. The threat of smoking may not be perceived as relevant for an individual, which would lead to a low likelihood of cessation.

Applications to Treatment Adherence. Protection motivation theory has been used to increase intentions to exercise (55), use condoms (56, 57), perform breast self-examination (58) and testicular self-examination (59), obtain genetic testing for breast cancer (60), floss (16, 61), stop smoking (62), reduce dietary fat (63), and decrease substance use (64). In addition, associations have been found between protection motivation theory variables and concurrent behavior, including dietary fat intake (63). Prospective studies have shown that protection motivation theory variables predicted subsequent breast self-exam (58), breast cancer screening (65), and adherence to a physiotherapist's recommendations (66).

In a meta-analysis that examined protection motivation theory applications to health behavior, Milne et al. (67) found that all threat and coping appraisal activities were associated with behavioral intentions. Among the specific appraisal components, self-efficacy showed the strongest relation (r = .33). In addition, all threat and coping appraisal activities except fear were associated with concurrent behavior. As predicted, the strongest correlate of concurrent behavior was behavioral intention ($r = .82$). Perceived vulnerability, self-efficacy, and response costs were the only appraisal variables that were significantly associated with subsequent behavior, with self-efficacy showing the strongest relation. Finally, as predicted, behavioral intentions were predictive of future behavior ($r = .40$).

Although this meta-analysis suggests a sizable relation between behavioral intentions and concurrent and subsequent behavior, there is room for improvement. The concept of implementation intentions, although developed in a theory of planned behavior framework, could be effectively applied to increase the relation between intentions and behavior in the protection motivation theory framework as well. To our knowledge, this has been done in only one study in the health domain: Milne et al. (48) demonstrated that supplementing protection motivation theory variables with implementation intentions strengthened the relationship between intentions to exercise and exercise participation.

Strategies Using Protection Motivation Theory. First, providers need to assess the patient's perceived susceptibility and severity of the outcome and frame the health message according to these perceptions. Providers can engage in this process by discussing with the patient his or her perception of pros and cons for engaging in the behavior, thus eliciting perceived barriers to the health behavior change in question, and discuss how to overcome these barriers. Providers could enhance perceived threat by stressing the possible negative consequences of the problem behavior and aspects of a patient's medical history that make them vulnerable to a health problem. For example, providers could emphasize that atherosclerosis can lead to stroke and point out that a patient's high cholesterol and blood pressure increase the likelihood of having atherosclerosis, and possibly a stroke later. This threat information should be balanced with information and strategies for helping patients cope. For instance, providers should assess the perceived benefits of engaging in exercise and medication adherence and incorporate these benefits as reinforcers of behavior (52). In addition, providers should stress the effectiveness of a particular response (e.g., smoking cessation can reverse lung damage). Finally, strategies for enhancing self-efficacy and strengthening the relation between intentions and behavior, discussed previously, should be used.

Health Belief Model

The most frequently used model in studies of health behavior and adherence (68), the health belief model was developed to explain why people fail to engage in disease prevention or screening tests before the onset of symptoms (69). The model proposes that the likelihood of one carrying out a particular health behavior (e.g., taking a medication) is a function of personal beliefs about perceived susceptibility, severity, benefits, and barriers (see Fig. 2.3). Perceived susceptibility refers to one's perception of the risk

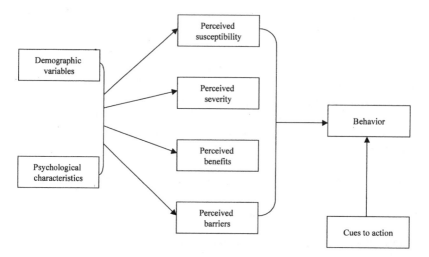

FIG. 2.3. Health belief model.

of contracting an illness. Perceived severity refers to the evaluation of the seriousness of contracting the illness and leaving it untreated and includes an evaluation of both social and medical/clinical consequences. The combination of perceived susceptibility and severity has been labeled perceived threat. In addition to deciding on perceived threat, an individual weighs the perceived benefits of an action (e.g., screening will detect problems at an early stage) against the perceived barriers to the action (e.g., difficulty in finding time to attend screening). The health belief model also stipulates that a cue or stimulus to action must trigger the behavior.

In sum, the model predicts that the likelihood of action is increased if the perceived threat of the disease is high, the benefits of the behavior outweigh the barriers, and certain cues are in place. Although the theoretical structure of the model has never been well specified, researchers suggest that the belief elements together produce some degree of psychological readiness to act in the face of threat. If these beliefs are above some threshold and environmental conditions permit, action is likely (70).

Several decades after the health belief model was conceptualized, it was revised. For instance, Bandura's (71) concept of self-efficacy was added to the model as a barrier (72). Other factors have been included as well, such as fairly nonspecific general health motivations, personal attributes that are stable across situations, resusceptibility to an illness previously contacted and currently under consideration, general orientation toward medicine, and characteristics of the patient–doctor relationship (73).

Review articles and meta-analyses have concluded that, in general, the constructs of the health belief model are good predictors of health behavior (74–76). However, inconsistencies in the way the constructs are measured have made it difficult to draw firm conclusions about the size of the effects (76, 77). Taken together, the findings of research on preventive medical behavior yield some of the strongest evidence for predictive usefulness of health beliefs, with the amount of variance explain between intention and behavior ranging from .25 to .50 (69).

Eraker et al.'s (78) health decision model was developed as an extension of the health belief model. It includes health belief model variables and patient preference, including decision analysis and behavioral decision theory. The health decision model includes bidirectional arrows and feedback loops, which suggest that adherence behavior can also change beliefs. To date, there is insufficient data on the validity and predictability of the health decision model.

Although the health belief model per se is not a theory about change, it has often been used in interventions involving health messages. In reality, the model may have its greatest use in developing and testing interventions. The components can serve as dimensions for defining the nature of a health threat in terms of different types of impact, risk for people, possible actions to take and their value, and what such actions might entail in terms of resources and skills. In addition, other parts of the communication process may be facilitated through health belief considerations; the attentional steps necessary for the process to occur can be affected by the way in which a health threat is presented and dramatized. The nature of existing beliefs about a health problem may also determine the value of different types of information (70).

The health belief model should fit best in the less repetitive realm where health considerations are clearly linked to the action. The model is also appropriate in the context of a decision about starting or stopping repetitive behaviors. The health belief model is likely to predict initiating the elimination of a habit because risky habits are often tied to a number of nonhealth considerations.

Applications to Treatment Adherence.   The evidence for health beliefs as causal factors in treatment adherence is not clear, particularly in relation to ongoing treatment of chronic disease. Hershey et al. (79) assessed treatment adherence among hypertensive patients attending a hypertensive clinic. None of the health belief model indexes differentiated levels of adherence to prescribed medications, with the exception of a six-item measure of barriers. A study by Cummings (80) on adherence among a group of hemodialysis patients included assessment of beliefs specific to various parts of the regimen. In general, beliefs about benefits and barriers were associated with adherence measures, particularly those self-reported. Among other beliefs, only susceptibility showed an association, but only for dietary restriction. Thus, the health belief model has not clearly demonstrated predictive validity in relation to adherence with medical recommendations.

One reason the model is difficult to apply is that different aspects of regimens are often unrelated (e.g., taking medication and keeping appointments) (81).

Strategies Using the Health Belief Model. The strategies for addressing barriers and benefits discussed under protection motivation theory are applicable to this theory as well. Another strategy would be creating cues to action, which could be accomplished by having patients form implementation intentions. For example, having patients decide to take medication after dinner every day should serve to create an association in memory between dinnertime and medication taking so that taking medication after dinner becomes routinized.

Self-Regulatory Model of Illness

Like social cognition models, the self-regulatory model (82) emphasizes the role of self-efficacy and cognitive representation of a threat. Where this model differs, however, is in its description of the interaction between cognitions, motivation, and behavior. Self-regulation refers to efforts to lessen the discrepancy between current status (i.e., ill) and a future goal state (i.e., less ill or not ill). The self-regulatory model breaks self-regulation down into three stages: representation of the illness, which may be activated by internal cues (e.g., symptoms) or external cues (e.g., information); development and implementation of a plan to cope with the illness; and evaluation of the coping mechanism (see Fig. 2.4). These stages serve to create a dynamic feedback loop; that is, a person moves from stage to stage, both forward and backward. For example, one could determine that one has a headache (representation), decide to ignore it (cope), realize that it is not going away on its own (evaluate), take medication (reenter coping stage), and feel better (reevaluate). As demonstrated in this example, the decision about whether to adhere is conceptualized as one of a number of possible procedures for coping with an illness threat.

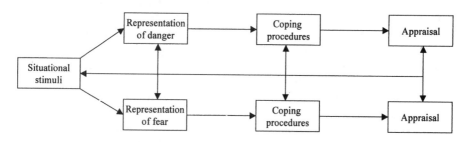

FIG. 2.4. Self-regulatory model of illness.

Important to note, this model stipulates that cognitive and affective processing occurs in parallel along the three stages. The cognitive component includes beliefs about the threat of illness, which give rise to coping mechanisms and an evaluation of those mechanisms for dealing with the threat. The affective component includes feelings about the illness, such as fear or distress, which give rise to coping mechanisms and an evaluation of those mechanisms for regulating emotion.

Applications to Treatment Adherence. One limitation to this model is that it is so complex that operationalizing the components is difficult. The lack of standardized instruments seems to be a barrier to the use of this model. In addition, the model is difficult to use because of its multivariate and transactional character. Thus, most empirical support for the model comes from studies highlighting the role of illness representations in behavior. Illness representations and beliefs have been shown to predict subsequent rehabilitation following myocardial infarction (83) and medication adherence for hypertension (84), asthma (85), and HIV (86).

The self-regulatory model is applicable to problems requiring a cognitive response to a threat that occurs with acute illness or episodic exacerbation of chronic disease. However, the self-regulatory model does not address maintaining sustained behavior in chronic diseases or prevention measures in which the threat is low. For example, many chronic diseases such as hypertension, hyperlipidemia, or osteoporosis are asymptomatic and thus have a silent impact on health. The model could be used to increase adherence to behaviors that help ameliorate or prevent such diseases, such as losing weight and exercising. For example, one could try to lose weight, evaluate one's efforts after a specified time period, adjust one's diet and exercise routine, and reevaluate the effort after another period of time. In the long run, this would reduce blood pressure and cholesterol levels.

Strategies Using the Self-Regulatory Model of Illness. Providers can help create accurate representations of illness using the strategies for inducing threat discussed under protection motivation theory. For example, patients need to be aware of the long-term effects of nonadherence to treatment regimens, such as increased risk of certain types of cancer and cardiovascular disease that results from obesity, smoking, hypertension, and hyperlipidemia. Providers can also help by suggesting coping strategies. Finally, providers can help patients appraise success or failure of their coping behaviors and help patients revise their coping behavior, if necessary. For instance, if a patient has been exercising three times per week but has not lost weight, the provider can help the patient adjust his or her exercise schedule and diet and then reevaluate at a follow-up visit.

STAGE THEORIES

Whereas the emphasis on intentions in the theory of reasoned action (24), the theory of planned behavior (25), and protection motivation theory (54) is fairly static (i.e., their primary focus is on learned predispositions retrieved from memory rather than on active processing of the implications of goal attainment), a number of quite similar health behavior models known as stage models have been proposed to describe the process of change (87, 88). Stage theories suggest that behavioral change occurs via progression through different stages. Stage theories have four key defining characteristics: a category system, whereby an individual can be in only one stage at one time; an ordering of categories; similar barriers to change within categories, such that people in the same category can be helped by similar interventions; and different barriers to change between categories (89). Thus, these models hold the most promise if interventions are tailored according to an individual's stage. Stage theories also have the advantage of drawing attention to the difference between adopting a behavior and maintaining it long term, which is frequently ignored in studies using continuum theories (90).

Transtheoretical Model

The transtheoretical model (87, 91) was originally developed for smoking cessation, but it has also been applied to adherence with other health behaviors, such as drug abuse, diet, exercise, seat belt use, avoidance of sun exposure, cancer self-exams, and condom use (92, 93). The crux of the model is that behavioral change occurs in a series of temporally ordered, discrete stages. Movement between stages is influenced by the ratio of pros and cons of the problem behavior, self-efficacy, temptations to revert to the problem behavior, and coping mechanisms used to change the problem behavior. The three organizing constructs of the model are stages of change, processes of change, and levels of change (93).

Stages of Change.   Six discrete stages reflect one's interest and motivation to alter a problem behavior. One is able to achieve successful behavioral change by moving through them in a predetermined temporal order (93), as follows:

1. *Precontemplation* is the stage in which there is an unwillingness to change a problem behavior or there is a lack of recognition of the problem. At this stage, patients either deny having or do not recognize consequences of a condition.

2. *Contemplation* involves consideration of change, with an evaluation of pros and cons of both the problem behavior and the change. Individuals frequently begin to weigh the consequences of action or inaction. At this point, patients are able to discuss the disadvantages and advantages associated with, for example, taking an antihypertensive medication to prevent a stroke. Usually, patients discuss changing their current behavior in the next 6 months.

3. *Preparation* is the period when there is a commitment to change in the near future—usually within 1 month. Patients express a high degree of motivation toward the desired behaviors and outcomes. Patients in the preparation stage have determined that the adverse costs of maintaining their current behavior exceed the benefits. Therefore, initiating a new behavior is more likely. Patients have moved from thinking about the issue to doing something about it.

4. *Action* involves altering behavior successfully for 1 day to 6 months.

5. *Maintenance* occurs when one has engaged in the new behavior for at least 6 months. During this stage, the focus is on lifestyle modification to stabilize the behavior change and avoid relapse (93).

6. *Termination* occurs when the problem behavior is no longer a concern for individuals. Therefore, this stage applies to some behaviors (e.g., smoking cessation) but not others (e.g., cancer screening). In the process of behavioral change, individuals often cycle through the first five stages before reaching termination or permanent behavior change (91, 94).

Processes of Change. The processes of change are the activities that take place as individuals move through the six stages. Ten processes have been identified that are responsible for movement (see Table 2.1) (93). Five of these processes are experiential or cognitive and include consciousness-raising, dramatic relief, environmental evaluation, self-evaluation, and self-liberation. These are internally mediated factors that are associated with an individual's emotions, values, and cognitions (95). Consciousness-raising is described as encouraging individuals to increase their level of awareness, seek new information, or gain an understanding about a problem. Dramatic relief refers to experiencing negative emotions about a problem behavior, after which time affect is reduced; it is a cathartic process. Environmental evaluation is assessing how one's problem affects the physical environment. Self-evaluation is assessing how one feels and thinks about oneself in relation to the problem. Self-liberation is when one believes in oneself and one's ability to change (96).

The remaining five processes are behavioral and include counterconditioning, helping relationships, reinforcement/contingency management, stimulus control, and social liberation (95, 96). Counterconditioning is

TABLE 2.1
Transtheoretical Model—Integration of Stages
of Change With Processes of Change

Process	Stage of Change				
	Precontemplation	Contemplation	Preparation	Action	Maintenance
Consciousness-raising	X	X			
Dramatic relief	X	X			
Environmental reevaluation	X	X			
Self-reevaluation		X			
Self-liberation			X		
Counterconditioning				X	X
Helping relationships				X	X
Reinforcement/Contingency management				X	X
Stimulus control				X	X
Social liberation				X	X

Note. From ref. 93.

substituting alternatives for problem behaviors (e.g., using meditation to cope with unpleasant emotions). Helping relationships are defined as those that provide trust, acceptance, and support (e.g., having a provider that listens when there is a need to discuss a problem). Reinforcement management is the use of positive reinforcements and appropriate goal setting with the patient. Stimulus control is helping the patient to restructure the environment so that the stimuli, or triggers, of the undesired behavior are controlled. Social liberation is increasing alternatives for nonproblem behaviors in society.

An integration of these processes with stages can be seen in Table 2.1. There is a match between the stage that the patient is in and the intervention that is used. Individuals in the contemplation stage would be most open to consciousness-raising, the use of dramatic relief, and environmental evaluation. In the action phase, effective use of behavioral processes would be particularly helpful (87, 96).

Levels of Change.   Individuals have multiple problems that often overlap. Poor blood pressure control, for example, may be associated with a lack of exercise, smoking, poor diet, and not taking medication as prescribed. With this recognition, the transtheoretical model incorporates five levels of change for consideration. These include changes that relate to the symptoms or situations, maladaptive cognition, interpersonal problems, family/systems problems, and intrapersonal conflicts. Treatment outcomes are often better when multiple problems are addressed (97).

The transtheoretical model incorporates the theory of decisional balance (98), which examines the pros and cons in decision making. The balance of perceived pros and cons of adopting a new behavior varies across the stages of change so that the cons of changing outweigh the pros in the precontemplation stage. At some point during the contemplation or preparation stage, the pros start outweighing the cons.

The concept of self-efficacy is also important to the model and has two components: *confidence,* which refers to the confidence people have that they can cope with high-risk situations without relapsing, and *temptation,* which refers to the intensity of an urge to revert to a problem behavior. In relation to the stages of change, self-efficacy is generally at its lowest point in the precontemplation stage and increases to its highest point in the maintenance stage. Studies have shown self-efficacy to be a predictor of movement into action and maintenance, but less so in the early stages where decision-making processes are more important. Once individuals have decided that taking medicines is worth the relative loss of freedom, doubt about their own ability to take the medications on a regular basis can be a barrier to change, causing them to continue to contemplate changing. As individuals become more confident in their ability, the likelihood of movement into action and taking the medication is greater.

Applications to Treatment Adherence. Support for the transtheoretical model has been accumulating over the past 20 years. The model has been applied successfully to preventive behaviors such as cancer screening (99), smoking (100, 101), diet (102, 103), exercise (104, 105), and contraceptive use (106). One of the most relevant findings for practice is that, typically, 40% of a population with an unhealthy behavior are in the precontemplation stage, 40% are in the contemplation stage, and fewer than 20% are in the preparation stage (107, 108). Several studies have focused on creating assessment tools to determine the level of motivation for change, which include the 12-item Readiness to Change Measure (109), the 20-item Alcohol Abstinence Self-Efficacy Scale (110), the University of Rhode Island Change Assessment (URICA) (111), the Stages of Change Readiness and Treatment Eagerness Scale (SOC-RATES) (112), and the Readiness Ruler (113).

Extensive relapse and recycling occurs in populations attempting to take action to change behavior. This appears to be the norm and has important implications for practice. Terms such as *noncompliant, nonadherent,* and *unmotivated* are frequent labels applied to patients who do not follow through on their treatment plans. This may reflect the norm of relapse or may reflect a poorly created treatment plan that does not consider a patient's stage of change. In labeling patients as such, the provider may be externalizing responsibility by placing blame rather than reflecting upon his or her own skills. Therefore, appreciating the stage of change the patient is in is imperative before one develops an optimal treatment plan.

Whereas the transtheoretical model has gained widespread popularity in health psychology, there is limited evidence of sequential movement through discrete stages in studies of specific behaviors. In addition, this model, like other stage theories, oversimplifies the complexities of behavioral change by imposing artificial categories on continuous processes (114–116). Although the transtheoretical model may have heuristic value, its practical utility is limited by concerns about the validity of stage assessments (117).

Strategies Using the Transtheoretical Model. Once a patient's stage of change is identified, the health care practitioner can help facilitate the patient's progression and movement through stages. Motivational interviewing is a framework that can help facilitate this movement. Motivational interviewing has been used extensively in the addiction field (118, 119); however, there has been considerable recent interest on the part of public health, health psychology, and medical professionals in adapting motivational interviewing to address other health behaviors and conditions such as regimen adherence (120).

Motivational interviewing is not a discrete intervention strategy but an amalgamation of principles and techniques drawn from several theoretical paradigms. A key goal of motivational interviewing is to assist individuals to work through their ambivalence about behavior change. Motivational interviewing assumes that, rather than trying to convince patients to change, providers would be more effective if they elicited arguments for change from patients themselves. Unlike many traditional patient-education paradigms, motivational interviewing usually does not involve providing information or advice unless the patient makes that request (121).

The technical aspects of motivational interviewing include three elements: (a) client-centered counseling skills, based on Rogerian counseling; (b) reflective listening statements, directive questions, and strategies to elicit internal motivation from the client, operationalized as self-motivating statements made by the client; and (c) strategies for ensuring that client resistance is minimized. Providers using motivational interviewing ask open-ended questions about the patient's values and goals and examine how they are discrepant with current behavior, respond with reflections to convey a sense of understanding, avoid arguments when encountering resistance, and convey hope that change is possible.

Support for the use of motivational interviewing has grown (see ref. 122 for a listing of studies involving motivational interviewing). Dunn and colleagues conducted a review to examine the effectiveness of brief behavioral interventions adapting the principles and techniques of motivational interviewing to four behavioral domains: smoking, substance abuse, HIV risk, and diet/exercise (118). They identified 29 randomized trials of motivational interviewing interventions. Sixty percent of the 29 studies yielded at least one significant behavior change effect size. No significant association between length of follow-up time and magnitude of effect sizes was found across studies.

Limited research has examined motivational interviewing–based interventions to promote medication adherence. However, Kemp and colleagues used motivational interviewing among people experiencing psychosis (123, 124), which resulted in improved observer-rated adherence compared to participants receiving nonspecific counseling. Furthermore, changes were retained over an 18-month follow-up period (123). It seems likely that motivational interviewing could be used successfully to improve adherence to various aspects of regimens, including medication, exercise, and diet.

Precaution Adoption Process Model

The precaution adoption process model's hypotheses were initially tested in prediction of home radon testing (125). The model consists of seven self-explanatory stages: unaware of the issue; aware of the issue but not personally engaged; engaged and deciding what to do; planning to act but not yet having acted; acting; having decided not to act; and maintenance.

This model differs from the transtheoretical model in a few ways. First, the precaution adoption process model distinguishes between people who have never thought about changing a behavior and those who have thought about it but decided not to, whereas the precontemplation stage of the transtheoretical model does not. The precaution adoption process model includes a stage in which people can be unaware of an issue. This is because it was developed to encourage behavior relevant to an issue about which people are unaware (i.e., that radon gas is in their homes), whereas the transtheoretical model was developed to change behavior that people are aware of (e.g., smoking). Second, the precaution adoption process model distinguishes people who are undecided and those who have already decided to act, whereas the contemplation stage does not. Finally, the precaution adoption process model does not describe the process by which cognitive and behavioral change takes place.

Although this model holds promise for understanding adherence, applications of it have been limited. It has been used to predict mammography (126), oral-contraceptive use (127), and osteoporosis prevention (128). Due to the overlap in conceptualization, the strategies developed in the transtheoretical model framework could be applied within the precaution adoption model framework as well.

CHALLENGES WITH EXISTING MODELS
AND THEORIES

There are many other models in literature that aim to predict adherence and further the field; space constraints prevent us from discussing all models in detail. Suffice it to say that no one unifying theory can encompass all aspects of behavior because no model explains completely an individual's interaction with the medical care system. In predicting relevant health behaviors such as treatment adherence, there are only a few clear rules for selection of the right framework. Data must exist that support the usefulness of a framework in predicting relevant health behavior or adherence. Often researchers will find data supporting the usefulness of a theoretical model, but not data on the specific behavior in question; therefore, the relevance of the model to the particular behavior is not known. Alternatively, supporting data may be obtained, but only in cross-sectional or longitudinal observational studies and not in randomized intervention studies, which precludes researchers from drawing conclusions about the usefulness of a model in a changing setting. In addition, there are few direct empirical comparisons of the predictive value of two or more models, making direct comparisons difficult.

The traditional models dominant in the study of patient adherence, such as the health belief model, are typically based on a rough cost–benefit calculus in which the patient considers the advantages and burdens of taking medications by weighing the probabilities of risks and benefits (69). Although these models have been useful as organizing frames, they have had limited predictive value. Furthermore, common problems using these models is that they often include cross-sectional designs to test predictive models and fail to explain how constructs are operationalized or validated (129). Moreover, many models allow us to examine only the patient's perspective, but adherence is clearly influenced by provider behavior as well. Therefore, it is necessary to go beyond the usual individual psychological focus of these models and give attention to contextual cues and reinforcements that are more amenable to intervention within treatment programs.

Considering maintenance is particularly important because intervention approaches have been identified that reliably elicit healthy changes in behavioral practices such as smoking, weight control, and exercise. Yet, rates of initial changes in behavior have not consistently translated into similar rates of behavioral maintenance. Some models, particularly the continuum models, make no direct reference to issues regarding behavioral maintenance, and empirical tests of these models have focused primarily on predicting a single behavioral outcome.

INTEGRATING MODELS TO PREDICT REGIMEN ADHERENCE

All of the theories reviewed earlier recognize the importance of motivation to change behavior and highlight the importance of strengthening the factors or processes that prompt behavioral change. In addition, it is clear from our review that the aforementioned models contain similar and overlapping components. For example, the concept of perceived behavioral control in the theory of reasoned action subsumes the concept of self-efficacy, which is incorporated in protection motivation theory, the health belief model, and the transtheoretical model. Likewise, the concept of behavioral intentions is found in many of the models. The overlap of concepts across models is one reason we believe the models should be integrated into interventions to increase treatment adherence.

Another reason for incorporating models is that it is difficult to operationally define some model components (especially in the self-regulatory model and health belief model) and examine each model as a whole. For instance, because the self-regulatory model is so complex, research has focused on illness representations and largely ignored the other components of the model and how they may work together to influence behavior.

Finally, integrating models is useful because it helps to explain behavior more accurately. For example, Ried and Christensen (130) examined relations between adherence to medication for urinary tract infections and variables from the health belief model (barriers and benefits) and the theory of reasoned action (belief strength, outcome evaluation, and behavioral intention). They found that health belief model variables explained 10% of the variance in adherence, whereas the theory of reasoned action variables explained an additional 19% of the variance. Thus, the amount of variance accounted for by variables from both models (29%) was greater than using either model alone. As another example, Senécal and colleagues (131) examined the relationship between constructs from social cognitive theory (self-efficacy) and self-determination theory (autonomy) and two outcomes—adherence and life satisfaction—among diabetics who managed their disease with self-care activities. Although constructs from both theories were significantly related to both outcomes, self-efficacy was more strongly related to adherence, whereas autonomy was more strongly related to life satisfaction. In sum, these findings suggest that interventions designed to increase adherence should utilize constructs from various theories of behavioral change.

How might various models be integrated? We made a distinction between theories of behavioral prediction (e.g., theory of planned behavior, health belief model) that "determine" the performance or nonperformance of any behavior at any given point in time and models of behavior change that focus on "stages" individuals may go through in their attempt to change behavior (e.g., transtheoretical model). Although behavioral prediction and behavior change theories often have different foci, they are complementary; the intensity and direction of the variables identified in behavioral prediction theories often serve as markers of a stage of change. The precontemplator has not formed an intention, may have low self-efficacy, and may perceive little social pressure. As one moves from strong negative through neutral through weak positive interventions, they may be moving from the precontemplation to the contemplation stage (87).

By integrating the theories, we can specify the conditions that must be met for behavioral change to occur. One must (a) have a strong positive intention or predisposition to perform a behavior, (b) perceive her or himself as having the requisite skills for the behavior, (c) not face physical, logistical, or social environmental barriers to performing the behavior, (d) believe that material, social, or other reinforcement will follow the behavior, (e) believe that there is normative pressure to perform and none sanctioning the behavior, (f) believe that the behavior is consistent with a person's self-image, (g) have a positive effect regarding the behavior, and (h) encounter cues or enablers to engage in the behavior at the appropriate time and place (52, 132). In general, for behavior to occur, the first three conditions must hold. The remaining five variables are viewed as influencing the strength and direction of intention.

The idea that models should be combined is at the heart of the collaborative-care paradigm. In contrast to the traditional medical model, in which providers tell patients what to do and nonadherence is viewed as the fault of the patient, the collaborative-care paradigm suggests that the provider and patient work together, in a partnership (133). This perspective acknowledges that patients can and do make decisions about whether and when to follow the suggested treatment regimen—in other words, they self-manage their disease. In the partnership, providers not only provide patients with technical information about their disease and treatment, but also help patients learn to problem solve. In this way, a patient can learn to work through different issues that may influence adherence to a treatment regimen.

One central feature of self-management education is that patients make short-term action plans—what we referred to earlier as forming implementation intentions. For example, a patient trying to adopt an exercise routine may decide to walk half a mile 3 days per week. Once the short-term goal has been reached, another action plan can be formed so that the amount of exercise gradually increases to an optimal level. Another feature of self-management is self-efficacy. If patients indicate that they are not confident they can carry out an action plan, the provider can work with them to instill confidence, perhaps by helping them rehearse a behavior or making their goal easier to achieve (e.g., start out by walking three times per week instead of every day). The key is for patients to participate in decisions about what they will do to manage their disease so that motivation will become more internal than external.

Self-management programs incorporating constructs from several theoretical models have proven successful for many diseases, including asthma, arthritis, and diabetes (133). Recently, Lorig and colleagues provided evidence for the efficacy of their Chronic Disease Self-Management Program (134). Patients with heart disease, lung disease, stroke, or arthritis participated in a group training program that met for 2½ hours weekly for 7 weeks. Peer leaders provided patients with information, trained them to problem solve, and used mastery techniques to increase self-efficacy. Two years after the program was initiated, patients had fewer emergency room/outpatient visits, less health distress, and greater self-efficacy and energy compared to their baseline values.

Self-management interventions will be most effective to the extent that they incorporate providers and patients and focus on environmental, individual, and interpersonal factors that influence behavior (135). Environmental factors include access to care, cost, insurance status, housing, and air quality. Individual differences include demographic, cognitive, knowledge, attitudinal (e.g., self-efficacy), affective (e.g., depression), and behavioral (e.g., skills) characteristics. At the interpersonal level, social support and communication are key factors for influencing adherence to physical activity as well as dietary and pharmacological interventions (136). Social support may come from a number of sources, including the health care provider, home (e.g., spouse, family), work, or within the treatment itself (e.g., fellow participants) and may be of emotional, informational, or instrumental nature. However, relatively little is known regarding how the nature of social support influences adherence. For example, in the dietary domain, support of an informational nature may be important (e.g., nutritional information), whereas instrumental support may be more important in the pharmacological domain (e.g., help with insulin administration for diabetes). The nature of the support may also vary depending on the duration of the behavior (i.e., how long the person has been adhering). For example, instrumental and informational support may be important predictors of adherence at the start of the behavior, whereas emotional support may begin to play a larger role after some time has elapsed and adherence has been maintained.

CONCLUSION

Further development and integration of theories to explain patient behavior will need to occur to improve treatment adherence. Adherence with lifestyle modifications, particularly toward the goal of primary prevention, is distressingly poor. Smoking cessation, exercise, and dietary modification can be extraordinarily difficult for patients to carry out and maintain successfully; failure rates are in the 75% to 80% range (137). Existing models of health behavior, such as the health belief model (69) and the theory of reasoned action (24), have found wide applicability in health behavior research but have not received as much attention in adherence research (138). For the state of the patient adherence literature to improve, further attention to the theoretical models that predict nonadherence is necessary.

ACKNOWLEDGMENTS

This research is supported by Grant R01 HL070713 from the National Heart, Lung, and Blood Institute.

REFERENCES

1. Manstead AS, Parker D. Evaluating and extending the theory of planned behavior. In: Stroebe M, Hewstone M, eds. *European Review of Social Psychology.* Chichester, England: John Wiley & Sons; 1995:69–95.

2. Thompson SC. Will it hurt less if I can control it? A complex answer to a simple question. *Psychol Bull.* 1981;90(1):89–101.

3. Seydel E, Taal E, Wiegman O. Risk appraisal, outcome and self-efficacy expectancies: cognitive factors in previous behavior related to cancer. *Psychol Health.* 1990;4:99–109.

4. Rotter JB. *Social Learning and Clinical Psychology.* Oxford, England: Prentice-Hall; 1954.

5. Rotter JB. Generalized expectancies for internal versus external control of reinforcement. *Psychological Monographs: General and Applied.* 1966;80(1):1–28.

6. Wurtele SK, Maddux JE. Relative contributions of protection motivation theory components in predicting exercise intentions and behavior. *Health Psychol.* 1987;5:453–466.

7. Wallston BD, Wallston KA. Locus of control and health: a review of the literature. *Health Educ Monogr.* 1978;6(2):107–117.

8. Norman P, Bennett P, Smith C, Murphy S. Health locus of control and health behaviour. *J Health Psychol.* 1997;3(2):171–180.

9. Molassiotis A, Nahas-Lopez V, Chung WY, et al. Factors associated with adherence to antiretroviral medication in HIV-infected patients. *Int J STD AIDS.* 2002;13(5):301–310.

10. Kirscht JP, Rosenstock IM. Patient adherence to antihypertensive medical regimens. *J Community Health.* 1977;3(2):115–124.

11. Nir Z, Neumann L. Relationship among self-esteem, internal–external locus of control, and weight change after participation in a weight reduction program. *J Clin Psychol.* 1995;51(4):482–490.

12. Schapira DV, Kumar NB, Lyman GH, Baile WF. The effect of duration of intervention and locus of control on dietary change. *Am J Prev Med.* 1991;7(6): 341–347.

13. Christensen AJ, Wiebe JS, Benotsch EG, Lawton WJ. Perceived health competence, health locus of control, and patient adherence in renal dialysis. *Cognit Ther Res.* 1996;20(4):411–421.

14. Voils CI, Steffens DC, Flint EP, Bosworth HB. Social support and locus of control as predictors of adherence to antidepressant medication in an elderly population. *Am J Geriatr Psychiatry.* In press.

15. Rippletoe PA, Rogers RW. Effects of components of protection motivation theory on adaptive and maladaptive coping with a health threat. *J Pers Social Psychol.* 1987;52:596–604.

16. Ronis DL, Antonakos CL, Lang WP. Usefulness of multiple equations for predicting preventive oral health behaviors. *Health Education Quarterly.* 1996;23: 512–527.

17. Desharnais R, Bouillon J, Godin G. Self-efficacy and outcome expectations as determinants of exercise adherence. *Psychol Rep.* 1986;59(1):155–159.

18. McAuley E, Jerome GJ, Marquez DX, et al. Exercise self-efficacy in older adults: social, affective, and behavioral influences. *Ann Behav Med.* 2003;25(1):1–7.

19. Gwaltney CJ, Schiffman S, Paty JA, et al. Using self-efficacy judgments to predict characteristics of lapses to smoking. *J Consult Clin Psychol.* 2002;70(5): 1140–1149.

20. Luszczynska A, Schwarzer R. Planning and self-efficacy in the adoption and maintenance of breast self-examination: a longitudinal study on self-regulatory cognitions. *Psychol Health.* 2003;18(1):93–108.

21. Safren SA, Otto MW, Worth JL, et al. Two strategies to increase adherence to HIV antiretroviral medication: life-steps and medication monitoring. *Behav Res Ther.* 2001;39:1151–1162.

22. Bandura A. *Social Foundation of Thoughts and Actions: A Social Cognitive Theory.* Englewood Cliffs, NJ: Prentice-Hall; 1986.

23. Woodard CM, Berry MJ. Enhancing adherence to prescribed exercise: structured behavioral interventions in clinical exercise programs. *J Cardiopulm Rehab.* 2001;21(4):201–209.

24. Ajzen I, Fishbein M. *Understanding Attitudes and Social Behavior.* Englewood Cliffs, NJ: Prentice-Hall; 1980.

25. Ajzen I. The theory of planned behavior. *Organizational Behavior and Human Decision Processes.* 1991;50:179–211.

26. Bandura A. Self-efficacy: toward a unifying theory of behavioral change. *Psychol Rev.* 1977;84(2):191–215.

27. Ajzen I. Perceived behavioral control, self-efficacy, locus of control, and the theory of planned behavior. *J Appl Social Psychol.* 2002;32:1–20.

28. Sutton S. Predicting and explaining intentions and behavior: How well are we doing? *J Appl Social Psychol.* 1998;28(15):1317–1338.

29. Mischel W, Cantor N, Feldman S. Principles of self-regulation: the nature of willpower and self-control. In: Higgins ET, Kruglanski, A, ed. *Social Psychology: Handbook of Basic Principles.* New York: Guilford Press; 1996:329–360.

30. Armitage CJ, Conner M. Efficacy of the theory of planned behaviour: a meta-analytic review. *Br J Soc Psychol.* 2001;40(Pt 4):471–499.

31. Sheeran P, Orbell S. Do intentions predict condom use? Meta-analysis and examination of six moderator variables. *Br J Soc Psychol.* 1998;37(Pt 2):231–250.

32. Godin G, Kok G. The theory of planned behavior: a review of its applications to health-related behaviors. *Am J Health Promot.* 1996;11(2):87–98.

33. Sheeran P. Intention–behavior relations: a conceptual and empirical review. In: Stroebe M, Hewstone M, eds. *European Review of Social Psychology.* Chichester, England: John Wiley & Sons; 2002:1–36.

34. Sheeran P, Orbell S. Using implementation intentions to increase attendance for cervical cancer screening. *Health Psychol.* 2000;19(3):283–289.

35. Bagozzi RP, Kimmel SK. A comparison of leading theories for the predicting of goal-directed behaviours. *Brit J Social Psychol.* 1995;34:437–461.

36. Bassili JN. Response latency versus certainty as indexes of the strength of voting intentions in a CATI survey. *Public Opinion Quarterly.* 1993;57:54–61.

37. Richard R, van der Pligt J, de Vries NK. Anticipated affect and behavioral choice. *Basic Appl Social Psychol.* 1996;18:111–129.

38. Sheeran P, Norman P, Orbell S. Evidence that intentions based on attitudes better predict behaviour than intentions based on subjective norms. *J Social Psychol.* 1999;29:403–406.

39. Sheeran P, Silverman M. Evaluation of three interventions to promote workplace health and safety: evidence for the utility of implementation intentions. *Soc Sci Med.* 2003;56(10):2153–2163.

40. Gollwitzer PM. *Goal Achievement: The Role of Intentions.* Chichester, England: John Wiley & Sons; 1993.

41. Gollwitzer PM, Brandstaetter V. Implementation intentions and effective goal pursuit. *J Person Soc Psychol.* 1997;73(1):186–199.

42. Gollwitzer PM. Implementation intentions: strong effects of simple plans. *Am Psychol.* 1999;54(7):493–503.

43. Bargh JA. Auto-motives: preconscious determinants of social interaction. In: Higgins ET, Sorrentino RM, eds. *Handbook of Motivation and Cognition: Foundations of Social Behavior.* Vol. 2. New York: Guilford Press; 1990:93–130.

44. Bargh JA. The four horsemen of automaticity: awareness, intention, efficiency, and control in social cognition. In: Wyer RS Jr, Srull TK, eds. *Handbook of Social Cognition.* 2nd ed. Hillsdale, NJ: Lawrence Erlbaum Associates; 1994:1–40.

45. Montano DE, Kasprzyk D, Taplin SH. The theory of reasoned action and the theory of planned behavior. In: Glanz K, Lewis F, Rimer B, eds. *Health Behavior and Health Education: Theory, Research, and Practice.* 2nd ed. San Francisco: Jossey-Bass; 1997:85–112.

46. Orbell S, Hodgkins S, Sheeran P. Implementation intentions and the theory of planned behavior. *Person Soc Psychol. Bull.* 1997;23(9):945–954.

47. Verplanken B, Faes S. Good intentions, bad habits, and effects of forming implementation intentions on healthy eating. *Eur J Soc Psychol.* 1999;29(5–6): 591–604.

48. Milne S, Orbell S, Sheeran P. Combining motivational and volitional interventions to promote exercise participation: protection motivation theory and implementation intentions. *Brit J Social Psychol.* 2002;7(2):163–184.

49. Sperry L. The ingredients of effective health counseling: health beliefs, compliance and relapse prevention. *Lancet.* 1986;42(2):279–287.

50. Lierman LM, Young HM, Kasprzyk D, Benoliel JQ. Predicting breast self-examination using the theory of reasoned action. *Nurs Res.* 1990;39(2):97–101.

51. Hash RB, Munna RK, Vogel RL, Bason JJ. Does physician weight affect perception of health advice? *Prev Med.* 2003;36(1):41–44.

52. Elder JP, Apodaca X, Parra-Medina D. Theoretical models of health education. In: Loue S, ed. *Handbook of Immigrant Health.* New York: Plenum Press; 1998.

53. Rogers RW. A protection motivation theory of fear appeals and attitude change. *J Psychol.* 1975;91(1):93–114.

54. Rogers RW. Cognitive and physiological processes in fear appeals and attitude change: a revised theory of protection motivation. In: Cacioppo JT, Petty RE, eds. *Social Psychophysiology: A Sourcebook.* New York: Guilford Press; 1983:153–176.

55. Fruin DJ, Pratt C, Owen N. Protection motivation theory and adolescents' perception of exercise. *J Appl Social Psychol.* 1991;22:55–69.

56. Abraham SCS, Sheeran P, Abrams D, Spears R. Exploring teenagers' adaptive and maladaptive thinking in relation to the threat of HIV infection. *Psychol Health.* 1994;9:253–272.

57. Tanner JF, Jr, Day E, Crask MR. Protection motivation theory: an extension of fear appeals theory in communication. *J Business Res.* 1989;19:267–276.

58. Hodgkins S, Orbell S. Can protection motivation theory predict behavior? A longitudinal test exploring the role of previous behavior. *Psychol Health.* 1998;13:237–251.

59. Steffen VJ. Men's motivation to perform the testicle self-exam: effects of prior knowledge and an educational brochure. *J Appl Social Psychol.* 1990;20:681–702.

60. Helmes AW. Application of the protection motivation theory to genetic testing for breast cancer risk. *Prev Med.* 2002;35(5):453–462.

61. Beck KH, Lund AK. The effects of health threat seriousness and personal efficacy upon intentions and behavior. *J Appl Social Psychol.* 1981;11:401–415.

62. Maddux JE, Rogers RW. Protection motivation theory and self-efficacy: a revised theory of fear appeals and attitude change. *J Exper Social Psychol.* 1983;19:242–253.

63. Plotkinoff RC, Higginbotham N. Predicting low-fat diet intentions and behaviors for the prevention of coronary heart disease: an application of protection motivation theory among an Australian population. *Psychol Health.* 1995;10: 397–408.

64. Ben-Ahron V, White D, Phillips K. Encouraging drinking at safe limits on single occasions: The potential contribution of protection motivation theory. *Alcohol Alcohol.* 1995;30:633–639.

65. Drossaert CC, Boer H, Seydel ER. Perceived risk, anxiety, mammogram uptake, and breast self-examination of women with a family history of breast cancer: the role of knowing to be at increased risk. *Cancer Detect Prev.* 1996;20(1):76–85.

66. Taylor AH, May S. Threat and coping appraisal as determinants of compliance with sports injury rehabilitation: an application of protection motivation theory. *J Sports Sci.* 1996;14(6):471–482.

67. Milne S, Sheeran P, Orbell S. Prediction and intervention in health-related behavior: a meta-analytic review of protection motivation theory. *J Appl Social Psychol.* 2000;30(1):106–143.

68. Leventhal H, Zimmerman R, Gutmann, M. Compliance: a self-regulation perspective. In: Gentry D, ed. *Handbook of Behavioral Medicine.* New York: The Free Press; 1984:369–436.

69. Rosenstock I. The health belief model and preventive health behavior. *Health Education Monographs.* 1974;2:354–386.

70. Kirscht JP. The health belief model and predictions of health actions. In: Gochman DS, ed. *Health Behavior: Emerging Research Perspectives.* New York: Plenum Press; 1988:27–41.

71. Bandura A, Reese LB, Adams NE. Microanalysis of action and fear arousal as a function of differential levels of perceived self-efficacy. *J Person Soc Psychol.* 1982;43:5–21.

72. Rosenstock I. Enhancing patient compliance with health recommendations. *J Pediat Health Care.* 1988;2:67–72.

73. Bosworth HB, Oddone EZ. A model of psychosocial and cultural antecedents of blood pressure control. *J Natl Med Assoc.* 2002;94(4):236–248.

74. Becker MH. The health belief model and personal health behavior. *Health Education Monographs.* 1974;2:324–508.

75. Janz NK, Becker MH. The health belief model: a decade later. *Health Education Quarterly.* 1984;11(1):1–47.

76. Harrison JA, Mullen PD, Green LW. A meta-analysis of studies of the health belief model with adults. *Health Education Research.* 1992;7(1):107–116.

77. Strecher VJ, Champion VL, Rosenstock IM. The health belief model and health behavior. In: Gochman, DS, ed. *Handbook of Health Behavior Research 1: Personal and Social Determinants.* New York: Plenum Press; 1997:71–91.

78. Eraker S, Kirscht JP, Becker MH. Understanding and improving patient compliance. *Ann Int Med.* 1984;100:258–268.

79. Hershey JC, Morton BG, Davis JB, Reichgott MJ. Patient compliance with antihypertensive medication. *Am J Public Health.* 1980;70(10):1081–1089.

80. Cummings KM, Becker MH, Kirscht JP, Levin NW. Psychosocial factors affecting adherence to medical regiments in a group of hemodialysis patients. *Med Care.* 1982;20(6):567–580.

81. Kirscht J, Rosenstock I. Patients' problems in following recommendations of health experts. In: Stone G, Cohen F, Adler N, eds. *Health Psychology*. San Francisco: Jossey-Bass; 1979:189–215.

82. Leventhal H, Diefenbach M, Leventhal EA. Illness cognition: Using common sense to understand treatment adherence and affect cognition interactions. *Cognit Ther Res*. 1992;16(2):143–163.

83. Petrie KJ, Weinman J, Sharp N, Buckley J. Role of patients' view of their illness in predicting return to work and functioning after myocardial infarction: longitudinal study. *BMJ*. 1996;312:1191–1194.

84. Meyer D, Leventhal H, Gutmann M. Common-sense models of illness: the example of hypertension. *Health Psychol*. 1985;4(2):115–135.

85. Horne R, Weinman J. Self-regulation and self-management in asthma: exploring the role of illness perceptions and treatment beliefs in explaining nonadherence to preventer medication. *Psychol Health*. 2002;17(1):17–32.

86. Reynolds NR. The problem of antiretroviral adherence: a self-regulatory model for intervention. *AIDS Care*. 2003;15(1):117–124.

87. Prochaska JO, DiClemente CC. Stages and processes of self-change of smoking: toward an integrative model of change. *J Consult Clin Psychol*. 1983;51(3): 390–395.

88. Weinstein ND. The precaution adoption process. *Health Psychol*. 1988;7(4): 355–386.

89. Weinstein ND, Rothman AJ, Sutton SR. Stage theories of health behavior: conceptual and methodological issues. *Health Psychol*. 1998;17(3):290–299.

90. Sonstroem R. Psychological models. In: Dishman RK, ed. *Exercise Adherence: Its Impact on Public Health*. Champagne, IL: Human Kinetics; 1988:125–153.

91. Prochaska JO, DiClemente CC. Stages of change in the modification of problem behaviors. *Prog Behav Modif*. 1992;28:183–218.

92. Nigg CR, Burbank PM, Padula C, et al. Stages of change across ten health risk behaviors for older adults. *Gerontologist*. 1999;39(4):473–482.

93. DiClemente CC, Prochaska J. Toward a comprehensive transtheoretical model of change. In: Healther WRMN, ed. *Treating Addictive Behaviors*. New York: Plenum Press; 1998:3–24.

94. Prochaska JO, Goldstein MG. Process of smoking cessation. Implications for clinicians. *Clin Chest Med*. 1991;12(4):727–735.

95. Cassidy CA. Facilitating behavior change. Use of the transtheoretical model in the occupational health setting. *AAOHN J*. 1997;45(5):239–246.

96. Prochaska JO, Diclemente CC, Norcross JC. In search of how people change: applications to addictive behaviors. *Am Psychol*. 1992;47(9):1102–1114.

97. DiClemente CC, Scott CW. Stages of change: interaction with treatment compliance and involvement. In: Onken LS, Blaine JD, Boren JJ, eds. *Beyond the Therapeutic Alliance: Keeping the Drug-Dependent Individual in Treatment*. NIDA Research Monograph No. 165. Rockville, MD: National Institute on Drug Abuse; 1997: 131–156.

98. Janis I, Mann L. *Decision Making*. New York: Macmillan; 1977.

99. Rakowski W, Ehrich B, Goldstein MG, et al. Increasing mammography among women aged 40–74 by use of a stage-matched, tailored intervention. *Prev Med.* 1998;27(5 Pt 1):748–756.

100. Plummer BA, Velicer WF, Redding CA, et al. Stage of change, decisional balance, and temptations for smoking: measurement and validation in a large, school-based population of adolescents. *Addict Behav.* 2001;26(4):551–571.

101. Clark MA, Rakowski W, Kviz FJ, Hogan JW. Age and stage of readiness for smoking cessation. *J Gerontol B Psychol Sci Soc Sci.* 1997;52(4):S212–S221.

102. Greene GW, Rossi SR, Reed GR, et al. Stages of change for reducing dietary fat to 30% of energy or less. *J Am Diet Assoc.* 1994;94(10):1105–1110.

103. Suris AM, Trapp MC, DiClemente CC, Cousins J. Application of the transtheoretical model of behavior change for obesity in Mexican American women. *Addict Behav.* 1998;23(5):655–668.

104. Jeffery RW, French SA, Rothman AJ. Stage of change as a predictor of success in weight control in adult women. *Health Psychol.* 1999;18(5):543–546.

105. Marcus BH, Rakowski W, Rossi JS. Assessing motivational readiness and decision making for exercise. *Health Psychol.* 1992;11(4):257–261.

106. Grimley DM, Riley GE, Bellis JM, Prochaska JO. Assessing the stages of change and decision-making for contraceptive use for the prevention of pregnancy, sexually transmitted diseases, and acquired immunodeficiency syndrome. *Health Education Quarterly.* 1993;20(4) · 455–470.

107. Dijkstra A, de Vries H, Bakker M. Pros and cons of quitting, self-efficacy, and the stages of change in smoking cessation. *J Consult Clin Psychol.* 1996;64(4): 758–763.

108. Fava JL, Velicer WF, Prochaska JO. Applying the transtheoretical model to a representative sample of smokers. *Addict Behav.* 1995;20(2):189–203.

109. Rollnick S, Heather N, Gold R, Hall W. Development of a short "readiness to change" questionnaire for use in brief, opportunistic interventions among excessive drinkers. *Br J Addict.* 1992;87(5):743–754.

110. DiClemente CC, Carbonari JP, Montgomery RP, Hughes SO. The Alcohol Abstinence Self-Efficacy scale. *J Stud Alcohol.* 1994;55(2):141–148.

111. McConnaughy EA, DiClemente CC, Prochaska JO, Velicer WF. Stages of change in psychotherapy: a follow-up report. *Psychotherapy: Theory, Research, and Practice.* 1989;4:494–503.

112. Miller WR, Rollnick, S. *Motivational Interviewing: Preparing People to Change Addictive Behaviors.* New York: Guilford Press; 1991.

113. D'Nofrio G, Bernstein E, Rollnick S. Motivating patients for change: a brief strategy for negotiation. In: Bernstein E, Bernstein J, eds. *Case Studies in Emergency Medicine and the Health of the Public.* Sudbury, MA: Jones and Bartlett Publishers; 1996:295–303.

114. Bandura A. *Self-Efficacy: The Exercise of Control.* New York: Freeman; 1997.

115. Bandura A. Health promotion from the perspective of social cognitive theory. *Psychology and Health.* 1998;13:623–649.

116. Davidson R. The transtheoretical model: a critical overview. In: Miller WR, Heather N, eds. *Treating Addictive Behaviors.* New York: Plenum Press; 1998: 25–38.

117. Littell JH, Girvin H. Stages of change. A critique. *Behav Modif.* 2002;26(2): 223–273.

118. Dunn C, Deroo L, Rivara FP. The use of brief interventions adapted from motivational interviewing across behavioral domains: a systematic review. *Addiction.* 2001;96(12):1725–1742.

119. Noonan W, Moyers T. Motivational interviewing: a review. *Journal of Substance Misuse.* 1997;2:8–16.

120. Emmons KM, Rollnick S. Motivational interviewing in health care settings. Opportunities and limitations. *Am J Prev Med.* 2001;20(1):68–74.

121. Rollnick S, Mason, P, Butler, C. *Health Behavior Change: A Guide for Practitioners.* London, England: Churchill Livingstone; 1999.

122. Accessed at October 20, 2004: http://motivationalinterview.org/library/biblio.html

123. Kemp R, Kirov G, Everitt B, et al. Randomised controlled trial of compliance therapy. 18-month follow-up. *Br J Psychiatry.* 1998;172:413–419.

124. Hayward P, Chan N, Kemp R, Youle S. Medication self-management: a preliminary report on an intervention to improve medication compliance. *J Ment Health.* 1995;4:511–517.

125. Weinstein ND, Sandman PM. A model of the precaution adoption process: evidence from home radon testing. *Health Psychol.* 1992;11(3):170–180.

126. Clemow L, Costanza ME, Haddad WP, et al. Underutilizers of mammography screening today: characteristics of women planning, undecided about, and not planning a mammogram. *Annals Behav Med.* 2000;22(1):80–88.

127. Emmett C, Ferguson E. Oral contraceptive pill use, decisional balance, risk perception and knowledge: an exploratory study. *J Reprod Infant Psychol.* 1999;17(4):327–343.

128. Blalock SJ, DeVellis RF, Giorgino KB, et al. Osteoporosis prevention in premenopausal women: Using a stage model approach to examine the predictors of behavior. *Health Psychol.* 1996;15:84–93.

129. Horne R, ed. *Adherence to Medication: A Review of Existing Research.* London: Harwood; 1998.

130. Ried LD, Christensen DB. A psychosocial perspective in the explanation of patients' drug-taking behavior. *Soc Sci Med.* 1988;27(3):277–285.

131. Senécal C, Nouwen A, White D. Motivation and dietary self-care in adults with diabetes: are self-efficacy and autonomous self-regulation complementary or competing constructs? *Health Psychol.* 2000;19(5):452–457.

132. Fishbein M, Triandis HC, Kanfer FH, et al. Factors influencing behavior and behavior change. In: Baum A, Revenson TA, Singer JE, eds. *Handbook of Health Psychology.* Mahwah, NJ: Lawrence Erlbaum Associates; 2001:3–18.

133. Bodenheimer T, Lorig K, Holman H, Grumbach K. Patient self-management of chronic disease in primary care. *JAMA.* 2002;288(19):2469–2475.

134. Lorig KR, Ritter P, Stewart AL, et al. Chronic disease self-management program: 2-year health status and health care utilization outcomes. *Med Care.* 2001;39(11):1217–1223.

135. Culos-Reed SN, Rejeski WJ, McAuley E, et al. Predictors of adherence to behavior change interventions in the elderly. *Control Clin Trials.* 2000;21(5 Suppl): 200S–205S.
136. Gallant MP. The influence of social support on chronic illness self-management: a review and directions for research. *Health Educ Behav.* 2003;30(2): 170–195.
137. Fiore MC, Smith SS, Jorenby DE, Baker TB. The effectiveness of the nicotine patch for smoking cessation. A meta-analysis. *JAMA.* 1994;271(24):1940–1947.
138. Mullen PD, Hersey JC, Iverson DC. Health behavior models compared. *Soc Sci Med.* 1987;24(11):973–981.

Part II

FACTORS INFLUENCING TREATMENT ADHERENCE

Chapter 3

Adherence to Physical Activity

Kelli L. Dominick
Miriam Morey

The aim of this chapter is to provide a synopsis of research related to physical activity adherence, with a primary focus on studies involving adults. We discuss evidence supporting the health benefits of physical activity and the widespread problem of nonadherence to physical activity recommendations. We provide an overview of studies examining factors related to physical activity adherence, then we focus on studies testing interventions to increase physical activity. Finally, we discuss clinical and policy implications of physical activity adherence research.

PHYSICAL FUNCTION/EXERCISE AND ADHERENCE

There is abundant evidence that physical activity results in positive health benefits. Early studies focused largely on cardiovascular risk factors, showing that physical activity is related to improvements in dyslipidemia, reduced blood pressure, decreased insulin resistance, reduced body fat, and an overall reduction in cardiovascular mortality (1–3). Research on the health benefits of physical activity has expanded widely to include a variety of outcomes. For example, physical activity is associated with improved psychological health (4) and functional status (5), reduced health care use and expenditures (6–9), and reduced risk for all-cause mortality (1, 10, 11). Physical activity is also associated with improvements in outcomes for many common conditions including hypertension (12), obesity (13), arthritis

(14), diabetes (15), depression (16), and chronic obstructive pulmonary disease (17).

There has been considerable debate and study regarding the amount of physical activity required for achieving health and fitness benefits. Although there is no clear consensus regarding the specific amount of physical activity required for health benefits, there is no doubt that physical activity must be performed regularly in order to achieve and maintain these benefits. The most widely disseminated physical activity guidelines come from a report of the Surgeon General. This report recommends that individuals set a goal of accumulating at least 30 minutes of moderate intensity physical activity on most, and preferably all, days of the week (18). Similarly, Healthy People 2010 guidelines recommend at least 30 minutes of moderate activity on 5 or more days per week or 20 minutes of vigorous activity three or more times per week (19). Current guidelines from the American College of Sports Medicine (ACSM) recommend that in order to develop and maintain cardiorespiratory fitness and body composition, individuals should perform physical activity 3–5 days per week, at an intensity of 55%–90% of maximum heart rate (or 40%–85% of maximum oxygen uptake or maximum heart rate reserve) for 20–60 minutes (20). Studies have shown that health benefits can be achieved when physical activity is performed intermittently, in shorter bouts that accumulate to the recommended total duration. However, these shorter bouts should be a minimum of 10 minutes each (20). Recent research has also shown that physical activity performed in the context of regular occupational, household, and leisure activities can produce benefits similar to those of structured exercise, as long as the frequency, intensity, and duration are sufficient (21–23).

Long-term adherence to physical activity is essential for the maintenance of health benefits. For example, Morey et al. reported that among older adults enrolled in a physical activity program for more than 10 years, participants classified as adherent had a long-term survival benefit by time compared to a nonadherent group (24). Other studies have shown that individuals who are more adherent to regular exercise programs, compared to those who are less adherent, experience greater improvements in fitness, physical function, quality of life, and disease-specific outcomes (25–27).

PROBLEM OF NONADHERENCE TO PHYSICAL ACTIVITY RECOMMENDATIONS

Despite the wealth of evidence regarding the health benefits of regular physical activity, nonadherence to physical activity recommendations is a significant problem. National data show that only 25% of Americans achieve recommended levels of physical activity, and 29% report getting no regular physical activity (28). This epidemic of physical inactivity has enormous public health implications. It has been estimated that the direct costs of physical inactivity, defined as the absence of leisure-time physical activity, are approximately $24 billion, or 2.4% of U.S. health care expenditures (8). During the past several decades, considerable efforts have been made to identify factors related to inactivity and to increase nationwide physical activity levels. Yet activity patterns in the United States have not improved significantly over the past 15 years (28–30). Even after individuals begin programs of regular physical activity, drop-out rates are very high. Specifically, studies suggest about 50% of adults who start a physical activity program will drop out within a few months (31).

FACTORS RELATED TO PHYSICAL ACTIVITY ADHERENCE

There have been several comprehensive reviews of the correlates and predictors of physical activity, covering more than 380 studies (32–37). This demonstrates the great amount of effort that has been directed at understanding individuals' physical activity behavior. This section describes the literature on correlates of physical activity, focusing on six categories of factors: demographic, health related and biological, cognitive and psychological, behavioral, social, program related, and environmental. Table 3.1 summarizes relationships of these factors to physical activity, focusing primarily on studies conducted within the past 5 years (1998–2003).

Demographic Factors

In general, demographic variables have been fairly strong correlates of physical activity. Demographic characteristics studied most widely have included age, gender, race and ethnicity, socioeconomic status (SES), and marital status.

Age. The benefits of physical activity for older adults have now been well established (38). Yet studies show that increasing age is still one of the most consistent predictors of decreased physical activity (32, 39). In the United States, more than 60% of older adults are not involved in regular physical activity (40, 41). Some data suggest physical activity levels increase slightly around the typical age of retirement (60–65), but then decline shortly afterward (42). Studies have also shown that there is a greater age-related decline in physical activity among older women in comparison to older men (29).

TABLE 3.1
Factors Associated With Physical Activity

Variable	Strength of Association	References
Demographic Factors		
Age	—	46, 50, 73, 80–82, 124, 129, 235–242
Gender	++	46, 50, 73, 124, 235–237, 239–241, 243
Non-White race/ethnicity	—	50, 60, 79–82, 121, 236, 242, 244
Income/socioeconomic status	++	46, 50, 73, 81, 235, 236, 240, 241, 245–247
Education	++	50, 60, 73, 79–82, 101, 129, 236, 238–241
Blue-collar occupation	-	73, 74
Married	+	73, 77–82
Childless	+	82
Health-Related and Biological Factors		
Poor Health	—	46, 97, 248
Injury History	+	242
Overweight/Obesity	—	81, 82, 240–242, 249
Heredity	++	83–88
Cognitive and Psychological Factors		
Barriers (perceived)	—	60, 80, 82, 97, 124, 238, 247, 248, 254, 255
Enjoyment of exercise	++	124, 237
Expected benefits of exercise	++	97, 217, 236, 242, 255–257
Intention to exercise	++	246, 247, 250–253, 258
Psychological health	+	232, 260, 261
Self-efficacy	++	46, 82, 89, 124, 132, 217, 236, 242, 244, 248, 254–257, 262–264
Self-motivation	++	82, 246
Self-schemata for exercise	++	262
Stage of change	++	132, 256, 264
Perceived health or fitness	++	46, 80, 82, 124, 236, 254
Attitudes	00	124, 246, 247, 250–253
Control over exercise	+	242, 246, 247, 251–253
Normative belief	00	77, 246, 247, 250, 251, 253
Knowledge of health and exercise	00	236, 238, 240
Stress	0	46, 256
Value of exercise outcomes	0	46, 256, 265
Behavioral Factors		
Activity history during childhood	00	266
Activity history during adulthood	++	246, 247, 254
Past exercise program	++	89, 246, 247, 251, 254
Smoking	-	73, 81, 82, 238–240, 267
Dietary habits (quality)	++	81, 238, 267
Alcohol use	0	267
Type A behavior	+	95, 268

(Continued)

TABLE 3.1
(Continued)

Variable	Strength of Association	References
Social Factors		
Group cohesion	+	99, 269, 270
Physician influence	++	46, 96, 236
Social isolation	-	101, 236, 242
Social support from friends/peers	++	60, 68, 79, 82, 97, 124, 132, 217, 237, 248, 253, 263, 265
Social support from spouse/family	++	60, 68, 79, 82, 97, 124, 132, 217, 238, 248, 253, 263
Program-Related Factors		
Exercise Intensity	-	104, 106, 118
Exercise Duration	-	107, 113
Exercise Frequency	0	104, 114
Home-based program (vs. center-based)	+	105, 116–118
Environmental Factors		
Access to facilities/walking locations	+	121–124, 129, 258
Neighborhood safety	+	60, 80, 121, 128, 239
Enjoyable scenery	+	60, 80, 235
Frequently observe others exercising	+	60, 80, 124
Hilly terrain	+	41, 80
Presence of sidewalks	0	60, 80, 121, 124, 258
Satisfaction with facilities	+	124, 129
Cost of program	0	124, 129
Heavy traffic	0	60, 80, 121, 258
Home equipment	+	80, 111, 124
"Sprawling" county	-	206
Urban location	-	60, 78, 80, 81, 235, 239, 245

Note. From ref. 32. Copyright 2002. Adapted by permission.

++ = repeated documentation of positive association with physical activity; + = weak or mixed evidence of positive association with physical activity; 00 = repeated documentation of no association with physical activity; 0 = weak or mixed evidence of no association with physical activity; — = repeated documentation of negative association with physical activity; - = weak or mixed evidence of negative association with physical activity.

Not surprisingly, poor health status is one of the most important and consistent correlates of inactivity among older individuals (36). Some specific health-related variables associated with reduced activity among older adults include poor perceptions of overall health, presence of chronic diseases, depressive symptoms, injuries, activity and mobility limitations, pain, and fear of pain (36, 43). Despite this strong association, low activity levels among older adults cannot be completely explained by poor health. For example, it has been estimated that more than half of older adults are healthy and fit enough to exercise (36). Other factors associated with physical activity among older adults include education level, prior exercise history, and social cognitive variables (such as exercise attitudes, self-efficacy, social support, and perceived benefits/barriers to exercise) (36, 43). These are all factors that have been related to physical activity levels in studies among the general adult population. Yet there may also be some factors that are particularly salient among older adults. First, some research suggests that social support for physical activity decreases substantially with age (44), and this may negatively affect activity among older adults. Second, older adults may be more likely than younger individuals to report lack of skill as a barrier to activity (45). Third, misconceptions about physical activity are problematic among older adults. Specifically, older adults may be deterred from physical activity because of beliefs that activity must be vigorous or uncomfortable to produce benefits (46, 47). Fourth, physicians are less likely to ask older adults about physical activity and less likely to counsel their patients to become more physically active (48).

Gender. Gender has also been a consistent predictor of physical activity, with men showing greater levels of activity than women (32, 34, 39). Data from the Third National Health and Nutrition Examination Survey (NHANES III) showed that the age-adjusted prevalence of reporting no leisure-time physical activity was 17% for men and 27% for women (49). Martin et al. reported that among a nationwide sample of households, 37% of men and 29% of women currently met the Centers for Disease Control and Prevention (CDC)/ACSM recommendations for physical activity (50). There is one context in which there have been discrepant findings regarding gender differences in physical activity adherence. Some research has shown that when individuals are enrolled in an exercise program for the treatment or prevention of a particular disease or condition (i.e., cardiovascular disease, osteoporosis), women may have greater adherence than men (51). However, other studies have found that women are also less adherent in disease-specific programs (52).

Though many barriers to physical activity are similarly influential among both women and men, there are some factors that are particularly relevant to women. First, the benefits of physical activity have historically not been as well studied or understood for women compared to men (53). This disparity in research has improved significantly over the past decade, and the health benefits of activity among women are now well documented. This increased knowledge may have a positive influence on women's activity levels over time. Second, previous physical activity guidelines emphasized fairly vigorous activity, which may have discouraged participation among women. Research has shown that only about 5% of women adopt vigorous activities (such as running) annually, but about 34% adopt moderate activities (such as walking) (54). Attrition rates from vigorous activity are also higher than from moderate activity among women. Newer physical activity guidelines focus more on moderate-level activities, and this change may also have a positive influence on women's activity levels as these recommendations continue to be conveyed. Third, women may experience a social environment that is not as supportive or conducive to activity as men. Women's frequent multiple roles, involving both work and family responsibilities, may be a particularly significant barrier to regular physical activity. For example, data show that women with young children at home are less active than women without young children (53).

Race and Ethnicity. Racial and ethnic minorities suffer disproportionately from chronic illnesses that are associated with physical inactivity, and elimination of these health disparities is a national health priority (55, 56). Yet studies show there are still considerable racial and ethnic differences in physical activity levels (56–58). Blacks, Hispanics, Asian and Pacific Islanders, and American Indians/Alaska Natives all report lower levels of physical activity compared to Whites (39, 55). Data from the National Health Interview Survey showed that the prevalence of reporting no leisure-time physical activity was 36% among non-Hispanic Whites, 52% among non-Hispanic Blacks, 54% among Hispanics, 46% among American Indians/Alaska Natives, and 42% among Asian/Pacific Islanders (55).

Low levels of physical activity among racial and ethic minorities may be confounded by SES (34, 51). However, some studies have controlled for income, work status, or education in statistical models and still observed racial differences in activity level (59, 60). Data from NHANES III show that African Americans and Mexican Americans have a higher level of leisure-time inactivity than White counterparts, even within specific SES categories (measured by education, income, occupation, employment, and poverty) (57). SES differences are likely to be influential, as they may limit resources or knowledge about physical activity. However, other psychological, social, physical, and environmental factors may also contribute to these differences.

Traditional predictive models of physical activity have not been sufficiently examined among ethnic and racial minorities, and factors influencing physical levels in these groups have not been well defined (61). However, these data are emerging, and in particular there is a growing literature on physical activity among racial and ethnic minority women (62–72). One study reported that whereas Anglo-American women valued the individual outcomes of physical activity, Mexican-American women often cited family responsibilities and attitudes as factors that either promoted or prevented them from being active (64). Other studies have shown that among African American women, family disapproval, family needs, and child care are particularly important barriers to activity (70–72). Greater understanding of physical barriers in other racial and ethnic groups is greatly needed for the development of successful interventions and public health strategies.

Socioeconomic Status.   Overall, SES has been a fairly consistent correlate of physical activity (32, 39). However, results vary based on the particular variable or facet of SES that is being examined. Blue-collar occupational status (typically manual and industrial labor), low income, and lower education level have all been associated with less physical activity (especially leisure-time physical activity) in some studies (32), but results have been weaker and more mixed for occupational status (34, 51). Some studies have shown little or no association between occupational status and leisure-time physical activity, and others have shown that individuals with blue-collar jobs report lower levels of leisure-time activity than white-collar workers. Yet individuals with blue-collar occupations may have total physical activity levels that are equal to or greater than individuals with white-collar jobs (51). For example, one recent population-based study found that leisure-time physical activity was lower among men and women who were less-skilled workers compared to professional workers (73). Among men, the inclusion of both occupational and home activity eliminated this disparity, but among women, this difference remained. These results show that women in blue-collar or less-skilled occupations may be at particular risk for low levels of overall physical activity. Ford et al. also reported that low-SES women spent significantly less time than higher-SES women in both leisure-time activity and job-related activity (74).

SES has also been a predictor of physical activity adherence in clinical samples. Specifically, blue-collar occupation and lower education level are associated with poorer physical activity adherence during and following completion of clinical programs such as cardiac rehabilitation (51, 52). Poorer adherence to clinical exercise programs may be related to financial constraints and limitations in health care coverage. Home-based and cost-modified programs are increasingly available, and this may improve adherence to clinical exercise programs among adults with lower SES.

There are several likely reasons that physical activity levels are lower among individuals with low SES. These individuals are more likely to live in communities that have fewer parks or recreational facilities, are more likely to lack financial resources to purchase home exercise equipment, may lack social support or encouragement to lead a physically active lifestyle, and may also lack understanding about the health benefits of activity (75). In addition, some research suggests that individuals with lower income levels receive less advice from their physicians about preventive health behaviors such as physical activity (76).

Marital Status.   Among studies that have examined the association of marital status with physical activity, results have been mixed. Some studies report a positive association between marriage and physical activity (77, 78), some report a negative association (73, 79), and others report no association (80–82). King et al. conducted a prospective study of marital transitions among a community sample and found that the transition from single to married resulted in positive changes in physical activity. However, a transition from being married to being single did not influence physical activity (77). Though marital status does not appear to be one of the strongest demographic predictors of research, marriage may result in a natural support system that can be utilized to promote activity within the dyad (77).

Health-Related and Biological Factors

Individuals with fewer chronic diseases and overall greater levels of health and physical function are more likely to be physically active (51). Overweight/obesity is another health-related factor that has been studied widely in the physical activity literature. Recent studies have reported a fairly consistent relationship between overweight/obesity and lower activity levels (32). For example, Brownson et al. found that among a national sample of women in the United States, those who were overweight were significantly less likely to report being regularly active (adjusted odds ratio [OR] = 0.69) and more likely to report having no leisure-time physical activity (adjusted OR = 1.50) compared to women who were not overweight (81).

There have also been several studies examining familial aggregation and genetic influences on physical activity (83–88). In general, these studies support that genetic factors are important contributors to physical activity and account for a substantial proportion of variation at the population level (35%–85%) (88). For example, a recent twin study showed that genetic factors explained a considerable amount of variance in both sports participation and leisure-time physical activity, especially among men (88). Among men in this study, genetic effects accounted for 68% of variation in sports participation and 63% of the variation in leisure-time physical activity. Corresponding numbers for women were 40% and 32%. Mechanisms by which genetic variations influence physical activity are not known, but they may be related to motor and somatic characteristics (88). Although these studies suggest that not all individuals are equally prone to engage in physical activity, it should be noted that environmental influences (which are modifiable through intervention) also contribute substantially to variation in physical activity behavior.

Cognitive and Psychological Factors

A wide array of cognitive and psychological variables have been examined as potential correlates of physical activity adherence (see Table 3.1) (32, 34, 37). Among these variables, studies have shown that the following are most consistently associated with greater physical activity levels: fewer perceived barriers, greater enjoyment of physical activity, greater expected benefits, better psychological health, greater self-efficacy for physical activity, greater self-motivation for physical activity, favorable self-schemata for exercise, intention to exercise, greater readiness to change, and better perceived health or fitness (32, 37). In a recent review of this literature, Trost et al. found that several constructs from the theory of reasoned action and theory of planned behavior (including attitudes, normative beliefs, and perceived control,) received relatively weak support as predictors of physical activity (32). (See chap. 2 for more details on the theory of reasoned action and the theory of planned behavior.) Knowledge of health and physical activity have also received weak support as a predictor of activity (32, 34, 37), confirming that interventions relying on health education alone (with no behavioral component) are not likely to induce change in physical activity.

Self-efficacy for physical activity, defined as an individual's confidence in his or her ability to be physically active on a regular basis, has been one of the strongest and most consistent cognitive correlates of activity level (32, 34, 37, 51). Self-efficacy is related to both adoption and maintenance of physical activity (54, 89, 90). It has been correlated with physical activity in a variety of settings, including large population-based community samples, exercise groups for healthy individuals, and clinical exercise programs (32, 51). Self-efficacy has also been shown to predict future physical activity levels in longitudinal studies (37). Furthermore, studies have shown that self-efficacy can be enhanced through training and feedback (91–93) and therefore may be a particularly important target for interventions.

Perceived barriers also correlate strongly with physical activity (32, 34, 37). The most commonly reported barrier to physical activity among U.S. samples is lack of time (34). Some other common barriers include lack of facilities, bad weather, safety, lack of exercise partner, fatigue or lack of energy, poor health, and self-consciousness about appearance (32). Like self-efficacy, perceived barriers have been shown to correlate with physical activity in many cross-sectional studies, and also to predict activity in prospective studies (34, 94). It is important to note that barriers may incorporate both subjective and objective components. However, both objective and subjective barriers are amenable to intervention. Objective barriers, such as lack of exercise facilities, may be modified by policy interventions, and subjective barriers may be modified through cognitive interventions that refute beliefs that hinder activity.

Behavioral Factors

A variety of behavior-related variables have been studied in the physical activity literature, the most common being prior physical activity history, smoking, alcohol use, and Type A behavior. Of these, prior activity history has shown the most consistent association with current activity level (32, 37). More specifically, prior activity history as an adult has been associated with current activity participation, whereas physical activity participation during childhood or youth has not been associated with current adulthood activity behavior (37).

Though there has been a popular belief that smoking is strongly and inversely correlated with physical activity, prior reviews have concluded that there is only a modest relationship between these variables and that not all studies have found an association (37, 51). However, among the most recent studies, all but one have found smoking to be negatively correlated with physical activity (32). For example, Brownson et al. found that among a national sample of women in the United States, those who smoked were significantly more likely than nonsmokers to report no leisure-time physical activity (adjusted OR = 1.42) (81). Among studies within clinical exercise programs such as cardiac rehabilitation, smoking has been a consistent predictor of poor adherence both during and after the formal program (51).

There have been only a few recent studies examining relationships of dietary habits and alcohol use with physical activity. Studies have generally shown that individuals with better dietary habits (i.e., consumption of fruits and vegetables, eating fewer fatty foods) are more likely to be physically active (32, 37). In contrast, studies have not shown any consistent relationship between alcohol use and physical activity (37). Type A behavior has been defined as a behavioral syndrome or style of living characterized by competitiveness, feelings of being under the pressures of time, striving for achievement, and aggressiveness (95). Studies have indicated that Type A behavior is associated with greater overall levels of physical activity but lower adherence within supervised exercise programs (34, 37). These results have important implications for interventions, suggesting that individuals with greater Type A behavior may be better suited to individual or home-based physical activity programs.

Social Factors

Social factors that have been studied as correlates of physical activity include exercise group cohesion, physician influence, and social support. Group cohesion has shown a modest positive correlation with adherence in some studies (37). However, physician influence and social support have been stronger and more consistent correlates of physical activity level and adherence (32, 37). Burton et al. reported that among a large sample of community-dwelling older adults, 40% of patients who had initiated exercise said their physician was a very important influence (46). Physician advice to exercise has also been reported a correlate of physical activity among the general adult population (96).

Social support has been significantly associated with physical activity in many cross-sectional studies (32). For example in the U.S. Women's Determinants study, women with high levels of social support for physical activity were about twice as likely to be active for at least 30 minutes a day on 5 or more days a week compared to women with low social support for physical activity (68). Social support has also been a predictor of physical activity adherence in prospective studies among community samples (94) and within organized exercise groups (97–100). Both family and friend support for physical activity appear to be influential (32, 37). However, some recent research has highlighted the particular importance of spousal support and involvement in physical activity (98, 101, 102). For example, Satariano et al. found that among a large community sample of adults, the leisure-time physical activity of the spouse was the strongest predictor of the leisure-time activity of the participant (101). Although studies have found very strong correlations between social support and physical activity, there have been few interventions aimed at enhancing friend or family support for activity among adults (103).

Program-Related Factors

In addition to person-level characteristics, there are program-related variables that influence individuals' physical activity adherence. Specific aspects of the activity regimen, including intensity, duration, and frequency, have been the focus of many studies. Studies of exercise intensity have shown that health benefits can be achieved with low- or moderate-intensity activity, and that adherence may be greater at these levels compared to high-intensity activity (104–106). For example, in the Training Levels Comparison Trial among individuals with coronary artery disease, subjects who exercised at a low intensity attended 64% of sessions during a 1-year period compared to 56% among the high-intensity group (106). With respect to exercise duration, recent evidence indicates that completing several shorter bouts of activity may result in greater adherence than one longer bout, while retaining some health benefits (107–110). However, for some health outcomes such as long-term weight loss and blood lipid changes, some studies indicate longer bouts may be more effective (111, 112). One recent study found that intermittent exercise was specifically beneficial for reducing rates of attrition at the beginning of an exercise program (113). This suggests intermittent activity should be at least provided as an option during initial phases of physical activity programs.

Frequency of physical activity has been less studied, and there have been some inconsistent findings. King et al. found higher rates of adherence among a group who exercised at high intensity 3 days per week compared to a group who exercised at lower intensity five times per week (114). In contrast, Perri et al. recently reported that the prescription of a higher frequency of exercise (5–7 days/week) was associated with greater adherence and completion of a greater amount of overall activity over a 6-month period compared to a lower frequency prescription (3–4 days/week) (104). The most recent guidelines for physical activity recommend that individuals complete some physical activity on "most, and preferably all, days of the week" (115). The latter study provides some support for this recommendation's feasibility among adults.

Studies have also compared group- or center-based programs versus home-based programs. Several studies have found that home-based exercise is associated with greater adherence and higher levels of activity (105, 114, 116, 117). However, a study among sedentary women concluded that a center-based program resulted in greater 18-month retention compared to a home-based program (118). Preferences for center-based versus home-based programs may vary according to a host of personal characteristics, and these relationships are not yet well understood. Individuals who are just beginning an activity program may benefit from some features of center-based programs, such as individualized instruction and the support of others who are initiating exercise. Home-based programs clearly offer increased flexibility, which may be essential for individuals with time or transportation limitations. Home- and center-based programs are both effective, and should be viewed as complementary approaches in the promotion of physical activity.

Within the context of group- or center-based programs, there are several factors that have been shown to enhance adherence. Some of these include: convenient time and location, reasonable cost, variety of exercise modalities, flexibility in exercise goals, and quality of the exercise leader (119). The latter has been cited as the most critical factor (119). Specifically, exercise leaders should be able to effectively educate participants about physical activity and to motivate participants to continue exercising using a variety of strategies. These qualities and abilities can have a substantial impact on adherence and dropout.

Environmental Factors

There is growing recognition that environmental factors have a tremendous influence on individuals' physical activity behavior (32, 120). Perhaps the most prominent theme to emerge in recent research involving environmental factors is that of convenient access. A number of studies show that simply having convenient access to parks, walking or biking trails, or other physical activity facilities is strongly associated with greater activity levels (121–127). King et al. reported that living within a 20-minute walking distance of a park or trail was related to higher pedometer readings (122).

Similarly, Powell et al. found that individuals who could walk to a place they would "feel safe walking for exercise or recreation" in 10 minutes or less were most likely to be physically active (123). The results from Powell et al. also highlight another theme of recent research—neighborhood safety (123, 124, 128). Data from the CDC show that higher levels of perceived neighborhood safety are associated with greater levels of physical activity, and that this relationship may be even more important among certain subgroups such as older adults, women, and individuals with lower education levels (128).

There are several other neighborhood environment factors that have been associated with physical activity levels. Some studies have found that aesthetic factors, such as pleasant neighborhood scenery, are related to greater levels of activity (60, 80, 120, 125). Other positive neighborhood factors include overall satisfaction with community recreation facilities (129) and being in an environment where others exercise regularly (80, 124). In addition to the neighborhood environment, studies have reported that the presence of exercise equipment in the home is positively associated with physical activity (120, 124, 130).

Some research has also focused on examining urban–rural differences in physical activity. Several studies have found lower levels of activity among adults living in rural areas compared to urban areas (32). However, many of these studies have assessed only leisure-time physical activity, which may not account for farming and other types of occupational activity that may be more common in rural areas. One study reported that rural women report more barriers to leisure-time physical activity, including caregiving responsibilities and access to facilities, compared to urban women (60). Studies are still needed to compare overall physical activity levels (including occupational activity) among urban and rural residents, but current data suggest rural residents may be at greater risk for physical inactivity.

Factors Related to Adoption Versus Maintenance of Physical Activity

Among studies of physical activity behavior, most studies examine correlates of physical activity using a cross-sectional design. Some studies examine predictors of maintenance and dropout in the context of structured exercise programs, but far fewer studies have used longitudinal designs to examine both adoption and maintenance of physical activity within large populations. Thus there is considerably less data concerning factors that predict adoption of activity compared to maintenance of activity, and little is known about whether predictors of adoption and maintenance differ considerably. Some research indicates that correlates of adoption and maintenance are similar (46, 131). For example, Burton et al. found that among a large sample of community-dwelling older adults, predictors of both activity adoption and maintenance included younger age, moderate to excellent health, and the belief that exercise is important for health (46). Other studies have found some differences in correlates of physical activity adoption and maintenance (54, 132). Litt et al. reported that among a group of older women, the best predictor of activity adoption was readiness to change, whereas maintenance was predicted by self-efficacy and social support (132). In contrast, other research has suggested that self-efficacy may be a more powerful predictor of adoption than maintenance of activity (133). Further research is needed to gain a clearer understanding of factors that influence different stages of exercise, because this information is important for designing interventions.

Future Directions for Studies Examining Factors Related to Physical Activity Adherence

There have been hundreds of studies on factors associated with adherence to physical activity recommendations. Although the methodology and scope of these studies has improved, there are still some key limitations that need to be addressed in future investigations:

1. The majority of studies are cross-sectional in design. These studies do not allow examination of causal factors or the identification of factors associated with adoption of activity. More longitudinal studies examining adoption and long-term maintenance of physical activity are needed to address these important issues.

2. There are limitations in the area of physical activity measurement. Differences in the measurement of activity are likely one reason for discrepant findings across some studies. Studies should employ comprehensive measures of physical activity that include occupational and home activity, as well as leisure-time activity. In addition, multiple measures should be used to capture a variety of process and outcome variables.

3. Although the literature regarding environmental variables is increasing, these data are still sparse in comparison to studies involving personal factors associated with physical activity. Additional studies are needed to examine environmental correlates of physical activity in a variety of populations and geographic regions.

4. Physical activity adherence is likely influenced by complex interactions among biological, physical, psychological, social, cultural, policy, and environmental factors. Therefore there is a need to employ a broader interdisciplinary focus to research in this area. In particular, studies should incorporate both personal and environmental variables and seek to study interactions between these factors.

5. Studies examining physical activity among racial and ethnic minorities are still sparse. More research is needed to identify the most important predictors of activity in a variety of racial and ethnic groups.

PHYSICAL ACTIVITY ADHERENCE INTERVENTION STUDIES

Because of the well-established health benefits of physical activity and the national goal of increasing activity levels (134), there have been many studies designed to identify successful physical activity adherence interventions. These studies have varied widely with respect to subject samples, settings, theoretical models, and intervention strategies. Intervention studies can be grouped into two main categories: individual-based interventions and public-health/environmental/policy interventions. The following sections summarize results of studies in each of these categories.

Individual Interventions

Individual interventions for physical activity adherence have been the most extensively studied by far. These interventions have been examined in the context of clinical physical activity programs, community settings, and work sites, and they have focused on both primary and secondary prevention of disease. The goal of these interventions is generally to affect cognitive, behavioral, and/or social variables that are thought to be related to individuals' physical activity levels (135). These interventions have been based on components from one or more theoretical models, most commonly social cognitive theory, the health belief model, and the transtheoretical model of change (103, 136). (See chap. 2, this volume, for more details on these models.) The majority of these interventions have been targeted directly toward the individual cognitions and behaviors, but there have also been studies that seek to enhance physical activity level through development of social support or group cohesion. Although the latter studies have a group-based component, they still target relatively small numbers of participants and seek to change behavior at the individual level. Therefore we discuss these studies in conjunction with individual-based interventions, rather than the large-scale public-health interventions reviewed later.

A recent systematic review concluded there is strong evidence to support the overall efficacy of individual interventions to increase physical activity (103). These studies have resulted in improvements in key outcomes, including time spent in physical activity, frequency of physical activity, attendance at exercise sessions, the percentage of individuals who start an exercise program, energy expenditure, and VO_2 max (an objective measure of fitness) (103). The following are brief descriptions of specific interventions that have been shown to enhance physical activity adherence:

1. *Health Education* (91, 137–142). Though studies indicate that health education alone is generally not sufficient to promote long-term changes in exercise adherence, this can be a critical component of broader interventions. It is important to provide individuals with information about the benefits of exercise, proper exercise techniques, and normal physiological responses that can be expected during exercise. This information helps to form a solid foundation for other behavioral strategies. Professional organizations such as the ACSM and the American Heart Association (AHA) provide educational tools that can be used in clinical, research, and community settings.

2. *Health Risk Appraisal* (140, 143). Health risk appraisals provide participants with information about various aspects of their current health, risk factors, and/or fitness level. This can be achieved simply through administering a brief questionnaire and providing feedback about responses. In addition, appraisals can include more involved assessments of body composition or exercise capacity (i.e., timed walking test or a treadmill test). Like health education, health risk appraisals are often not sufficient to engender long-term behavior change. Yet they can enhance motivation and also be used to monitor changes in health and fitness throughout a program.

3. *Goal Setting* (91, 137–140, 142–148). This intervention involves asking participants to identify and document personal goals related to their physical activity behavior. There are several important principles of effective goal-setting interventions. First, participants should be encouraged to set goals that are specific and relatively short term. This allows participants to readily assess progress. Second, participants should also be instructed to set realistic goals. This increases the likelihood of early success, which can enhance participants' self-efficacy for physical activity. Third, it is important to ask participants to think through and document specific steps they will take toward meeting their goal(s). Fourth, it is helpful to combine goal setting with some type of feedback or accountability from another individual.

4. *Contracts* (142, 149–153). This strategy involves asking participants to write out specific physical behaviors they intend to do. In addition, participants identify individuals who will be responsible for verifying that they have fulfilled their contract. Verification may be conducted by either clinical/research staff members or a friend or family member identified by the participants. This strategy can also be combined with reinforcements and incentives.

5. *Self-Monitoring* (138, 140, 142, 144, 145, 150, 151, 154–158). This is one of the most commonly used intervention components. Self-monitoring involves asking participants to observe and document their physical activity

behavior. Participants can be asked to record a variety of variables, including the mode of activity, duration, frequency, heart rates, perceived exertion level, and psychological responses to activity. Participants are often asked to turn in their self-monitoring records to group leaders or other participants, which facilitates consistency and completeness of records.

6. *Reinforcement and Incentives* (139, 149, 153, 154, 159–161). These strategies are often combined with self-monitoring and/or goal setting. In general, these strategies reward participants for attaining some activity-related goal. Some common rewards include money, T-shirts, fitness equipment, and reductions in health insurance (within workplace settings). Some incentive strategies require participants to contribute money at the beginning of a program. Then some money is forfeited (sometimes to other groups or group members) if participants fail to achieve a specified goal.

7. *Problem Solving* (91, 137, 139, 148, 157, 158). There are many potential obstacles associated with adhering to physical activity. For example, some individuals may need to find child care or identify ways to involve their children in their activity. Some obstacles may be environmental, including access to facilities or a safe exercise environment. Problem-solving interventions teach individuals to identify obstacles that hinder them, generate potential solutions, select a solution to implement, evaluate the outcome, and choose another solution if needed.

8. *Relapse Prevention* (91, 137, 138, 140, 142, 145, 155, 159, 162, 163). Similar to problem solving, this intervention involves instructing participants to identify future situations that may lead to lapses in adherence. There are some common triggers of relapse (i.e., changes in schedule, vacations), but participants should be instructed to anticipate situations that may be particularly salient for them. Participants are then taught to develop specific strategies to deal with these potential situations.

9. *Stimulus Control* (91, 142, 145, 164). This strategy is built on the principle that environmental cues exert an important influence on behavior. Stimulus control interventions involve teaching participants to structure their environment in ways that encourage physical activity or, conversely, discourage inactivity. For example, participants may be encouraged to place exercise equipment in easily accessible locations. Communities and workplaces can also have an important role in stimulus control interventions by structuring the physical environment to promote activity.

10. *Cognitive Restructuring* (142, 145, 148). Maladaptive thoughts and beliefs can contribute to nonadherence. For example, individuals may believe that exercise must be vigorous or painful to produce any health benefit. Individuals may also have negative self-statements related to physical activity (e.g., "I will never be able to maintain a regular exercise program"). Many times individuals are not aware of these thoughts and beliefs, and they do not recognize that such thoughts directly influence behavior. Cognitive re-

structuring is a process of teaching individuals to recognize these thoughts and replace them with more positive self-statements that can help to promote regular physical activity.

11. *Enhancing Social Support* (91, 137–139, 142, 151, 155, 157, 163, 165–167). Group exercise programs are an excellent source for developing social support for physical activity. There are also ways that social support can be enhanced in the context of individual and home-based programs. One strategy is to provide support through interactions with personal trainers, nurses, or other health professionals (160, 168, 169) Another important strategy is to foster support for physical activity within participants' natural social contacts. For example, participants can be encouraged to seek out a person who will exercise with them regularly or provide feedback and encouragement about their exercise behavior. Friends or family members can be provided with specific instructions about how they can provide support to the participant for their physical activity goals.

12. *Modeling* (142, 148, 170). Social modeling is one important strategy for enhancing self-efficacy for physical activity. This strategy involves providing examples of individuals who are similar to participants and who are successfully engaging in physical activity. Social modeling often occurs naturally within group exercise programs. Videos or other media may also be used to provide participants with examples of social modeling.

13. *Motivational Interviewing* (169, 171, 172). This intervention is based on the transtheoretical model (see chap. 2, this volume) and explores stage-specific motivational conflicts. Motivational interviewing developed as a technique for negotiating behavior changes with people who are reluctant or ambivalent about changing (173). The goal of this method is to increase individuals' intrinsic motivation for physical activity, so that changes arise internally rather than being imposed from an external source.

Studies have not indicated that any specific intervention is optimal for enhancing physical activity adherence in all settings and populations. Rather, the strategies just described should be considered a "toolbox" of methods that can be employed in clinical and research settings. Interventions involving multiple components are generally more successful than those employing a single strategy, and many studies and clinical programs now use combinations of these approaches (91, 138, 142, 148). Regardless of the specific strategies chosen, research indicates there are some general principles that can lead to effective adherence interventions:

1. *Intervention Intensity.* Studies have shown that brief interventions (such as a one-time health risk appraisals or fitness testing) are generally not a sufficient stimulus to promote behavior change (135, 174, 175). Although brief interventions may seem attractive with respect to cost and time

commitments, there is strong evidence that successful promotion of long-term exercise adherence typically require considerable and sustained intervention (171).

2. *Tailored Approach.* There has been recent interest comparing standardized behavioral interventions with interventions that are tailored to participants' needs, goals, or readiness to change. Several studies have provided evidence that tailoring interventions may result in better outcomes and improved adherence (176–179). Whereas tailored interventions may require more effort to disseminate than standardized protocols, computer programs now make tailoring increasingly feasible (180). (See chap. 17, this volume, for additional details on the use of tailoring and adherence.)

3. *Lifestyle Approach.* Traditional methods of prescribing exercise, which are based on a specified frequency, intensity, duration, and mode of activity, often fail to elicit long-term adherence. Therefore there has been a recent shift of focus toward encouraging lifestyle physical activity (181). Recommendations for lifestyle physical activity involve "daily accumulation of at least 30 minutes of self-selected activities, which includes all leisure, occupational, or household activities that are at least moderate to vigorous in their intensity and could be planned or unplanned activities that are a part of everyday life" (181). Several studies have now shown that interventions designed to enhance lifestyle physical activity produce health and fitness benefits similar to those of structured physical activity (21–23). Furthermore, research suggests lifestyle physical activity interventions are associated with greater adherence and levels of activity compared to structured programs (182).

Channels of Delivery for Individual Interventions. In addition to identifying physical activity interventions that are efficacious, it is critical to determine effective ways of delivering these programs. In general, interventions can be delivered in person, via some form of media (telephone, mail, Internet), or a combination of these two approaches. Interventions to enhance physical activity adherence were first developed and implemented on a face-to-face basis. There are clear advantages to this method of delivery. Perhaps most important, this type of interaction permits meaningful interaction and dialogue about participants' needs, preferences, and perceived barriers to physical activity. However, there are also clear limitations to this method. Because of the time and financial burdens associated with face-to-face interventions, this approach is limited with respect to reaching large numbers of individuals.

One specific method of in-person delivery involves health care providers. This is an attractive strategy for two main reasons. First, the majority of adults have contact with physicians on at least a yearly basis and average more than three office visits per year (183). Therefore this method has the potential to reach a larger number of individuals than other in-person strategies. Second, clinicians' recommendations regarding health behaviors are generally valued and trusted by patients, and research shows that patients want to receive information about physical activity from their physicians (184). The AHA (185), National Heart, Lung, and Blood Institute (186), and U.S. Preventive Services Task Force (187) have recommend that all primary-care providers counsel patients regarding regular physical activity as part of routine health examinations. However, studies show that physicians provide physical activity counseling infrequently and typically do not spend more than 3–5 minutes providing this type of counseling (188–193). One clear drawback to in-person delivery in the health care setting is overburdened clinicians. Physicians have also reported the following barriers to physical activity counseling: lack of significant reimbursement, lack of counseling training, perceived ineffectiveness of counseling, lack of organizational support, limited availability of materials, and lack of standardized protocols (191, 194, 195). These issues must be addressed if physical activity counseling is to be a regular component of primary health care delivery.

Studies examining the health care provider–based physical activity counseling have varied considerably in methodology, particularly with respect to the intensity of the intervention. For example, one intervention involved 3–5 minutes of in-person structured physical activity counseling and one brief follow-up telephone call (196), whereas another intervention involved provision of an exercise prescription and an in-person follow-up visit to adjust this prescription (197). Results of provider-based studies have been mixed, with some showing increases in participants' physical activity levels and some showing no effect. Even systematic reviews of these studies have drawn differing conclusions, reporting these interventions have no effects to moderate effects (198–200).

Despite ongoing questions about the effectiveness of primary-care provider–based interventions, studies have provided insight into some characteristics of successful interventions. First, studies suggest that written exercise prescriptions are more effective than advice alone (201). Second, more intensive interventions involving multiple contacts are more effective than brief, single-visit interventions (137, 171). Future provider-based interventions should incorporate these important characteristics. Specifically, further study is needed on methods to supplement brief face-to-face physician- or nurse-delivered counseling with long-term telephone and/or mail follow-up (202). This type of strategy may be a feasible, fairly low-cost way of reaching a large number of individuals with an intervention that is intensive enough to promote long-term physical activity adherence.

Whereas the majority of physical activity adherence studies have examined face-to-face interventions (or have at least involved some in-person component), there has been growing interest in alternative methods of delivery. Programs delivered via media (i.e., telephone, mail, Internet) can reach larger groups of individuals than in-person interventions, with lower cost and effort. Reviews of media-based studies have found that overall, these approaches are effective in increasing participants' physical activity levels (203, 204). Some research has even suggested adherence rates may be higher in telephone-assisted, home-based interventions compared to programs involving face-to-face contact (105, 117). One recent study found that a totally computer automated, behaviorally based intervention produced short-term changes in physical activity levels (205). However, this program failed to elicit long-term changes, which may require some type of more intensive or direct human interaction. Additional research is needed to compare in-person and home-based, media-delivered programs during adoption and maintenance phases of physical activity. Studies are also needed to compare the feasibility, efficacy, and cost-effectiveness of different telephone, mail, and Internet-based interventions among various populations. Though optimal strategies for media-delivered physical activity interventions are not yet clear, these interventions may play a critical role in improving national rates of physical activity adherence. These interventions may become increasingly essential in the midst of a health care climate that limits physicians' time for individual counseling, as well as reimbursement for programs such as cardiac rehabilitation (117). In addition, these interventions are crucial for reaching underserved groups who may not have access to in-person programs.

Public Health, Environmental, and Policy Interventions

Individualized interventions clearly play a critical role in enhancing adherence to physical activity recommendations. However, the problem of inactivity is widespread, and large-scale, population-based strategies to this problem are an essential counterpart to intensive individualized interventions. Recent studies have emphasized the importance of environmental and community factors in the prediction of individuals' physical activity levels (121–123, 206, 207). Yet population-based environmental and policy interventions have not been nearly as well studied or widely implemented as individualized approaches (208, 209).

Public health, environmental, and policy strategies to enhance physical activity adherence can range from very simple, low-cost interventions to complex policies involving budget allocation and transportation restructuring (208). Some studies have focused exclusively on large-scale, mass media approaches to increasing physical activity. These interventions frequently target other cardiovascular disease risk factors as well. Most of these campaigns have included multiple delivery methods, including television, radio, printed materials, and community events. A review of these studies noted that recall of campaign messages is fairly high—approximately 70%

of survey respondents across studies (203). However, these interventions have generally had little influence on physical activity levels within communities. These types of interventions may be useful in settings where the benefits of physical activity are not as well known, but repeating these mass-media campaigns in areas that have already been targeted does not further increase activity levels (210).

Other types of environmental and policy interventions have shown promising results (211–214). Two studies examined a simple intervention of posting signs in public areas to encourage the use of stairways (212, 213). In both studies, rates of stairway use approximately doubled, but these rates declined again after the signs were taken down. These studies highlight the potential impact of low-cost public-health strategies that are able to reach a large number of individuals. Other studies have involved more complex interventions. Linenger et al. (214) examined the impact of both environmental and policy changes related to physical activity on a military base. Environmental changes included bicycle trails, new equipment and facilities, and the organization of running and cycling clubs. Policy changes included enhancing the budget for environmental changes and implementing release time for physical activity. During the course of this intervention, there were significant improvements in fitness among military personnel at the base, but there were no improvements in a control military base during the same time period. Roberts et al. reported positive results from an extensive policy and environmental intervention in Northern Ireland (215). This intervention involved the creation of 14 publicly funded leisure centers over a 7-year period. Activity among individuals in this city increased during this time period, compared to a sample of individuals from throughout the United Kingdom.

There are significant challenges in both the study and implementation of environmental and policy interventions for physical activity. Studies of this magnitude can be extremely expensive, requiring substantial financial resources and cooperation of multiple agencies (208). In addition, it is difficult to evaluate interventions that occur at a community level. Despite these limitations, further efforts in this area are critical. Without amenable environments, other interventions aimed at increasing activity may be impeded. Experience in other countries has shown that widespread policies to enhance simple activities such as walking and cycling can have a significant impact (207), and similar efforts are greatly needed in the United States.

PHYSICAL ACTIVITY ADHERENCE INTERVENTIONS
IN SPECIAL POPULATIONS

There are several demographic groups known to have lower levels of physical activity, including older adults, women, ethnic and racial minorities, and individuals with low SES (56, 58). Though these groups have been understudied with respect to physical activity adherence, there have been recent efforts to develop and test interventions in these specific groups. The following sections summarize physical activity adherence research among each of these groups.

Older Adults

The health status of older adults varies widely, creating a challenge in devising adherence strategies for this segment of the population. In a comprehensive review of the effectiveness of physical activity interventions for older adults, van der Bij et al. found that most short-term interventions were successful and had high rates of participation. However, participation declined as the length of the intervention declined (216). Of particular importance to the older adult is the effect of cognitive mediators, such as self-efficacy in adherence patterns. Brassington et al. found that changes in self-efficacy and fitness outcome realizations were related to 12-month exercise adherence whereas social mediators, such as exercise-related social support, were not (217). This should not minimize the potential impact of social support but should emphasize the importance of including building cognitive mediators and other self-regulatory skills as part of an ongoing process aimed at sustained physical activity (218, 219).

Some research has been directed at identifying personal preferences for physical activity interventions that may enhance adherence among subgroups of older adults. For example, in a random sample of middle-aged and older, well-educated adults in California, older men appeared to prefer exercising on their own compared to older women. Although women in general preferred to exercise on their own, those who were younger and less-educated preferred a class setting for exercise (220). Equally challenging is the fact that predictors of adherence are not necessarily consistent across different types of physical activities and may fluctuate with life transitions to different situations or settings (221). A recent review suggests that older adults require individually tailored interventions to incorporate strategies that address unique barriers, such as intermittent illness and the burden of caregiving, with social problem-solving models of behavior change (43). One of the most promising efforts to date is the creation of The National Blueprint Project, which consists of a coalition of national organizations committed to develop a national strategy for the promotion of physically active lifestyles among the older adult. A major goal of the National Blueprint is to facilitate strategic partnerships in which organizations come together to develop joint initiatives among home, community, public-policy agencies, and national advocacy in the areas of physical activity and aging (222).

Ethnic and Racial Minorities

Although there are limited data in this important area of research, it is clear that exercise adherence interventions for racial and minority groups must be tailored to meet specific cultural concerns, perspectives, and values (223). It is essential to involve communities directly in the development and implementation of physical activity programs. Interventions that rely heavily on community involvement are known to be more effective and well accepted than those imposed on a community exclusively from an outside organization (61). Some recent studies have examined physical activity promotion programs in the context of churches in the African American community (224–226). For example, Yanek et al. (226) examined a church-based health promotion intervention that combined spiritual strategies with standard behavioral methods and found that this strategy improved health outcomes among African American women. There is a clear need to develop, test, and implement similar strategies within the existing community and social structures of other racial and ethnic minority groups.

Individuals With Low Socioeconomic Status

Very few studies have examined physical activity interventions specifically among low-SES groups or communities (61). Because individuals with low SES are often not represented in clinical trials of exercise adherence, it is not clear whether these interventions are appropriate for this demographic group. However, some recent data support the efficacy of several common interventions in this population. Lowther et al. examined fitness assessment and exercise consultations, two commonly used interventions, among a large sample from a socially and economically deprived community (227). Results showed that individuals who received both the assessment and consultation significantly increased physical activity levels, even at 1-year follow-up. Rimmer et al. examined the effects of a highly structured, center-based, 12-week exercise program among African Americans with disabilities who resided in difficult social environments (75). Adherence was 87% in this study, and participants in the exercise group had significant improvements in strength, body composition, and VO_2 max compared to a control group.

Although these studies demonstrate that some traditional interventions improve exercise adherence among low-SES samples, many individuals with low SES do not have access to the types of interventions studied. Additional studies should test methods of disseminating these programs widely within lower-SES communities. Also, further work is needed to define critical barriers to activity and to compare different types of interventions (i.e., home-based vs. center-based, different cognitive and behavioral strategies) among individuals with lower SES. This is a demographic group that has been vastly understudied and could benefit greatly from effective physical activity interventions.

Women

Interventions to enhance physical activity adherence were developed primarily on the basis of studies involving either all male or mixed-gender samples (53). However, recent studies have provided important data on the effectiveness of specific adherence interventions among women (26, 100, 118, 182, 228–233). Data from the Activity Counseling Trial revealed important gender differences in the response to primary care–based physical activity interventions (137). This study compared "recommended care" (including physician advice to exercise and written education material), assistance (interactive mail and behavioral counseling at physician visits), and counseling (all components of the assistance intervention, plus regular telephone counseling and behavioral classes). Among men in this study, the assistance and counseling interventions were not more effective than recommended care. Among women, both assistance and counseling resulted in better physical activity outcomes compared to the recommended care group. These results suggest women are particularly responsive to intensive behavioral counseling and should be targeted for such interventions.

Another important focus of physical activity adherence research among women has been the examination of interventions that consider or incorporate family and caregiving responsibilities (100, 231, 232, 234). For example, King et al. examined a home-based exercise program specifically for sedentary women who were caring for relatives with dementia (234). The average adherence rate in this study was 74%, and participants in the exercise group showed significant improvements in physical activity level and stress-related outcomes compared to an attention control group (232). Miller et al. examined two physical activity interventions (printed material about overcoming exercise barriers and printed material plus discussion groups) among mothers of preschool-age children (100). Compared to women in a control group, women in the printed-material and discussion group were significantly more likely to meet physical activity recommendations following the intervention. Miller et al. also found that partner support and self-efficacy attenuated this group effect, suggesting that these variables may be mediators of physical activity behavior change among women.

These studies demonstrate the efficacy of several different physical activity adherence interventions among women. They also highlight key components. Interventions for women should incorporate social support from groups or family members, and future studies should examine ways that social support for activity may be enhanced among women. Because women often have multiple roles involving both family responsibilities and work outside the home, future interventions should also seek to encourage physical activity within women's normal daily routines.

Future Directions for Physical Activity Intervention Research

Physical activity interventions have advanced in methodology, use of media and technology for dissemination, and incorporation of some at-risk subgroups. The following are some key limitations that should be considered in future interventions:

1. Most physical activity intervention studies examine only short-term outcomes, and there is little information about how well specific interventions may promote long-term physical activity adherence. This is critical, because long-term adherence is important for maintaining health benefits.

2. Few studies have examined adherence as a primary outcome measure. Most exercise studies employ behavioral components to enhance adherence, but the primary outcome is often change in exercise capacity. This makes it difficult to rigorously examine adherence as a specific outcome.

3. Most interventions involve personal and interpersonal approaches, and these studies typically attract individuals who are reasonably motivated to exercise, have a history of physical activity, and have access to health care or exercise facilities. There is a need for more interventions at organizational, environmental, and societal levels. These approaches are important for reaching a wider segment of the population.

4. There is a still need for more studies involving groups who are at greatest risk for inactivity—that is, older adults, women, those who are overweight, ethnic minorities, individuals with low SES, and persons with disabilities.

5. Studies have largely focused on encouraging structured exercise. In light of the shift in focus toward lifestyle physical activities, studies should examine interventions that encourage incorporation of activity into daily routines and the effectiveness of these approaches within certain segments of the population. For example, it is not known if the lifestyle approach is suitable for functionally frail older adults.

CLINICAL AND POLICY IMPLICATIONS

Research has confirmed the importance of physician influence on patients' physical activity. Studies have not yet identified an optimal strategy for enhancing physical activity within the primary-care setting. However, research does suggest that clinicians can improve patients' adherence simply by assessing and encouraging physical activity on a regular and repeated basis. Current rates of physical activity recommendation by physicians are low and must be increased. There are several specific steps that may improve current practice in this area. First, more attention could be given to training medical students regarding physical activity (and other health behavior) recommendations and counseling. Because physical activity guidelines change over time, continuing education for clinicians at all stages of their career would also be valuable. Second, physical activity assessment and recommendations could be included as a quality indicator within medical systems. This would provide both a reminder system and accountability for physicians to speak with patients about their physical activity. Third, physicians should be informed about local resources related to physical activity, including both clinical and community facilities. This would allow easy referral for patients who are interested in group activities, specific types of facilities, or more intensive exercise counseling. Fourth, physicians' time with patients is clearly limited, and there is a need to develop programs that enhance physician recommendations with more detailed behavioral counseling, delivered by a nurse or health educator.

Recent research has also highlighted the significant influence of the environment on physical activity behavior. Public health initiatives and policies that enhance opportunities for physical activity within communities may have a tremendous impact on nationwide activity levels. There is a need to increase the number, safety, and accessibility of parks and recreational facilities within communities. There is also a need to improve the availability and safety of biking and walking routes that can be used for regular transportation. In addition to community-based efforts, work sites can play an important role in encouraging physical activity. Work site programs may be particularly important for large organizations that can influence greater numbers of employees. Some practical strategies for work sites include on-site exercise groups, provision of on-site shower facilities for employees, and financial incentives that encourage physical activity (such as reduced costs for health club memberships).

SUMMARY

Physical activity is associated with many physical and psychological health benefits. Yet despite decades of effort to improve physical activity levels, only about a quarter of Americans achieve recommended levels of physical activity and about 30% report getting no regular activity. Research has identified a number of factors associated with lower physical activity levels, including demographic characteristics (female gender, older age, low SES, racial and ethnic minorities), poor physical health, social and cognitive variables (particularly low social support for activity, low physical activity self-efficacy, and greater perceived barriers to activity), and environmental characteristics (especially lack of convenient access to safe recreational areas). Studies are still needed to examine predictors of physical activity in some understudied populations, especially racial and ethnic minorities. A variety of behavioral interventions have demonstrated efficacy in enhancing physical activity levels among communities and improving adherence within structured programs. However, further work is needed to examine whether such interventions enhance long-term adherence to physical activity recommendations. The low national rates of physical activity also signal a need for greater dissemination of physical activity interventions that have shown efficacy. Improving rates of physical activity will require a broad transdisciplinary focus and development of strategic partnerships among community, medical, environmental, and public-policy agencies.

REFERENCES

1. Bijnen FC, Caspersen CJ, Feskens EJ, Saris WH, Mosterd WL, Kromhout D. Physical activity and 10-year mortality from cardiovascular diseases and all causes: The Zutphen Elderly Study. *Arch Intern Med.* 1998;158:1499–1505.
2. Berlin JA, Colditz GA. A meta-analysis of physical activity in the prevention of coronary heart disease. *Am J Epidemiol.* 1990;132(4):612–628.
3. McKechnie R, Mosca L. Physical activity and coronary heart disease: prevention and effect on risk factors. *Cardiovascular Reviews.* 2003;11(1):21–25.
4. Paluska SA, Schwenk TL. Physical activity and mental health: current concepts. *Sports Med.* 2000;29(3):167–180.
5. Singh MA. Exercise to prevent and treat functional disability. *Clin Geriatr Med.* 2002;18(3):431–462.
6. Wang G, Helmick CG, Macera C, Zhang P, Pratt M. Inactivity-associated medical costs among US adults with arthritis. *Arthritis Rheum.* 2001;45(5):439–445.
7. Perkins AJ, Clark DO. Assessing the association of walking with health services use and costs among socioeconomically disadvantaged older adults. *Prev Med.* 2001;32(6):492–501.
8. Colditz GA. Economic costs of obesity and inactivity. *Med Sci Sports Exerc.* 1999;31(11):S663–S667.
9. Pratt M, Macera C, Wang G. Higher direct medical costs associated with physical inactivity. *The Physician and Sportsmedicine.* 2000;28(10):63–70.
10. Lee IM, Paffenbarger RS, Hennekens CH. Physical activity, fitness, and longevity. *Aging (Milano).* 1997;9:2–11.
11. Lee IM, Skerrett PJ. Physical activity and all-cause mortality: what is the dose–response relation? *Medicine & Science in Sports & Exercise.* 2001;33(6 Suppl): S459–S471.

12. Wallace JP. Exercise in hypertension: a clinical review. *Sports Med.* 2003;33(8): 585–598.

13. Thompson PD, Buchner D, Pina IL, et al. Exercise and physical activity in the prevention and treatment of atherosclerotic cardiovascular disease: a statement from the Council on Clinical Cardiology (Subcommittee on Exercise, Rehabilitation and Prevention) and the Council on Nutrition, Physical Activity, and Metabolism (Subcommittee on Physical Activity). *Circulation.* 2003;107(24): 3109–3116.

14. Bischoff HA, Roos EM. Effectiveness and safety of strengthening, aerobic, and coordination exercises for patients with osteoarthritis. *Curr Opin Rheumatol.* 2003;15(2):141–144.

15. Hamdy O, Goodyear LJ, Horton ES. Diet and exercise in type 2 diabetes mellitus. *Endocrinol Metab Clin North Am.* 2001;30(4):883–907.

16. Brosse AL, Sheets ES, Lett HS, Blumenthal JA. Exercise and the treatment of clinical depression in adults: recent findings and future directions. *Sports Med.* 2002;32(12):741–760.

17. Bourjeily G, Rochester CL. Exercise training in chronic obstructive pulmonary disease. *Clin Chest Med.* 2000;21(4):763–781.

18. U.S. Department of Health and Human Services. *Physical Activity and Health: A Report of the Surgeon General.* Atlanta, GA: U.S. Department of Health and Human Services, Centers for Disease Control and Prevention, National Center for Chronic Disease Prevention and Health Promotion; 1996.

19. U.S. Department of Health and Human Services. *Healthy People 2010: Understanding and Improving Health.* 2nd ed. Washington, DC: U.S. Government Printing Office; 2000.

20. American College of Sports Medicine. The recommended quantity and quality of exercise for developing and maintaining cardiorespiratory and muscular fitness, and flexibility in healthy adults. *Med Sci Sports Exerc.* 1998;30(6):1–36.

21. Dunn AL, Gracia ME, Marcus BH, Kampert JB, Kohl HW, Blair SN. Six-month physical activity and fitness changes in Project Active, a randomized trial. *Med Sci Sports Exerc.* 1998;30(7):1076–1083.

22. Dunn AL, Marcus BH, Kampert JB, Garcia ME, Kohl HW, Blair SN. Comparison of lifestyle and structured interventions to increase physical activity and cardiorespiratory fitness: a randomized trial. *JAMA.* 1999;281:327–334.

23. Andersen RE, Bartlett SJ, Moser CD, Evangelisti MI, Verde TJ. Lifestyle or aerobic exercise to treat obesity in dieting women. *Med Sci Sports Exerc.* 1997;29 (Suppl 5):S46.

24. Morey MC, Pieper CF, Crowley GM, Sullivan RJ, Puglisi CM. Exercise adherence and 10-year mortality in chronically ill older adults [comment]. *J Am Geriatr Soc.* 2002;50(12):1929–1933.

25. Belza B, Topolski T, Kinne S, Patrick DL, Ramsey SD. Does adherence make a difference? Results from a community-based aquatic exercise program. *Nurs Res.* 2002;51(5):285–291.

26. Clark DO, Stump TE, Damush TM. Outcomes of an exercise program for older women recruited through primary care. *J Aging Health.* 2003;15(3):567–585.

27. Wallace ES, White JA, Downie A, Dalzell G, Doran D. Influence of exercise adherence level on modifiable coronary heart disease risk factors and functional-fitness levels in middle-aged men. *Br J Sports Med.* 1993;27(2):101–106.

28. Centers for Disease Control and Prevention. Physical activity trends—United States, 1990–1998. *MMWR.* 2001;50(9):166–169.

29. Caspersen CJ, Merritt RK, Stephens T. International physical activity patterns: a methodological perspective. In: Dishman RK, ed. *Advances in Exercise Adherence.* Champaign, IL: Human Kinetics; 1994:71–108.

30. U.S. Department of Health and Human Services. *Health People 2000: National health promotion and disease prevention objectives.* Washington DC: U.S. Department of Health and Human Services; 2000.

31. Dishman RK. Overview. In: Dishman RK, ed. *Exercise Adherence: Its Impact on Public Health.* Champaign, IL: Human Kinetics; 1988.

32. Trost SG, Owen N, Bauman AE, Sallis JF, Brown W. Correlates of adults' participation in physical activity: review and update. *Med Sci Sports Exerc.* 2002;34(12): 1996–2001.

33. Dishman RK. Determinants of participation in physical activity. In: Bouchard C, Shephard RJ, Stephens T, Sutton JR, McPherson BD, eds. *Exercise, Fitness, and Health: A Consensus of Current Knowledge.* Champaign, IL: Human Kinetics; 1990: 75–102.

34. Dishman RK, Sallis JF. Determinants and interventions for physical activity and exercise. In: Bouchard C, Shephard RJ, Stephens T, eds. *Physical Activity, Fitness and Health: International Proceedings and Consensus Statement.* Champaign, IL: Human Kinetics; 1994:214–238.

35. Dishman RK, Sallis JF, Orenstein DR. The determinants of physical activity and exercise. *Public Health Rep.* 1985;100:158–171.

36. Rhodes RE, Martin AD, Taunton JE, Rhodes EC, Donnelly M, Elliot J. Factors associated with exercise adherence among older adults. An individual perspective. *Sports Med.* 1999;28(6):397–411.

37. Sallis JF, Owen N. *Physical Activity and Behavioral Medicine.* Thousand Oaks, CA: Sage Publications; 1999:110–134.

38. Agency for Healthcare Research and Quality, Centers for Disease Control. *Physical Activity and Older Americans.* Washington, DC: U.S. Department of Health and Human Services; 2002.

39. Barnes PM, Schoenborn CA. *Physical Activity Among Adults: United States 2000. Advance Data From Vital and Health Statistics; no. 333.* Hyattsville, MD: National Center for Health Statistics; 2003.

40. Davis MA, Neuhaus JM, Moritz DJ, Lein D, Barclay JD, Murphy SP. Health behaviors and survival among middle-aged and older men and women in NHANES I Epidemiologic Follow-Up Study. *Prev Med.* 1994;23:369–376.

41. U.S. Department of Health and Human Services. *Physical Activity and Health: A Report to the Surgeon General.* Atlanta, GA: U.S. Department of Health and Human Services; 1996.

42. Stephens T, Caspersen CJ. The demography of physical activity. In: Bouchard C, Shephard RJ, Stephens T, eds. *Physical Activity, Fitness, and Health.* Champaign, IL: Human Kinetics; 1995:204–213.

43. Brawley LR, Rejeski WJ, King AC. Promoting physical activity for older adults: the challenges for changing behavior. *Am J Prev Med.* 2003;25(3Sii):172–183.

44. Stephens T, Craig CL. *The Well-Being of Canadians: Highlights From the 1988 Campbell's Soup Survey.* Ottowa: Canadian Fitness and Lifestyle Research Institute; 1990.

45. Craig CL, Russell SJ, Cameron C, Beaulieu A. *1997 Physical Activity Benchmarks Report.* Ottowa: Canadian Fitness and Lifestyle Research Institute; 1998.

46. Burton LC, Shapiro S, German PS. Determinants of physical activity and maintenance among community-dwelling older persons. *Prev Med.* 1999;29:422–430.

47. Lee C. Factors related to the adoption of exercise among older women. *J Behav Med.* 1993;16:323–334.

48. Morey MC, Sullivan RJ. Medical assessment for health advocacy and practical strategies for exercise initiation. *Am J Prev Med.* 2003;25 (3Sii):204–208.

49. Crespo CJ, Ketejiah SJ, Heath GW, Sempos CT. Leisure-time physical activity among US adults: results from the Third National Health and Nutrition Examination Survey. *Arch Intern Med.* 1996;156:93–98.

50. Martin SB, Morrow JR, Jackson JW, Dunn AL. Variables related to meeting the CDC/ACSM physical activity guidelines. *Med Sci Sports Exerc.* 2000;32:2087–2092.

51. King AC, Blair SN, Bild DE, et al. Determinants of physical activity and interventions in adults. *Med Sci Sports Exerc.* 1992;24(6):S221–S236.

52. Daly J, Sindone AP, Thompson DR, Hancock K, Chang E, Davidson P. Barriers to participation in and adherence to cardiac rehabilitation programs: a critical literature review. *Prog Cardiovasc Nurs.* 2002;17(1):8–17.

53. Pinto BM, Marcus BH, Clark MM. Promoting physical activity in women: the new challenges. *Am J Prev Med.* 1996;12(5):395–400.

54. Sallis JF, Haskell WL, Fortmann SP, Vranizan KM, Taylor CB, Solomon DS. Predictors of adoption and maintenance of physical activity in a community sample. *Prev Med.* 1986;15:331–341.

55. Crespo CJ. Encouraging physical activity in minorities: eliminating disparities by 2010. *The Physician and Sportsmedicine.* 2000;28(10):36–51.

56. Jones DA, Ainsworth BE, Croft JB, Macera CA, Lloyd EE, Yusuf HR. Moderate leisure-time physical activity: who is meeting the public health recommendations? A national cross-sectional study. *Arch Fam Med.* 1998;7(3):285–289.

57. Crespo CJ, Smit E, Andersen RE, Carter-Pokras O, Ainsworth BE. Race/Ethnicity, social class and their relation to physical activity during leisure time: results from the Third National Health and Nutrition Examination Survey, 1988–94. *Am J Prev Med.* 2000;18(1):46–53.

58. Centers for Disease Control and Prevention. Prevalence of leisure time and occupational physical activity among employed adults—United States, 1990. *MMWR.* 2000;49(19):420–424.

59. Washburn RA, Kline G, Lackland DT, Wheeler FC. Leisure time physical activity: are there black/white differences? *Prev Med.* 1992;21:127–135.

60. Wilcox S, Castro C, King AC, Housemann R, Brownson RC. Determinants of leisure time physical activity in rural compared to urban older and ethnically di-

verse women in the United States. *J Epidemiol Community Health.* 2000;54: 667–672.

61. Taylor WC, Baranowski T, Young DR. Physical activity interventions in low-income, ethnic minority, and populations with disability. *Am J Prev Med.* 1998;15(4):334–313.

62. Henderson KA, Ainsworth BE. Sociocultural perspectives on physical activity in the lives of older African American and American Indian women: a cross cultural activity participation study. *Women Health.* 2000;31(1):1–20.

63. Whitt MC, Kumanyika SK. Tailoring counseling on physical activity and inactivity for African-American women. *Ethn Dis.* 2002;12(4):62–71.

64. Berg JA, Cromwell SL, Arnett M. Physical activity: perspectives of Mexican American and Anglo American midlife women. *Health Care for Women International.* 2002;23(8):894–904.

65. Dergance JM, Calmbach WL, Dhanda R, Miles TP, Hazuda HP, Mouton CP. Barriers and benefits of leisure time physical activity in the elderly: differences across cultures. *J Am Geriatr Soc.* 2003;51(6):863–868.

66. Masse LC, Anderson CB. Ethnic differences among correlates of physical activity in women. *Am J Health Promot.* 2003;17(6):357–360.

67. Henderson KA, Ainsworth BE. A synthesis of perceptions about physical activity among older African American and American Indian women. *Am J Public Health.* 2003;93(2):313–317.

68. Eyler AA, Brownson RC, Donatelle RJ, King AC, Brown D, Sallis JF. Physical activity social support and middle- and older-aged minority women: results from a U.S. survey. *Soc Sci Med.* 1999;49(6):781–789.

69. James AS, Hudson MA, Campbell MK. Demographic and psychosocial correlates of physical activity among African Americans. *Am J Health Behav.* 2003; 27(4):421–431.

70. Richter DL, Wilcox S, Greaney ML, Henderson KA, Ainsworth BE. Environmental, policy, and cultural factors related to physical activity in African American women. *Women Health.* 2002;36(2):91–109.

71. Wilcox S, Richter DL, Henderson KA, Greaney ML, Ainsworth BE. Perceptions of physical activity and personal barriers and enablers in African American women. *Ethn Dis.* 2002;12(3):353–362.

72. Felton GM, Boyd MD, Bartoces MG, Tavakoli AS. Physical activity in young African American women. *Health Care for Women International.* 2002;23(8):905–918.

73. Salmon JW, Owen N, Bauman A, Schmitz MKH, Booth M. Leisure-time, occupational, and household activity among professional, skilled, and less-skilled workers and homemakers. *Prev Med.* 2000;30:191–199.

74. Ford ES, Merritt RK, Heath GW, et al. Physical activity behaviors in lower and higher socioeconomic status populations. *Am J Epidemiol.* 1991;133(12): 1246–1256.

75. Rimmer JH, Nicola T, Riley B, Creviston T. Exercise training for African Americans with disabilities residing in difficult social environments. *Am J Prev Med.* 2002;23(4):290–295.

76. Billings J, Zeitel L, Lukomnik J, Carey T, Blank A, Newman L. Impact of socio-economic status on hospital use in New York City. *Health Aff (Millwood).* 1993;12: 162–173.

77. King AC, Kiernan M, Ahn DK, Wilcox S. The effects of marital transitions on changes in physical activity: results from a 10-year community study. *Ann Behav Med.* 1998;20:64–69.

78. Brown WJ, Young AF, Byles JE. Tyranny of distance? The health of mid-age women living in five geographical areas of Australia. *Aust J Rural Health.* 1999;7: 148–154.

79. Dowda M, Ainsworth BE, Addy CL, Saunders R, Riner W. The correlates of physical activity among U.S. young adults, 18 to 30 years of age, from NHANES III. *Ann Behav Med.* 2033;26(1):15–23.

80. King AC, Castro C, Wilcox S, Eyler AA, Sallis JF, Brownson RC. Personal and environmental factors associated with physical inactivity among different racial-ethnic groups of US middle-aged and older ages adults. *Health Psychol.* 2000;19: 354–364.

81. Brownson RC, Eyler AA, King AC, Brown DR, Shyu YL, Sallis JF. Patterns and correlates of physical activity among US women 40 years and older. *Am J Public Health.* 2000;90:267–270.

82. Sternfeld B, Ainsworth BE, Queensberry CP. Physical activity in a diverse population of women. *Prev Med.* 1999;28:313–323.

83. Perusse L, Leblanc C, Bouchard C. Familial resemblance in lifestyle components: Results from the Canada fitness survey. *Can J Public Health.* 1988;79: 201–205.

84. Lauderdale DS, Fabsitz R, Meyer JM, Sholinsky P, Ramakrishanan V, Goldberg J. Familial determinants of moderate and intense physical activity: a twin study. *Med Sci Sports Exerc.* 1997;29:1062–1068.

85. Aarnio M, Winter T, Kujala UM, Kaprio J. Familial aggregation of leisure-time physical activity—a three-generation study. *Int J Sports Med.* 1997;18:549–556.

86. Beunen G, Thomis M. Genetic determinants of sports participation and daily physical activity. *Int J Obes.* 1999;3:1–9.

87. Perusse L, Tremblay A, Leblanc C, Bouchard C. Genetic and familial environmental influences on level of habitual physical activity. *Am J Epidemiol.* 1989;129: 1012–1022.

88. Maia JAR, Thomis M, Beunen G. Genetic factors in physical activity levels: a twin study. *Am J Prev Med.* 2002;23(2S):87–91.

89. Oman RF, King AC. Predicting the adoption and maintenance of exercise participation using self-efficacy and previous exercise participation rates. *Am J Health Promot.* 1998;12(3):154–161.

90. McAuley E. The role of efficacy cognitions in the prediction of exercise behavior in middle-aged adults. *J Behav Med.* 1992;15(1):65–88.

91. Rejeski WJ, Brawley LR, Ambrosius WT, et al. Older adults with chronic disease: benefits of group-mediated counseling in the promotion of physically active lifestyles. *Health Psychol.* 2003;22(4):414–423.

92. McAuley E, Jerome GJ, Marquez DX, Elavsky S, Blissmer B. Exercise self-efficacy in older adults: social, affective, and behavioral influences. *Ann Behav Med.* 2003;25(1):1–7.

93. McAuley E, Talbot HM, Martinez S. Manipulating self-efficacy in the exercise environment in women: influences on affective responses. *Health Psychol.* 1999;18(3):288–294.

94. Sallis JF, Hovell MF, Hofstetter CR, Barrington E. Explanation of vigourous physical activity during two years using social learning variables. *Soc Sci Med.* 1992;34(1):25–32.

95. Pargman D, Green L. The Type A behavior pattern and adherence to a regular running program by adult males ages 25 to 39 years. *Percept Mot Skills.* 1990;70(3 Pt 1):1040–1042.

96. Kreuter MW, Chheda SG, Bull FC. How does physician advice influence patient behavior? Evidence for a priming effect. *Arch Fam Med.* 2000;9(5): 426–433.

97. Moore SM, Dolansky MA, Ruland CM, Pashkow FJ, Blackburn GG. Predictors of women's exercise maintenance after cardiac rehabilitation. *J Cardpulm Rehabil.* 2003;23(1):40–49.

98. Wallace JP, Raglin JS, Jastremski CA. Twelve month adherence of adults who joined a fitness program with a spouse vs without a spouse. *J Sports Med Phys Fitness.* 1995;35(3):206–213.

99. Fraser SN, Spink KS. Examining the role of social support and group cohesion in exercise compliance. *J Behav Med.* 2002;25(3):233–249.

100. Miller YD, Trost SG, Brown WJ. Mediators of physical activity behavior changes among women with young children. *Am J Prev Med.* 2002;23(2S):98–103.

101. Satariano WA, Haight TJ, Tager IB. Living arrangements and participation in leisure-time physical activities in an older population. *J Aging Health.* 2002; 14(4):427–451.

102. Macken LC, Yates B, Blancher S. Concordance of risk factors in female spouses of male patients with coronary heart disease. *J Cardpulm Rehabil.* 2000;20(6): 361–368.

103. Kahn EB, Ramsey LT, Brownson RC, et al. The effectiveness of interventions to increase physical activity: a systematic review. *Am J Prev Med.* 2002;22(4S): 73–107.

104. Perri MG, Anton SD, Durning PE, et al. Adherence to exercise prescriptions: effects of prescribing moderate versus higher levels of intensity and frequency. *Health Psychol.* 2002;21(5):452–458.

105. King AC, Haskell WL, Taylor CB, Kraemer HC, DeBusk RF. Group- vs home-based exercise training in healthy older men and women. A community-based clinical trial. *JAMA.* 1991;266(11):1535–1542.

106. Lee JY, Jensen BE, Oberman A, Fletcher GF, Fletcher BJ, Raczynski JM. Adherence in the training levels comparison trial. *Med Sci Sports Exerc.* 1996;28(1): 47–52.

107. Jakicic JM, Wing RR, Butler BA, Robertson RJ. Prescribing exercise in multiple short bouts versus one continuous bout: effects on adherence, cardiorespi-

ratory fitness, and weight loss in overweight women. *Int J Obes Relat Metab Disord.* 1995;19(12):893–901.

108. DeBusk RF, Stenestrand U, Sheehan M, Haskell WL. Training effects of long versus short bouts of exercise in healthy subjects. *Am J Cardiol.* 1990;65(15): 1010–1013.

109. Murphy MH, Hardman AE. Training effects of short and long bouts of brisk walking in sedentary women. *Med Sci Sports Exerc.* 1998;30(1):152–157.

110. Hansen CJ, Stevens LC, Coast JR. Exercise duration and mood state: how much is enough to feel better? *Health Psychol.* 2001;20(4):267–275.

111. Jakicic JM, Winters C, Lang W, Wing RR. Effects of intermittent exercise and use of home exercise equipment on adherence, weight loss, and fitness in overweight women: a randomized trial. *JAMA.* 1999;282(16):1554–1560.

112. Woolf-May K, Kearney EM, Owen A, Jones DW, Davison RC, Bird SR. The efficacy of accumulated short bouts versus single daily bout of brisk walking in improving aerobic fitness and blood lipid profiles. *Health Educ Res.* 1999;14(6): 803–815.

113. Jacobsen DJ, Donnelly JE, Snyder-Heelan K, Livingston K. Adherence and attrition with intermittent and continuous exercise in overweight women. *Int J Sports Med.* 2003;24(6):459–464.

114. King AC, Haskell WL, Young DR, Oka RK, Stefanick ML. Long-term effects of varying intensities and formats of physical activity on participation rates, fitness, and lipoproteins in men and women aged 50 to 65 years. *Circulation.* 1995;91(10):2596–2604.

115. National Institutes of Health Consensus Development Panel on Physical Activity and Cardiovascular Health. Physical activity and cardiovascular health. *JAMA.* 1996;276(3):241–246.

116. Perri MG, Martin AD, Leermakers EA, Sears SF, Notelovitz M. Effects of group-versus home-based exercise in the treatment of obesity. *J Consult Clin Psychol.* 1997;65(2):278–285.

117. Carlson JJ, Johnson JA, Franklin BA, VanderLaan RL. Program participation, exercise adherence, cardiovascular outcomes, and program cost of traditional versus modified cardiac rehabilitation. *Am J Cardiol.* 2000;86(1):17–23.

118. Cox KL, Burke V, Gorely TJ, Beilin LJ, Puddey IB. Controlled comparison of retention and adherence in home- vs center-initiated exercise interventions in women ages 40–65 years: The S.W.E.A.T. Study (Sedentary Women Exercise Adherence Trial). *Prev Med.* 2003;36(1):17–29.

119. Franklin BA. Program factors that influence exercise adherence: practical adherence for the clinical staff. In: Dishman RK, ed. *Exercise Adherence: Its Impact on Public Health.* Champaign, IL: Human Kinetics; 1988:237–258.

120. Humpel N, Owen N, Leslie E. Environmental factors associated with adults' participation in physical activity. *Am J Prev Med.* 2002;22(3):188–199.

121. Huston SJ, Evenson KR, Bors P, Gizlice Z. Neighborhood environment, access to places for activity, and leisure time physical activity in a diverse North Carolina population. *Am J Health Promot.* 2003;Sept/Oct:58–69.

122. King WC, Brach JS, Belle S, Killingsworth R, Fenton M, Kriska AM. The relationship between convenience of destination and walking levels in older women. *Am J Health Promot.* 2003;Sept/Oct:74–82.

123. Powell KE, Martin LM, Chowdhury PP. Places to walk: convenience and regular physical activity. *Am J Public Health.* 2003;93(9):1519–1521.

124. Booth M, Owen N, Bauman A, Clavisi O, Leslie E. Social-cognitive and perceived environment influences associated with physical activity in older Australians. *Prev Med.* 2000;31:15–22.

125. Ball KT, Bauman A, Leslie E, Owen N. Perceived environmental and social influences on walking for exercise in Australian adults. *Prev Med.* 2001;33: 434–440.

126. Troped PJ, Saunders RP, Pate RR, Reininger B, Ureda JR, Shompson SJ. Associations between self-reported and objective physical environment factors and use of a community rail-trail. *Prev Med.* 2001;32:191–200.

127. Sallis JF, Hovell MF, Hofstetter CR, et al. Distance between homes and exercise facilities related to frequency of exercise among San Diego residents. *Public Health Rep.* 1990;105:179–185.

128. Centers for Disease Control and Prevention. Neighborhood safety and the prevalence of physical inactivity—selected states, 1996. *MMWR.* 1999;48: 143–146.

129. MacDougall C, Cooke R, Owen N, Wilson K, Bauman A. Relating physical activity to health status, social connections and community facilities. *Aust N Z J Public Health.* 1997;21:631–637.

130. Jakicic JM, Wing RR, Butler BA, Jeffery RW. The relationship between presence of exercise equipment in the home and physical activity level. *Am J Health Promot.* 1997;11:363–365.

131. Sallis JF, Hovell MF, Hofstetter CR. Predictors of adoption and maintenance of vigorous physical activity in men and women. *Prev Med.* 1992;21:237–251.

132. Litt MD, Kleppinger A, Judge JO. Initiation and maintenance of exercise behavior in older women: predictors from the social learning model. *J Behav Med.* 2002;25(1):83–97.

133. McAuley E, Blissmer B. Self-efficacy determinants and consequences of physical activity. *Exerc Sport Sci Rev.* 2000;28(2):85–88.

134. U.S. Department of Health and Human Services. *Healthy People 2010: Conference Edition.* Washington, DC: U.S. Department of Health and Human Services; 2000.

135. King AC. Clinical and community interventions to promote and support physical activity participation. In: Dishman RK, ed. *Advances in Exercise Adherence.* Champaign, IL: Human Kinetics; 1994:183–212.

136. Marcus BH, King TK, Clark NM, Pinto BM, Bock BC. Theories and techniques for promoting physical activity behaviors. *Sports Med.* 1996;22(5):321–333.

137. The Writing Group for the Activity Counseling Trial Research Group. Effects of physical activity counseling in primary care: the Activity Counseling Trial: a randomized controlled trial. *JAMA.* 2001;286:677–687.

138. Hallam J, Petosa R. A worksite intervention to enhance social cognitive theory constructs to promote exercise adherence. *Am J Health Promot.* 1998;13(1):4–7.

139. Heesch KC, Masse LC, Dunn AL, Frankowski RF, Mullen D. Does adherence to a lifestyle physical activity intervention predict changes in physical activity. *J Behav Med.* 2003;26(4):333–348.

140. Friedman RH. Automated telephone conversations to assess health behavior and deliver behavioral interventions. *J Med Syst.* 1998;22(2):95–102.

141. Kerse NM, L. F, Jolley D, Arroll B, Young D. Improving the health behaviours of elderly people: randomised controlled trial of a general practice education programme. *BMJ.* 1999;319:683–687.

142. Sullivan T, Allegrante JP, Peterson MG, Kovar PA, MacKenzie CR. One-year followup of patients with osteoarthritis of the knee who participated in a program of supervised fitness walking and supportive patient education. *Arthritis Care & Research.* 1998;11(4):228–233.

143. Elder JP, Williams SJ, Drew JA, Wright BL, Boulan TE. Longitudinal effects of preventive services on health behaviors among an elderly cohort. *Am J Prev Med.* 1995;11:354–359.

144. Martin JE, Dubbert PM, Katell AD, et al. Behavioral control of exercise in sedentary adults: Studies 1 through 6. *J Consult Clin Psychol.* 1984;52:795–811.

145. Owen N, Lee C, Naccarella L, Haag K. Exercise by mail: a mediated behavior-change program for aerobic exercise. *J Sport Psychol.* 1987;9:346–357.

146. Mayer JA, Jermanovich A, Wright BL, Elder JP, Drew JA, Williams SJ. Changes in health behaviors of older adults: the San Diego Medicare Preventive Health Project. *Prev Med.* 1994;23:127–133.

147. Proper KI, Hildebrandt VH, van der Beek AJ, Twisk JW, van Mechele W. Effect of individualized counseling on physical activity, fitness and health: a randomized controlled trial in a workplace setting. *Am J Prev Med.* 2003;24(3):218–226.

148. Lorig KR, Sobel DS, Stewart A, et al. Evidence suggesting that a chronic disease self-management program can improve health status while reducing hospitalization. *Med Care.* 1999;37(1):5–14.

149. Robison JI, Rogers MA, Carlson JJ, et al. Effects of a 6-month incentive-based exercise program on adherence and work capacity. *Med Sci Sports Exerc.* 1992;24(1):85–93.

150. Oldridge NB, Jones NL. Improving patient compliance in cardiac rehabilitation. Effects of written agreement and self-monitoring. *J Cardpulm Rehabil.* 1983;3:257–262.

151. Stoffelmayr BE, Mavis BE, Stachnik T, et al. A program model to enhance adherence in work-site-based fitness programs. *J Occup Med.* 1992;34(2):156–161.

152. Wysocki T, Hall G, Iwata BA, Riordon M. Behavioral management of exercise: contracting for aerobic points. *J Appl Behav Anal.* 1979;12:55–64.

153. Epstein LH, Wing RR, Thompson JK, Griffin W. Attendance and fitness in aerobics exercise: the effects of contract and lottery procedures. *Behav Modif.* 1980;4:465–479.

154. Noland MP. The effects of self-monitoring and reinforcement on exercise adherence. *Res Q Exerc Sport.* 1989;60(3):216–224.

155. King AC, Taylor CB, Haskell WL, Debusk RF. Strategies for increasing early adherence to and long-term maintenance of home-based exercise training in healthy middle-aged men and women. *Am J Cardiol.* 1988;61(8):628–632.

156. Juneau M, Rogers F, De Santos V, et al. Effectiveness of self-monitored, home-based, moderate-intensity exercise training in middle-aged men and women. *Am J Cardiol.* 1987;60(1):66–70.

157. Castro CM, King AC, Brassington GS. Telephone versus mail interventions for maintenance of physical activity in older adults. *Health Psychol.* 2001;20(6): 438–444.

158. King AC, Pruitt LA, Phillips W, Oka R, Rodenburg A, Haskell WL. Comparative effects of two physical activity programs on measured and perceived physical functioning and other health-related quality of life outcomes in older adults. *J Gerontol A Biol Sci Med Sci.* 2000;55(2):M74–M83.

159. Marcus BH, Stanton AL. Evaluation of relapse prevention and reinforcement interventions to promote exercise adherence in sedentary females. *Res Q Exerc Sport.* 1993;64(4):447–452.

160. Jeffery RW, Wing RR, Thorson C, Burton LR. Use of personal trainers and financial incentives to increase exercise in a behavioral weight-loss program. *J Consult Clin Psychol.* 1998;66(5):777–783.

161. Kravitz L, Furst D. Influence of reward and social support on exercise adherence in aerobic dance class. *Psychol Rep.* 1991;69:423–426.

162. Belisle M, Roskies E, Levesque JM. Improving adherence to physical activity. *Health Psychol.* 1987;6(2):159–172.

163. King AC, Frederiksen LW. Low-cost strategies for increasing exercise behavior. *Behav Modif.* 1984;8:3–21.

164. Keefe FJ, Blumenthal JA. The life fitness program: a behavioral approach to making exercise a habit. *J Behav Ther Exp Psychiatry.* 1980;11:31–34.

165. Wankel LM, Yardley JK, Graham J. The effects of motivational interventions upon the exercise adherence of high and low self-motivated adults. *Canadian Journal of Applied Sport Sciences.* 1985;10(3):147–156.

166. Heinzelmann F, Bagley RW. Response to physical activity programs and their effects on health behavior. *Public Health Rep.* 1970;85:905–911.

167. Toobert DJ, Strycker LA, Glasgow RE, Barrera M, Bagdade JD. Enhancing support for health behavior change among women at risk for heart disease: the Mediterranean Lifestyle Trial. *Health Educ Res.* 2002;17(2):574–585.

168. Wing RR, Jeffery RW, Pronk N, Hellerstedt WL. Effects of a personal trainer and financial incentives on exercise adherence in overweight women in a behavioral weight loss program. *Obes Res.* 1996;4(5):457–462.

169. Sims J, Smith F, Duffy A, Hilton S. Can practice nurses increase physical activity in the over 65s? Methodological considerations from a pilot study. *Br J Gen Pract.* 1998;48:1249–1250.

170. McAuley E, Courneya KS, Rudolph DL, Lox CL. Enhancing exercise adherence in middle-aged males and females. *Prev Med.* 1994;23(4):498–506.

171. Harland J, White M, Drinkwater C, Chinn D, Farr L, Howel D. The Newcastle exercise project: a randomised controlled trial of methods to promote physical activity in primary care [comment]. *BMJ.* 1999;319(7213):828–832.

172. Wilson DK, Friend R, Teasley N, Green S, Reaves IL, Sica D. Motivational versus social cognitive interventions for promoting fruit and vegetable intake and physical activity in African American adolescents. *Ann Behav Med.* 2002;24(4): 310–319.

173. Miller WC, Pollock S. *Motivational Interviewing: Preparing People to Change Addictive Behaviour.* London: Guilford Press; 1991.

174. Simons-Morton DG, Calfas KJ, Oldenburg B, Burton NW. Effects of interventions in health care settings on physical activity or cardiorespiratory fitness. *Am J Prev Med.* 1998;15(4):413–430.

175. Hillsdon M, Thorogood M, Anstiss T, Morris JA. Randomised controlled trials of physical activity promotion in free living populations: a review. *J Epidemiol Community Health.* 1995;49(5):448–453.

176. Peterson TR, Aldana SG. Improving exercise behavior: an application of the stages of change model in a worksite setting. *Am J Health Promot.* 1999;13: 229–232.

177. Marcus B, Emmons KM, Simkin-Silverman LR, et al. Evaluation of motivationally tailored vs. standard self-help physical activity interventions at the workplace. *Am J Health Promot.* 1998;12:246–253.

178. Marcus BH, Bock BC, Pinto BM, Forsyth LH, Roberts MB, Traficante RM. Efficacy of an individualized, motivationally-tailored physical activity intervention. *Ann Behav Med.* 1998;20(3):174–180.

179. Blissmer B, McAuley E. Testing the requirements of stages of physical activity among adults: the comparative effectiveness of stage-matched, mismatched, standard care, and control interventions. *Ann Behav Med.* 2002;24(3):181–189.

180. Vandelanotte C, De Bourdeaudhuij I. Acceptability and feasibility of a computer-tailored physical activity intervention using stages of change: project FAITH. *Health Educ Res.* 2003;18(3):304–317.

181. Dunn AL, Andersen RE, Jakicic JM. Lifestyle physical activity interventions: history, short- and long-term effects, and recommendations. *Am J Prev Med.* 1998;15(4):398–412.

182. Cardinal BJ, Sachs ML. Effects of a mail-mediated, stage-matched exercise behavior change strategies on female adults' leisure-time exercise behavior. *J Sports Med Phys Fitness.* 1996;36(2):100–107.

183. Schappert SM. *National Ambulatory Medical Care Survey: 1991. 230th ed.* Hyattsville, MD: National Center for Health Statistics; 1993.

184. Godin G, Shephard R. An evaluation of the potential role of the physician in influencing community exercise behavior. *Am J Health Promot.* 1990;4:225–229.

185. American Heart Association. *1999 Heart and Stroke Statistical Update.* Dallas, TX: American Heart Association; 1998.

186. National High Blood Pressure Education Program. *The Sixth Report of the Joint National Committee on Prevention, Detection, and Treatment of High Blood Pressure.* 6th ed. Bethesda, MD: National Institutes of Health, National Heart, Lung, and Blood Institute, National High Blood Pressure Education Program; 1997.

187. U.S. Preventive Services Task Force. *Guide to Clinical Preventive Services.* 2nd ed. Baltimore: Williams & Wilkins; 1996.

188. Reed BD, Jensen JD, Gorenflo DW. Physicians and exercise promotion. *Am J Prev Med.* 1991;7:410–415.

189. Wee CC, McCarthy EP, Davis RB, Phillips RS. Physician counseling about exercise. *JAMA.* 1999;282(16):1583–1588.

190. Centers for Disease Control and Prevention. Physician advice and individual behaviors about cardiovascular disease risk reduction—seven states and Puerto Rico, 1997. *MMWR.* 1999;48:74–77.

191. Lewis CE, Clancy C, Leake B, Schwartz JS. The counseling practices of internists. *Ann Intern Med.* 1991;114:54–58.

192. Centers for Disease Control and Prevention. Missed opportunities in preventive counseling for cardiovascular disease—United States, 1995. *MMWR.* 1998;47:91–95.

193. Damush TM, Stewart AL, Mill KM, King AC, Ritter PL. Prevalence and correlates of physician recommendations to exercise among older adults. *J Gerontol A Biol Sci Med Sci.* 1999;54:M423–M427.

194. Lewis CE, Wells KB, Ware J. A model for predicting the counseling practices of physicians. *J Gen Intern Med.* 1986;1:14–19.

195. Orleans CT, George LK, Houpt JL, Brodie KH. Health promotion in primary care: a survey of U.S. family practitioners. *Prev Med.* 1985;14:636–647.

196. Calfas KJ, Long BJ, Sallis JF, Wooten WJ, Pratt M, Patrick K. A controlled trial of physician counseling to promote the adoption of physical activity. *Prev Med.* 1996;25(3):225–233.

197. Goldstein MG, Pinto BM, Marcus BH, Lynn H, Jette AM, Rakowski W. Physician-based physical activity counseling for middle-aged and older adults: a randomized trial. *Ann Behav Med.* 1999;21:40–47.

198. Eaton CB, Menard LM. A systematic review of physical activity promotion in primary care office settings. *Br J Sports Med.* 1998;32:11–16.

199. Eden KB, Orleans CT, Mulrow CD, Pender NJ, Teutsch SM. Does counseling by clinicians improve physical activity? A summary of the evidence for the U.S. Preventive Services Task Force. *Ann Intern Med.* 2002;137:208–215.

200. Eakin EG, Glasgow RE, Riley KM. Review of primary care-based physical activity intervention studies: effectiveness and implications for practice and future research. *J Fam Pract.* 2000;49:158–168.

201. Swinburn BA, Walter LG, Arroll B, Tilyard MW, Russell DG. The green prescription study: a randomized controlled trial of written exercise advice provided by general practitioners. *Am J Public Health.* 1998;88:288–291.

202. Green BB, McAfee T, Hindmarsh M, Madsen L, Caplow M, Buist D. Effectiveness of telephone support in increasing physical activity levels in primary care patients. *Am J Prev Med.* 2002;22(3):177–183.

203. Marcus BH, Owen N, Forsyth LH, Cavill NA, Fridinger F. Physical activity interventions using mass media, print media, and information technology. *Am J Prev Med.* 1998;15(4):362–378.

204. Castro CM, King AC. Telephone-assisted counseling for physical activity. *Exerc Sport Sci Rev.* 2002;30(2):64–68.

205. Pinto BM, Friedman R, Marcus BH, Kelley H, Tennestedt S, Gillman MW. Effects of a computer-based, telephone-counseling system on physical activity. *Am J Prev Med.* 2002;23(2):113–120.

206. Ewing R, Schmid T, Killingsworth R, Zlot A, Raudenbush S. Relationship between urban sprawl and physical activity, obesity, and morbidity. *Am J Health Promot.* 2003;Sept/Oct:47–57.

207. Pucher J, Dijkstra L. Promoting safe walking and cycling to improve public health: lessons from The Netherlands and Germany. *Am J Public Health.* 2003;93(9):1509–1516.

208. Sallis JF, Bauman A, Pratt M. Environmental and policy interventions to promote physical activity. *Am J Prev Med.* 1998;15(4):379–397.

209. King AC, Jefferey RW, Fridinger F, et al. Environmental and policy approaches to cardiovascular disease prevention through physical activity: issues and opportunities. *Health Education Quarterly.* 1995;22:499–511.

210 Owen N, Bauman A, Booth M, Oldenburg B, Magnus P. Serial mass-media campaigns to promote physical activity: reinforcing or redundant. *Am J Public Health.* 1995;85:244–248.

211. Vuori IM, Oja P, Paronen O. Physically active commuting to work: testing its potential for exercise promotion. *Med Sci Sports Exerc.* 1994;26:844–850.

212. Blamey A, Mutrie N, Aitchison T. Health promotion by encouraged use of stairs. *BMJ.* 1995;311:289–290.

213. Brownell KD, Stunkard AJ, Albaum JM. Evaluation and modification of exercise patterns in the natural environment. *Am J Psychiatry.* 1980;137:1540–1545.

214. Linenger JM, Chesson CV, Nice DS. Physical fitness gains following simple environmental change. *Am J Prev Med.* 1991;7:298–310.

215. Roberts K, Dench S, Minten J, York C. *Community Response to Leisure Centre Provision in Belfast.* London: Sports Council; 1989.

216. van der Bij AK, Laurant MGH, Wesing M. Effectiveness of physical activity interventions for older adults. *Am J Prev Med.* 2001;22(2):120–133.

217. Brassington GS, Atienza AA, Perczek RE, DiLorenzo TM, King AC. Intervention-related cognitive versus social mediators of exercise adherence in the elderly. *Am J Prev Med.* 2002;23(2 Suppl):80–86.

218. Chao D, Foy CG, Farmer D. Exercise adherence among older adults: challenges and strategies. *Control Clin Trials.* 2000;21(5 Suppl):212S–217S.

219. Rejeski WJ, Focht BC. Aging and physical disability: on integrating group and individuals counseling with the promotion of physical activity. *Exerc Sport Sci Rev.* 2002;30(4):166–170.

220. Wilcox S, King AC, Brassington GS, Ahn DK. Physical activity preferences of middle-aged and older adults: a community analysis. *Journal of Aging and Physical Activity.* 1999;7(4):386–399.

221. Rejeski WJ, Brawley LR, Ettinger W, Morgan T, Thompson C. Compliance to exercise therapy in older participants with knee osteoarthritis: implications for treating disability. *Med Sci Sports Exerc.* 1997;29(8):977–985.

222. Sheppard L, Senior J, Park CH, Mockenhaupt R, Chodzko-Zajko W, Bazzarre T. The National Blueprint Consensus Conference Summary report: strategic

priorities for increasing physical activity among adults aged >=50. *Am J Prev Med.* 2003;25(2):209–213.

223. Pasick RJ, D'Onofrio CN, Otero-Sabogal R. Similarities and differences across cultures: questions to inform a third generation for health promotion research. *Health Education Quarterly.* 1996;23:S142–S161.

224. Kumanyika SK, Charleston JB. Lose weight and win: a church-based weight loss program for blood pressure control among black women. *Patient Education & Counseling.* 1992;19:19–32.

225. Resnicow K, Jackson A, Braithwaite R, et al. Healthy Body/Healthy Spirit: a church-based nutrition and physical activity intervention. *Health Educ Res.* 2002;17(5):562–573.

226. Yanek LR, Becker DM, Moy TF, Gittelsohn J, Koffman DM. Project Joy: Faith based cardiovascular health promotion for African American women. *Public Health Rep.* 2001;116:68–81.

227. Lowther M, Mutrie N, Scott EM. Promoting physical activity in a socially and economically deprived community: a 12 month randomized control trial of fitness assessment and exercise consultation. *J Sports Sci.* 2002;20(7):577–588.

228. Toobert DJ, Glasgow RE, Radcliffe JL. Physiologic and related behavioral outcomes from the Women's Lifestyle Heart Trial. *Ann Behav Med.* 2000;22(1): 1–9.

229. Toobert DJ, Glasgow RE, Nettekoven LA, Brown JE. Behavioral and psychosocial effects of intensive lifestyle management for women with coronary heart disease. *Patient Education & Counseling.* 1998;35(3):177–188.

230. Toobert DJ, Strycker LA, Glasgow RE, Bagdade JD. If you build it, will they come? Reach and Adoption associated with a comprehensive lifestyle management program for women with type 2 diabetes. *Patient Education & Counseling.* 2002;48(2):99–105.

231. Ransdell LB, Taylor A, Oakland D, Schmidt J, Moyer-Mileur L, Shultz B. Daughters and mothers exercising together: effects of home- and community-based programs. *Med Sci Sports Exerc.* 2003;35(2):286–296.

232. Castro CM, Wilcox S, O'Sullivan P, Baumann K, King AC. An exercise program for women who are caring for relatives with dementia. *Psychosom Med.* 2002; 64(3):458–468.

233. Carter ND, Khan KM, McKay HA, et al. Community-based exercise program reduces risk factors for falls in 65- to 75-year-old women with osteoporosis: randomized controlled trial. *CMAJ.* 2002;167(9):997–1004.

234. King AC, Baumann K, O'Sullivan P, Wilcox S, Castro C. Effects of moderate-intensity exercise on physiological, behavioral, and emotional responses to family caregiving: a randomized controlled trial. *J Gerontol A Biol Sci Med Sci.* 2002;57(1):M26–M36.

235. Bauman A, Smith BA, Stoker L, Bellew B, Booth M. Geographical influences upon physical activity participation: evidence of a "coastal effect." *Aust N Z J Public Health.* 1991;23:322–324.

236. Clark DO. Physical activity and its correlates among urban primary care patients aged 55 and older. *J Gerontol B Psychol Sci Soc Sci.* 1999;54:41–48.

237. Leslie E, Owen N, Salmon JW, Bauman A, Sallis JF, Lo SK. Insufficiently active Australian college students: perceived personal, social, and environmental influences. *Prev Med.* 1999;28:20–27.

238. Lian WM, Gan GL, Phi H, Wee S, Ye HC. Correlates of leisure-time physical activity in an elderly population in Singapore. *Am J Public Health.* 1999;89: 1578–1580.

239. Ross CE. Walking, exercise, and smoking: does neighborhood matter? *Soc Sci Med.* 2000;51:265–274.

240. Ruchlin HS, Lachs MS. Prevalence and correlates of exercise among older adults. *J Appl Gerontol.* 1999;18:341–357.

241. Salmon JW, Bauman A, Crawford D, Timperio A, Owen N. The association between television viewing and overweight among Australian adults participating in varying levels of leisure time physical activity. *Int J Obes.* 2000;24:600–606.

242. Simonsick E, Guralnik JM, Fried LP. Who walks? Factors associated with walking behavior in disabled older women with and without self-reported walking difficulty. *J Am Geriatr Soc.* 1999;47:672–680.

243. Talbot LA, Fleg JL, Metter EJ. Secular trends in leisure-time physical activity in men and women across four decades. *Prev Med.* 2003;37:52–60.

244. Wilbur J, Michaels Miller A, Chandler P, McDevitt J. Determinants of physical activity and adherence to a 24-week home-based walking program in African American and Caucasian women. *Res Nurs Health.* 2003;26(3):213–224.

245. Parks SE, Housemann RA, Brownson RC. Differential correlates of physical activity in urban and rural adults of various socioeconomic backgrounds in the United States. *J Epidemiol Community Health.* 2003;57(1):29–35.

246. Brenes GA, Strube MJ, Storandt M. An application of the theory of planned behavior to exercise among older adults. *Journal of Applied Social Psychology.* 1998;28:2274–2290.

247. Bozionelos G, Bennett P. The theory of planned behavior as predictor of exercise: the moderating influence of beliefs and personality variables. *J Health Psychol.* 1999;4:517–529.

248. Eyler AA, Brownson RC, Bacak RJ, Housemann RA. The epidemiology of walking for physical activity in the United States. *Med Sci Sports Exerc.* 2003;35(9): 1529–1536.

249. Martinez-Gonzalez MA, Martinez JA, Hu FB, Gibney MJ, Kearney J. Physical inactivity, sedentary lifestyle and obesity in the European Union. *Int J Obes.* 1999;23:1192–1201.

250. Courneya KS, Bobick TM, Schinke RJ. Does the theory of planned behavior mediate the relation between personality and exercise behavior. *Basic and Applied Social Psychology.* 1999;21:317–324.

251. Kerner MS, Grossman AH. Attitudinal, social, and practical correlates to fitness behavior: a test of the theory of planned behavior. *Percept Mot Skills.* 1998;87:1139–1154.

252. Michels TC. Predicting exercise in older Americans: using the theory of planned behavior. *Mil Med.* 1998;163:524–529.

253. Courneya KS, Plotnikoff RC, Hotz SB, Birkett NJ. Social support and the theory of planned behavior in the exercise domain. *Am J Health Behav.* 2000;24: 300–308.

254. Clark DO, Northwehr F. Exercise self-efficacy and its correlates among socioeconomically disadvantaged older adults. *Health Educ Behav.* 1999;26:535–546.

255. Mitchell SA, Olds RS. Psychological and perceived situational predictors of physical activity: a cross-sectional analysis. *Health Educ Res.* 1999;14:305–313.

256. Rodgers WM, Gauvin L. Heterogeneity of incentives for physical activity and self-efficacy in highly active and moderately active women exercisers. *Journal of Applied Social Psychology.* 1998;28:1016–1029.

257. Sears SR, Stanton AL. Expectancy-value constructs and expectancy violation as predictors of exercise adherence in previously sedentary women. *Health Psychol.* 2001;20(5):326–333.

258. Giles-Corti B, Donovan RJ. Relative influences of individuals, social environmental, and physical environmental correlates of walking. *Am J Public Health.* 2003;93(9):1583–1589.

259. Kiernan M, King AC, Kraemer HC, Stefanick ML, Killen JD. Characteristics of successful and unsuccessful dieters: an application of signal detection methodology. *Ann Behav Med.* 1998;20(1):1–6.

260. Ziegelstein RC, Fauerbach JA, Stevens SS, Romanelli J, Richter DP, Bush DE. Patients with depression are less likely to follow recommendations to reduce cardiac risk during recovery from a myocardial infarction. *Arch Intern Med.* 2000;160(12):1818–1823.

261. Glazer KM, Emery CF, Frid DJ, Banyasz RE. Psychological predictors of adherence and outcomes among patients in cardiac rehabilitation. *J Cardpulm Rehabil.* 2002;22(1):40–46.

262. Yin Z, Boyd MP. Behavioral and cognitive correlates of exercise self-schemata. *J Psychol.* 2000;134(3):269–282.

263. Castro CM, Sallis JF, Hickman SA, Lee RE, Chen AH. A prospective study of psychological correlates of physical activity for ethnic minority women. *Psychology and Health.* 1999;14:277–293.

264. Sullum J, Clark MM, King TK. Predictors of exercise relapse in a college population. *J Am Coll Health Assoc.* 2000;48:175–180.

265. Caserta MS, Gillett PA. Older women's feelings about exercise and their adherence to an aerobic regimen over time. *Gerontologist.* 1998;38(5):602–609.

266. Taylor WC, Blair SN, Cummings SS, Wun CC, Malina RM. Childhood and adolescent physical activity patterns and adult physical activity. *Med Sci Sports Exerc.* 1999;31:118–123.

267. Johnson MF, Nichols JF, Sallis JF, Calfas KJ, Hovell MF. Interrelationships between physical activity and other health behaviors among university women and men. *Prev Med.* 1998;27:536–544.

268. Albright CL, King AC, Taylor CB, Haskell WL. Effect of a six-month aerobic exercise training program on cardiovascular responsivity in health middle-aged adults. *J Psychosom Res.* 1992;36(1):25–36.

269. Estabrooks PA. Sustaining exercise participation through group cohesion. *Exerc Sport Sci Rev.* 2000;28(2):63–67.

270. Estabrooks PA, Carron AV. Group cohesion in older adult exercisers: prediction and intervention effects. *J Behav Med.* 1999;22(6):575–588.

Chapter 4

Adherence to Diet Recommendations

William S. Yancy, Jr.
Jarol Boan

The association between diet and health is ubiquitous. It can be found in daily conversation, advertisements, and television programs. We read about it in cartoons, magazine articles, and self-help books. Since the publication of the Surgeon General's report on diet and health in 1977, diet's relationship with health has become increasingly prevalent in the health care arena (1). Many a patient has dreaded the upcoming lecture on diet at the next doctor's appointment. Of course, there are good reasons that our society is obsessed with what we eat. After tobacco use, diet (combined with activity) pattern is considered the most prominent contributor to mortality in the United States (2).

The major intermediary between diet and mortality is obesity. In fact, the preceding statement can be altered slightly to state that, after tobacco use, obesity is the second-leading preventable cause of death in the United States (3). If one views obesity as an extension of an unhealthy diet, then a host of acute and chronic illnesses can be judged as diet related, including: diabetes mellitus (DM), hypertension, coronary heart disease (CHD), congestive heart failure, hyperlipidemia, cancer, gall bladder disease, osteoarthritis, gastroesophageal reflux disease (GERD), and obstructive sleep apnea (4–6). The strong association of obesity with these diseases has become more important in the past 20 years as the prevalence of obesity (defined as body mass index [BMI] ≥ 30 kg/m^2) (7) has increased from 14.5% in 1980 to 30.5% in 2000 (8, 9). If overweight individuals (BMI 25–29.9 kg/

m²) are also considered, then the proportion of Americans who are above recommended weight rises to nearly 65% (9).

Obesity is the prime reason that the word *diet* is more commonly used to connote a prescribed therapy than its original meaning of "food and drink regularly provided or consumed" (10). In a nationwide survey of adults in 1996, 29% of men and 44% of women were trying to lose weight (11). If one includes those actively trying to maintain their current weight (i.e., avoid weight gain), then nearly 65% of men and 80% of women were attempting to alter their daily habits in some way (11). Unfortunately, in this study, most people were not following current recommendations for weight loss. Dieting was the most commonly reported strategy for weight loss but only about 50% of those trying to lose weight reported actually consuming fewer calories, the best proven method for losing weight. Adherence to a diet regimen (especially a reduction in calories) is so difficult that it is often likened to cessation of addictive behaviors (e.g., cigarette smoking). However, "addiction" to food is more complex than addictions to other substances because everyone needs nourishment to survive.

Many diet and weight loss interventions have been proven effective over short durations. Even more difficult than initiating a weight loss diet, however, is maintaining weight loss once this onerous task has been achieved. Adherence to dietary interventions tends to wane over longer durations. Overall, patients who adhere to weight loss programs of various types typically lose approximately 10% of original body weight, but one third to two thirds of this weight is regained at 1 year, and nearly all of it is regained at 5 years (12). Due to these depressing statistics on long-term effectiveness, patients and health professionals are quick to discount these interventions.

Therapeutic diets are recommended for a wide range of illnesses in addition to obesity, including DM, hypertension, hyperlipidemia, GERD, celiac disease, chronic kidney disease, and multiple metabolic deficiencies. For some of these diseases (e.g., DM, hypertension, hyperlipidemia), diet therapy prevents future complications whereas for others (e.g., GERD, celiac disease, metabolic deficiencies, in-born errors of metabolism) the beneficial effects are immediate. However, even dietary interventions with immediate beneficial impact lack perfect adherence. For example, a gluten-free diet for the treatment of celiac disease is associated with alleviation of symptoms and high motivation for adherence (13). Although adherence to a gluten-free diet is better than with other dietary recommendations, dietary indiscretions in this population do occur. In one survey, 36% of patients with celiac disease reported difficulty in complying with the gluten-free diet (14). Dietary interventions without immediate benefit understandably have even lower adherence rates.

Nevertheless, dietary intervention is an important, often first-line, therapeutic option because it is less expensive than medical interventions, has fewer side effects, and frequently has multiple benefits. However, because adherence to these interventions wanes over longer durations, patients and health professionals often resort to second-line therapies such as medication and even surgery. These second-line interventions are useful in certain situations, but first-line diet interventions should not be neglected simply because, on average, they are ineffective in the long run. Some patients are able to make permanent dietary changes and enjoy lifelong successful outcomes. For other patients, we might yet develop new approaches that improve their long-term adherence. For these reasons, it is important to give diet recommendations adequate consideration before discarding them in a refractory patient. Understanding the barriers and predictors of dietary adherence, as well as which interventions are effective, can increase the chance of success. Additionally, it is crucial that we continue our research of methods that can improve adherence to diet recommendations.

The aim of this chapter is to summarize the literature regarding patient adherence to diet recommendations, focusing mainly on the adult population. We have used diet interventions for obesity as the primary source of data but also have considered diet interventions for other common primary care problems such as hypertension and hyperlipidemia; diet recommendations for each of these problems generally apply to the majority of people. We have not reviewed interventions for special disease populations (e.g., patients with chronic kidney failure or metabolic deficiencies) because diet recommendations for these health problems are frequently not generalizable. In addition, because transient adherence to diet is not therapeutic, this chapter emphasizes studies of durations of at least 1 year, when available. Our summary includes discussions of predictive factors for diet adherence and of interventions to improve diet adherence. We also provide occasional practical clinical pearls and recommendations for areas of further research.

BARRIERS TO DIET ADHERENCE

Identifying barriers to diet adherence can be an important step toward a successful diet intervention. Unfortunately, many barriers to diet adherence exist (see Table 4.1), and it is clear that they are very difficult for people to overcome. For example, recent recommendations from both the U.S. Department of Agriculture (Dietary Guidelines) (15) and the National Heart, Lung, and Blood Institute (NHLBI) of the National Institutes of Health (NIH; Clinical Guidelines) (16) recommend a decrease in total caloric intake, including reducing portion sizes, to achieve weight loss. To examine adherence to current recommendations, Neilsen and Popkin examined consumer surveys from 1977 to 1996 and found that food portion sizes

TABLE 4.1
Barriers to Diet Adherence

Inadequate dietary knowledge	Poor availability of healthy food choices
Inability to interpret food labels	High availability of unhealthy food choices
Inability to estimate portion sizes	Behavioral/psychological issues
Inconsistent public recommendations	Low self-esteem
Cultural and ethnic factors	Lack of motivation
Occupation/workplace environment	Eating disorders
Low income/lack of resources	Lack of empathy from health care provider

increased both inside and outside the home for all food categories except pizza (17). These data have given rise to the concept of a toxic environment that "pervasively surrounds [Americans] with inexpensive, convenient foods high in both fat and calories" (18).

One barrier that has unique issues regarding diet, but also is common to many interventions, is lack of patient knowledge. Educating the patient is a common means of improving adherence to any intervention. Similarly, educating the patient is the main goal of diet counseling, and effectiveness of learning is important for a patient to adhere effectively to a diet. Unfortunately, learning is quite difficult given the complexities of nutrition information and of food choices available to a patient. Moreover, learning the healthiest food selections has never been as difficult as it is today when even renowned nutrition researchers stage debates in prominent medical journals over what types of foods should be eaten (19, 20).

Despite multiple studies, clinical guidelines, and public recommendations in support of lowering dietary fat, evidence from a systematic review suggests that low-fat diets are no better than other types of weight-reducing diets in achieving and maintaining weight loss over a 12- to 18-month period (21). Recently, greater weight loss and improvement in serum lipids has been reported with a low-carbohydrate/high-fat diet (Atkins-type diet) (22–27), suggesting that the role of dietary fat requires reevaluation. With these data in mind, and the controversy they have created, it is not surprising that patients receive streams of conflicting diet information from health professionals, friends, television, radio, newspapers, and magazines. In fact, the recent interest in these diets by researchers and consumers has resulted in a sudden shift in the food industry, which previously promoted low-fat products but now is promulgating low-carbohydrate products.

Expanding a patient's knowledge of nutrition, however, is only one of the barriers to overcome when trying to improve diet adherence. In order for a patient to change eating behaviors, the patient must be motivated to do so. Similar to other lifestyle modifications, several psychological models can be used to assess patient motivation to change and predict success, including the stages of change (transtheoretical) (28), health belief (29), locus of control (30), and self-efficacy (31) models (see chap. 2, this volume, for more details on theoretical models). These models emphasize certain methods for helping to motivate patients but have been used infrequently in diet intervention studies (32).

Other barriers to diet modification include resource constraints, environmental factors, and cultural/social factors. A healthy diet may be considered more expensive and time consuming to prepare than a less healthy diet (33). Similarly, low socioeconomic communities may have less access to healthy food options and more access to unhealthy food options (34). Even the wealthiest communities, however, are bombarded with the environmental pressures of unhealthy food options and advertising in today's world. Intermingled among these issues are cultural, ethnic, and social factors, which can make healthy diet changes very difficult for patients, and can challenge health practitioners trying to assist patients in these endeavors (35). As an example of culture's powerful influence on diet, eating habits are one of the latest of the features assimilated from the new culture in individuals who relocate from one country to another (36). Meal size is another example of how social factors influence diet changes; the size of the meal is positively correlated with the number of people present at the meal (37).

Behavioral or psychological issues may constitute some of the greatest barriers to modifying diet. With maturation, one's eating habits become ingrained as a part of one's behavior. For some people, food is often used to relieve stress or to adapt to difficult situations. When these behaviors become maladaptive, eating disorders might result. Not surprisingly, obese people have a higher prevalence of two distinct eating disorders: binge-eating syndrome and night-eating syndrome. Binge eating is a feeling of loss of control while consuming an amount of food that is larger than most people would eat. Binge eating is twice as prevalent in obese patients than in nonobese patients (38). Moreover, relative to obese patients who do not binge eat, binge eaters have higher BMIs as well as higher rates of comorbid depression and anxiety (38). Among bariatric-surgery patients, the prevalence of preoperative binge eating ranges from 13% to 49% (39). Night-eating syndrome, first recognized by Stunkard in 1955, is defined by ingestion of 50% of the daily caloric intake after the evening meal, awakening at least once a night for three nights a week to eat, and morning anorexia. In morbidly obese patients, the prevalence of night-eating syndrome may be as high as 26% (40). Dieting or chronic restrained eating may be important triggers for these disorders, which often go unrecognized due to the surreptitious manner in which patients binge. These disorders are complex psychological illnesses; further studies are needed to define appropriate therapies in obese patients with these problems.

In addition to eating disorders, another psychological disorder that can be a barrier to dietary adherence is depression, especially in obese patients.

Obese people are particularly vulnerable to symptoms of low self-esteem and depression, and depression has been linked strongly with nonadherence (41–44). (See chap. 9, this volume, for more details on depression and adherence.) Possible contributors to low self-esteem include repeated unsuccessful weight loss attempts, failure to measure up to the thin ideal promoted by the media, discrimination, increased physical pain, and decreased physical ability (45–47). Health care providers must be aware of the possibility of depressive symptoms in obese patients, and should avoid stereotyping their patients as having personality disorders responsible for their obesity. Health professionals are not immune to discrimination of obese people (48); discrimination has even been demonstrated in obesity specialists (48, 49). This discrimination might constitute yet another barrier to dietary adherence. Therefore, when working with obese patients, it is important for health care providers to maintain an empathetic attitude; avoid accusatory, derogatory, or nihilistic remarks; and rather, work with the patient to identify barriers to adherence and work to overcome these barriers.

MEASURES OF DIET ADHERENCE

Dietitians, nurses, physicians, and researchers struggle frequently with the difficult task of measuring adherence to diet recommendations. The ultimate goal of altering diet intake is to reduce morbidity and mortality. Generally, the ultimate measures of adherence to diet recommendations are intermediate clinical outcomes, such as blood pressure or serum lipids, which can predict morbidity and mortality. However, if these measures do not change, or if the health practitioner wishes to determine adherence early in the intervention before clinical outcomes are measured, other tools are employed. Additionally, other methods of examining diet adherence are needed in population-based analyses of food intake at a single time point (e.g., cross-sectional studies). In these situations, various instruments are used, including food records, diet recall, food frequency questionnaires, and biomarkers (50).

Food Records

Food records have been, until recently, the "gold standard" for assessing adherence to diet recommendations. Basically, the patient records all food and liquid consumed over a specified time period, usually 3–7 days. The more information that the patient provides (e.g., type, brand, cut, amount, method of preparation) the more accurate will be the assessment of what nutrients were consumed. Data from food records can be analyzed using computer software (e.g., Nutritionist Pro from First DataBank, Inc.; Nutri-Base from CyberSoft, Inc.; Food Processor from ESHA Research) to produce estimates of nutrient intake. Suggestions for increasing the estimates' representativeness of actual nutrient intake include: collecting food records from both week and weekend days, providing food record training (e.g., how to estimate portion sizes, extent of detail to record) to patients, have patients actually measure or weigh foods prior to consuming, and having a registered dietitian perform the interface with the software program. An advantage to food records is that the process of recording what is eaten can be educational to the patient and result in beneficial diet modifications. In addition, multiple days can be recorded so the impact of day-to-day variation is minimized. One problem with food records is that patients might adhere strictly to the diet recommendations only during the period they are recording food intake. Therefore, food records might not accurately reflect their adherence over longer durations. Other drawbacks include the inconvenience that food records place on the patient, and the necessity of the patient being literate (51).

24-Hour Diet Recall

A method of diet assessment that is less burdensome to the patient is the 24-hour diet recall. With this method, patients recall all food and drink consumed over the past 24 hours. This can be performed in approximately 20 minutes, and can be done in person or over the phone, thereby increasing the convenience to the patient. Accuracy of the 24-hour diet recall can be improved by using a multiple-pass method, which uses five successive approaches to questioning the patient about what was eaten. The approaches are designed to elicit information from the subject in different ways in order to avoid missing certain foods that might otherwise be forgotten. Even with this method, energy intake might be underestimated by up to 13% (52). In addition, pictures of foods of different portion sizes can improve accuracy but also increase the complexity and duration of the assessment. Because only 24 hours are covered, the 24-hour diet recall may not accurately reflect what one patient eats on a day-to-day basis (51, 53). Another drawback is that trained personnel might be necessary to obtain accurate recording of diet intake. Generally, this strategy is used to assess diet adherence in a large sample of subjects (51). However, it can also be clinically useful at the individual level because, if done unannounced, it might be more likely than food records to pick up diet indiscretions.

Food Frequency Questionnaire

In contrast to diet recall, food frequency questionnaires (FFQs) can be self-administered by the patient and scored by personnel who do not have a nutrition background. These instruments ask patients detailed questions about what types and amounts of foods they have eaten, and at what frequencies, over long time periods. They are typically used in cross-sectional or cohort studies to determine eating patterns in subjects who are part of a large population-based sample, rather than to determine adherence to a focused dietary intervention. Because these questionnaires are self-administered and ask about specific foods, they must be culturally appropriate for the targeted patients in order to be accurate. Because FFQs are designed as self-administered instruments to escape the need for a nutritionally knowledgeable facilitator, the more comprehensive ones are typically quite long (100–180 questions) and can take more than an hour to complete.

Other Methods

Food records, diet recall, and FFQs suffer from one other significant problem—bias. Bias becomes most apparent when trying to estimate energy intake from these instruments. Though it had long been suspected that these instruments might not measure energy intake perfectly, it was not until certain technologies became available that this could be proved. One of these technologies, doubly labeled water, is an elaborate method used by a limited number of research facilities to estimate total energy expenditure (54). In patients who are neither gaining nor losing weight, total energy expenditure is balanced with total energy intake (55). Researchers found that patients typically underestimate energy intake on diet assessment instruments in comparison with total energy expenditure as measured by doubly labeled water (55–59). Using this and other methods to validate self-report of diet intake, researchers have found that obese patients and patients trying to lose weight underestimate their energy intake (by as much as 50%; see ref. 56) to a greater extent than do others (55–57, 60–62). Interestingly, the foods that are typically underreported are desserts and snack-type foods that are typically eaten between meals (63).

To increase the accuracy of adherence assessments, some studies have begun to use other biochemical markers in addition to diet assessments. Biochemical markers include serum or urine measurements that can be used to determine adherence to certain diet recommendations. For example, the urinary sodium level can be used to monitor adherence in patients following a low-salt diet (64, 65). Similarly, fatty acid composition of serum cholesterol esters (66) or fat tissue (67) can be used to assess adherence to diets of differing fat contents. Other examples include urine ketones for ketogenic diets (27, 68), urinary nitrogen for protein intake (65, 69, 70), and various serum vitamin and mineral levels (65, 70–72). Unfortunately, there is not a simple, reliable marker for energy intake. Other methods that are used in research studies or clinical care include weighing all food that is eaten, taking pictures of food plates before and after eating, and diet assessment by a dietitian or interactive computer software (55, 73–77). For clinical and research purposes, it is important to recognize the shortcomings of each of these diet assessment methods, and use validation techniques when available.

Future Directions for Studies Examining Measures of Diet Adherence

Measures of diet adherence have been extensively studied, quite simply because researchers and clinicians have continually struggled to improve upon the accuracy of existing measures. Diet analysis methods such as food records, 24-hour diet recall, and FFQs are still of use, especially when other options for monitoring dietary intake are not available. The following are key issues that should be considered in future research:

1. Researchers should recognize the limitations of data derived from diet records obtained by patient self-report (e.g., food records, 24-hour diet recall, FFQ, diet interview) when interpreting such data.
2. Biomarkers and clinical endpoints should be used in research studies to validate diet assessments when feasible.

PREDICTORS OF DIET ADHERENCE

When attempting to tailor a diet intervention to an individual, identifying predictors of adherence can be as important as recognizing barriers to adherence. Predictors of diet adherence are frequently the same factors associated with adherence to health interventions in general. Unfortunately, factors associated with diet adherence have not been reviewed systematically. Moreover, depending on the research study, many of these factors have been shown to have both positive and negative associations with diet adherence; only a few factors have demonstrated unambiguous association in one direction (see Table 4.2).

Two of the factors most consistently associated with dietary adherence include attendance at follow-up sessions and self-monitoring (of dietary intake, but also of body weight for weight loss interventions) (64, 78–83). Another predictor, duration of intervention, is actually derived more by com-

TABLE 4.2
Predictors of Adherence to Diet Recommendations

Variable	Direction of Association	References
Demographic Factors		
Age	+	89, 90
Female gender	+	64, 91
	-	90, 92
African American race	-	89, 93
Education	+	79, 80
	-	92
Health-Related and Biological Factors		
Overweight/obese	-	89, 90
Prior weight control program	-	81, 90
Poor health	-	88
Psychiatric illness	-	90
Cognitive and Psychological Factors		
Patient complaints regarding prescribed diet	-	64
Feelings of deprivation	-	79
Multiple life stressors	-	89
Belief in diet–health connection	+	94
Hunger	-	95
Expectation of efficacy of intervention	+	81
Disinhibition	-	88
Restraint	+	88, 96
Behavioral Factors		
Patient prepares own meals	+	64
Attendance of counseling sessions	+	64, 78–81
Self-monitoring	+	78, 82, 83
Eating away from home	-	89
Smoking	-	89
Drinking alcohol	-	89
Social Factors		
Spousal support	+	97, 98
	-	81
Marital satisfaction	+	97
	-	99
Satisfactory home/work environment	+	100
Perceived social support	+	81
Intervention-Related Factors		
Monetary cost of diet	-	79
Time consumed following diet	-	79
Duration of intervention	+	84

Note. Some of these factors also had *no* association with adherence in some studies, but these are not cited.

paring longer duration interventions with shorter ones, as opposed to examining factors within one intervention (84). These factors are reflected in many current successful interventions, which have frequent follow-up over long durations and emphasize patient involvement in monitoring as well as in menu and food preparation (64, 85, 86). As one would expect, predictors of poor adherence include prior attempts at weight loss, poor health, psychiatric illness, and multiple life stressors (81, 87, 88). Patients with these factors should therefore be targeted for more aggressive and supportive interventions to improve their chances of success. Additionally, adherence might be enhanced if counseling is directed toward reducing the cost and inconvenience of the prescribed diet, and toward helping patients make healthier food selections when eating out (79, 89).

Future Directions for Studies Examining Predictors of Diet Adherence

From the current literature, it is difficult to isolate consistent predictors of diet adherence because there are few articles concentrating on this topic. The best candidates from the articles reviewed include attendance at counseling sessions, certain types of social support, and involvement in the food preparation process. Not only are these factors found most consistently in the literature, but also they have face validity and are actionable items that can be addressed in an intervention. A few key issues that should be considered in future research include:

1. Large clinical trials and prospective observational studies are the best designs to examine predictors of diet adherence because they are most likely to produce valid and generalizable results. These investigations should be encouraged to collect appropriate data prospectively for this specific purpose. Of course, the results of some clinical studies might not be generalizable because of the strict inclusion criteria often associated with these studies.

2. Potential predictive variables should be chosen carefully such that useful predictors are examined and bias is avoided. For example, examining fat intake only (but not other macronutrients) as a predictor of weight loss might lead to biased conclusions about the effect of macronutrients on obesity.

3. Similarly, interpretation of predictors should also be done carefully. For example, in studies examining low-fat diets, identification of lower fat intake as a predictor of weight loss does not mean that lower fat intake is *generally* a predictor of weight loss but rather only in the setting of these types of interventions.

4. The adherence outcome measure should be reliable and useful, and various measures should be considered to strengthen validity. For example, in a weight loss trial, it is not useful to identify predictors of diet adherence as measured by food records if the food record results do not predict weight loss.

STRATEGIES TO IMPROVE DIET ADHERENCE

Education

Though most experts agree that patient education alone is not adequately effective for sustained changes in diet behavior (32), education remains an important part of most diet interventions. The best evidence for both of these statements exists in the multitude of diet modification clinical trials that use education alone as a so-called "active" control intervention that typically results in minimal dietary change or improvement in clinical endpoints. Meanwhile the treatment group classically receives education *plus* another intervention (or perhaps several), and the combination is found to be effective in comparison to the control intervention (101, 102).

One reason education alone might be ineffective in these studies is that it is commonly delivered to patients in such a minimalist fashion. The educational intervention provided to control patients might constitute a simple printed handout or a single lecture. As with any educational process, learning might be enhanced by using a more interactive approach. An essential first step to patient education in the clinical setting is an assessment of the patient's current dietary intake and knowledge about nutrition. A common oversight made by clinical practitioners is advising dietary modifications without initially determining the status quo. An easy and insightful way to do this is to ask the patient a brief recall of recent meals (24-hour diet recall). Next have the *patient* identify foods that should have been avoided *and* propose healthier alternatives. This helps the patient to learn how to modify the diet without the health professional "preaching" to the patient. Moreover, this baseline assessment allows the health professional the opportunity to tailor advice to the patient.

Behavioral and Cognitive Therapy

After education, behavioral therapy is the next most commonly employed strategy to improve adherence to diet recommendations. Given that eating is a behavior practiced thousands of times by the time a patient reaches adulthood, a technique to change behavior is a logical choice to effect diet modification. Behavior techniques (see Table 4.3) range from the intro-

TABLE 4.3
Behavioral Techniques for Adhering to a Weight Control Diet

Keep an eating diary.	Shop from a list.
Maximize awareness of eating.	Buy foods that require preparation.
Examine patterns in your eating.	Keep problem foods out of sight.
Prevent automatic eating.	Keep healthy foods visible.
Identify triggers for eating.	Remove serving dishes from the table.
Weigh yourself regularly.	Leave the table after eating.
Keep a weight graph.	Serve and eat one portion at a time.
Alter the antecedents to eating.	Avoid being a food dispenser.
Do nothing else while eating.	Use alternatives to eating.
Follow an eating schedule.	Use techniques for eating away from home.
Eat in one place.	Prepare in advance for special events.
Do not clean your plate.	Plan in advance for high-risk situations.
Put your fork down between bites.	Identify your behavior chains.
Pause during the meal.	Interrupt your behavior chains.
Shop on a full stomach.	

Note.   From ref. 104. Copyright 1994 by American Health Publishing. Adapted by permission.

spective (e.g., increase awareness of eating, examine eating patterns, identify and control stimuli that provoke overeating) to the concrete (e.g., shop on a full stomach or put your fork down between bites) (103, 104). The introspective techniques will be more useful in patients who are both observant and open-minded to change; in other words, patients who are more likely to recognize unfavorable eating patterns and develop methods for interrupting these patterns. The introspective types of behavioral interventions utilize behavioral strategies (e.g., self-monitoring) but can lead to the development of cognitive strategies (e.g., recognizing situations that lead to unhealthy food choices, then formulating a plan to avoid these situations or find an alternative to the unhealthy foods). The more concrete behavioral techniques will be useful in all patients but may be particularly suited to patients who are less educated or more resistant to change.

Cognitive therapy is another cornerstone to diet modification and is especially useful for helping the patient to recognize maladaptive eating behaviors and what changes need to be made to improve their diet (see Table 4.4). More important, cognitive therapy has been used to help patients recognize how to maintain new eating behaviors and prevent relapse into previous behaviors (32). As mentioned previously, cognitive techniques are often combined with behavioral techniques to strengthen the intervention. Because these techniques are frequently combined, it is difficult to tease out the independent effects of each in the scientific literature.

A recent systematic review of the literature regarding obesity treatment is the most recent compilation of data regarding behavioral interventions for weight loss (not maintenance) (105). This review, by McTigue et al., was

TABLE 4.4
Cognitive Techniques for Adhering to a Weight Control Diet

Weigh advantages and disadvantages of losing weight.	Stop dichotomous thinking.
Realize complex causes of obesity.	Counter impossible dream thinking.
Distinguish hunger from cravings.	Focus on behavior rather than weight.
Confront or ignore cravings.	Banish imperatives from vocabulary.
Set realistic goals.	Be aware of high-risk situations.
Counter food and weight fantasies.	Distinguish lapse and relapse.
Ban perfectionist attitudes.	Outlast urges to eat.
Beware of attitude traps.	Cope positively with slips and lapses.

Note. From ref. 104. Copyright 1994 by American Health Publishing. Adapted by permission.

limited to randomized controlled trials (RCTs) of duration 1 year or longer, and found three previous systematic reviews (16, 106, 107) showing that behavioral therapy and/or counseling (diet and/or exercise) resulted in average weight loss of 3–6 kg over 12–60 months. The weight loss was, on average, 2–3 kg more than that experienced by controls. The review by McTigue et al. also identified 17 additional RCTs published since 1995, which had similar weight loss results. In these studies, interventions were most likely to be successful if they were high-intensity (contact with the participant more often than monthly) and included more than one component (i.e., diet education, exercise education, behavioral therapy). Moderate-intensity (monthly contact) and low-intensity (less frequent contact than monthly) interventions showed mixed results.

Intensive Interventions. One example of a successful high-intensity intervention was the Diabetes Prevention Program, a multicenter, three-arm trial that randomized 3,234 people at risk for diabetes to either a placebo pill, metformin plus minimal diet and exercise education (yearly individual sessions with handouts), or an intensive lifestyle intervention (diet, exercise, and behavioral education in a 16-lesson, 24-week curriculum, followed by monthly sessions, with both individual and group sessions) (101). The intensive-lifestyle group lost more weight (−5.6 kg vs. −2.1 kg vs. 0.1 kg) and had lower diabetes incidence (14.4% vs. 21.7% vs. 28.9%) than the metformin group and the control group, respectively. Interestingly, these results were seen even though only 50% of participants in the intensive group achieved the goal of 7% or more weight loss at 24 weeks, and only 58% were adherent to the exercise recommendation (150 minutes per week) at the most recent visit (mean follow-up 2.8 years). The intensive group successfully reduced energy intake by an average of 150–200 kcal per day compared with the other groups. This study emphasizes the importance of measuring clinical outcomes (e.g., incidence of diabetes) because the intensive intervention might have been considered only mildly successful if only adherence or weight loss were measured.

Another successful high-intensity intervention was the Women's Healthy Lifestyle Project Clinical Trial (108). It randomized 535 premenopausal-age women to either assessment only (control) or a 5-year (intensive group sessions for the first 6 months) cognitive-behavioral program aimed at reducing saturated fat and energy intake, and increasing physical activity. Compared with the control group, the intervention group had smaller increases in body weight (0.2 lb vs. 5.2 lb), and serum low-density lipoprotein cholesterol (LDL-C), triglycerides, and glucose over 54 months. In regard to dietary changes, the intervention group successfully reduced fat and cholesterol intake compared with controls at each of the five time points that diet was assessed by an FFQ.

Incremental Effects of Behavioral or Cognitive Interventions. A few studies have attempted to examine the incremental effect of several strategies on adherence to diet recommendations. For example, one study compared the following interventions: (a) behavior therapy plus cognitive therapy, (b) behavioral therapy plus nutrition education, (c) behavior therapy plus cognitive therapy plus nutrition education, or (d) behavior therapy plus social support for weight loss (109). The interventions were reportedly successful for weight loss over time (p values were given but weight change was not actually reported) but no one intervention was superior to another in this small sample ($n = 69$) of patients. In another randomized study, 63 overweight subjects were assigned to either a behavioral intervention or a behavioral intervention plus a cognitive intervention "focused on changing specific maladaptive self-statements related to weight loss" (110). Over a 3-month period, both groups lost a similar amount of weight.

Diet Assessment. Though it is true that accurate diet assessment can be difficult and often unreliable when used to monitor adherence in research studies (see previous section on Measures Of Diet Adherence), a simple 24-hour diet recall (or several-day food record) may be one of the most useful tools a clinician can use to improve adherence for several reasons. First, by assessing a patient's current diet rather than simply providing diet recommendations, the clinician often learns valuable information about the patient's socioeconomic, educational, and psychological background, which can guide future diet recommendations. Socioeconomic status can be revealed by types of food eaten and restaurants visited. Educational background may be obvious from the manner in which the patient details what was eaten and by the patient's knowledge of nutritional information. Psychological issues (depression, binging, night-eating syndrome) can frequently be elicited by examining the patient's eating patterns. Second, the act of assessing diet sends a message of importance to the patient because the clinician is dedicating extra time to perform the assessment and must listen to the patient. Third, diet assessment will almost always reveal diet indiscretions and misinformation. For example, a brief diet assessment of a diabetic patient with suddenly poorly controlled blood glucose revealed that the patient had been drinking large quantities of fruit juice at the recommendation of an acquaintance.

Financial Incentives.   One particular behavioral approach that has been examined in some detail is the use of financial or other incentives to enhance adherence to diet recommendations. One method encouraged in some weight loss programs advises the individual to reward herself (e.g., with a frivolous gift) for reaching certain goals. However, most studies have looked at the effect of rewards from outside sources (e.g., the employer or research project itself). Several studies have included various methods of financial incentives, but some did not actually test this strategy against a control group—either all study groups received the incentive or no control group was included (111, 112). In these two work site studies, money was deducted from the subject's paycheck and returned to the subject contingent on reaching weight loss goals. In another study, monetary incentive was examined by comparing the following study arms: no treatment, standard behavioral treatment, standard behavioral treatment plus food provision, and standard behavioral treatment plus food provision and incentives (113). At 6, 12, and 18 months, food provision enhanced weight loss in comparison with standard behavioral treatment, but incentives did not enhance weight loss further. Aside from the transparent reasons that food provision would be successful (e.g., appropriate food selections and quantities are made available to the subject, food preparation is simplified allowing a more structured eating schedule), the authors also found that subjects in groups that were provided food became better than other groups at estimating caloric content of foods. Unfortunately, 12 more months after the interventions had ceased, all treated groups had gained back weight and maintained only slightly better weight loss than the no-treatment control group (87).

Food provision as an incentive was examined further in a subsequent study that compared the following groups: standard behavioral therapy (control), written meal plans including weekly grocery lists, food provision that was free, and food provision that cost $25 per week (114). The interventions lasted 6 months with follow-up at 18 months. Interestingly, all three treatment groups lost similar amounts of weight at 6 months and maintained over half of this weight loss at 18 months. This finding was important because food provision is not an economically practical weight loss intervention in the real world. Food provision for a fee or meal plans might be viable alternatives.

Social Support

Eating is commonly associated with social interaction, and eating behavior can be profoundly influenced by the interpersonal environment (37). Therefore, support from family members, friends, and coworkers can be effective for assisting patients to change eating habits. Social support is frequently employed by clinical interventions and commercial programs to improve adherence to diet recommendations. For example, involving the spouse in educational and counseling sessions can augment diet adherence, especially if the spouse takes an active role in buying and preparing food for the patient (115). The spouse can also provide motivation for the patient and assist the patient in avoiding relapses, but this should be done in a supportive manner.

Unfortunately, studies of the effect of spousal involvement on dietary adherence have demonstrated mixed results. In regard to weight loss, a systematic review identified four long-term (1 year or greater) studies that examined this issue (97, 116–119). Subjects in the spousal-involvement arm maintained greater long-term weight loss than the control group in only one of these trials (116). As with almost all interventions for weight loss, interim analyses at early time points and studies of shorter duration yielded more positive results (117, 120). This pattern of positive effect immediately after the intervention or after early (2–3 months) follow-up, but not with longer follow-up, was confirmed by a meta-analysis of studies examining spousal involvement (121).

One reason that spousal involvement might not have improved diet adherence in many of these trials is that several of these studies included multiple intervention arms, possibly reducing the power to examine the efficacy of spousal involvement. Another criticism of some of these studies is that the spouse did not necessarily play an active role in the intervention but rather simply observed during educational sessions and/or simply provided psychological support (115). Interventions that have the spouse actively involved in food choices and preparation might be more successful.

Spousal involvement has also been examined in studies looking at other outcomes besides weight loss. For example, spousal involvement had a positive influence on dietary adherence to low-fat diets aimed at reducing serum lipids, but food record assessments, as opposed to actual serum lipid measurements, were used to measure success in two studies (115, 122). In a third study (123), new couples (living together <2 years) were randomized to either (a) usual care, or (b) a low-intensity or (c) a high-intensity 16-week program of lifestyle modifications, including diet recommendations. The low-intensity group participants met with a facilitator initially, and then were mailed printed modules every 2 weeks. The high-intensity group received the same modules but met every 4 weeks with facilitators who explained the modules and provided feedback. In the high-intensity group, LDL-C decreased significantly compared with the usual care group immediately after the 16-week couple intervention. Differences remained between these two groups at the end of 1 year, but LDL-C had increased from baseline in the usual care group and returned to baseline in the high-intensity group.

Other means of social support are commonly used in weight loss interventions. For example, one study found that weight loss and maintenance was greater in subjects who entered an intervention with three friends or family members compared with subjects who were recruited alone (124). In addition, in a factorial design type of analysis, this study compared standard behavioral therapy (SBT) with SBT plus social support strategies and found that the latter intervention appeared more effective for weight maintenance.

The beneficial impact of social support is often utilized by commercial weight loss programs. Some of these programs schedule patients to attend frequent (up to weekly) educational and interactive group sessions that allow exchange of diet tips, recipes, and behavioral techniques. These group sessions foster the development of new social relationships among patients who have a common goal, dietary change. Motivation is enhanced by weighing each participant during these sessions creating a sort of accountability among peers. Several reports of these programs, including one randomized controlled trial, indicate that this approach can successfully induce moderate weight loss (125–127).

In the randomized controlled trial, 423 subjects from six U.S. clinical centers received either (a) a self-help program with minimal exposure to a nutritionist or (b) vouchers to attend sessions at Weight Watchers for free (127). The Weight Watchers program provides diet (low-fat, reduced-calorie) and activity plans; a behavior intervention based on cognitive restructuring (i.e., teaches participants "to identify, challenge, and correct the irrational thoughts that frequently undermine weight control efforts"; ref. 84), and weekly group meetings led by a successful former graduate of the program and consisting of social support, a weigh-in, and written educational materials. Similar proportions (~75%) of subjects from each group completed the 2-year study with the Weight Watchers subjects experiencing more weight loss at 1 year (−4.3 kg vs. −1.3 kg) and 2 years (−2.9 vs. −0.2 kg). This study confirms that a multifaceted approach (education, behavior, social support) can improve weight loss but also confirms how difficult it can be to achieve substantial weight loss, even with an intensive, comprehensive program.

Alternative Diet Composition Approaches

In attempt to confirm or refute anecdotal reports of successful weight loss from popular carbohydrate-restricted diets, and to examine the safety of these diets, several recent clinical trials have examined this alternative approach to the low-fat diet (22–27). Interestingly, a systematic review found that low-fat diets are no more effective for weight loss (at 6 months or greater follow-up) than control diets (21). In contrast, each of the five randomized clinical trials found that a carbohydrate-restricted diet modeled after the Atkins diet (128) resulted in significantly greater weight loss than a low-fat, energy-restricted control diet over 3–6 months, with weight loss ranging from 5.8 to 12.0 kg in the test groups. However, in the two studies that carried follow-up to 1 year, the between-groups comparison was no longer statistically significant (22). In one of these studies, retention was greater in the carbohydrate-restricted diet group (76%) than in the control group (57%) (27). Each of the other studies had similar discrepancies in retention (i.e., greater retention in the carbohydrate-restricted diet group) but the comparisons were not statistically significant or not examined statistically (22–26).

These results indicate that adherence to the carbohydrate-restricted diet is easier than a low-fat, energy-restricted diet, at least over 6 months duration. There are several potential reasons for this. First, the carbohydrate-restricted diet might be simpler to understand. It restricts only carbohydrates, as compared with the low-fat diet, which restricts fat, saturated fat, cholesterol, and calories. In addition, it is fairly easy to restrict carbohydrates to the recommended level simply by focusing on certain foods (i.e., meat, eggs, nonstarchy vegetables, and cheese) and avoiding starchy and sugary foods, negating the need to count even carbohydrate grams. Second, compared with a low-fat diet, a carbohydrate-restricted diet may result in less hunger. This satiating effect was demonstrated in three of the studies, in which the test diet subjects substantially reduced energy intake despite the instruction to eat low-carbohydrate foods until satiated and to disregard calories (24, 26, 27). A possible explanation may be the high protein content of these diets (24, 26, 27). Of the macronutrients, protein appears to be the most satiating in controlled feeding studies (129). Finally, subjects on the carbohydrate-restricted diet might have been more motivated to adhere to the diet because of the greater weight loss they experienced. Multiple trials already in progress will study these diets for longer durations, examine mechanisms of weight loss, and consider adherence more comprehensively.

Future Directions for Studies Examining Strategies to Improve Diet Adherence

As discussed earlier in this chapter, diet adherence is extremely difficult for patients and research subjects, especially for long durations. Though studies have clearly shown that diet changes can result in significant therapeutic effects such as weight loss, blood pressure control, and serum lipid reduction, these effects are difficult to maintain. Practitioners frequently resort to other therapies such as medication and even surgery. They might even skip first-line diet interventions in favor of second- and third-line therapies if their previous experience with the former has resulted in infrequent and modest success. Therefore, future research must examine innovative strategies for enhancing diet adherence, including:

- Use of technology to maximize the intensity of the intervention, while minimizing the inconvenience to the patient and practitioner.
- Consideration of new diet approaches to which patients might adhere more easily.
- Tailoring the diet approach to the patient's metabolic problems and food preferences to maximize therapeutic effect and diet adherence, respectively.

LIMITATIONS IN DESIGNS OF RANDOMIZED CONTROLLED TRIALS FOR DIETARY INTERVENTIONS

Clinical trials aimed at improving diet adherence are numerous, and diverse, in both methods and goals. Diet studies suffer from many limitations, several of which are unique to diet interventions (see Table 4.5). We list these to inform the reader of issues that should be considered when interpreting the results of a study, but also to make the reader aware of the difficulties researchers face when designing a study. These problems should be considered carefully and minimized to the extent possible during the design process of new diet trials.

PRACTICAL STRATEGIES FOR IMPROVING DIET ADHERENCE

We have compiled several strategies that can be effective for improving diet adherence in the clinical setting (see Table 4.6). These suggestions pertain especially to weight-reducing diets but may also be applicable for diets used

TABLE 4.5
Limitations in Designs of Randomized Controlled
Trials for Dietary Interventions

Lack of blinding to the diet
Randomization limited by consent and compliance issues
Lack of a gold-standard intervention to achieve weight loss
Effects of interventions confounded by changes in exercise and behavior
High attrition rates
Lack of intention-to-treat analyses
Lack of long-term follow-up

TABLE 4.6
Practical Strategies for Improving Diet Adherence

Use self-monitoring (e.g., diet records, weighing).
Identify and employ alternatives to eating (e.g., exercise, hobbies).
Diet with a partner(s).
Avoid triggers for eating (especially high-risk foods).
Keep acceptable foods accessible and unacceptable foods inaccessible.
Keep a regular eating schedule and eat frequent small amounts rather than infrequent binges.
Practice responses to hosts/acquaintances who urge you to indulge or eat more.
Follow an eating schedule.
Use a shopping list and stick to the list.
Do not grocery shop when hungry.
Become involved in food preparation.
Eat slowly.
Do not feel compelled to clean your plate.
Indulge infrequently in small amounts.
Give away or sell clothes that are too big after losing weight.
Realize that lapses will occur and return to diet after lapses.

---

for other purposes. Some of these tips have been confirmed in research studies whereas others have been utilized regularly with good effect despite a lack of empirical evidence. Obviously, these strategies should be adapted to the individual to maximize success.

In addition to these specific practical strategies for improving dietary adherence, health care practitioners can maximize their interactions with patients and improve therapeutic response if they are aware of certain general issues related to obesity. Adherence to dietary recommendations by obese patients requires that physicians:

- Understand that the current obesity epidemic is the result of interactions between genes and the environment (i.e., diet and exercise habits) as well as metabolic, social, behavioral, and psychological factors.
- Understand that obesity is a chronic disease, and a chronic-disease model should be undertaken in treatment.
- Understand that some patients may have to do much more than others to maintain a healthy weight.
- Identify barriers to adherence.
- Validate the difficulties that their patients face.
- Develop techniques to motivate positive health behaviors.
- Identify eating disorders and know when to refer patients appropriately.
- Avoid stereotyping their obese patients with specific personality disorders that they think may be responsible for their obesity.

- Avoid criticizing or judging patients when they do not achieve their weight goals.

CONCLUSION

Diet is one of the most widely discussed and debated topics in our society, and with good reason—diet is considered the second most common cause of preventable death in the United States. The barriers to diet adherence are numerous, many of which can be extremely difficult for patients to overcome. In addition, practitioners face countless challenges measuring, predicting, and improving diet adherence for their patients. Despite these hurdles, diet remains the first-line therapy for many common disorders, including obesity, hypertension, and hyperlipidemia (7, 130, 131). In fact, better adherence to diet recommendations would greatly reduce the morbidity and mortality associated with these and many other disorders. However, because adherence to diet can be so difficult and restrictive, patients and practitioners frequently abandon diet interventions in favor of medications and even surgery, despite the many adverse effects and complications, not to mention cost, inherent to these latter therapies.

Research to date has identified several factors that predict successful diet adherence, including patient self-monitoring, social support, and increased program duration, and has incorporated these into successful diet interventions. However, future research needs to identify more predictors, as well as determine which are strongest and most consistent. Moreover, researchers must continue to examine the incremental effects of certain interventions on diet adherence. Researchers should also continue to consider alternative diet and diet delivery approaches. Only with these goals in mind can researchers devise the most effective and efficient diet interventions.

REFERENCES

1. Anonymous. Food and nutrition in health and disease. *Ann N Y Acad Sci.* 1977;300:1–437.
2. McGinnis JM, Foege WH. Actual causes of death in the United States. *JAMA.* 1993;270(18):2207–2212.
3. Allison DB, Fontaine KR, Manson JE, Stevens J, VanItallie TB. Annual deaths attributable to obesity in the United States. *JAMA.* 1999;282(16):1530–1538.
4. Nilsson M, Johnsen R, Ye W, Hveem K, Lagergren J. Obesity and estrogen as risk factors for gastroesophageal reflux symptoms. *JAMA.* 2003;290(1):66–72.

5. Pi-Sunyer FX. Medical hazards of obesity. *Ann Intern Med.* 1993;119(7 Pt 2): 655–660.

6. Kenchaiah S, Evans JC, Levy D, et al. Obesity and the risk of heart failure. *N Engl J Med.* 2002;347(5):305–313.

7. National Institutes of Health, National Heart Lung and Blood Institute, North American Association for the Study of Obesity. *The Practical Guide: Identification, Evaluation and Treatment of Overweight and Obesity in Adults.* NIH Publication No. 00-4084. Rockville, MD: U.S. Department of Health and Human Services, Public Health Service; 2000.

8. Flegal KM, Carroll MD, Kuczmarski RJ, Johnson CL. Overweight and obesity in the United States: prevalence and trends, 1960–1994. *Int J Obes Relat Metab Disord.* 1998;22(1):39–47.

9. Flegal KM, Carroll MD, Ogden CL, Johnson CL. Prevalence and trends in obesity among US adults, 1999–2000. *JAMA.* 2002;288(14):1723–1727.

10. Mish FC, ed. *Webster's Ninth New Collegiate Dictionary.* Springfield, MA: Merriam-Webster, Inc.; 1985.

11. Serdula MK, Mokdad AH, Williamson DF, Galuska DA, Mendlein JM, Heath GW. Prevalence of attempting weight loss and strategies for controlling weight. *JAMA.* 1999;282(14):1353–1358.

12. Methods for voluntary weight loss and control. NIH Technology Assessment Conference Panel. Consensus Development Conference, 30 March to 1 April 1992. *Ann Intern Med.* 1993;119(7 Pt 2):764–770.

13. Dissanayake AS, Truelove SC, Whitehead R. Jejunal mucosal recovery in coeliac disease in relation to the degree of adherence to a gluten-free diet. *Q J Med.* 1974;43(170):161–185.

14. Lamontagne P, West GE, Galibois I. Quebecers with celiac disease: analysis of dietary problems. *Can J Diet Pract Res.* 2001;62(4):175–181.

15. Dietary Guidelines Advisory Committee. *Report of the Dietary Guidelines Advisory Committee on the Dietary Guidelines for Americans, 1995.* Washington, DC: U.S. Department of Agriculture, Agricultural Research Services; 1995.

16. NHLBI Obesity Education Initiative. *Clinical Guidelines on the Identification, Evaluation, and Treatment of Overweight and Obesity in Adults: The Evidence Report.* NIH Publication No. 98-4083. Bethesda, MD: U.S. Department of Health and Human Services, Public Health Service, National Institutes of Health, National Heart, Lung, and Blood Institute; 1998.

17. Nielsen SJ, Popkin BM. Patterns and trends in food portion sizes, 1977–1998. *JAMA.* 2003;289(4):450–453.

18. Wadden TA, Brownell KD, Foster GD. Obesity: responding to the global epidemic. *J Consult Clin Psychol.* 2002;70(3):510–525.

19. Connor WE, Connor SL. Should a low-fat, high-carbohydrate diet be recommended for everyone? The case for a low-fat, high-carbohydrate diet. *N Engl J Med.* 1997;337(8):562–563.

20. Katan MB, Grundy SM, Willett WC. Should a low-fat, high-carbohydrate diet be recommended for everyone? Beyond low-fat diets. *N Engl J Med.* 1997;337(8): 563–566.

21. Pirozzo S, Summerbell C, Cameron C, Glasziou P. Advice on low-fat diets for obesity. *Cochrane Database System Rev.* 2003;3.

22. Foster GD, Wyatt HR, Hill JO, et al. A randomized trial of a low-carbohydrate diet for obesity. *N Engl J Med.* 2003;348:2082–2090.

23. Stern L, Iqbal, N, Sheshadri P, et al. The effects of low-carbohydrate versus conventional weight loss diets in severely obese adults: one-year follow-up of a randomized trial. *Ann Intern Med.* 2004;140:778–785.

24. Brehm BJ, Seeley RJ, Daniels SR, D'Alessio DA. A randomized trial comparing a very low carbohydrate diet and a calorie- restricted low fat diet on body weight and cardiovascular risk factors in healthy women. *J Clin Endocrinol Metab.* 2003;88(4):1617–1623.

25. Sondike SB, Copperman N, Jacobson MS. Effects of a low-carbohydrate diet on weight loss and cardiovascular risk factor in overweight adolescents. *J Pediatr.* 2003;142(3):253–258.

26. Samaha FF, Iqbal N, Seshadri P, et al. A low-carbohydrate as compared with a low-fat diet in severe obesity. *N Engl J Med.* 2003;348:2074–2081.

27. Yancy Jr. WS, Guyton JR, Bakst RP, Westman EC. A randomized, controlled trial of a low-carbohydrate, ketogenic diet versus a low-fat diet for obesity and hyperlipidemia. *Ann Intern Med.* 2004;140:769–777.

28. DiClemente CC, Prochaska JO. Self-change and therapy change of smoking behavior: a comparison of processes of change in cessation and maintenance. *Addict Behav.* 1982;7(2):133–142.

29. Becker M. *The Health Belief Model and Personal Health Behavior.* Thorofare, NJ: Stock; 1974.

30. Wallston K, Wallston B. Development of the multidimensional health locus of control (MHLC) scales. *Health Educ Monographs.* 1978;6:160–170.

31. Bandura A. Self-efficacy: toward a unifying theory of behavioral change. *Psychol Rev.* 1977;84:191–215.

32. Brownell KD, Cohen LR. Adherence to dietary regimens. 2: Components of effective interventions. *Behav Med.* 1995;20(4):155–164.

33. Sherman AM, Bowen DJ, Vitolins M, et al. Dietary adherence: characteristics and interventions. *Control Clin Trials.* 2000;21(5 Suppl):206S–211S.

34. Morland K, Wing S, Diez Roux A, Poole C. Neighborhood characteristics associated with the location of food stores and food service places. *Am J Prev Med.* 2002;22(1):23–29.

35. Thomas J. Nutrition intervention in ethnic minority groups. *Proc Nutr Soc.* 2002;61(4):559–567.

36. Brownell KD, Cohen LR. Adherence to dietary regimens. 1: An overview of research. *Behav Med.* 1995;20(4):149–154.

37. de Castro JM, de Castro ES. Spontaneous meal patterns of humans: influence of the presence of other people. *Am J Clin Nutr.* 1989;50(2):237–247.

38. Smith DE, Marcus MD, Lewis CE, Fitzgibbon M, Schreiner P. Prevalence of binge eating disorder, obesity, and depression in a biracial cohort of young adults. *Ann Behav Med.* 1998;20(3):227–232.

39. Powers PS, Perez A, Boyd F, Rosemurgy A. Eating pathology before and after bariatric surgery: a prospective study. *Int J Eat Disord.* 1999;25(3):293–300.
40. Rand CS, Macgregor AM, Stunkard AJ. The night eating syndrome in the general population and among postoperative obesity surgery patients. *Int J Eat Disord.* 1997;22(1):65–69.
41. Sheslow D, Hassink S, Wallace W, DeLancey E. The relationship between self-esteem and depression in obese children. *Ann N Y Acad Sci.* 1993;699:289–291.
42. Goldstein LT, Goldsmith SJ, Anger K, Leon AC. Psychiatric symptoms in clients presenting for commercial weight reduction treatment. *Int J Eat Disord.* 1996;20(2):191–197.
43. Carpenter KM, Hasin DS, Allison DB, Faith MS. Relationships between obesity and DSM–IV major depressive disorder, suicide ideation, and suicide attempts: results from a general population study. *Am J Public Health.* 2000;90(2):251–257.
44. DiMatteo MR, Lepper HS, Croghan TW. Depression is a risk factor for noncompliance with medical treatment: meta-analysis of the effects of anxiety and depression on patient adherence. *Arch Intern Med.* 2000;160(14):2101–2107.
45. Rand CS, Macgregor AM. Morbidly obese patients' perceptions of social discrimination before and after surgery for obesity. *South Med J.* 1990;83(12):1390–1395.
46. Yancy WS, Jr., Olsen MK, Westman EC, Bosworth HB, Edelman D. Relationship between obesity and health-related quality of life in men. *Obes Res.* 2002;10(10):1057–1064.
47. Wooley SC, Garner DM. Obesity treatment: the high cost of false hope. *J Am Diet Assoc.* 1991;91(10):1248–1251.
48. Kaminsky J, Gadaleta D. A study of discrimination within the medical community as viewed by obese patients. *Obes Surg.* 2002;12(1):14–18.
49. Schwartz MB, Chambliss HO, Brownell KD, Blair SN, Billington C. Weight bias among health professionals specializing in obesity. *Obes Res.* 2003;11(9):1033–1039.
50. Johnson RK. Dietary intake—how do we measure what people are really eating? *Obes Res.* 2002;10 Suppl 1:63S–68S.
51. Vitolins MZ, Rand CS, Rapp SR, Ribisl PM, Sevick MA. Measuring adherence to behavioral and medical interventions. *Control Clin Trials.* 2000;21(5 Suppl):188S–194S.
52. Jonnalagadda SS, Mitchell DC, Smiciklas-Wright H, et al. Accuracy of energy intake data estimated by a multiple-pass, 24-hour dietary recall technique. *J Am Diet Assoc.* 2000;100(3):303–308.
53. Forster JL, Jeffery RW, VanNatta M, Pirie P. Hypertension prevention trial: do 24-h food records capture usual eating behavior in a dietary change study? *Am J Clin Nutr.* 1990;51(2):253–257.
54. Schoeller DA. Measurement of energy expenditure in free-living humans by using doubly labeled water. *J Nutr.* 1988;118(11):1278–1289.
55. Black AE, Prentice AM, Goldberg GR, et al. Measurements of total energy expenditure provide insights into the validity of dietary measurements of energy intake. *J Am Diet Assoc.* 1993;93(5):572–579.

56. Schoeller DA, Bandini LG, Dietz WH. Inaccuracies in self-reported intake identified by comparison with the doubly labelled water method. *Can J Physiol Pharmacol.* 1990;68(7):941–949.

57. Bandini LG, Schoeller DA, Cyr HN, Dietz WH. Validity of reported energy intake in obese and nonobese adolescents. *Am J Clin Nutr.* 1990;52(3):421–425.

58. Livingstone MB, Prentice AM, Strain JJ, et al. Accuracy of weighed dietary records in studies of diet and health. *BMJ.* 1990;300(6726):708–712.

59. Schoeller DA. How accurate is self-reported dietary energy intake? *Nutr Rev.* 1990;48(10):373–379.

60. Prentice AM, Black AE, Coward WA, et al. High levels of energy expenditure in obese women. *Br Med J (Clin Res Ed).* 1986;292(6526):983–987.

61. Briefel RR, Sempos CT, McDowell MA, Chien S, Alaimo K. Dietary methods research in the third National Health and Nutrition Examination Survey: underreporting of energy intake. *Am J Clin Nutr.* 1997;65(4 Suppl):1203S–1209S.

62. Lichtman SW, Pisarska K, Berman ER, et al. Discrepancy between self-reported and actual caloric intake and exercise in obese subjects. *N Engl J Med.* 1992;327(27):1893–1898.

63. Poppitt SD, Swann D, Black AE, Prentice AM. Assessment of selective underreporting of food intake by both obese and non-obese women in a metabolic facility. *Int J Obes Relat Metab Disord.* 1998;22(4):303–311.

64. Schmid TL, Jeffery RW, Onstad L, Corrigan SA. Demographic, knowledge, physiological, and behavioral variables as predictors of compliance with dietary treatment goals in hypertension. *Addict Behav.* 1991;16(3–4):151–160.

65. Sacks FM, Svetkey LP, Vollmer WM, et al. Effects on blood pressure of reduced dietary sodium and the Dietary Approaches to Stop Hypertension (DASH) diet. DASH-Sodium Collaborative Research Group. *N Engl J Med.* 2001;344(1):3–10.

66. Sarkkinen ES, Agren JJ, Ahola I, Ovaskainen ML, Uusitupa MI. Fatty acid composition of serum cholesterol esters, and erythrocyte and platelet membranes as indicators of long-term adherence to fat-modified diets. *Am J Clin Nutr.* 1994;59(2):364–370.

67. van Staveren WA, Deurenberg P, Katan MB, Burema J, de Groot LC, Hoffmans MD. Validity of the fatty acid composition of subcutaneous fat tissue microbiopsies as an estimate of the long-term average fatty acid composition of the diet of separate individuals. *Am J Epidemiol.* 1986;123(3):455–463.

68. Westman EC. A review of very low carbohydrate diets. *J Clin Outcomes Management.* 1999;6:36–40.

69. Isaksson B. Urinary nitrogen output as a validity test in dietary surveys. *Am J Clin Nutr.* 1980;33(1):4–5.

70. Bingham SA, Day NE. Using biochemical markers to assess the validity of prospective dietary assessment methods and the effect of energy adjustment. *Am J Clin Nutr.* 1997;65(4 Suppl):1130S–1137S.

71. Bingham SA, Cummings JH. Urine nitrogen as an independent validatory measure of dietary intake: a study of nitrogen balance in individuals consuming their normal diet. *Am J Clin Nutr.* 1985;42(6):1276–1289.

72. Le Marchand L, Hankin JH, Carter FS, et al. A pilot study on the use of plasma carotenoids and ascorbic acid as markers of compliance to a high fruit and vegetable dietary intervention. *Cancer Epidemiol Biomarkers Prev.* 1994;3(3):245–251.

73. Kretsch MJ, Fong AK. Validation of a new computerized technique for quantitating individual dietary intake: the Nutrition Evaluation Scale System (NESSy) vs the weighed food record. *Am J Clin Nutr.* 1990;51(3):477–484.

74. Fong AK, Kretsch MJ. Nutrition Evaluation Scale System reduces time and labor in recording quantitative dietary intake. *J Am Diet Assoc.* 1990;90(5):664–670.

75. Iwaoka F, Yoshiike N, Date C, Shimada T, Tanaka H. A validation study on a method to estimate nutrient intake by family members through a household-based food-weighing survey. *J Nutr Sci Vitaminol (Tokyo).* 2001;47(3):222–227.

76. Williamson DA, Allen HR, Martin PD, Alfonso AJ, Gerald B, Hunt A. Comparison of digital photography to weighed and visual estimation of portion sizes. *J Am Diet Assoc.* 2003;103(9):1139–1145.

77. Heetderks-Cox MJ, Alford BB, Bednar CM, Heiss CJ, Tauai LA, Edgren KK. CD-ROM nutrient analysis database assists self-monitoring behavior of active duty Air Force personnel receiving nutrition counseling for weight loss. *J Am Diet Assoc.* 2001;101(9):1041–1046.

78. Wylie-Rosett J, Swencionis C, Ginsberg M, et al. Computerized weight loss intervention optimizes staff time: the clinical and cost results of a controlled clinical trial conducted in a managed care setting. *J Am Diet Assoc.* 2001;101(10): 1155–1162.

79. Urban N, White E, Anderson GL, Curry S, Kristal AR. Correlates of maintenance of a low-fat diet among women in the Women's Health Trial. *Prev Med.* 1992;21(3):279–291.

80. Tinker LF, Perri MG, Patterson RE, et al. The effects of physical and emotional status on adherence to a low-fat dietary pattern in the Women's Health Initiative. *J Am Diet Assoc.* 2002;102(6):789–800, 888.

81. Jeffery RW, Bjornson-Benson WM, Rosenthal BS, Lindquist RA, Kurth CL, Johnson SL. Correlates of weight loss and its maintenance over two years of follow-up among middle-aged men. *Prev Med.* 1984;13(2):155–168.

82. Boutelle KN, Kirschenbaum DS. Further support for consistent self-monitoring as a vital component of successful weight control. *Obes Res.* 1998;6(3):219–224.

83. Wing RR, Hill JO. Successful weight loss maintenance. *Annu Rev Nutr.* 2001;21: 323–341.

84. Wadden TA, Foster GD. Behavioral treatment of obesity. *Med Clin North Am.* 2000;84(2):441–461, vii.

85. Perri MG, McAdoo WG, McAllister DA, et al. Effects of peer support and therapist contact on long-term weight loss. *J Consult Clin Psychol.* 1987;55(4):615–617.

86. Wing RR. Behavioral Weight Control. In: Wadden TA, Stunkard AJ, eds. *Handbook of Obesity Treatment.* New York: Guilford Press; 2002.

87. Jeffery RW, Wing RR. Long-term effects of interventions for weight loss using food provision and monetary incentives. *J Consult Clin Psychol.* 1995;63(5): 793–796.

88. Karlsson J, Hallgren P, Kral J, Lindroos AK, Sjostrom L, Sullivan M. Predictors and effects of long-term dieting on mental well-being and weight loss in obese women. *Appetite*. 1994;23(1):15–26.

89. Van Horn L, Dolecek TA, Grandits GA, Skweres L. Adherence to dietary recommendations in the special intervention group in the Multiple Risk Factor Intervention Trial. *Am J Clin Nutr*. 1997;65(1 Suppl):289S–304S.

90. Jeffery RW, Sherwood NE, Brelje K, et al. Mail and phone interventions for weight loss in a managed-care setting: Weigh-To-Be one-year outcomes. *Int J Obes Relat Metab Disord*. 2003;27(12):1584–1592.

91. Jeffery RW, Hellerstedt WL, French SA, Baxter JE. A randomized trial of counseling for fat restriction versus calorie restriction in the treatment of obesity. *Int J Obes Relat Metab Disord*. 1995;19(2):132–137.

92. Evers SE, Bass M, Donner A, McWhinney IR. Lack of impact of salt restriction advice on hypertensive patients. *Prev Med*. 1987;16(2):213–220.

93. Kumanyika SK, Obarzanek E, Stevens VJ, Hebert PR, Whelton PK, Kumanyaka SK. Weight-loss experience of Black and White participants in NHLBI-sponsored clinical trials. *Am J Clin Nutr*. 1991;53(6 Suppl):1631S–1638S.

94. Patterson RE, Kristal AR, White E. Do beliefs, knowledge, and perceived norms about diet and cancer predict dietary change? *Am J Public Health*. 1996;86(10):1394–1400.

95. LaPorte DJ, Stunkard AJ. Predicting attrition and adherence to a very low calorie diet: a prospective investigation of the eating inventory. *Int J Obes*. 1990;14(3):197–206.

96. McGuire MT, Wing RR, Klem ML, Hill JO. Behavioral strategies of individuals who have maintained long-term weight losses. *Obes Res*. 1999;7(4):334–341.

97. Dubbert PM, Wilson GT. Goal-setting and spouse involvement in the treatment of obesity. *Behav Res Ther*. 1984;22(3):227–242.

98. Streja DA, Boyko E, Rabkin SW. Predictors of outcome in a risk factor intervention trial using behavior modification. *Prev Med*. 1982;11(3):291–303.

99. Black DR. Weight changes in a couples program: negative association of marital adjustment. *J Behav Ther Exp Psychiatry*. 1988;19(2):103–111.

100. Dolecek TA, Milas NC, Van Horn LV, et al. A long-term nutrition intervention experience: lipid responses and dietary adherence patterns in the Multiple Risk Factor Intervention Trial. *J Am Diet Assoc*. 1986;86(6):752–758.

101. Knowler WC, Barrett-Connor E, Fowler SE, et al. Reduction in the incidence of type 2 diabetes with lifestyle intervention or metformin. *N Engl J Med*. 2002;346(6):393–403.

102. Tuomilehto J, Lindstrom J, Eriksson JG, et al. Prevention of type 2 diabetes mellitus by changes in lifestyle among subjects with impaired glucose tolerance. *N Engl J Med*. 2001;344(18):1343–1350.

103. Serdula MK, Khan LK, Dietz WH. Weight loss counseling revisited. *JAMA*. 2003;289(14):1747–1750.

104. Brownell KD. *The LEARN program for weight control*. 6th ed. Dallas, TX: American Health Publishing; 1994.

105. McTigue KM, Harris R, Hemphill B, et al. Screening and interventions for obesity in adults: summary of the evidence for the U.S. Preventive Services Task Force. *Ann Intern Med.* 2003;139(11):933–949.

106. NHS Centre for Reviews and Dissemination University of York. The prevention and treatment of obesity. *Eff Health Care.* 1997;3:1–12.

107. Douketis JD, Feightner JW, Attia J, Feldman WF. Periodic health examination, 1999 update: 1. Detection, prevention and treatment of obesity. Canadian Task Force on Preventive Health Care. *CMAJ.* 1999;160(4):513–525.

108. Kuller LH, Simkin-Silverman LR, Wing RR, Meilahn EN, Ives DG. Women's Healthy Lifestyle Project: A randomized clinical trial: results at 54 months. *Circulation.* 2001;103(1):32–37.

109. Kalodner CR, DeLucia JL. The individual and combined effects of cognitive therapy and nutrition education as additions to a behavior modification program for weight loss. *Addict Behav.* 1991;16(5):255–263.

110. DeLucia JL, Kalodner CR. An individualized cognitive intervention: does it increase the efficacy of behavioral interventions for obesity? *Addict Behav.* 1990;15(5):473–479.

111. Jeffery RW, Forster JL, Snell MK. Promoting weight control at the worksite: a pilot program of self-motivation using payroll-based incentives. *Prev Med.* 1985;14(2):187–194.

112. Forster JL, Jeffery RW, Sullivan S, Snell MK. A work-site weight control program using financial incentives collected through payroll deduction. *J Occup Med.* 1985;27(11):804–808.

113. Jeffery RW, Wing RR, Thorson C, et al. Strengthening behavioral interventions for weight loss: a randomized trial of food provision and monetary incentives. *J Consult Clin Psychol.* 1993;61(6):1038–1045.

114. Wing RR, Jeffery RW, Burton LR, Thorson C, Nissinoff KS, Baxter JE. Food provision vs structured meal plans in the behavioral treatment of obesity. *Int J Obes Relat Metab Disord.* 1996;20(1):56–62.

115. McCann BS, Retzlaff BM, Dowdy AA, Walden CE, Knopp RH. Promoting adherence to low-fat, low-cholesterol diets: review and recommendations. *J Am Diet Assoc.* 1990;90(10):1408–1414, 1417.

116. Pearce JW, LeBow MD, Orchard J. Role of spouse involvement in the behavioral treatment of overweight women. *J Consult Clin Psychol.* 1981;49(2):236–244.

117. Rosenthal B, Allen GJ, Winter C. Husband involvement in the behavioral treatment of overweight women: initial effects and long-term follow-up. *Int J Obes.* 1980;4(2):165–173.

118. Black DR, Lantz CE. Spouse involvement and a possible long-term follow-up trap in weight loss. *Behav Res Ther.* 1984;22(5):557–562.

119. Glenny AM, O'Meara S, Melville A, Sheldon TA, Wilson C. The treatment and prevention of obesity: a systematic review of the literature. *Int J Obes Relat Metab Disord.* 1997;21(9):715–737.

120. Brownell KD, Heckerman CL, Westlake RJ, Hayes SC, Monti PM. The effect of couples training and partner co-operativeness in the behavioral treatment of obesity. *Behav Res Ther.* 1978;16(5):323–333.

121. Black DR, Gleser LJ, Kooyers KJ. A meta-analytic evaluation of couples weight-loss programs. *Health Psychol.* 1990;9(3):330–347.

122. Bovbjerg VE, McCann BS, Brief DJ, et al. Spouse support and long-term adherence to lipid-lowering diets. *Am J Epidemiol.* 1995;141(5):451–460.

123. Burke V, Giangiulio N, Gillam HF, Beilin LJ, Houghton S. Physical activity and nutrition programs for couples: a randomized controlled trial. *J Clin Epidemiol.* 2003;56(5):421–432.

124. Wing RR, Jeffery RW. Benefits of recruiting participants with friends and increasing social support for weight loss and maintenance. *J Consult Clin Psychol.* 1999;67(1):132–138.

125. Lowe MR, Miller-Kovach K, Phelan S. Weight-loss maintenance in overweight individuals one to five years following successful completion of a commercial weight loss program. *Int J Obes Relat Metab Disord.* 2001;25(3):325–331.

126. Gosselin C, Cote G. Weight loss maintenance in women two to eleven years after participating in a commercial program: a survey. *BMC Women's Health.* 2001;1(1):2.

127. Heshka S, Anderson JW, Atkinson RL, et al. Weight loss with self-help compared with a structured commercial program: a randomized trial. *JAMA.* 2003;289(14):1792–1798.

128. Atkins RC. *Dr. Atkins' New Diet Revolution.* New York: Simon & Schuster; 1998.

129. Stubbs J, Ferres S, Horgan G. Energy density of foods: effects on energy intake. *Critical Reviews in Food Science & Nutrition.* 2000;40(6):481–515.

130. Chobanian AV, Bakris GL, Black HR, et al. The seventh report of the Joint National Committee on Prevention, Detection, Evaluation, and Treatment of High Blood Pressure: the JNC 7 report. *JAMA.* 2003;289(19):2560–2572.

131. Executive Summary of the Third Report of the National Cholesterol Education Program (NCEP) Expert Panel on Detection, Evaluation, and Treatment of High Blood Cholesterol in Adults (Adult Treatment Panel III). *JAMA.* 2001;285(19):2486–2497.

Chapter 5

Smoking Cessation and Adherence

Lori A. Bastian
Stephanie L. Molner
Laura J. Fish
Colleen M. McBride

This chapter addresses the problem of adherence to smoking cessation. Several types of interventions targeting smokers have been successful at promoting short-term cessation, but fewer studies have shown long-term adherence to cessation. In this review, we provide examples of successful interventions that have predominantly evaluated short-term cessation. We also discuss some novel interventions that may be more successful at achieving long-term cessation (abstinence).

Statement of the Problem

Cigarette smoking is the leading cause of preventable death in the United States. It is known to cause cancer, heart disease, peripheral vascular disease, and chronic pulmonary disease. According to estimates, 22.8% of adults in the United States continue to smoke despite awareness of the causal association between smoking and disease (1). Smoking cessation confers appreciable reductions in risk for lung cancer and cardiovascular disease, with risk reduced to that of a nonsmoker within 12 months postcessation (1, 2). Thus, encouraging smoking cessation is necessary to reduce incidence rates of lung cancer and other smoking-related health outcomes.

The prevalence of smoking and cessation rates vary notably by socioeconomic indicators. In fact, smoking prevalence rates are increasing in low-income, less educated, minority, and adolescent populations (3). In England, the prevalence of smoking among unskilled workers' households is twice as high as that in professionals' households (4). Smoking has risen among the poor, and studies have demonstrated that poor women have greater difficulty quitting (4). Smoking prevalence is almost three times higher among women who have only 9 to 11 years of education (33%) than among women with college graduation or more years of education (11%) (5). Finally, Blacks may begin smoking at a later age and are less likely to quit smoking than Whites (6).

Rates of adolescent smokers have increased by 80% in the past decade and this group has proven to have low cessation rates (7). For example, school-based cessation programs have difficulty recruiting, high attrition rates, and low cessation rates for those who do participate (8, 9). The poor results of many teen cessation programs may be due to the lack of fit between the needs of teens and the interventions utilized. A focus group of teenagers reported that participants prefer nonjudgmental and confidential support from cessation counselors (8). In this focus group study, the teens preferred private, computer-based programs and personalized telephone counseling.

Some patient populations are motivated to stop smoking and are reasonably successful. A cardiovascular event such as a myocardial infarction, bypass surgery, or stroke among smokers is associated with significant cessation rates. Some studies have shown 50%–60% quit rates at 6 months for patients who are advised to quit after having a heart attack (10, 11). Among smokers hospitalized for heart disease, a stepped-care intervention that included starting with a low-intensity intervention and then exposing treatment failures to successively more intense intervention demonstrated cessation rates of 53% compared to 42% for the minimal intervention group (12). However, this differential effect was not statistically significant at the 1-year follow-up survey (39% vs. 36% cessation rates). Even among smokers admitted to a hospital for serious heart disease events, up to 70% start smoking again within a year (13).

Despite the highest prevalence of smoking occurring among patients with substance abuse (14), schizophrenia (14), and alcoholism (15), these individuals have low rates of cessation. Compared with nonalcoholics, individuals with a history of alcoholism report higher levels of nicotine dependence and are generally less likely to stop smoking following cessation interventions (16, 17). Several have proposed this is related to the comorbidity of alcohol dependence and depression (18). Schizophrenic patients also have high rates of smoking (58%–88%) and are often nicotine-dependent smokers who have great difficulty with cessation (19). These groups require more pharmacotherapy-based research.

Other serious medical conditions such as cancer and subarachnoid hemorrhage are associated with intermediate cessation rates. For example, in a study of 152 smokers surviving a subarachnoid hemorrhage, more than 33% continued to smoke 3 months after diagnosis (20). Likewise, more than 30% of smokers diagnosed with head, neck, or lung cancer continue to smoke after their diagnosis (21).

A meta-analysis was performed to examine whether history of depression is associated with failure to quit smoking (22). No difference in either short-term or long-term abstinence was observed between smokers with or without a history of depression (23). These results are in contrast to smokers with current depression. Glassman et al. reported a quit rate of 14% for study subjects meeting criteria for major depression, whereas 31% of subjects without depression successfully quit (24). Depressed smokers appear to experience more withdrawal symptoms on quitting, are less likely to be successful at quitting, and are more likely to relapse (25). Nicotine replacement therapy (NRT) may be particularly important prior to initiating a quit attempt in this population.

To review, adherence to smoking cessation (abstinence rates) is relatively low in the general population and very low in special populations that have very high rates of smoking. Overall, rates of 6- and 12-month abstinence are 8%–27% in the more successful interventions and 0%–19% for control groups (26). Although relapse is the most frequent outcome of cessation, with reported rates as high as 83%–89% depending on the intervention, understanding the factors associated with relapse is complicated.

INTERVENTIONS

Examples of Methods used in Successful Interventions

Interventions that combine physician recommendation, generic self-help guides, tailored print materials, telephone counseling, and pharmacotherapy have been shown to increase the likelihood of smoking cessation when compared to control groups or generic self-help guides alone (27–31). Quit rates for these programs are modest, ranging from 6%–26%, with multicomponent interventions achieving the highest cessation rates (28, 32, 33).

Physician Recommendation. The unique role of the primary-care physician in enhancing smoking cessation is obvious. More than 75% of smokers have contact with their physician each year (34). Thus physicians have enormous potential opportunities to counsel their patients regarding cessation. And, it has been well established that physicians can have a significant effect on the smoking behavior of their patients (35, 36). Simple advice by one's physician to stop smoking is more effective than no advice at all, and the effectiveness of physicians' advice increases with the "dose" of the intervention (ranging from 50 seconds to 15 minutes of counseling) (37, 38). A single 3-minute physician counseling session produces a cessation rate of about 10% at 1 year (37). Involving two or more health care providers (e.g., physician, nurse, pharmacist) can raise the cessation rate to about 20% (37). Follow-up phone calls from office staff and individualized letters signed by a physician have been shown to improve cessation rates (37).

Current evidence-based recommendations promote physician counseling based on the transtheoretical model (39). Briefly, smokers go through stages during a cessation attempt: precontemplation (not ready to quit), contemplation (concerned but not ready to stop), preparation (decided to quit), and action (have stopped). Smokers' motivation to stop may change over time, so it is important for physicians to address smoking cessation at each visit. Counseling from a physician can help speed the transition to the preparation phase. Physicians should note that hospitalization affords a unique time to intervene, because patients are in a smoke-free environment and motivated to preserve their health (40).

In a systematic review of cessation interventions, about half of the clinic-based studies incorporated system-directed interventions aimed at prompting providers to counsel or changing the health care environment to facilitate provider counseling (26). These interventions incorporated medical record prompts into office procedures. An example of a clinic-based intervention with cessation rates of 14% at 2-month follow-up, used a combination of system-directed support, a follow-up physician letter, and a telephone call that addressed specific barriers reported by the subject (41).

Generic Self-Help Guides. Self-help cessation programs that can include printed cessation guides and NRTs are used and preferred by the majority of smokers who are trying to quit (32). These modalities enable individuals to engage in the cessation process at their own pace and to avoid the logistical barriers of group-based programs. Additionally, these modalities can be proactively provided to smokers who are not motivated to quit and likely would not seek assistance to do so (27). Self-help guides can offer information and specific skills needed to quit smoking and be developed to be appropriate for specific target groups (e.g., those with low reading levels, older smokers, African Americans, etc.) (42). Thus, self-help interventions are recommended for widespread dissemination by the Agency for Healthcare Research and Quality (AHRQ).

The majority of smokers quit on their own, without the help of a physician or therapist (43). Therefore, smoking cessation materials that smokers can use on their own have the potential to reach a large number of smokers in a cost-effective manner. The purpose of self-help interventions is to provide a structured approach to smoking cessation without the need for person to person contact. Self-help interventions, in the form of written materials, videotapes, audiotapes, or Web-based programs, have the potential to bridge the gap between the clinical approach to smoking cessation oriented toward individuals and public-health approaches that target populations (27). Self-regulatory skills required to withstand the urge to smoke may be better learned and retained through face-to-face contact than through the simple modeling offered by self-help materials (44).

Self-Help Interventions With Tailoring.   There is increasing evidence that tailoring self-help materials to individual characteristics increases the effectiveness of the materials (45). According to Skinner et al., "tailored print communications have demonstrated an enhanced ability to attract notice and readership . . . are more effective than non-tailored communications for influencing health behavior change . . . [and] can be an important adjunct to other intervention components" (46). Selection of tailoring variables should be theoretically based. Individualized data is collected via a baseline interview or data previously collected. Tailored materials can vary by individual characteristics such as stage of readiness, self-efficacy for quitting, risk perception, and barriers to quitting.

Tailoring begins with the development of message objectives, the translation of those objectives into message elements (e.g., text, illustrations, and graphic-design characteristics) and assignment of the elements to participant variables (e.g., relationship to patient, stage of readiness to quit). Individual responses to questionnaires are used to select relevant message elements from the computer-based library of possible text and graphical pieces. Using word processing packages, clip art, and a high-grade color printer, these graphics and text are placed into a graphical layout to yield a highly customized printed health communication. The materials have a similar look but include content and graphics that are customized to each individual's needs and characteristics (see chap. 17, this volume, for more details on tailoring).

Etter et al. conducted a randomized trial among a sample of 2,000 daily smokers in French-speaking Switzerland to test the effectiveness of a computer-tailored smoking cessation program as compared to a usual-care control group (47). The outcome measure was self-reported abstinence (no puff of tobacco in the last 4 weeks) at 7 months after enrollment. The intervention consisted of an eight-page tailored counseling letter, tailored to stage of readiness, level of dependence, attitudes toward smoking, self-efficacy, and previous quit experience, and two 16-page stage-matched booklets. Self-reported abstinence was 2.6 times greater in the intervention group than in the control group (5.8% vs. 2.2%, $p < .001$). In multivariate analysis, significant predictors of cessation were participation in the program, a previous quit attempt in the past year, stage of readiness, and tobacco dependence. The authors concluded that the program was effective among smokers in a general population, including smokers typically resistant to change such as precontemplators and heavy smokers (47).

Shiffman et al. evaluated the efficacy of the Committed Quitters Program (CQP), a computer-tailored set of printed behavioral-support materials offered free to purchasers of the NicoDerm CQ patches, which comes with a users guide and audiotape (48). Callers to the CQP enrollment were randomized to receive either the users guide or CQP. CQP consisted of three to five mailings over a 10-week period. The materials included a calendar booklet, two trifold brochures, a newsletter, and an award certificate. The materials were tailored on demographics, smoking history, motives for quitting, expected difficulties quitting, and potential high-risk situations. Abstinence and use of program materials were assessed by telephone interview at 6 and 12 weeks. Overall, abstinence rates did not differ significantly between the two groups. However, participants who reported using the program materials (80% of the sample) were more likely to report quitting at 6 weeks (38.8% vs. 30.7%) and 12 weeks (18.2% vs. 11.1%) than the users guide group. The authors concluded that the CQP program was an effective behavioral treatment, improving quit rates over NRT and brief nontailored materials.

Strecher reviewed 10 trials that examined the effectiveness of tailored print communications as compared to standard materials (49). In the majority of studies, tailored materials had a significant impact ($p < .01$) and an additional study found significant effects for light and moderate smokers. Significant positive effects were also seen among precontemplators.

Telephone Counseling. Telephone counseling is a cost-effective intervention that broadens the reach of health interventions by efficiently providing individual assistance to a large population, including those in isolated communities (50, 51). Telephone counseling may be proactive, in which one or more calls are initiated by the counselor, or it may be reactive in which a smokers calls a quit-line or a help-line. Smokers may access proactive counseling by calling a help-line and scheduling calls with a counselor who will contact them at an established time (52). Telephone counseling may serve as the main intervention, or as an adjunct to face-to-face counseling or NRT (52).

A meta-analysis of trials comparing proactive counseling as the main intervention or as a supplement to self-help materials to a less intensive intervention found telephone counseling increases quit rates by 60% (52). Proactive counseling is particularly effective when it supplements self-help materials as it encourages the use of self-help materials and recommended quitting strategies (50–54). Orleans et al. found that telephone counseling increased quit rates and adherence to the quitting protocol included in the self-help materials given to the smokers (54). The counseling had a long-term effect on smoking cessation that was evident at both an 8-month and 16-month follow-up. Counseling also increased the number of serious quit attempts made, and nonquitters reported a greater mean reduction in daily nicotine intake. Borland et al. also found that telephone counseling facilitated smoking cessation as compared to those who only received self-help materials (50). The counseling increased quit attempts and reduced the rate of relapse for those who did quit.

There is weak evidence that telephone counseling increases success rates as a follow-up to a face-to-face intervention. Analysis of four studies comparing proactive counseling as an adjunct treatment to NRT versus NRT alone found no statistically significant effect of the addition of telephone support. There is some evidence, however, that the support and advice telephone counseling provides to smokers using NRT may be somewhat beneficial (52).

Multiple telephone calls are more effective than single telephone counseling calls, and the flexibility of telephone counseling allows for the counseling calls to be scheduled according to the needs of the recipient (51, 52). Zhu et al. examined the effectiveness of multiple- and single-session phone calls to a control group that received a smoking quit kit (55). Multiple-session counseling calls had higher quit rates than single-session calls, and both counseling interventions had higher abstinent rates than the control group. The phone calls for the multiple-session intervention were structured so that three of the five calls occurred during the first week post quit attempt. This relapse-sensitive schedule fostered accountability and provided additional social support for the quitter when needed most. Zhu et al. also found a dose–response relation between the number of calls and abstinence rates, which was achieved by reducing the relapse rates (55). It may be beneficial to exploit the flexibility of telephone counseling calls and schedule calls when the risk of relapse is highest and the needs of the quitter may be the greatest (50, 52, 55, 56).

Proactive telephone counseling is most effective as a main intervention. The calls encourage use of self-help materials, support adherence to quitting protocols, and initiate change (51). Successful interventions involve multiple phone calls that take advantage of the flexibility of telephone counseling and schedule the calls when they are most needed (52).

Nicotine Replacement Therapy. Pharmacotherapy is a safe and effective treatment for nicotine dependence (37, 57). It is recommended that NRT be considered a part of treatment for every smoker unless pregnant or breast-feeding, the smoker is an adolescent or smokes less than 10 cigarettes a day, or there is a medical contraindication (37). By replacing the nicotine from cigarettes, NRT effectively relieves withdrawal symptoms and reduces the urge to smoke, which facilitates behavior modification (5, 57).

The U.S. Department of Health and Human Services identifies nicotine gum, nicotine patch, nicotine inhaler, nicotine nasal spray, and sustained-release bupropion as first-line medications in the treatment of nicotine dependence (5). NRT is also available as a sublingual tablet/lozenge.

A meta-analysis of the effectiveness of the gum, patch, nasal spray, nasal inhaler, and nicotine tablets found all forms of NRT to be significantly more effective than placebo in achieving abstinence (57). NRT increased long-term quit rates 1.5- to twofold (57). The 2-mg nicotine gum (nicotine polarcrilex) improves long-term abstinence rates 30% to 80% compared to placebo (37). For the most dependent smokers, the 4-mg gum is more effective than the 2-mg gum (5, 57). Meta-analysis of the transdermal nicotine patch found that smokers who used the patch were more than twice as likely to quit smoking as were those who wore a placebo patch (58). The nicotine inhaler and nicotine nasal spray both double long-term abstinence rates when compared to placebo (37). Abstinence rates after 12 months for smokers using nasal spray and inhaler were 24% and 17% respectively (57). Compared to placebo, use of nicotine lozenges to stop smoking resulted in 2.1 to 3.7 greater odds of being abstinent after 6 weeks, and abstinence was maintained 1 year after quitting (59). Silagy et al. found that 20% of smokers who used the tablet were abstinent after 12 months (57).

Sustained-release bupropion is the first non-nicotine medication approved by the Food and Drug Administration (FDA) for smoking cessation (37). Studies examining the effectiveness of bupropion indicate that bupropion increases 12-month smoking abstinence twofold compared to placebo (60). Results from one study associates bupropion with higher quitting rates than the nicotine patch (61). Bupropion is considered an effective therapy for relapsed smokers and for smokers with a history of depression, as well as preventive treatment in smokers who have successfully quit (60, 61). In an actual practice setting (Group Health Cooperative) the combination of bupropion and minimal or moderate counseling was associated with 1-year quit rates of 24% and 33% (62). In one study, bupropion combined with NRT increased quit rates compared to single therapies (63).

A comparison of the nicotine gum, patch, spray, and inhaler found no difference in effects on withdrawal symptoms or abstinence rates (64). Abuse liability of the NRTs plus the lozenge is also demonstrated to be low (65). The nicotine patch diffuses nicotine through the skin at a constant rate, and it is recognized as the easiest form of NRT to use (5, 57, 64). The patch is effective whether worn 16 hours/day or 24 hours/day, and there is no evidence that weaning from treatment is better than abrupt withdrawal (58). Hajek et al. found that the patch had the highest adherence rates compared to the gum, spray, and inhaler, which were used less than the recommended amount (64). The nasal spray has the fastest nicotine delivery, however 75% to 100% of smokers who use the spray experience adverse effects (59, 64). For smokers who prefer acute oral administration of nicotine, but find the spray and inhaler irritating or feel uncomfortable with chewing gum, the sublingual tablet/lozenge may be an effective form of NRT (59).

Examples of Novel Intervention Methods

Teachable Moment. A loved one's diagnosis of late-stage lung cancer may prompt relatives who smoke to consider smoking cessation (66). The diagnosis of cancer has been shown to have a strong emotional impact on the social network of the cancer patient (67, 68). Serious illness and death of a close loved one are widely considered to be major life events that can signal a shift in priorities, increase awareness of one's mortality, and in turn, can have broad-reaching influences on life choices and lifestyle (68, 69). Reactions of fear, anxiety, sadness, and existential concerns are commonly reported and may be greater for family members than for the patient (70, 71). Others have suggested that, in the initial time following the diagnosis, relatives may be especially distressed, often more so than the patient (72–74). This is also a time of rallying and mobilization of extended family and friends when illness-related issues become a major focus of the family's thinking (75). Relatives can become intimately aware of the patient's day-to-day symptoms, treatment side effects, and the long-term prognosis, an experience described as the "intimate reciprocity of suffering" (76).

The diagnosis of lung cancer and general awareness of its association to smoking may have a particularly powerful impact on relatives who smoke. A recent study of 47 newly diagnosed lung cancer patients and their relatives who smoke ($n = 109$) indicated that relatives reported distress related to the patient's lung cancer diagnosis, and 79% of relatives who smoked reported that the diagnosis had increased their desire to quit (77). Despite their relatively strong desire to quit, 71% of relatives in this study continued to smoke after their loved one's diagnosis. Sarna, in a descriptive evaluation of lung cancer patients and their relatives, reported that some relatives (in particular, adult daughters) who smoked were prompted to quit immediately following their loved one's diagnosis of lung cancer (78). Sarna also noted that the majority of relatives (74%) continued to smoke after their loved one's diagnosis of lung cancer (78). This may be due, in part, to the lack of smoking cessation programs for family members. Thus, relatives who smoke are in the unfortunate situation of being acutely distressed, wanting to quit smoking, and lacking formal assistance to support their cessation efforts. This may make it difficult, if not impossible, for relatives to be successful at any efforts they take to quit smoking. In fact, there is consistent evidence that high levels of stress and depression undermine efforts at smoking cessation and moreover that smoking cessation (without appropriate NRT) may increase depression (24). Thus, novel interventions that offer these relatives formalized assistance in taking steps toward quitting and provide a forum for them to discuss fears and concerns about smoking are needed. Also, if the family does not stop, it makes it harder for the patient to quit—contextual influence.

Stress and Coping Interventions.   The transactional model of stress and coping could guide the development of smoking cessation interventions timed to coincide with a loved one's diagnosis of lung cancer. How individuals experience and cope with stress can promote or inhibit healthful practices and outcomes (79–81). The transactional model of stress and coping provides a framework for understanding and shaping individuals' efforts to cope with a stressful experience (80). This framework suggests that when confronted with a stressful event, individuals' judgment about the cause of the event, whether it is controllable, the degree of harm or threat to themselves (primary appraisals), and their ability to change the situation (secondary appraisals) influence whether individuals will adopt a behavior change such as smoking cessation. Cognitive appraisals can increase or decrease distress and, in turn, influence coping responses, both what the individual thinks (cognitive) and the actions they take (behavioral). Coping responses can be approach or avoidance oriented (82). Approach-oriented coping includes cognitive and behavioral efforts to manage or change the person–environment relationship that is the source of the distress. This could include steps taken to remediate threat or emotional processing that enables individuals to reappraise the situation or their ability to influence the outcome. For example, individuals may seek to reinterpret the stressful situation as a positive experience or seek out the support of others to help them cope with their distress (83). By contrast avoidant patterns of coping including denial, escape (e.g., use of drugs and alcohol), and behavioral disengagement (e.g., give up trying to attain goals) may be used to distance the event (84). Coping responses are neither inherently adaptive nor maladaptive, with adaptive referring to coping efforts that are associated with improved health and social functioning (82, 85). However, avoidance-oriented coping patterns have been associated consistently with greater distress and dysfunction, and approach-oriented coping has predicted positive health outcomes (84, 86). Thus, increasing approach-oriented strategies and minimizing avoidance-oriented coping responses has been encouraged.

Lazarus and others have argued that coping responses are moderated by other factors linked to the psychological magnitude of the stressful event (85, 87, 88). Events that elicit strong negative emotional responses such as fear, anxiety, or sadness alert the individual to personal threat, which in turn prompts greater coping responses. Accordingly, in a study of 668 cancer patients, higher levels of appraised stress prompted greater coping responses among patients (89). Individuals' dispositional traits such as optimism—the tendency to have positive rather than negative expectancies for outcomes—motivation to change, available social support, and affect also can play a significant role in determining coping responses (79).

Taken together the stress and coping model suggests that the likelihood of cessation and sustained abstinence is increased to the degree that the relative is psychologically impacted by the diagnosis, believes that the outcome can be prevented, and adopts adaptive (take steps to quit smoking) rather than avoidant (smoking more to alleviate stress and depression) coping strategies. Thus, an intervention program that encourages cognitive appraisals that the loved one's diagnosis is a "wake-up" call, that lung cancer is a preventable outcome, and raises awareness of approach and avoidant coping strategies, could increase the likelihood of long-term abstinence from smoking.

A growing literature describes interventions that have been developed based on the transactional model. Several have been targeted to those living with HIV (90, 91), those coping with osteoarthritis (92), infertile women (93), and women who were deciding about genetic testing for breast cancer (79). Results suggest that interventions that encourage cognitive and behavioral skills development can decrease levels of depression and associated maladaptive strategies such as self-blaming among persons living with HIV (90), levels of pain and physical disability among patients with osteoarthritis (92) as well as distress among infertile women (93) and women at risk for breast cancer (94), and improve understanding of information needed for informed decision making (94). By and large, these interventions have been multisession and group based and have focused exclusively on the coping responses of individuals who themselves are experiencing the health event. None of these interventions have targeted those indirectly impacted by a loved one's diagnosis of cancer to influence coping responses and encourage lifestyle changes. The transactional model suggests that stressful life events and associated appraisals can prompt coping strategies that may or may not be conducive to adaptive behavior change. Novel interventions could be used to encourage adaptive coping efforts directed to smoking cessation.

Kinship Network Interventions.   Kinship networks are an innovative context for smoking cessation interventions. Behavior change interventions targeting families who share a residence have shown significant improvements in dietary change (95–98). Less often considered for behavior change interventions are broader kinship networks, that is, relationships between adult persons who are related by blood, adoption, or marriage but who do not necessarily live together (99). Like families who share a household, these systems are characterized by a nexus of long-term relationships that can be among the most proximal and influential of social influences. Several studies have suggested that up to 40% of individuals cited kin as their closest relationships (100, 101). Moreover, a substantial body of work shows that aged parents and their adult children have strong bonds even when they do not live in close geographic proximity or see each other frequently (100). Prior research also shows that adult sibling relationships take on greater importance with increasing age (102, 103). McBride's data support this; over half of the relatives of lung cancer patients reported talking by telephone on a weekly basis after the diagnosis (77).

Certainly, kinship networks vary in size, stage of the life cycle, frequency of contact, relationship quality, and geographical proximity, which may be important in determining the potential influence of these networks on behavior change. Yet, common to these networks are the patterns of shared meaning and transactional relationships of power, coercion, conformity, expectation, affection, and support. Kinship networks often share ideas or hypotheses about how the world operates and how the family should cope with situations (104). It has been argued that kinship-based prevention interventions could be used effectively to support and expand relatives' natural coping abilities. However, interventions to promote smoking cessation have targeted almost exclusively cancer patients (105). These interventions have shown promising cessation outcomes among patients with head and neck cancers, but family members have been enlisted only to support the patient's efforts to quit smoking. Only one other study to date has evaluated smoking cessation services provided to family members of cancer patients, of whom only 23% were lung cancer patients (106). In the study by McBride et al., patients ($N = 47$) identified their family members who smoke and then were asked to give their relative a letter from the medical oncologist and a written smoking cessation guide to encourage cessation (77). Patients and family members were highly receptive to this protocol (80% of patients contacted at least one relative who smoked), and subgroup analyses suggested higher cessation rates among relatives of the lung cancer patients (16%) than among relatives of those with other cancers (8%). However, the study did not include a control group to assess intervention effects. Thus, despite the potential of kinship networks for promoting behavior change, interventions that target these broader networks have not been evaluated for promoting smoking cessation.

Internet Interventions.   The Internet can be accessed 24 hours a day from almost anywhere including home, work, libraries, and even coffee shops and airports. The easy access from anywhere and by anyone makes the Internet a cost-effective and efficient method to provide smoking cessation information to large numbers of smokers. Numerous smoking cessation programs are available on the Internet today including sites supported by the American

Lung Association (www.lungusa.org), the National Cancer Institute (www.smokefree.gov) and the U.S. Department of Health and Human Services Office on Women's Health (www.4woman.gov/QuitSmoking). These Web-based smoking cessation programs, as well as the many others that are available, may comprise a step-by-step cessation guide, instant messaging, support communities, links to other online resources, and information regarding local, state, and national telephone quit-lines. Enrollment in these programs is easy and anonymous, and smokers are allowed to progress at their own rate and visit the intervention site as often or as little as they like. Multiple contacts can be made with the smoker via e-mail, and assistance may be personalized to meet the needs of the smoker (107).

Despite the numbers of Web-based smoking cessation programs available today, there is little information about the effectiveness of these programs (107–109). Bessell et al. systematically reviewed 10 health-related comparative studies that used the Internet to deliver an intervention (110). One smoking cessation program was included in the review. Although there was evidence that the Internet may be a useful and cost-effective intervention method, they concluded that considerable research needs to be done to determine the impact of Internet use on health outcomes (110). Both Feil et al. and Lenert et al. developed and evaluated an Internet smoking cessation program, and both found encouraging results in the behavior of the smokers that suggest that the Internet may be useful in smoking cessation programs (107, 109). Lenert et al. suggest that e-mail may be used to supplement and enhance Web-based materials (107). Future Internet interventions may examine the impact of tailoring messages to promote smoking cessation.

There are several problems inherent in evaluating the Web-based smoking cessation programs. The anonymity of the Internet-based programs may be part of the appeal to smokers, however it makes it challenging to track participants; requesting specific identification from smokers may influence the decision to participate and thus bias the sample (109). E-mail may be used to assist with tracking participants; however it is easy to change an e-mail address as well as to ignore messages (107, 109). The anonymity of participants as well as the ease of using the Internet may pose a problem to a thorough evaluation of Web-based programs as it is difficult to verify that participants are not utilizing other alternative Web sites or obtaining additional information elsewhere (109).

APPROPRIATE OUTCOMES TO MEASURE

Follow-Up Length. In a systematic review of cessation interventions in minority populations, the number of follow-ups reported by researchers and the length of time between these contacts varied greatly (8–260 weeks)

(26). The most common follow-up period was 1 year. To make the distinction between short-term (less than 6 months) and long-term (at least 12 months) cessation both of these time points are valuable to measure.

Outcome Measures. An appropriate outcome measures is the 7-day point prevalent abstinence. Subjects are asked whether they have smoked a cigarette, even a puff, in the past 7 days. If they endorse the 7-day abstinence, then it is appropriate to measure a more prolonged abstinence period. This can be measured by asking subjects, "Have you had a cigarette, even a puff, since the last time you were surveyed [date of prior survey is provided]." If they report smoking since the last survey, they can be asked if they have smoked for 7 days in a row since the last survey. They also can be asked if there were ever 3 weeks in a row in which they smoked at least one day of that week since the last survey.

Biochemical Verification. The issue of biochemical verification in smoking cessation research is controversial. Some researchers feel that biochemical measures are essential because subjects typically underreport cigarette consumption, whereas other researchers favor the use of self-report because of logistical difficulties of biochemical validation (111). The decision to use biochemical validation should be based on the needs of the particular study. Studies that compare cessation rates in intervention groups compared to control groups may require biochemical validation to overcome the potential for a response bias related to "pleasing" the investigator. Collecting biochemical samples in large intervention trials or large observation studies may not be as feasible as it is in smaller scale, clinical studies (112). The refusal rates in larger studies are generally high. Because subjects who refuse are typically classified as smokers, this classification can lead to an overestimate in smoking rates (113). Study samples that are made of volunteers tend to have very low false-negative rates whereas high-risk or patient samples tend to have high false-negative rates (111). Thus, biochemical validation may have limited impact in volunteer samples. Finally, there is some evidence that use of biochemical validation in certain populations such as adolescents is important to decrease the likelihood of false self-reports (114).

The two biochemical measures most often used in smoking cessation research are carbon monoxide (CO) and cotinine. CO is absorbed rapidly into the bloodstream during smoking and has a half-life of 4–5 hours in sedentary adults (115). The sensitivity of exhaled CO for identifying active smoking is between 80% and 85% meaning that the rate of false positives is between 15% and 20% (116). Measures of exhaled CO can be influenced by the time of day, recency of last cigarette, environmental tobacco smoke, air pollution, and indoor combustion sources (111). Cotinine, a metabolite of nicotine, is present in bodily fluids such as urine and saliva and has a half-life between 15 and 40 hours (116, 117). Saliva sampling is the recommended method of biochemical validation because it is fairly simple to implement and the results tend to be highly accurate with a less than 2% rate of false negatives (118, 119).

CLINICAL AND RESEARCH IMPLICATIONS

Stopping smoking prolongs life and reduces morbidity. With one quarter of the population continuing to smoke and rising rates of smoking initiation in adolescents, more interventions need to be developed and disseminated broadly. Research is needed to evaluate both short-term and long-term cessation rates and to better understand the factors contributing to relapse. The presence of multiple smokers in a household contributes to relapse but also exposes vulnerable children to passive smoking (120, 121). From a public-health perspective, more emphasis needs to be placed on the negative effects of passive smoking.

To date, the most successful interventions (cessation rates over 50%) incorporate multiple components (tailored print materials, telephone counseling, and NRT) and target special populations such as those with a recent diagnosis of heart disease or cancer (11, 21, 122). Future interventions can attempt to promote cessation among specific target groups capitalizing on the "teachable moment" and utilizing multicomponent interventions (66).

Clearly, physicians and other health care providers play an important role in the campaign against smoking. Despite this enormous potential many physicians do not follow clinical recommendations to counsel based on the transtheoretical model (123). Time and lack of reimbursement are major obstacles to integrating smoking cessation services. Novel ways to provides these services in a busy office practice are being explored and may include the use of federally funded centralized counseling services such as those provided by the American Cancer Society and National Cancer Institute.

ACKNOWLEDGMENTS

This research is supported by Grant R01-CA-92622 from the National Cancer Institute.

REFERENCES

1. American Cancer Society. *Cancer Facts and Figures 2004.* Available at: http://www.cancer.org. Accessed 10/06/04.
2. Peto R, Darby S, Deo H, Silcocks P, Whitley E, Doll R. Smoking, smoking cessation, and lung cancer in the UK since 1950: combination of national statistics with two case-control studies. *BMJ.* 2000;321:323–329.

3. Watson JM, Scarinci IC, Klesges RC, et al. Relationships among smoking status, ethnicity, socioeconomic indicators, and lifestyle variables in a biracial sample of women. *Prev Med.* 2003;37:138–147.

4. Graham H. Patterns and predictors of smoking cessation among British women. *Health Promot Int.* 1999;14:231–239.

5. U.S. Department of Health and Human Services. *Reducing Tobacco Use: A Report of the Surgeon General.* Atlanta, Georgia: U.S. Department of Health and Human Services, Centers for Disease Control and Prevention, National Center for Chronic Disease Prevention and Health Promotion, Office on Smoking and Health; 2000.

6. Kiefe CI, Williams OD, Greenlund KJ, Ulene V, Gardin JM, Raczynski JM. Health care access and seven-year change in cigarette smoking. The CARDIA Study. *Am J Prev Med.* 1998;47:229–233.

7. McWhorter WP, Boyd GM, Mattson ME. Predictors of quitting smoking: the NHANES1 follow up experience. *J Clin Epidemiol.* 1993;43:1399–1405.

8. Vuckovic N, Polen MR, Hollis JF. The problem is getting us to stop. What teens say about smoking cessation. *Prev Med.* 2003;37:209–218.

9. Digiusto E. Pros and cons of cessation interventions for adolescent smokers at school. In: Richmond R, ed. *Interventions for Smokers: An International Perspective.* Baltimore: Williams & Wilkins; 1994:107–136.

10. DeBusk R, Houston M, Superko H, et al. A case management system for coronary risk factor modification after acute MI. *Ann Intern Med.* 1994;120:721–729.

11. Ockene J, Kristeller J, Goldberg R, et al. Smoking cessation and severity of disease: the Coronary Artery Smoking Intervention Study. *Health Psychol.* 1992;11:119–126.

12. Reid R, Pipe A, Higginson L, et al. Stepped-care approach to smoking cessation in patients hospitalized for CAD. *J Cardiopulm Rehabil.* 2003;23:176–182.

13. Rigotti NA, Singer DE, Mulley AG, et al. Smoking cessation following admission to a cardiac care unit. *J Gen Int Med.* 1991;6:305–311.

14. Gariti P, Alterman AI, Mulvaney FD, Epperson L. The relationship between psychopathology and smoking cessation treatment response. *Drug Alcohol Depend.* 2000;60:267–273.

15. Hurt RD, Eberman KM, Croghan KP, Morse RM, Palmen MA, Bruce BK. Nicotine dependence treatment during inpatient treatment for other addictions: a prospective intervention trial. *Alcohol Clin Exp Res.* 1994;18:867–872.

16. Hays JT, Offord KP, Croghan IT, et al. Smoking cessation rates in active and recovering alcoholics treated for recovering nicotine dependence. *Ann Behav Med.* 1999;21:1–8.

17. Hymowitz N, Cummings KM, Hyland A, Lynn WR, Pechacek TF, Hartwell TD. Predictors of smoking cessation in a cohort of adult smokers followed for five years. *Tob Control.* 1997;6:S57–S62.

18. Patten CA, Drews AA, Myers MG, et al. Effects of depressive symptoms on smoking abstinence and treatment adherence among smokers with a history of alcohol dependence. *Psychol Addict Behav.* 2002;16:135–142.

19. George TP, Vessicchio JC, Termine A, et al. A placebo controlled trial of Bupropion for smoking cessation in schizophrenics. *Biol Psych.* 2002;52:53–61.

20. Ballard J, Kreiter KT, Claasen J, Kowalski RG, Connolly ES, Mayer SA. Risk factors for continued cigarette use after subarachnoid hemorrhage. *Stroke.* 2003; 34:1859–1863.

21. Schnoll RA, Malstrom JC, Rothman RL, et al. Longitudinal predictors of continued tobacco use among patients diagnosed with cancer. *Ann Behav Med.* 2003;25:214–222.

22. Hitsman B, Borrelli B, McChargue DE, Spring B, Niaura R. History of depression and smoking cessation outcome: a meta-analysis. *J Consult Clin Psychol.* 2003;71:657–663.

23. Ginsberg JP, Klesges RC, Johnson KC, Eck LH, Meyers AW, Winders SA. The relationship between a history of depression and adherence to a multicomponent smoking-cessation program. *Addict Behav.* 1997;22:783–787.

24. Glassman AH, Helzer JE, Covey LS, et al. Smoking, smoking cessation, and major depression. *JAMA.* 1990;264:1546–1549.

25. Hall SM, Munoz RF, Reus VI, Sees KL. Nicotine, negative affect, and depression. *J Consult Clinic Psychol.* 1993;61:761–767.

26. Lawrence D, Graber JE, Mills SL, et al. Smoking and intervention in U.S. racial/ethnic minority populations: an assessment of the literature. *Prev Med.* 2003;36: 204–216.

27. Curry SJ. Self-help interventions for smoking cessation. *J Consult Clinl Psychol.* 1993;61:790–803.

28. Velicer WF, Prochaska JO, Fava JL, Laforge RG, Rossi JS. Interactive versus non-interactive interventions and dose–response relationships for stage-matched smoking cessation programs in a managed care setting. *Health Psychol.* 1999;18: 21–28.

29. Rimer BK, Orleans CT. Tailoring smoking cessation for older adults. *Cancer.* 1994;74:2051–2054.

30. Strecher VJ, Kreuter M, Den Boer DJ, Kobrin S, Hospers HJ, Skinner CS. The effects of computer-tailored smoking cessation messages in family practice settings. *J Fam Pract.* 1994;39:262–270.

31. Rimer BK, Conaway M, Lyna P, et al. The impact of tailored interventions on a community health center population. *Patient Education and Counseling.* 1999;37: 125–140.

32. AHCPR. Smoking cessation clinical practice guideline. *JAMA.* 1996;275:1270–1280.

33. Curry SJ, McBride C, Grothaus LC, Louie D, Wagner EH. A randomized trial of self-help materials, personalized feedback, and telephone counseling with non-volunteer smokers. *J Consul Clin Psychol.* 1995;63:1005–1014.

34. Davis RM. Uniting physicians against smoking: the need for a coordinated national strategy. *JAMA.* 1988;259:2900–2901.

35. Russell M, Wilson C, Taylor C, Baker C. Effects of general practitioners' advice against smoking. *BMJ.* 1979;2:231–235.

36. Ockene JK, Zapka JG. Physician-based smoking intervention: a rededication to a five-step strategy to smoking research. *Addict Behav.* 1997;22:835–848.

37. Fiore MC, Bailey WC, Cohen SJ, et al. *Treating Tobacco Use and Dependence. A Clinical Practice Guideline.* AHRQ publication No. 00-0032. Rockville, MD: U.S. Department of Health and Human Services; 2000.

38. Hollis J, Lichenstein E, Vogt T, Stevens VJ, Biglan A. Nurse-assisted counseling for smokers in primary care. *Ann Int Med.* 193;118:521–525.

39. Prochaska JO, DiClemente CC. Stages and processes of self-change of smoking: toward an integrative model of change. *J Consult Clin Psychol.* 1983;51:390–395.

40. Grable JC, Ternullo S. Smoking cessation from office to bedside. *Postgrad Med J.* 2003;114:45–52.

41. Manfredi C, Crittenden K, Warnecke, et al. Evaluation of motivational smoking cessation interventions for women in public health clinics. *Prev Med.* 1999;28: 51–60.

42. Resnicow K, Vaughan R, Futterman R, et al. A self-help smoking cessation program for inner-city African Americans: results from the Harlem Health Connection Project. *Health Edu Behav.* 1997;24:201–217.

43. Fiore MC, Novotny TE, Pierce JP, et al. Methods used to quit smoking in the United States. Do cessation programs help? *JAMA.* 1990;263(20):2760–2765.

44. Killen JD, Fortman SP, David L, Varady A. Nicotine patch and self-help video for cigarette smoking cessation. *J Consult Clin Psychol.* 1997;65:663–672.

45. Lancaster T, Stead LF. Self-help interventions for smoking cessation. *Cochrane Database Syst Rev.* 2003;3.

46. Skinner CS, Campbell MK, Rimer BK, Curry S, Prochaska JO. How effective is tailored print communication? *Ann Behav Med.* 1999;21:290–298.

47. Etter J, Perneger TV. Effectiveness of a computer-tailored smoking cessation intervention. *Arch Intern Med.* 2001;161:2596–2601.

48. Shiffman S, Paty JA, Rohay JM, et al. The efficacy of computer-tailored smoking cessation materials as a supplement to nicotine patch therapy. *Drug Alcohol Depen.* 2001;64:35–46.

49. Strecher VJ. Computer-tailored smoking cessation materials: a review and discussion. *Patient Education and Counseling.* 1999;36:107–117.

50. Borland R, Segan C, Livingston P, Owen N. The effectiveness of callback counselling for smoking cessation: a randomized trial. *Addiction.* 2001;96:881–889.

51. McBride C, Rimer B. Using the telephone to improve health behavior and health service delivery. *Patient Education and Counseling.* 1999;37:3–18.

52. Stead LF, Lancaster T, Perera R. Telephone counseling for smoking cessation (Cochrane Review). In: *The Cochrane Library,* Issue 3, 2003. Oxford: Update Software.

53. Curry SJ, McBride C, Grothaus L, Louie D, Wagner EH. A randomized trial of self-help materials, personalized feedback, and telephone counseling with nonvolunteer smokers. *J Consult Clin Psychol.* 1995;63(6):1005–1014.

54. Orleans CT, Shoenbach V, Wagner E, Quade D. Self-help quit smoking interventions: effects of self-help materials, social support instructions, and telephone counseling. *J Consult Clin Psychol.* 1991;59(3):439–448.

55. Zhu SH, Stretch V, Balabanis M, Rosbrook B, Sadler G, Pierce JP. Telephone counseling for smoking cessation: effects of single-session and multiple-session interventions. *J Consult Clin Psychol.* 1996;64(1):202–211.

56. Miller CE, Ratner PA, Johnson JL. Reducing cardiovascular risk: identifying predictors of smoking relapse. *Can J Cardiovasc Nurs.* 2003;7–12.

57. Silagy C, Lancaster T, Stead L, Mant D, Fowler G. Nicotine replacement therapy for smoking cessation (Cochrane Review). In: *The Cochrane Library.* Issue 3. Oxford: Update Software; 2003.

58. Fiore M, Smith S, Jorenby D, Baker TB. The effectiveness of the nicotine patch for smoking cessation: a meta-analysis. *JAMA.* 1994;271(24):1940–1947.

59. Shiffman S, Dresler C, Hajek P, Gilburt SJA, Targett DA, Strahs KR. (2002). Efficacy of a nicotine lozenge for smoking cessation. *Arch Intern Med.* 2002;162: 1267–1276.

60. Jorenby D. Clinical efficacy of bupropion in the management of smoking cessation. *Drugs.* 2002;62(Suppl 2):25–35.

61. Holm K, Spencer C. Bupropion: a review of its use in the management of smoking cessation. *Drugs.* 2000;59(4):1007–1024.

62. Swan GE, McAfee T, Curry SJ, et al. Effectiveness of bupropion SR for smoking cessation in a health care setting. *Arch Intern Med.* 2003;163:2337–2344.

63. Jorenby DE, Leischow SJ, Nides MA, et al. A controlled trial of sustained-release bupropion, a nicotine patch, or both for smoking cessation. *N Engl J Med.* 1999;340:685–691.

64. Hajek P, West R, Foulds J, Nilsson F, Burrows S, Meadow A. Randomized comparative trial of nicotine polacrilex, a transdermal patch, nasal spray, and an inhaler. *Arch Intern Med.* 1999;159:2033–2038.

65. Houtsmuller E, Henningerfield J, Stitzer M. Subjective effects of the nicotine lozenge: assessment of abuse liability. *Psychopharmacology.* 2003;167:20–27.

66. McBride CM, Emmons K, Lipkus I. Understanding the potential of teachable moments for motivating smoking cessation. *Health Educ Res.* 2003;18:156–170.

67. Kristjanson LJ, Ashcroft T. The family's cancer journey: a literature review. *Cancer Nurs.* 1994;17:1–17.

68. Lewis FM. The impact of cancer on the family: a critical analysis of the research literature. *Patient Education and Counseling.* 1986;8:269–289.

69. Galloway SC. Young adults' reactions to the death of a parent. *Oncol Nurs Forum.* 1990;17:899–904.

70. Weisman AD, Worden JW. The existential plight in cancer: significance of the first 100 days. *Int J Psych Med.* 1976;7:1–15.

71. Rait D, Lederberg M. The family of the cancer patient. In: Holland JC, Rowland JH, eds. *Handbook of Psychology: Psychological Care of the Patient With Cancer.* New York: Oxford University Press; 1989:585–597.

72. Sarna L. Lung cancer. In: Holland JC, ed. *Psycho-Oncology.* New York: Oxford University Press; 1998:340–348.

73. Baider L, Koch U, Esacson R, De-Nour AK. Prospective study of cancer patients and their spouses: the weakness of marital strength. *Psycho Oncol.* 1998;7:49–56.

74. Kaye JM, Gracely EJ. Psychological distress in cancer patients and their spouses. *J Cancer Edu.* 1993;8:47–52.

75. Cassileth BR, Lusk EJ, Brown LL, Cross PA. Psychosocial status of cancer patients and next of kin: normative data from the Profile of Mood States. *J Psychosoc Oncol.* 1985;3:99–105.

76. Sutherland AM. Psychological impact of cancer and its therapy. *Med Clin North Am.* 1956;40:705–720.

77. McBride CM, Pollak KI, Garst J, et al. Distress and motivation for smoking cessation among lung cancer patients' relatives who smoke. *J Cancer Educ.* 2003;18: 150–156.

78. Sarna L. Smoking behaviors of women after diagnosis with lung cancer. *Image J Nurs Sch.* 1995;27:35–41.

79. Lerman C, Glanz K. Stress coping and health behavior. In: Glanz K, Lewis FM, Rimer BK, eds. *Health Behavior and Health Education: Theory, Research and Practice.* San Francisco: Jossey-Bass; 1997:113–138.

80. Lazarus RS, Folkman S. *Stress, Appraisal, and Coping.* New York: Springer; 1984.

81. Bagozzi RP, Baumgartner H, Pieters R. Goal-directed emotions. *Cognitive Emotions.* 1998;12:1–26.

82. Stanton AL, Kirk SB, Cameron CL, Danoff-Burg S. Coping through emotional approach: scale construction and validation. *J Person Soc Psychol.* 2000;78: 1150–1169.

83. Folkman S. Positive psychological states and coping with severe stress. *Soc Sci Med.* 1997;45:1207–1221.

84. Carver CS, Scheier MF, Weintraub JK. Assessing coping strategies: a theoretically based approach. *J Person Soc Psychol.* 1989;56:267–283.

85. Lazarus RS. Coping theory and research: past, present, and future. *Psychosom Med.* 1993;55:234–247.

86. McCaul KD, Sandgren AK, King B, et al. Coping and adjustment to breast cancer. *Psycho Oncol.* 1999;8:230–236.

87. Aspinwall LG, Taylor SE. A stitch in time: self-regulation and proactive coping. *Psychol Bull.* 1997;121:417–436.

88. Bagozzi RP, Gopinath M, Nyer PU. The role of emotions in marketing. *J Acad Market Sci.* 1999;27:184–206.

89. Dunkel-Schetter C, Feinstein LG, Taylor SE, Falk RL. Patterns of coping with cancer. *Health Psychol.* 1992;11:79–87.

90. Folkman S, Chesney MA, Collette L, Boccellari A, Cooke M. Caregiver burden in HIV-positive and HIV-negative partners of men with AIDS. *J Consult Clinl Psychol.* 1994;62:746–756.

91. Heckman TG, Kalichman SC, Roffman RR, et al. A telephoned-delivered coping improvement intervention for persons living with HIV/AIDS in rural areas. *Soc Work Groups.* 1999;21:49–60.

92. Keefe FJ, Caldwell DS, Baucom D, et al. Spouse-assisted coping skills training in the management of knee pain in osteoarthritis: long-term follow-up results. *Arthritis Care Res.* 1999;12:101–111.

93. McQueeney DA, Stanton AL, Sigmon S. Efficacy of emotion-focused and prob-lem-focused group therapies for women with fertility problems. *J Behav Med.* 1997;20:313–331.

94. Lerman C, Lustbader E, Rimer B, et al. Effects of individualized breast cancer risk counseling: a randomized trial. *J Natl Cancer Instit.* 1995;87:286–292.

95. Fitzgibbon ML, Stolley MR, Kirschenbaum DS. An obesity prevention pilot program for African American mothers and daughters. *J Nutr Edu.* 1995;27: 93–99.

96. Fitzgibbon ML, Stolley MR, Avellone ME, Sugerman S, Chavez N. Involving parents in cancer risk reduction: a program for Hispanic American families. *Health Psychol.* 1996;15:413–422.

97. Perry CL, Luepker RV, Murray DM, et al. Parent involvement with children's health promotion: the Minnesota Home Team. *Am J Public Health.* 1988;78: 1156–1160.

98. Witschi JC, Singer M, Wu-Lee M, et al. Family cooperation and effectiveness in a cholesterol-lowering diet. *J Am Diet Assoc.* 1978;72:384–389.

99. Broderick CB. *Understanding Family Process: Basics of Family Systems Theory.* Newbury Park, CA: Sage Publications, Inc.; 1993:269.

100. Hoyt DR, Babchuk N. Adult kinship networks: the selective formation of inti-mate ties with kin. *Social Forces.* 1983;62:84–101.

101. Shulman N. Life cycle variation in patterns of close relationships. *J Marriage Fam.* 1975;37:813–822.

102. Cumming E, Schneider DM. Sibling solidarity: a property of American kinship. *Am Anthropol.* 1961;63:498–507.

103. Bultena GL. Rural-urban differences in the familial interaction of the aged. *Rural Sociol.* 1969;34:5–15.

104. Lederberg MS, Jacobs J, Ostroff J, et al. Part XIII: psychological issues for the family. In: Loscalzo M, ed. *Psycho-Oncology.* New York: Oxford University Press; 1998:1189.

105. Gritz ER, Carr CR, Rapkin D, et al. Predictors of long-term smoking cessation in head and neck cancer patients. *Cancer Epidemiol Biomarkers Prev.* 1993;2: 261–270.

106. Schilling A, Conaway MR, Wingate PJ, et al. Recruiting cancer patients to par-ticipate in motivating their relatives to quit smoking. A cancer control study of the Cancer and Leukemia Group B (CALGB 9072). *Cancer.* 1997;79:152–160.

107. Lenert L, Munoz R, Stoddard J, et al. Design and pilot evaluation of an Internet smoking cessation program. *J Am Med Inform Assn.* 2003;10:16–20.

108. Curry S, Ludman E, McClure J. Self-administered treatment for smoking cessa-tion. *J Clin Psychol.* 2003;59(3):305–319.

109. Feil E, Noell J, Lichtenstein E, Boles SM, McKay HG. Evaluation of an Internet-based smoking cessation program: lessons learned from a pilot study. *Nicotine Tob Res.* 2003;5:189–194.

110. Bessell T, McDonald S, Silagy C, Anderson JN, Hiller JE, Sansom LN. Do Internet interventions for consumers cause more harm than good? A system-atic review. *Health Expectations.* 2002;5:28–37.

111. Velicer WF, Prochaska JO, Rossi JS, Snow MG. Assessing outcome in smoking cessation studies. *Psychol Bull.* 1992;111(1):23–41.

112. Ockene JK, Kuller LH, Svensden KH, Meilahn E. The relationship of smoking cessation to coronary heart disease and lung cancer in the Multiple Risk Factor Intervention Trial. *Am J Public Health.* 1990;80(8):954–958.

113. Windsor RA, Orleans CT. Guidelines and methodological standards for smoking cessation intervention research among pregnant women: improving the science and art. *Health Education Quarterly.* 1986;13:131–161.

114. Murray DM, Perry CL. The measurement of substance use among adolescents: when is the bogus pipeline method needed? *Addict Behav.* 1987;12:225–233.

115. Stewart RD. The effect of carbon monoxide on humans. *Annual Review of Pharmacology.* 1975;15:409–425.

116. Benowitz NL. The use of biological fluid samples in assessing tobacco smoke consumption. *NIDA Research Monograph Series.* 1983;48:6–26.

117. Murray DM, McBride CM, Lindquist R, Belcher JD. Sensitivity and specificity of saliva thiocyanate and cotinine for cigarette smoking: a comparison of two collection models *Addict Behav.* 1991;16:161–166.

118. Abrams DB, Follick MJ, Biener L, Carey KB, Hitti J. Saliva cotinine as a measure of smoking status in field settings. *Am J Public Health.* 1987;77:846–848.

119. Haddow JE, Paloman GE, Knight GJ. Use of serum cotinine to assess the accuracy of self reported nonsmoking. *BMJ.* 1986;293:1306.

120. Stoddard JJ, Gray B. Maternal smoking and medical expenditures for childhood respiratory illness. *Am J Public Health.* 1997;87:205–209.

121. Aligne CA, Stoddard JJ. Tobacco and children. An economic evaluation of the medical effects of parental smoking. *Arch Pediatr Adolesc Med.* 1997;151: 648–653.

122. Haustein KO. What can we do in secondary prevention of cigarette smoking? *European Journal of Cardiovascular Prevention and Rehabilitation.* 2003;10: 476–485.

123. Curry SJ, Grothaus LC, McAfee T, Pabiniak C. Use and cost effectiveness of smoking-cessation services under four insurance plans in a health maintenance organization. *New Engl J Med.* 1998;339:673–679.

Chapter 6

Medication Treatment Adherence

Hayden B. Bosworth

SIGNIFICANCE OF MEDICATION ADHERENCE: PREVALENCE OF NONADHERENCE

Medications are the most common forms of medical intervention. In 1998–1999, more than 80% of the adult population took at least one medication in the preceding week, and 25% took at least five. These rates translate into 169 million and 52 million individuals, respectively (1) and more than 3.3 billion prescription drugs dispensed (2). Nonadherence with medication regimens leads to suboptimal outcomes and higher health care costs. In fact, it is estimated that the cost of medication nonadherence in the United States exceeds $100 billion annually (3), primarily as a result of lost productivity and preventable hospital admissions and emergency room visits. Nonadherence with therapeutic medication recommendations is prevalent. Across different definitions of nonadherence, approximately 50% of patients do not take their prescribed medication as recommended (4–7). The true rate of nonadherence may be higher as patients with a history of nonadherence are likely underrepresented in outcomes research. Moreover, because medication nonadherence is closely associated with treatment dropout, patients who are prone to nonadherence are difficult to recruit and retain in clinical care and research protocols.

Examples of rates of poor medication adherence include highly active antiretroviral therapy (HAART). In order to effectively suppress viral replication, HAART medications must be taken 90% to 100% of the time (8);

however, adherence rates to prescribed HAART therapies vary from 22% to 80%, in both clinical trials and clinical practice settings (9–13). In fact, in one study, no individuals with adherence greater than 90% progressed to AIDS, whereas 38% and 8% of those with adherence rates ≥50% and 51%–89%, respectively, progressed to AIDS (14). Similar rates of non-adherence are observed in transplant patients who are screened for high motivation (15, 16). These rates of poor medication adherence to medication are remarkably similar for various chronic diseases and have remained relatively consistent over the last three decades. This is disturbing given the advances in pharmaceutical treatment of various diseases and disorders.

Though medication adherence rates may be similar for different diseases, the consequence of nonadherence differs across diseases. Patients with diabetes or hypertension who take only half of their prescribed doses will receive the full benefit of those medications as soon as adherence improves. In contrast, transplant recipients may suffer organ rejection. Similarly, patients with HIV who take only half of their prescribed doses most likely compromise the future effectiveness of those and related medications, forfeiting the opportunity to benefit from these therapies. Even if these patients later attain perfect adherence, the virus may have developed resistance to the prescribed medications and possibly to other drugs in the same class.

Chronic diseases, particularly asymptomatic ones, such as hypertension and hyperlipidemia, tend to carry an even higher rate of medication non-adherence than short-term acute illnesses. When patients must take medication regularly without an end in sight, about 50% of them fail to follow the regimen as prescribed. For example, newly prescribed antihypertensive drugs were stopped within 6 months by about 55% of patients in the United Kingdom (17) and within 1 year by about 44% of patients in the United States (18). Other diseases like asthma are chronic with an inflammatory component that requires prophylactic daily medication for some even when individuals do not have symptoms. Adherence with asthma medication guidelines in the Nurses Health Study was 57% for mild persistent asthma, 55% for moderate persistent asthma, and 32% for severe persistent asthma (19). Similar nonadherence has been reported among individuals with rheumatoid arthritis: 36% were consistently adherent and 24% reported consistently nonadherent (20).

Medication adherence for short-term/acute problems is different from chronic diseases. The estimated nonadherence rate is about 20% to 30% under circumstances in which patients are given a short-term course of medication (e.g., a 10-day course of antibiotics for a urinary tract infection). Unfortunately, patients often discontinue the medication as soon as the distressing symptoms disappear and potentially inducing antibiotic resistance.

Some diseases like depression can be short term as well as long term. Among the few studies that have examined medication adherence for depression, it is estimated that 20% to 80% of patients who have antidepressant medications prescribed fail to adhere to the prescription at 1 month (21–24). In general, adherence is greater in clinical studies than in clinical practice (25).

The implications of medication nonadherence are vast. At least 10% of all hospitalizations are associated with patients' nonadherence with medications (26) and over half of asthma emergency room visits (27) may be related to medication nonadherence. Patients who are nonadherent with antipsychotic medications have 3.7 times greater risk of relapse than adherent patients. Relapse due to nonadherence of antipsychotic medications may also be more severe and dangerous (28). Conversely, patients who adhere to medication treatment have demonstrated fewer psychiatric hospitalizations (29) and hospitalization days (30). Among the few studies that have examined the effects of long-term continuation of antidepressant medications, patients who discontinued antidepressant treatment early have a significantly increased risk of a relapse/recurrence (risk ratio = 1.77) (31).

The consequences of partial adherence depend on the disease state, patient population, and pharmacokinetics and pharamacodynamics of a drug. If medication adherence is not taken into account, therapeutic and toxic drug effects can be substantiality underestimated, and dosing requirements for optimal efficacy may be overestimated. In clinical practice, medication nonadherence can lead to additional diagnostic and treatment procedures that may be costly and countertherapeutic. From a research perspective, poor medication adherence in a trial increases the required sample size needed in order to maintain the same power (32).

The substantial variation in estimates of nonadherence and the failure to recognize nonadherence when it occurs are likely the result of two serious shortcomings discussed in the next section: imprecise measurement of medication adherence and limitations in understanding the factors that contribute to adherence and nonadherence.

Measurement of Medication Adherence

The estimation of the magnitude of adherence, the identification of predictors and impact of predictors, and the evaluation of clinical interventions, are all dependent on adequate measurement of adherence. Medication nonadherence has been defined as not having a prescription filled, not taking enough medication, taking too much medication, not observing the correct interval between doses, not observing the correct duration of treatment, and taking additional nonprescribed medication. There are no clear indications of patient nonadherence and the identification of poor medicinal adherence is difficult because except in extreme circumstances, direct observation of medication use is usually impractical (33).

COMMON FORMS OF MEDICATION NONADHERENCE

The distinction between unintentional and intentional medication adherence is important. At one time or another, most patients make unintentional errors in taking medications, usually because of forgetfulness or misunderstanding of instructions. However, the literature suggests that intentional nonadherence is also a significant problem, particularly among patients with chronic disorders requiring long-term therapy, such as asthma, hypertension, HIV infection, and diabetes (4–6). One of the most common reasons for missing medications is that individuals feel good and decide not to take their medications.

Once a patient obtains a medication, the two most common nonadherent behaviors include omitting one or more doses or taking a medication at the wrong time (34). Consumption of extra doses is less common (35, 36). Comprehension of the prescribed regimen is the first step in successfully complying with the regimen. Studies have reported that one fifth to one half of elderly patients have difficulty understanding or lack knowledge about their medication regimen (37–39). Patients may confuse the role and use of their medications, particularly with more complicated regimens. For example, patients with moderate to severe asthma are typically prescribed two forms of medication, a daily anti-inflammatory medication and a "use as needed" bronchodilator to administer when they have symptoms. When patients are interviewed about their understanding of these two medications, there are often gaps in their knowledge about which of these medications is prescribed to treat the symptoms of an asthma attack. A written medication schedule or figure with instructions can often enhance adherence (40).

Rudd (34) has termed the behavior of inconsistent adherers as "partial compliance." Electronic medication monitors indicate that about 50%–60% of patients achieve near-optimal or excellent adherence (34), and 5%–10% of patients display low levels of adherence, with long periods of taking no medications at all. Partial compliers, who represent the remaining 30%–40% of patients, display highly variable adherence, with day-to-day and week-to-week inconsistencies. For example, for some patients, Monday–Friday adherence presents no problem, but weekends or holidays disrupt medication routines. Partial compliers appear to understand their regimen and the need for pill taking; yet they skip doses or sometimes take "drug holidays" for up to weeks at a time. This is particularly the case among HIV/AIDS patients where interruptions of antiretroviral treatment are increasingly being used for treatment failure and to help manage the toxic effects of therapy. However, recent research has found that these drug holidays are associated with greater progression of disease and do not confer immunologic or virologic benefits of patients (41).

Whereas partial adherence is intentional in some patients, in others, it may be unintentional. Forgetting to take a medication is the most common cause of underdosing. Cognition and memory plays an important role in adherence (42–44), particularly among older adults (45). In data from the Framingham Heart Study, a strong graded relation between cognitive performance, including memory, and the probability of having stopped antihypertensive medication use was reported (46); those in the lowest 10th percentile of education-adjusted cognitive performance were more than three times as likely to have stopped treatment than those in the normal performance group.

Partial unintentional adherence often occurs in the scheduling of when to take a medication. When patients skip or are off schedule with doses, for example, they often skip or are off schedule with all medications taken at that time (47). If a patient sleeps through a morning dose of medication(s) or is late taking an evening dose because of being delayed at work, for example, all medications taken at that time are missed or delayed. Partial adherence or nonadherence may also be affected by such factors as using more than one pharmacy, seeing a number of different physicians, confusion about the regimen, inaccurately labeled containers, and among older adults and those with problems with arthritis, the inability to open childproof containers (48). Each of these behaviors must be considered in formulating strategies to enhance medication treatment adherence for patients (26).

CORRELATES OF MEDICATION NONADHERENCE

Despite the magnitude and importance of treatment nonadherence, there are relatively few consistent predictors of pharmacological adherence. In a review of potential predictors of patient adherence, Dunbar-Jacobs and colleagues reported that most of the data are unclear and inconclusive (49). In addition, adherence in one area does not predict adherence in another area. However, correlates of medication adherence can be characterized by five factors: patient characteristics, clinical characteristics, provider characteristics, the social environment, and policy. The fifth area, policy, which includes factors such as financial coverage of medication and drug benefits, is not discussed here (50).

Patient Characteristics

Demographic Factors. Treatment nonadherence tends to increase as the number of medications taken increases, which suggests that nonadherence may be a greater problem for the elderly. The elderly potentially are at increased risk of poor medication adherence due to the increased likelihood of multiple medication usage because of worse severity and number of diseases.

Less understood is the relationship of medication adherence among children, which often involves parental involvement. Adolescence by itself is not a reason for nonadherence; medication adherence rates are comparable to those of adults (51). However, treatment adherence in childhood and adolescence is characterized by specific challenges that are related to biological, psychological, and social development. For example, changes in physical appearance and increased comparisons of physical attributes with friends heighten awareness of potentially constraining physical and social side effects of treatment and may lead to questioning the necessity of medical instructions. For instance, 25% of adolescents with diabetes were found to fail to take insulin injections or required blood tests because they did not believe the treatment was necessary (52). In addition, unlike adults, parental psychological well-being is related to adherence with medical regimens. Increased parental supervision has been quite effective in the improvement of general adherence among adolescents with diabetes (52). Age of the child, chronicity of illness, and coping skills of the child are related to medication adherence (53). In addition, disintegrated family structure and functioning are associated with poor medication adherence in children and adolescents with chronic disorders (54, 55).

Individuals with low socioeconomic status including low income and low levels of education (56) are more likely to be nonadherent with their medication regimen. Among individuals with low income, spending money on medications often becomes a low priority because of competing needs and limited resources. Additional socioeconomic factors related to poor medication adherence include: increased barriers to care such as lack of insurance (57), decreased likelihood of having a regular source of care (58, 59), or cost of medications (59, 60). In a 2-year period more than 2 million elderly Medicare beneficiaries did not adhere to drug treatment regimens because of cost. This poor adherence tended to be more common among beneficiaries with no or partial medication coverage and was associated with poorer health and higher rates of hospitalization (61).

Cognitive Factors. To fully understand instructions for taking medications, patients must pay attention to the health professional, encode or learn the treatment plan so that it can be recalled accurately from long-term memory at a later time, and integrate this new regimen into their daily activities. In his seminal work, Herbert Simon demonstrated that human beings, on average, can maintain seven bits of information in their short-term memory. Many chronic-disease management regimens require the manipulation of complex information. For example, patients with type II diabetes are instructed to minimize calories and control intake of carbohydrates. Most are instructed to test their capillary blood glucose at least twice a day—before their first meal of the day and 2 hours after their largest meal of the day. Many type II diabetics also take multiple oral medications to control their blood glucose, and some take insulin, which requires careful balance of energy expenditure, energy intake, and medication dose. This regimen does not account for additional treatments to treat and control the complications of diabetes. Considering the complexity of the regimen and the consequent demands for information processing, it is not surprising that about half of individuals with type II diabetes have inadequate glucose control.

In addition to the role processing information has on adherence, cognition and memory play an important role in medication adherence (42–44), particularly among older adults where declines in memory function contribute to forgetting to take medications (45). Cognitive declines among older adults may also be problematic because of the increased cognitive demands required for organizing and maintaining their complex medical regimens (42–44). In fact, it has been estimated that patients recall only 50% of what they are told by their providers (62, 63). Patients must follow the regimen prospectively and remember that, at some time in the near future, a specific dose must be taken—often under certain conditions (e.g., with food or an empty stomach). They also must be able to monitor their own adherence behavior over the course of a day by updating their "working memory" efficiently and thereby remembering, for example, that they already took their big blue pill in the morning, but did not take the little red pill. Furthermore, individuals must use inductive reasoning to determine when to take the next appropriate dosage. For instance, if an individual awoke at 8:00 a.m. and she had to take the medication three times a day, the individual must determine that the next time the medication is to be taken is 4:00 p.m.

Psychiatric and Mental Factors. Though adherence has little relation to sociodemographic factors such as age, gender, and race, patients with psychiatric disorders including dementia (37, 64) and substance use problems (65–67) are less likely to adhere to medication regimens. For example, high levels of nonadherence to highly active antiretroviral therapy have been associated with former or current injection drug use. Malow et al. (68) reported adherence rates of only 17% in a group of 290 street-recruited

HIV-positive drug users. In addition, lack of social support and lack of material resources such as stable housing also are related to nonadherence (69).

There is little support for psychological characteristics as predictors of adherence such as personality, but certain states may influence adherence (e.g., depression decreases and optimism increases adherence) (see chap. 8 for more details on the impact of depression and depressive symptoms on treatment adherence). In addition, though anxiety is usually associated with decreased adherence, how an individual actually copes with the anxiety is more likely to be a better predictor of medication adherence (49).

Attitudes and Adherence.   People with a negative view of medicines, perceiving them to be generally harmful substances that are overused by doctors, are less likely to be adherent. For example, Bosworth et al. reported that the perception that menopause is natural led to a greater likelihood of discontinuing hormone replacement therapy over a 9-month period of time (70).

Decisions about taking medication are likely to be informed by beliefs about medicines as well as beliefs about the illness, which the medication is intended to treat or prevent (71). Research suggests that medication adherence is related to personal perception so that necessity of medication and concerns about potential adverse effects are weighed. That is, for a particular medication, individuals balance the perceived benefits (necessity beliefs) against perceived risks (concerns) (72). Among 324 patients from four chronic-illness groups (asthma, renal, cardiac, and oncology), most patients (89%) believed that their prescribed medication was necessary for maintaining health. However, more than a third had strong concerns about their medication based on beliefs about the dangers of dependence or long-term effects. In the same study, Horne et al. reported a higher belief in the *necessity* correlated with higher reported adherence ($r = 0.21$) and higher *concerns* of medication correlated with lower reported adherence ($r = -0.33$) (72).

Knowledge, Risk Perception, and Adherence.   Knowledge is essential for treatment adherence, but information alone is not enough to promote behavioral changes required as part of the management of the disease (73). Knowledge has three specific meanings; all contribute to improving the likelihood of following a prescribed regimen: specific information about the regimen, general medical information, and the rationale for treatment. As stated in the health belief model, patients must believe they are vulnerable or susceptible to the disease or its consequences. Patients must believe that, by following a particular set of health recommendations, they will abolish or at least reduce the threat or severity of the particular disease and its consequences. Finally, patients must believe in the efficacy of the treatment (74, 75) (see chap. 2 for more details on theoretical models that incorporate risk perception). It has been found, for instance, that among adolescents with diabetes, poor glycemic control is linked to a lack of illness- and treatment-related knowledge (76).

Clinical Characteristics

A factor that is unique to pharmacological interventions concerns the complexity of the drug regimen. Adherence to prescribed medications decreases with increasing dosing frequency (77). Complexity of medication regimen is particularly an issue for current treatment strategies for patients infected with HIV, which involve the use of multiple drugs because of the rapid emergence of resistance to antiretroviral monotherapy and development of opportunistic diseases (78, 79). Consequently, patients with HIV/AIDS are likely to require complex dosing schedules involving a combination of active drugs, together with other medications, including prophylaxis for opportunistic infections and other routinely prescribed medications.

Complexity of medication regimen is also related to increased comorbidity and age. Cramer (80) observed that the number of medications is not as important as the number of times a day doses must be remembered. The more often a dose must be taken per day, the less likely the patient is going to take the medication correctly. Gatley (81) showed that patients whose medication was to be taken once daily had an adherence rate of almost 70%. If the medication was prescribed twice daily adherence fell to less than 50%, with three times daily to just over 40% and with four times daily to almost 20%.

Medication Adherence Trends. Though data suggest that as many as 30% of persons fail to fill medication prescriptions (82), among those who remain on treatment, medication adherence typically decreases with time (83). Studies suggest that adherence during the first month of treatment is one of the most powerful predictors of long-term adherence (84, 85). For example, depression medication adherence has been shown to be 68% after 3 weeks of treatments, but this percentage decreased after 12 weeks to 40% (86). A meta-analysis of studies with tricyclics versus fluoxetine demonstrated that the percentage of dropouts over 4- to 8-week-lasting trials was 38% and 30%, respectively (87). In addition, adherence improves immediately before a scheduled clinic visit, perhaps owing to heightened awareness (88), remains high for several days after the visit, and then wanes within a month (89). Increased frequency of office visits, therefore, may improve medication adherence (89).

Side Effects. Intolerance of side effects is often a significant cause of nonadherence. Donovan (90) reported that the most common reason for not taking drugs or dosages prescribed is patients' fear of side effects. For example, in a sample of 190 patients undergoing protease inhibitor treatment, side effects was the most frequent explanation for nonadherence (35%) (79). In addition, side effects play a particularly important role in asymptomatic diseases such as hypertension where the treatment may make the individual feel worse than the actual disease.

Physicians rarely assess patients' experience with medication side effects. A recent study reported that nearly half of all patients in a primary-care setting were not asked about how their medications were helping, and that more than two thirds of the patients were not asked any questions about barriers to taking medications or side effects related to medication (91). These results have important clinical implications, especially because many patients are reluctant to ask physicians about their medication (91). Older adults may be at increased risk for side effects from medications, based on differences in pharmacokinetics (i.e., drug metabolism) and pharmacodynamics (i.e., increased sensitivity) (92).

The proportion of patients who change or discontinue treatment because of side effects is difficult to estimate. Among hypertensive patients, for instance, data from clinical trials suggest that discontinuation occurs in approximately 15% of patients randomized to ACE inhibitors, 15%–20% of those taking diuretics, 20%–25% of those taking beta-blockers after 6 months to 1 year of treatment (93), and 20% using calcium channel blockers after 4 years of treatment (94). There are few effectiveness data about medication side effects as reasons for discontinuation of treatment. The rates of discontinuation, however, are likely to be higher in practice than they are in clinical trials.

Asymptomatic Diseases. Hyperlipidemia and hypertension have been coined asymptomatic "silent diseases." As a result, adherence problems are important for these diseases because patients may perceive no immediate benefit of treatment. Without appreciating the long-term consequences, patients often adhere poorly to or completely disengage in their provider-initiated cholesterol or hypertension management therapy. Two recent studies used drug database refills as a measurement of adherence and showed that statin therapy persistence declines remarkably over time in elderly cohorts. Benner (95) found that after 5 years of statin treatment only 25% of patients maintained an adherence rate (proportion of days covered) of at least 80%. Jackevicius (96) and colleagues observed also in a retrospective cohort study that within 6 months of statin initiation at least 25% of the patients discontinued therapy. In terms of hypertension, as many as 30% to 60% of hypertensive patients discontinue their treatment within the first year of care, and fewer than 20% remain in therapy after 5 years (97).

Of those remaining in treatment, antihypertensive medication adherence is approximately 40% to 70% (98–100).

Provider Characteristics

Most treatment adherence interventions have focused on the patient and medical environment levels (e.g., patient adherence with medications and medical follow-up). These intervention strategies often assume that the provider is treating patients appropriately, a potentially flawed assumption. Some patients may follow the advice exactly but do not benefit from treatment possibly as a result of under prescribing on the part of the provider. For example, Berlowitz (101) reported that approximately 40% of a sample of veteran patients had poor blood pressure control ($\geq$160/90 mm Hg) despite an average of more than six hypertension-related visits per year. They reported that providers frequently failed to increase the dose of antihypertensive medications or try new agents in patients with persistently elevated blood pressure. Although knowledge about a disease and familiarity with its treatment is necessary, this is insufficient to ensure a high degree of adherence (102). When patients are encouraged to actively participate in care decisions, they are likely to be more committed to those decisions and ultimately achieve higher levels of adherence (103). Thus, providers can and must play a major role in achieving patient treatment adherence and subsequent control of chronic diseases and health promotion in their patients (104, 105). Provider skills, including the ability to communicate openly, have a nonjudgmental attitude, and the ability to transfer knowledge and teach skills, are required to ensure medication adherence.

Social Environment

Barriers to care, such as a lack of transportation or physical disabilities, may limit patients' ability to see their primary-care provider, obtain medication, and subsequently result in poor medication adherence (58, 99, 106, 107). In addition, time required away from work, long travel times, and waiting for appointments are barriers to adequate treatment adherence (24, 87, 88). People must have the knowledge and means to obtain social services that may enhance medication adherence.

Summary of Nonadherence Correlates

In summarizing the risk factors for medication adherence, much of this research has been obtained through cross-sectional studies. Because adherence is likely to decline over time, longitudinal investigations of predictors of short- and long-term adherence will be of maximum benefit (108). The development of "risk profiles" may alert clinicians to circumstances requiring enhanced interventions or education, or modified dosing regimens (109). Risk profiles include memory deficits, complex medication regimens, substance or alcohol abuse, and concerns regarding medications. Additional factors that are related to adherence include the patient's knowledge, confidence in ability to follow recommended behaviors, perceptions of health and benefits of therapy or behavior, and availability of social support.

MEDICATION ADHERENCE MEASURES

The absence of a singular conceptual basis of medication adherence is problematic. Strategies to improve adherence can be evaluated only within the context of a given definition. Furthermore, comparative assessment of the adherence literature is difficult across studies using different definitions and methods of operationalizing adherence. A commonly used, but arbitrary measure of optimal adherence has been 80% (102, 110). This level has not been validated in all circumstances and may well vary depending on several factors, including, for example, the half-life of the prescribed compound (111). Adherence to medication is not a dichotomy and as discussed earlier patients can demonstrate a wide variety of patterns of medication use.

The assessment of adherence is a complex task that requires a creative approach to measure the levels of patients' adherence to treatment. There is no gold standard with the exception of actually observing an individual taking their medication. Dunbar-Jacob (112), for example, reported discrepant adherent rates; self-report based on a 7-day recall interview was 97%; pill count was 94%; and Medication Event Monitoring System (MEMS) was 84%. In another study for the treatment of alcohol dependence, pill count yielded a higher estimate of adherence (88%) than MEMS caps (80%) (113).

Researchers interested in measuring medication adherence often rely on one of six measures of adherence: pharmacy refills, pill counts, electronic measures (e.g., MEMS caps), biological indices, self-report, and physician judgments. Unfortunately, because of the disparate metrics employed by investigators, comparison across methodology (e.g., self-report vs. pharmacy records), or even across studies within methodology is difficult. Although there may not be the "best" measurement strategy to obtain an approximation of adherence behavior, strategies employed must meet basic psychometric standards or acceptable reliability and validity properties.

Direct Methods

Direct methods for assessing medication adherence include those that are more objective and require limited interpretation. Five general direct methods exist for assessing medication adherence: pharmacy refills, pill counts, electronic measurement devices, biological indices, and direct observation.

Pharmacy Refills. Assessing adherence using pharmacy refills consist of examining pharmacy refill data for individual patients from a centralized pharmacy after a specified follow-up period. Most pharmacy refill reports include a calculation of the date on which the stock will be finished. From this refill report, the regularity of the refill pattern can be deduced. Pharmacy refill records provide a reliable and nonintrusive longitudinal measure of medication adherence. However, it is necessary that all patients obtain their medication from a centralized pharmacy such as the Department of Veterans' Affairs (VA) or a health maintenance organization in order to keep track of medication refills. In addition, this method of assessing medication adherence requires extensive data-tracking programs. Furthermore, pharmacy refill data have primarily been used to estimate adherence with medications taken for chronic illnesses (114, 115) and may not provide accurate estimates for medications taken for a short period, such as antibiotics. Another limitation of pharmacy refills is that there is no information on when the medication was taken or by whom. In addition, it is possible that there are overlaps in refills such that refills may not always be accurate. Though pill refill data is available, coding the data and operationalizing adherence can be time consuming. Dunbar-Jacob (99) suggested that pharmacy refills may be as reasonable as self-report in measuring medication adherence, but are likely to provide an overestimate of true adherence because simply refilling a medication prescription does not necessarily mean the patient uses the medication as prescribed.

Pill Counts. At each visit, patients are asked to bring their medication to a clinic or research visit and their unused medications are assessed over a prespecified time period. Pill count adherence rate is often defined as the [(Number of pills dispensed − Number of pill returned) / Number of pills prescribed] * 100. This reflects the percentage of doses presumably taken. Pill counts can be useful (e.g., clinical trials) and this method typically yields higher estimates of medication nonadherence compared with self-report measures and electronically monitored adherence (correlation with electronic monitor was $r = 0.24$ in one study; see ref. 116). The problem with pill counts, apart from being intrusive, is that it does not give any indication of when the medication was taken or whether it was thrown away and thus may result in overestimation of adherence. It is possible that pills are dispensed and pills from a previous prescription are added to the container, patients may share their pills with others, or have some of their supplies in other locations. Several studies have noted patients engaging in "pill dumping" as a means of preventing acknowledgment of poor adherence behavior (117). In addition, for patients with chronic conditions, there may be a tendency to refill prescriptions before the current supply runs out. Consequently, the use of dispensed date may result in erroneous estimates of nonadherence. Pill counts are also not suitable for medications administered in nondiscrete dosages or taken on an as-needed basis.

Electronic Measurement Devices or Microelectric Event Monitoring. Electronic monitors, including the MEMS (AARDEX USA, APREX, a division of AARDEX, Union City, CA), consist of a microprocessor placed in a medication container with a switch that is activated by the interruption of an electrical current. When activated, the microprocessor records the date and time the bottle was opened. Several months of data can be stored on these units before they need to be downloaded onto a computer. These medication monitors can provide information on the pattern of drug intake, including the frequency and timing of medication dosing over a fairly extended period of time. Measures of adherence computed using data obtained by MEMS caps are described as follows:

1. MEMS adherence rate = (Number of days on which MEMS cap was opened at least once / Number of days of monitoring by MEMS) * 100. This reflects the percentage of days on which at least one dose was presumed taken. If an individual does not open the pill bottle on particular day, that day is coded as a nonadherence day.
2. Prescribed intervals method that quantitates the fraction of doses taken at the prescribed dosing intervals. If the prescribed dosing frequency was 12 hours (for a twice-a-day regimen), then a dosing event is considered adherent if it occurred within 8 to 14 hours of the previous dosing event. Prescribed intervals = Number of prescribed dosing intervals +/− 2 hr / total number of possible intervals (116).

Other electronic monitors can be used to assess medication adherence including tablet blister packs, pill rings, eye drop solution bottles, and aerosol spray nebulizers. Variations on electronic monitors are being developed. Devices have been developed, for example, that report medication patterns to a provider via telephone and modems and related information can be used to reorder medications. Devices are also being tested that not only record when a medication cap is open, but are able to be programmed to inform the user through various methods (i.e., noise or flashing light) that a medication dosage is due.

Electronic monitors are not widely available and are relatively expensive. In addition, patients often are aware that their medication use is being monitored. Adherence assessment via electronic devices may produce "reactivity" (i.e., the assessment activity itself tends to move the behavior in the socially desirable or therapeutic direction). In addition, electronic monitors preclude the use of a pill box to organize the medication being monitored by the electronic cap and some patients remove more than one dose per bottle opening to avoid carrying around the medication bottle when leaving home. Additional limitations of this technology include the need for accompanying technology to interpret the readings of the computer chip, patient acceptance and accurate use of the computerized caps, and inaccurate interpretations if multiple doses are removed at once. These limitations may result in electronic monitoring underestimating a patient's actual adherence. Electronic monitored adherence rates consistently range between 10% and 20% lower than rates assessed by other methods, including self-reports (118) and pill counts (119).

Biological Indices.   Another option is to monitor pharmacological markers such as blood drug levels, drug assays, or biological markers. As a measure of medication adherence, these markers often are confounded with physiological differences among patients and with patient–drug interactions. For example, there are genetic differences in how individuals absorb, metabolize, and excrete drugs. Drugs and urine levels can be assessed only during clinic visits. In addition, these assays can be expensive and the measurements can be misleading if the medication has a short serum half-life as the patient may have taken their pills only just before the time of determination or may have misused just that dose. In response to such limitations, biological tracer substances with minimal interindividual variation and long half-lives have been added to drugs (120, 121), but this process presents ethical concerns.

Supervised Dosing.   Supervised dosing of patient has seldom been used, with the exception of antitubercular treatment (122, 123), methadone for treatment of narcotic addiction, and monitoring glycemic adherence in children with diabetes. Up to half the people with tuberculosis do not complete their treatment. A Cochrane review that compared policies of directly observed therapy with self-treatment requiring treatment for tuberculosis, found in six studies ($N = 1,910$) that patients allocated to observed therapy had similar outcomes in relation to cure as did self-monitored patients (relative risk 1.06; 95% confidence interval [CI] 0.98–1.14). The obvious drawback of supervised dosing is its expense for the health system and inconvenience for patients. It has been advocated only in extreme cases where societal costs of nonadherence are obvious. Though not reviewed here, there are also ethical issues related to supervised dosing.

Indirect Methods

Indirect methods for measuring medication adherence involve more subjective interpretations and are often based on an individual's perception of adherence. Indirect measurements of adherence are more frequently reported in the literature, possibly due to the relative ease by which these measures are obtained.

Provider Assessment

Health care provider–rated adherence is an easy and inexpensive measure of medication adherence, however it appears to be the least accurate measure (124, 125). This type of assessment is particularly problematic because a provider typically interacts with the patient for only a brief period of time at unpredictable intervals. Furthermore, there is evidence that providers tend to substantially overestimate medication adherence in their own patients (125). Actual patient adherence as measured by use of MEMS cap as compared to physicians' predictions of patient adherence revealed that physicians incorrectly classified the patients' adherence ability 41% of the time (125). Thus, health care providers are limited by the extent to which individuals know how to obtain adherence information from patients. It may be worth considering using other health care providers' judgment such as nurses because it has been reported that they may be more accurate at rating patient adherence (126).

Self-Report Measures

Self-report assessments of patients' adherence continue to be the most commonly used measure because they are simple, inexpensive, and convenient to use (97). Unlike serum drug concentration assays and electronic monitoring, self-report measures of adherence offer a convenient "spot check" estimate of medication adherence behavior. Self-report measures have proven to be efficient and effective in determining medication adherence (127), and have been correlated with pill counts (128) and blood pressure control (129), and virological outcome (130). Fleece et al. (129) found that correlations between self-report, using self-monitoring, were reasonable compared with blood pressure control (partial correlation = −0.56 with systolic blood pressure and −0.51 with diastolic blood pressure). Fong et al. (131) reported that patients who reported they were in full adherence with their HAART regimen were more likely to have undetectable (<500 copies/mL) plasma virus level (adjusted OR, 4.22; 95% CI, 1.75–12.33). Self-report scores as measured by the Morisky scale (127) had a sensitivity of 72% and specificity of 74% for ≥80% adherence with antidepressant medication (132). Others have found that self-reported measures of medication adherence have a sensitivity of 55% and specificity of 87% compared with pill counts (133).

There are three basic types of patient self-report: questionnaires, interviews (in person or by phone), and self-monitoring logs (e.g., diaries). Questionnaire-based measures include multi-item scales (summarized later), visual-analog scales, or reports of missed doses. The status of self-report as a measure of adherence appears to be as reasonable as other measures, particularly when used in conjunction with another assessment procedure. In studies for which ecological (external) validity is extremely important, self-report measures offer the closest approximation of everyday patient–provider interactions concerning medication taking. Maintaining confidentiality of the data and promoting a cooperative relationship between patients and the study team who collect the data can maximize the accuracy of patients' self-reported adherence. These procedures make it less likely that patients will be defensive and deliberately distort their responses or that communication problems would otherwise render assessments inaccurate, as is particularly a concern when patient adherence reports are collected by health professionals themselves (134).

There are inherent self-reported biases such as halo effects (e.g., over-reporting adherence) that are likely to exist (128) and the information is limited by recall bias. Self-reported adherence represents "an upper limit" of the estimate of actual adherence due to social desirability. For example, one study indicated that approximately 40% of hypertensive patients who reported taking 100% of their antihypertensive medications were, in fact, taking less than 75% of their medication as indicated by pill count (135). Caregivers of children also are likely to feel obligated to report higher adherence because of demand characteristics of the adherence interview (i.e., interviewer expectations of good adherence), or may fear that accurate reporting of poor adherence may result in undesirable consequences (i.e., loss of custody of the child due to medical neglect) (53).

Despite the biases using self-report measures of medication adherence, studies have tended to show that patients are accurate when they say that they have not taken their medication (136). Because reports of nonadherence may be more accurate than reports of adherence, self-report tends to underestimate the true extent of nonadherence by approximately 20% (128). Reasons for overreporting adherence may include: Individuals might wish to intentionally deceive the researcher, they might not understand their regimen and therefore not realize that they are not adhering, they might forget instances of nonadherence, or the patient does not accurately recall whether he or she has adhered.

We examined adherence in a sample of 108 currently treated geriatric depressed patients using the Morisky self-reported measure of medication adherence (127). Among this sample, 33% reported that they did not take their antidepressant as prescribed in the last week. Among the individual items, forgetfulness was the most common endorsed item: 28% reported that they forgot to take their depression medicine in the last week. In a sample of 588 hypertensive patients, 29% reported that they sometimes forget to take their blood pressure medication, 15% reported that they sometimes were careless taking their blood pressure medication, 6% reported they sometimes stop taking their blood pressure medication because they feel better, and 6% reported they stop taking their medication because they feel worse (137).

Measures of Self-Report Adherence.   In the case of self-report measures of medication adherence, mode of administration needs to be considered. For example, patients are likely to be more honest in anonymous modes of administration such as mailed surveys, but there is an increase likelihood of missing data and poor response rates. In contrast, patients may be more subject to social desirability if administered a survey in person, but there are potentially fewer missing data. Another consideration is the time frame for assessing nonadherence. Measures that assesses prior medication adherence over the last day, week, or month will likely result in different findings. Though medication adherence in the last day or week is less influenced by recall bias, the responses may not necessarily reflect general adherence. However, an assessment of medication adherence over a longer period of time, such as a month, may be more influenced by recall biases and may not be appropriate for certain individuals (i.e., older adults, increased co-morbidity), but may give an overall rating of medication adherence.

Investigators recommend triangulation such that the use of various methods for assessing medication adherence eventually captures the construct. In fact, one can consider using factor analysis to create a latent variable to represent medication adherence. However, the downside is that this often makes it difficult to easily interpret and operationalize medication adherence. If a latent model is not used and the investigator includes multiple measures of medication adherence, the investigator needs to be prepared to handle discrepancies in measures of medication adherence.

The following are descriptions of examples of both generic and disease specific self-report medication adherence instruments. One of the most commonly used and adapted measures of self-reported adherence was created by Morisky et al. (127) (see Table 6.1). Scores for each of the four items are summed to give a scale score ranging from 4 to 20 or 0–4 depending on what anchors are used, where higher scores indicate higher levels of reported adherence. This measure has been used to measure adherence with asthma medications (138), hypertension (127), and other chronic diseases (139).

In addition to examining generic measures of self-reported adherence, consideration should be given to assessing patients' beliefs about medica-

TABLE 6.1
Morisky et al.'s Self-Rated Measure of Medication Adherence

- "Some people forget to take their medicines. How often does this happen to you?"
- "Some people miss out a dose of their medication or adjust it to suit their own needs. How often do you do this?"
- "Some people stop taking their medication when they feel better. How often do you do this?"
- "Some people stop taking their medication when they feel worse. How often do you do this?"

Note. Item responses score on a 5-point scale where 5 = never, 4 = rarely, 3 = sometimes, 2 = often, and 1 = very often. Adapted from ref. 127.

tions. Patients' beliefs about their medicines has been assessed using the Beliefs about Medicines Questionnaire (BMQ), which has been validated for use in the chronic illness groups asthma, renal, cardiac, and oncology (71). The BMQ comprises two 5-item scales assessing patients' beliefs about the *necessity* of prescribed medication for controlling their illness and their *concerns* about the potential adverse consequences of taking it. Examples of items from the *necessity* scale include: "My health, at present, depends on my medicines" and "My medicines protect me from becoming worse." Examples of items from the *concerns* scale include: "I sometimes worry about the long-term effects of my medicines" and "I sometimes worry about becoming too dependent on my medicines." Respondents indicate their degree of agreement with each individual statement about medicines on a 5-point Likert scale, ranging from 1 = strongly disagree to 5 = strongly agree. Scores obtained for the individual items within each scale are summed to give a scale score. Thus, total scores for the *necessity* and *concerns* scales range from 5 to 25 where higher scores indicate stronger beliefs in the concepts represented by the scale. Beliefs about medicines were related to reported adherence (71).

Two examples of asthma adherence scales include one for oral medications and a second scale to monitor inhaler use. Each scale consists of four items that ask simple yes–no questions about adherence. For each item the "no" response indicated better adherence. This procedure was used to negate any "yes-saying" response bias in obtaining disclosures of nonadherence. The scales were able to detect the impact of an intervention designed to improve adherence and score distributions were relatively wide enough to discriminate among individual levels of adherence. Both adherence scales can be completed in less than 5 minutes and their reliability is high. The predictive validity of the measure has not been examined (140).

Two examples of self-report measures of medication adherence for HIV/AIDS include the Simplified Medication Adherence Questionnaire (SMAQ) and the Adult AIDS Clinical Trial Group questionnaire (AACTG).

The SMAQ is a six-item self-report measure of adherence developed by clinicians and based on the Morisky scale (127). Additional questions were incorporated, with the aim of obtaining more adherence-specific measurements. A modified version of a question used by Samet et al. (141) to determine the number of missed doses over the previous 24 hours was employed. Although such a limited time frame may reflect the accuracy of patient recall, it may not reflect the overall trend of patient medication adherence. Therefore, the authors added three additional questions: (a) Thinking about the last week, how often have you not taken your medicine? (b) Did you not take any of your medicine over the last weekend? (c) Over the past 3 months, how many days have you not taken any medicine at all? The SMAQ was considered "positive" when a nonadherent patient was detected, that is, when there was a positive response to any of the questions. The SMAQ showed 72% sensitivity, 91% specificity, and a likelihood ratio of 7.94 to identify nonadherent patients, compared with the MEMS. The Cronbach alpha coefficient of the SMAQ was 0.75 (142).

The AACTG questionnaire assesses adherence to antiretrovirals (67). Question A investigates adherence over the previous days and asks for how many days the patient has missed all the medication doses. The answers could be none, 1, 2, 3, or 4 days. Question B asks how many times the patient has been off schedule with any medication doses over the previous 4 days. The answer are never, sometimes, half of the time, most of the time, or all the time. Question C investigates whether the patient has skipped any medication doses during the previous weekend, and the answer is scored as yes or no. Question D investigates the last time the patient has missed any medication doses, and the answer can be the last week, 2 weeks ago, >2–4 weeks ago, 1–3 months ago, longer than 3 months, or never. If the patient skipped at least one medication dose anytime, he or she is asked to explain the reasons for that according to a 13-item questionnaire that considers the most frequently reported causes of missing doses in HIV patients. The items are: problems with schedule, too many pills, fell asleep, change in routine, forgot, being busy, feeling bad, did not want to be seen, thought it was toxic, and fear of adverse events. For each item, the answer about the reason for missing medication can be never, seldom, sometimes, or frequently. The patient is considered to be adherent to treatment if he or she has not skipped doses nor been off schedule over the previous 4 days and if he or she has not skipped any medication doses during the previous weekend and has not missed doses over the previous 3 months. If a patient, answering the first question, reports full adherence to treatment (no missed medication doses over the previous 4 days) but has inconsistent responses to questions B through D, he or she is considered nonadherent.

The Hill–Bone Compliance to High Blood Pressure Therapy Scale (143) assesses patient behaviors for three important behavioral domains of high blood pressure treatment: (a) reduced sodium intake, (b) appointment keeping, and (c) medication taking. This scale is composed of 14 items in three subscales. Each item is a 4-point Likert-type scale. Internal consistency reliability and predictive validity of the scale were evaluated using two community-based samples of hypertensive adults enrolled in clinical trials of high blood pressure care and control. The Cronbach alpha for the total scale were 0.74 and 0.84, respectively. High adherence scale scores predicted significantly lower levels of blood pressure and blood pressure control. Moreover, high adherence scale scores at the baseline were significantly associated with blood pressure control at both baseline and at follow-up in the two independent samples. This brief instrument provides a simple method for clinicians in various settings to assess patients' self-reported adherence levels and to plan appropriate interventions.

In summary, when considering measures of medication adherence, investigators need to consider the use of generic versus disease-specific measures of adherence. A disease-specific measure of adherence is likely to be more sensitive to change and relevant to clinicians. A generic measure of medication adherence permits comparison of medication adherence rates across various diseases, medications, and studies and is potentially useful for policymakers and resource allocation; however, generic measures of medication adherence may lack sensitivity to detect changes.

RESEARCH INTERVENTIONS

Almost all research on medication adherence focuses on a health outcome and presumes that adherence to selected recommendations mediates or facilitates achievement of the desired outcome. Compared with the many thousands of trials for individual drugs, there are only a handful of rigorous trials of medication adherence interventions. This is unfortunate given the astounding advances in medical therapeutics during the past decades, yet limited attention given to improving adherence to these therapeutics. Although studies have examined efforts to raise individual adherence, few are randomized controlled trials with adherence as the primary outcome (144, 145). Still fewer have addressed efforts to remediate adherence when patients have difficulty implementing recommended behaviors or to improve long-term adherence. A systematic review of the literature notes the paucity of effective interventions to enhance medication adherence (7).

Haynes et al. (145) identified 3 short-term and 36 long-term studies that involved randomized controlled trials to improve medication adherence, measured both adherence and treatment outcome, and had at least 80% follow-up of each group studied. Among short-term treatments, one of three interventions showed an effect on both adherence and clinical outcome. Eighteen of 36 interventions among long-term treatments reported in 30 randomized control trials were associated with improvements in medication adherence, but only 16 of the 30 interventions led to improvements in treatment outcomes. Almost all of the interventions that were effective for long-term care were complex, including combinations of more convenient care, information, reminders, self-monitoring, reinforcement, counseling, family therapy, and other forms of additional supervision or attention by a health care provider (physician, nurse, pharmacist, or other). Even the most effective interventions did not lead to large improvements in adherence and treatment outcomes. In general, many of the interventions for long-term medications were complex and labor intensive.

Roter et al. (146) examined treatment adherence in a broader manner and included 153 studies published between 1977 and 1994 in a meta-analysis that synthesized the literature examining the effectiveness of adherence interventions. This meta-analysis included 116 randomized trials addressing both acute and chronic disorders. Regardless of the adherence measure used, the interventions yielded mean effect sizes ranging from small to large that were highly significant. An examination of the focus of the intervention (educational, behavioral, affective, or some combination) showed that a combined focus resulted in larger effects than did the single-focus interventions. These researchers pointed out that intervention studies examining adherence should include additional outcomes, such as quality of life, patient satisfaction, understanding, and functional status in order to have a more comprehensive picture of adherence.

Zygmunt et al. (147) reviewed psychosocial intervention for improving adherence with antipsychotic medications. They reported that 13 (33%) of 39 identified studies that involved random assignment and included adherence as a primary or secondary variable, reported significant interventions effects of improving treatment adherence. Psychoeducational interventions whether individual or family therapy programs that focused on attitudinal and behavioral change were largely unsuccessful in improving adherence. Concrete problem solving such as reminders, self-monitoring tools, cues, reinforcements, or motivational techniques were common features of successful programs. Interventions targeted specifically to problems of nonadherence were more likely to be effective (55%) than were more broadly based treatment interventions (26%). Despite these promising trends, Zygmunt et al. (147) concluded that most studies rely on dichotomous subjective reports of pill taking to measure adherence, an approach that overestimates adherence and reduces the likelihood of detecting intervention effects (28). A majority (62%) of the studies in the review that employed specific, objective measures of adherence such as pill counts and plasma levels found improved adherence in the intervention group, even when the intervention was not specifically targeted toward adherence.

SPECIFIC TYPES OF MEDICATION ADHERENCE STRATEGIES

Medication adherence–enhancing strategies may be implemented concurrent with the introduction of treatment, later in the course as a remediation measure, or as a technique to maintain adherence. The majority of strategies to influence medication adherence have been directed at correction and include contingency contracting (148), social support (149, 150), and multiple behavioral strategies (151). These strategies have proved successful in remediation of medication nonadherence but have not been effective in maintenance (51). Less attention has been given to the evaluation of strategies that might be effective at maintaining adherence. The maintenance-directed intervention strategies used most consistently have been educational or behavioral in nature. Summaries of educational and behavioral interventions are presented next.

Educational Interventions

Educational interventions include written and/or verbal instructions delivered individually, in a group, or by telephone, as well as the use of audiovisual material. Numerous studies have shown a direct relationship between medication adherence and the patient's understanding of the regimen. In a meta-analysis of articles written between 1961 and 1984 on intervention strategies, written interventions, except for patient package inserts, were shown to produce increased knowledge and decreased medication utilization errors. The studies on patient package inserts resulted in an average effect size value near zero for both knowledge and medication utilization errors (152). Thus, knowledge alone will not change behavior. Following are a few examples of well-designed educational interventions.

Levy (153) reported that an intervention involving asthma education from hospital-based specialist asthma nurses improved adherence and clinical outcomes in asthmatic patients. Self-reported adherence was significantly higher in the intervention group for use of inhaled topical steroids and rescue medication for severe asthmatic attacks. In terms of clinical outcomes, intervention patients had significantly higher peak expiratory flow values and significantly fewer symptoms at 6 months than patients in the control group.

A randomized clinical trial to improve self-management practices in a sample of 267 adults with asthma reported significant improvements in self-reported adherence as measured by the Morisky scale (127) among those randomized to the intervention as opposed to usual care (154). Improvements in adherence were documented at 12-month follow-up and whereas visits to emergency department or hospitalization for asthma in the past 12 months decreased, there were no significant differences across groups. The intervention included a skill-oriented workbook and a one-to-one counseling session involving discussing the workbook and adherence-enhancing strategies. Information on the various types of asthma medications, including precautions for using them, and forms were provided to assist users in understanding and adhering to medication schedules.

In a study evaluating a psychoeducative intervention to improve patients' knowledge and customs in handling medication to increase self-efficacy, Tuldra (155) assessed effects among HIV patients prescribed HAART. In an intention to treat analysis, no improvements were found in adherence or clinical outcomes (the p values were slightly above the 0.05 significance level). Self-reported adherence and pill refills of $\geq 95\%$ of medication prescribed were reported. However, when a per protocol analysis was conducted, the intervention resulted in improvements in adherence to HAART at 48 weeks and an increase in the proportion of patients with a viral load less than 400 copies/ml. Overall, 85% of patients with adherence $\geq 95\%$ but only 45% of those with adherence <95% had viral load <400 copies/ml ($p = .008$).

Literacy.   The effectiveness of written education materials is influenced by the reading ability of the target group or individual. Owen and colleagues (156) reported that the mean readability of 445 patient education materials was at the 10th-grade level. Two populations who are often disadvantaged in terms of benefiting from education interventions are individuals with low literacy skills and the elderly. Approximately 50 million U.S. citizens are undereducated, which may limit their ability to understand medication labels and instructions, organize their thoughts and perceptions about the purpose of their medications, and understand how to administer their medications (157). In the National Adult Literacy Study, a cross-sectional study of the U.S. population, the proportion of Americans who read at the lowest reading level ranged from 16% among those 45–54 years old to 26% among those 55–64 years old to 44% among those age 65 and older (158). In terms of health-related issues, Williams (159) found that only 42% of the patients in two public hospitals understood directions for taking medication on an empty stomach, and 26% were unable to understand information regarding when a next appointment was scheduled. Basic skills in reading are particularly important in the health care setting where patient participation in planning and implementing therapeutic regimens is critical for success. Functional health literacy means being able to read and understand health-related materials such as prescriptions, appointment cards, medicine labels, and directions for home health care (160). Besides being prevalent, functional health illiteracy is related to poorer health status (161, 162), fewer health-promoting behaviors (163), and poorer health knowledge (164).

It cannot be overemphasized that educational programs should be based on an appraisal of each individual's needs rather than relying upon the application of a package suitable for all. Providers must establish what is known before offering the patient new knowledge. Providers should aim to build in and develop simple points into more complex ideas. Also concrete examples to support or explain concepts should be provided. This is important given the increased reliance on patient literature to supplement educational sessions because of reduced length of hospital stays and fewer follow-up contacts.

Ways of Presenting Written Information. Written instructions about the medication regimen should be a core part of every interaction with the patient. A series of studies by Morrow and colleagues has focused on effective instruction formats for older patients that are generalizable to all literate patients. Comprehension and recall of medication information is facilitated significantly when medication-taking instructions are clear (165) and structured in lists rather than paragraphs (166). The use of picture charts, color-coded medication schedules, and large print may enhance older and functionally illiterate adults' level of understanding (48, 157). Combined use of written and verbal instruction may enhance treatment adherence (167). Patients' lack of understanding of medications relates to technical words, incomplete written instructions, and lack of knowledge of regimen duration.

Return demonstration of information (i.e., how to take pills) is a method to ensure patients understand relevant information. Package inserts are important to individuals for risk–benefit information but often fail to provide benefits of treatment and have little effect on self-reported behavior (168). Research has shown that it is better to provide limited amounts of materials, and these materials should relate to and reinforce what is covered in the visit (169).

Behavioral Interventions

Behavioral strategies, including self-monitoring, cueing, chaining (associating new behaviors with established ones), positive reinforcement, and patient contracting, have been used to enhance medication adherence (102, 154). A contingency contract is wherein both providers and patients set forth a treatment goal and the specific obligations of each in attempting to accomplish this goal and a time limit for its achievement. Beyond increasing the likelihood of adherence to medication therapy, contracts offer a written outline of the expected behavior, the involvement of the patient in the decision-making process concerning the regimen and the opportunity to discuss potential problems and solutions with the provider, a formal commitment to the problem from the patient, and rewards that create incentives for adherence goals.

The use of social support interventions (i.e., nurses, pharmacists, family members) for instruction/follow-up is essential to ensure adequate treatment adherence (99, 157). Nurses, by virtue of their numbers and amount of patient contact, have great potential for impacting patient health behavior. In addition, there is support for the value of involving pharmacists in attempts to increase patient cooperation with prescribed therapies. The family can also enhance supervision of the patient, as well as assist and encourage patient adherence. Social support is crucial to long-term treatment plans that require continuous action on the part of the patient.

Additional strategies include developing prompts and reminder systems, identifying a potential relapse into old behavior, setting appropriate and realistic goals, and rewarding achievement of new behaviors. Other behavioral methods that have improved medication adherence have included simplifying regimens to once or twice daily and eliminating unnecessary medications (34). Maintenance of most behaviors declines over time; constant questioning and follow-up are essential to ensure adequate adherence (99). Following are suggested behavioral maneuvers and physical devices to enhance medication adherence:

1. Patients can be instructed to identify a medication-reminder cue and place medication taking in their habitual daily routine. The cues can be activities, such as personal toilet, meals, coffee, or bedtime. An example of a physical cue is the medication container placed prominently in the center of the daily activity cue. The National Heart, Lung, and Blood Institute Web site provides other additional helpful medication reminder cues: http://www.nhlbi.nih.gov/hbp/treat/tips.htm.

2. A written medication description with instructions on starting the prescription is given to the patient. This includes the drug's name, strength, and form; medical condition treated or purpose; number of doses per day and their time of day; the relationship to food, beverages, and other medications; and any special instructions such as potential drug–drug interactions.

3. The patient self-records a daily medication record of each dose taken or missed with relevant comments. The clinician or health care extender can review with the patient this medication diary over the telephone or at the next clinic visit.

4. A variety of simple medication containers with compartments for each day's dose for 1 or several weeks are available and are popular with patients.

5. Electronic monitoring devices providing comprehensive descriptions of adherence behavior, which record the date and time of medication-taking events.

Incentives. As in other areas of human psychology, positive reinforcement in various forms to encourage or improve adherence may be more beneficial than chastising the patient for poor adherence. In a study (170) of renal transplant patients, provision of free immunosuppressive medications resulted in short-term improvements in adherence, but there was no benefit beyond the first year after transplantation. Use of financial incentives to improve adherence has also been advocated but remains controversial. In a literature review (171), 10 of 11 studies showed improvements in patient adherence with use of financial incentives, particularly for treatment of infectious diseases like tuberculosis. Using monetary incentives to improve adherence has been condemned by some as coercion and contrary to the "mutual participation principle" of decision making advocated by some (172).

Examples of some well-developed behavioral interventions to improve medication adherence are now discussed. Piette (173) evaluated the effect of biweekly automated telephone assessment and self-care education calls with nurse follow-up on the management of diabetes. Compared with usual care, patients in the intervention group reported fewer problems with medication adherence and more frequent glucose monitoring (both $p < 0.03$). Patients in the intervention group also had lower glycated hemoglobin levels, lower serum glucose levels, and fewer diabetic symptoms than those in the control group.

Incomplete adherence is one of several possible causes of uncontrolled hypertension. Yet, nonadherence remains largely unrecognized and is falsely interpreted as treatment resistance, because it is difficult to confirm or exclude objectively. In one study involving hypertensive patients resistant to a three-drug regimen, the use of electronic monitors resulted in improvement in both systolic and diastolic blood pressure over 2 months as a result of adapting drug therapy. In addition, the overt monitoring of adherence stimulated about one third of previously uncontrolled patients to improve their adherence and achieve blood pressure control (174).

Multifaceted Interventions

We are conducting the Veterans Study to Improve the Control of Hypertension (V-STITCH) (175) which consists of two interventions, a provider- and nurse-administered patient-tailored intervention to improve blood pressure control. This 4-year randomized controlled trial is being conducted in a primary-care setting among hypertensive veterans and their providers.

The provider intervention includes a well-developed electronically generated hypertension decision support system (DSS) delivered to the provider at each patient's visit. The DSS includes a compilation of all the patient's blood pressure readings over the last 12 months, highlighting those ≥140/90 mm/Hg based on all primary-care clinic visits. The DSS also includes a list of the patient's active antihypertensive medications, current dose, last fill, and maximum suggested dose. Providers are reminded to take action based on Joint National Committee on Prevention, Detection, Evaluation, and Treatment of High Blood Pressure (JNC VI) (176) and VA treatment guidelines for hypertension. The intervention is designed to improve guideline concordant therapy. Providers not randomized to receive the intervention receive a menu listing patients' recent blood pressure and allows them to include the most recent reading.

The patient intervention involves eight standardized telephone modules administered by a nurse case manager every 2 months for 24 months to improve medication adherence and self-management and subsequent blood pressure control. The modules consist of literacy, hypertension knowledge, memory, social support, patient–provider communication, missed appointments, side effects, and health behaviors; all modules are related to medication adherence and blood pressure control (175, 177). The database consists of algorithms to ensure that each module is tailored to the patients' needs. For example, the literacy module is activated at every medication change for patients who are known to be functionally illiterate. The database allows the nurse case manager to consistently assess patients' hypertension needs and if a problem is determined, that particular module is activated at the next call. The intervention database informs the nurse when the patient needs to be called again as well as what transpired during the past phone conversation. At the conclusion of the study, the database will contain an entire record for each patient describing what occurred (i.e., decision made, answers to questions) during the intervention. Outcomes will consist of whether patients' blood pressure is controlled or not at each outpatient visit over 24 months. In addition, medication adherence will also be assessed using two methods. The Morisky scale will be administered at baseline, 6 months, and 24 months, and antihypertensive refill over the 24 months will be collected.

CLINICAL IMPLICATIONS

Though a combination of appropriate educational, behavioral, and communication strategies is known to enhance medication adherence, additional research employing different intervention strategies needs to be conducted. The notion that the provider is solely responsible for the patient's behavior and outcome is no longer tenable in the health care system, particularly because studies have shown that physicians and nurses tend to underestimate the extent of nonadherence and are generally unable to identify those patient who do not adhere with prescribed medication regimens (178).

Clinicians' Assessment of Medication Adherence

One of the important difficulties in managing poor medication adherence is a lack of accurate and affordable measures. Clinicians must frequently rely on their own judgment but unfortunately demonstrate no better than chance accuracy in predicting the adherence of their patients (133). In general, patients tend to overestimate their medication adherence (99) and unless a patient is not responding to therapy, it may be extremely difficult to identify poor medication adherence. In research settings, pill counts, drug levels, pharmacy dispensing records, and electronic medication monitors are available to measure medicinal adherence but these methods may be susceptible to overestimating adherence (179). In many nonresearch situations these approaches may be difficult to implement due to their obtrusiveness, cost, or complexity. In the clinical setting asking patients about their medication use is often the most practical means of ascertainment, but it is prone to inaccuracy. A key validated question is "Have you missed any pills in the past week?" and any indication of having missed one or more pills signals a problem with low adherence (180). Asking nonresponders about their medication adherence will detect more than 50% of those with low adherence, with a specificity of 87% (133). Other practical measures to assess adherence include watching for those who do not respond to increments in treatment intensity and patients who fail to attend appointments.

Education and training of medical personnel in adherence diagnosis and management is not readily available in the current medical education. Authoritative textbooks on general medicine, medical therapies, pharmacology, and patient interviewing do not typically address adherence and its management. Drug industry publications for health care professionals occasionally have brief descriptions of the rudiments of adherence management. Most clinicians learn adherence management by self-instruction from clinical experience. A variety of medical care personnel can be trained to assist clinicians as effective adherence counselors, including nurses, physician's assistants, dietitians, psychologists, and nondegreed office staff.

Behaviors such as a provider making direct eye contact, transmitting interest in what the patient says, explaining recommendations thoroughly and clearly, praising treatment adherence and problem solving, and expressing willingness to modify the treatment plan in accordance with the patient's concerns have been demonstrated as ways to promote adherence (181). Additional methods to improve the interaction of the provider with patients include expressing empathy and acceptance through the use of active listening and reflective responses. Providers should also resist entering into conflict with the patient and avoid the imposition of values or beliefs onto the patient.

Patients should be provided with a clear rationale for the necessity of a particular treatment and their concerns should be elicited and addressed. To ensure that the necessary information has been understood, key instructions should be provided both verbally and in written form, asking the patient to verify that they understand the instructions (182). Common misperceptions should be anticipated and avoided, including that the medication can be stopped when the prescription runs out or the condition comes under control, that different medications cannot be taken together at the same time of the day, and that symptoms are guides to when to take the medication.

At the heart of simple instructions is a simple regimen. Medications that can be given once a day are best (183). For patients who require more than one medication, all should be prescribed to be taken at the same time if this is consistent with therapeutic activity. Whenever possible, negotiating a therapy that the patient is able to follow should be a first priority. Besides simplifying the dosing regimen, some examples of ways to tailor the therapy include exploring the patient's schedule, beliefs, and preferences, altering the administration route, and using adherence aids (4, 184).

Several ethical issues must be addressed when considering and attempting to improve patient adherence to medication regimens (185). First, before adherence becomes a legitimate concern, the clinical diagnosis must be correctly established. Second, the treatment being prescribed must be of known efficacy for this diagnosis and appropriate for the patient's circumstances. Third, methods for helping the patient to follow the treatment must be of established effectiveness. Fourth, in the end, the patient's right to refuse treatment must be respected.

Adherence and Initiation of Treatment

Adherence management starts with instructing the patient at the initiation of treatment with careful monitoring and support during the critical first 2 weeks of treatment (186, 187). Adherence problems encountered at the start of treatment or during the course of treatment can be addressed by a five-step problem-solving approach: (a) specifying the problem in concrete terms, (b) identifying possible solutions, (c) developing a plan for implementing the solutions, (d) trying out the solutions, and (e) evaluating the results (187). The five most common strategies of adherence problems have been identified and clinical management procedures developed for them: (a) The patient lacks knowledge of the disease and its treatment; (b) the patient rejects the diagnosis; (c) the patient rejects the prescribed drug; (d) the patient lacks the skills to establish self-medication as a habit; and (e) the patient engages in frequent self-debate regarding the decision to follow prescribed regimen (186). Clinical management for the first three is by patient education, and for the last two is by behavioral counseling.

The simplest adherence management available to clinician is a time-efficient, problem-solving process based on questioning the patient. The process aims to determine if an adherence problem is present, to define the problem, and to design and test a solution by collaborative negotiation with the patient. Asking the patient open-ended questions to describe their adherence practices starts the process and the search for adherence problems. The questions must be asked in a manner that is nonjudgmental and nonthreatening to gain the patient's trust and truthfulness. Usually the patient's answers provide information that quickly makes the next logical question obvious to the clinician. The major obstacle to adherence management is getting the process started. To facilitate the start, five questions directed to the patient are frequently cited: "Please describe for me how you remember to take your medicine." "Many patients find it difficult to take their medicine regularly. Do you ever miss or forget to take your medicine?" "How do you remember to take your medicine on the weekend, when you eat out, when you visit, when you travel, and so on?" "What do you think you could do to solve the problem of missing doses?" "Are there any future events that may interfere with taking your medication, and how do you plan to cope?" See Table 6.2 for techniques of questioning and promoting medication adherence.

Goal setting must be implemented as part of the initiation of the treatment regimen. Working toward a goal that is specific, attainable, and proximal in time heightens self-efficacy and promotes behavioral change. A time frame should be included in the goals (e.g., in 2 weeks or at the time of the next visit in 4 weeks). Telephone contacts may be used to review progress toward the goal when the patient is not seen on a frequent basis. When the goal is attained, reinforcement is provided for the success, and the next level of the goals is set. When the patient is unsuccessful in attaining the behavior, the provider can encourage the patient to continue.

Encouraging patients to access social support can play a significant role in the successful initiation of medication regimen. Social support includes the involvement of others (family, friends, or coworkers) in the knowledge and treatment of the condition. The goal of these strategies is to develop an ally who can help ease the behavioral change, reduce obstacles to maintenance, and be supportive during failures and successes (see Table 6.2).

TABLE 6.2
Techniques of Questioning That Promote Medication Adherence

Technique	Sample Questions
Do not criticize	• Most of us miss doses at times. What has been your experience?
Be specific	• Were you able to take your medications as intended this morning?
	• Can you tell me what the purpose of the medication is and when did you take it last?
	• When did you last miss a dose? Why? How can you avoid doing that?
Ask about the medications' effects on the patient's quality of life	• How do you feel about taking these pills?
Ask about side effects	• Have you experienced any side effects?
	• How have side effects affected the way you take your medications?
Identify the problem	• What medications do you find the most difficult to take?
	• What causes difficulty?
Identify sources of support	• Who can help you take these medications?

Note. From ref. 209. Copyright 2001 by LWW Business Office. Adapted by permission.

Patients need information in order to feel committed to the course of treatment to which they are expected to adhere. Use of medical jargon is likely to leave patients feeling disengaged and devoid of responsibility for their care. Effective communication between medical practitioners and patients takes time, a rare commodity in the clinical setting (see chap. 11 for more details on methods for improving patient–provider communication).

Patients are often influenced by the approval or disapproval of others, such as close friends and loved ones, as well as by the social and cultural group to which they belong. Such influence can provide support for health actions or conversely can interfere with and jeopardize methods for preventing and treating disease. The medical professional may need to work within the constraints of these norms in order to win the patient's cooperation.

Telephone counseling is an effective and potentially cost-effective mechanism for the simultaneous addressing of education, psychosocial, and practical barriers to adherence (188). In two ongoing studies (the Take Control of Your Blood Pressure [TCYB] study and the Veterans Study to Improve the Control of Hypertension [V-STITCH study]) (175, 177), we have chosen to test a nurse-delivered, telephone-based intervention. Nurse-delivered interventions have been found to significantly improve patient outcomes for multiple diseases (i.e., diabetes, heart failure) (189–192). Telephone-based interventions have several important features. First, telephone reminders are quite effective in changing behavior. A meta-analysis, for example, examined the effectiveness of patient reminder systems in primary-care settings for immunization; immunization rates due to reminders increased from 5 to 20 percentage points (193). Second, telephone interventions are relatively easy to implement. Third, patients generally appreciate being reminded by a health care provider, and such reminder systems may actually improve the patient–provider relationship (193). Fourth, delivering a patient intervention administered by a nurse-case manager by telephone may enhance the intervention's cost-effectiveness because patients may require fewer clinic visits (194, 195).

Organizational Factors

Missing appointments is correlated with lower adherence rates to prescribed regimens, is the first sign of dropping out of care entirely, and the most severe form of nonadherence. Telephone or appointment reminders by letter or telephone provide a relatively easy method to overcome this problem, by contracting with patients to keep appointments, and by contacting patients immediately if appointments are missed. Calling patients who miss appointments is logically the most important method of helping patients adhere to prescribed regimens, because reminding or recalling patients is effective and relatively inexpensive (196) and dropping out of care results in total nonadherence to prescribed medications. Additional organizational factors include reducing the time between screening and follow-up appointments, and the amount of waiting time at clinical visits.

Future Directions of Medication Adherence Research. The methodological rigor of medication adherence studies has been questioned. One explanation for this situation may be that health care researchers empirically test potential factors that might overcome low adherence regardless of any theoretical framework. Researchers have attempted to identify causal relationships between variables, assuming that the variables can be treated as independent. However, the phenomenon of medication-taking behavior involves variables that are interrelated with the possibility of feedback loops. The years of research on medication adherence provide little consistent information other than the fact that people do not follow provider's recommendations. Further research is needed to investigate how patients administer their medications and their decision-making process.

Additional explanation for the limited success of these interventions is that they attempt to overcome intentional nonadherence (e.g., by issuing reminders or clear instructions), but fail to address the perceptions of treatment that may lead to intentional nonadherence. In addition, many measures of adherence are imprecise (see the section Medication Adherence

Measures). Other problems with medication adherence studies are that existing interventions are limited because they focus on patients who are willing to participate in research studies. Investigators may be missing the key problems or beneficiaries of intervention, including those who have not sought care and those who dropped out of care. In fact, the first task facing many health care providers may be improving patient attendance to medical appointments.

An additional problem with previous research is that many studies are underpowered to detect differences. As a general guide, studies with a single intervention and control group need to include at least 50 participants per group if they are to have at least 60% power to detect an absolute difference of 25% in the proportion of patients judged to have adequate adherence. McDonald et al. (144) reported that only 11 of the 33 randomized control trials met this standard. In addition, among the 33 studies reviewed, none examined major clinical endpoints and the follow-up was relatively short term in all, the longest being 24 months.

The most promising strategies are combinations of interventions, including patient education, behavioral strategies (e.g., medication charts and pill organizers), contracts, and telephone follow-up (148, 197). Management of risk factors by multidisciplinary teams within systems designed to modify health care delivery and respond to patient and provider needs have been more successful than physicians alone providing interventions in a traditional, minimally structured environment (192, 198). In addition, the use of tailored interventions, a recent advancement, has been demonstrated to be effective in the areas of smoking cessation, reducing dietary fat intake, and increasing mammography use (199–202). (See chap. 17 for more details on the use of tailored interventions.) Finally, cost-effectiveness of interventions need to be conducted to improve the likelihood of translating and disseminating findings into the clinical environment.

RESEARCH CONCLUSIONS

The cost of nonadherence in the United States is estimated to be more than $100 billion (26). These potentially unnecessary expenses increase the financial burden for families and society in general, including higher insurance premiums and taxes. Nonadherence with medications is a significant problem and is seen in almost half of the patients treated for chronic conditions. Identifying patients more likely to be nonadherent with treatment has been the subject of many studies. Although there are many factors related to poor adherence, there are relatively few consistently reported factors. These consistent factors include complexity of the treatment regimen and patient beliefs and motivation. However, several studies have shown that nonadherence with one aspect of treatment does not predict non-adherence with other aspects. This review of the medication adherence literature has revealed several areas where gaps in knowledge exist and more research is needed.

Methodology

Many studies lack generalizability because of small samples, descriptive study designs, and inadequate reporting of demographic information. Future research should include studies that seek to increase our understanding of adherence from the patient's perspective. Qualitative studies may be useful in revealing some important elements of adherence that otherwise would be difficult to elicit.

Monitoring Devices

Use of microelectric devices has been a major advance in medication monitoring and useful in clinical research. Not only do they help providers determine whether medications are taken as prescribed, but they also provide information on medication-taking behavior, allowing providers to provide feedback to the patient. Additional studies need to address the following: (a) Does use of these devices actually improve patient adherence? (b) Can their high cost be justified in terms of medical expense savings? (c) Should patients be informed when these devices are used?

Individualized, tailor-made care planning and personal goal setting should be emphasized. Pharmacist-led interventions have led to improved adherence (203, 204). The combination of traditional methods with newer technologies, such as e-mail communication by pharmacists with physicians, represents an innovative approach to improving adherence (205).

CLINICAL CONCLUSIONS

As appointment nonadherence can be easily checked, it should serve as a warning signal for medication nonadherence: If patients do not always keep follow-up appointments, their taking the medication should be scrutinized so that subclinical nonadherence can be identified as fast as possible. Anticipating the most common adverse events as well as when they are likely to occur, and what can be done to ameliorate them also can improve medication adherence. It is useful to ask patients what they already know and believe about the medications before and after explaining these points.

FUTURE DIRECTIONS

Medication treatment adherence must be addressed on several levels, including the patient, the provider, and the health care system. Patients need the knowledge, attitude, and skills to follow an appropriately prescribed regimen (206). Similarly, providers need to follow established guidelines in prescribing regimen; ensure that patients understand the reason for the prescribed drugs and possible side effects, the interactions with other agents, and the manner in which the drug is to be taken; and ensure that the recommended regimen is as simple as possible. Finally, the system or organization within which providers work needs to provide resources and set policies that support optimal practices, particularly prevention-oriented activities (207). There is substantial evidence that the involvement of other health care professionals to support treatment plans improves the effectiveness of interventions and increases the prevalence of patient behavior change or adherence (208).

Improving medication adherence will only become more important as the cost of medications continues to increase, advances in medication treatment for various diseases continues, and the use of these medications increases as the population ages.

ACKNOWLEDGMENTS

This research is supported by Grant R01 HL070713 from the National Heart, Lung, and Blood Institute and a grant from the Department of Veterans Affairs, Veterans Health Administration, HSR&D Service (investigator initiative research grant 20-034). In addition, this research is supported by a grant from the Pfizer Foundation Health Communication Initiative.

REFERENCES

1. Kaufman DW, Kelly JP, Rosenberg L, Anderson TE, Mitchell AA. Recent patterns of medication use in the ambulatory adult population of the United States: the Slone survey. *JAMA*. 2002;287(3):337–344.
2. Prescription drug trends—a chart book update (#3112). Kaiser Family Foundation, 2003. Available at http://www.kff.org. Accessed July 21, 2003.
3. Lewis A. Non-compliance: A $100 billion problem. *Remington Report*. 1997;5(4): 14–15.
4. Feldman R, Bacher M, Campbell N, Drover A, Chockalingam A. Adherence to pharmacologic management of hypertension. *Can J Public Health*. 1998;89(5): I16–I18.
5. Flack J, Novikov SV, Ferrario CM. Benefits of adherence to antihypertensive drug therapy. *Eur Soc Cardiol*. 1996;17(Suppl A):16–20.

6. Mallion JM, Baguet JP, Siche JP, Tremel F, de Gaudemaris R. Compliance, electronic monitoring and antihypertensive drugs. *J Hypertens Suppl.* 1998;16(1): S75–S79.

7. Haynes RB, McKibbon KA, Kanani R. Systematic review of randomised trials of interventions to assist patients to follow prescriptions for medications. *Lancet.* 1996;348(9024):383–386.

8. Mehta S, Moore RD, Graham NM. Potential factors affecting adherence with HIV therapy. *AIDS.* 1997;11(14):1665–1670.

9. Montaner J, Reiss P, Cooper D, et al. A randomized, double-blind trial comparing combinations of nevirapine, didanosine, and zidovudine for HIV-infected patients: the INCAS Trial. *JAMA.* 1998;279:930–937.

10. Kaufmann D, Pantaleo G, Sudre P, Telenti A. CD4-cell count in HIV-1-infected individuals remaining viraemic with highly active antiretroviral therapy (HAART). Swiss HIV Cohort Study. *Lancet.* 1998;351(9104):723–724.

11. Rodriguez-Rosado R, Jimenez-Nacher I, Soriano V, Anton P, Gonzalez-Lahoz J. Virological failure and adherence to antiretroviral therapy in HIV-infected patients. *AIDS.* 1998;12(9):1112–1113.

12. Tuldra A, Ferrer MJ, Fumaz CR, et al. Monitoring adherence to HIV therapy. *Arch Intern Med.* 1999;159(12):1376–1377.

13. Turner BJ, Laine C, Cosler L, Hauck WW. Relationship of gender, depression, and health care delivery with antiretroviral adherence in HIV-infected drug users. *J Gen Intern Med.* 2003;18(4):248–257.

14. Bangsberg DR, Hecht FM, Charlebois ED, et al. Adherence to protease inhibitors, HIV-1 viral load, and development of drug resistance in an indigent population. *AIDS.* 2000;14(4):357–366.

15. De Geest S, Borgermans L, Gemoets H, et al. Incidence, determinants, and consequences of subclinical noncompliance with immunosuppressive therapy in renal transplant recipients. *Transplantation.* 1995;59(3):340–347.

16. Dew MA, Roth LH, Thompson ME, Kormos RL, Griffith BP. Medical compliance and its predictors in the first year after heart transplantation. *J Heart Lung Transplant.* 1996;15(6):631–645.

17. Jones J, Gorkin L, Lian JF, Staffa JA, Fletcher AP. Discontinuation of and changes in treatment after start of new courses of antihypertensive drugs: a study of the United Kingdom population. *BMJ.* 1995;311:293–295.

18. Bloom S. Continuation of initial antihypertensive medication after 1 year of therapy. *Clin Ther.* 1998;20:671–681.

19. Barr RG, Somers SC, Speizer FE, Camargo CA Jr. Patient factors and medication guideline adherence among older women with asthma. *Arch Intern Med.* 2002;162(15):1761–1768.

20. Viller F, Guillemin F, Briancon S, Moum T, Saurmeijer T, van den Heuvel W. Compliance to drug treatment of patients with rheumatoid arthritis: a 3 year longitudinal study. *J Rheumatol.* 1999;26(10):2114–2122.

21. Katon W, Von Korff M, Lin E, Bush T, Ormel J. Adequacy and duration of antidepressant treatment in primary care. *Med Care.* 1992;30:67–76.

22. Lin EH, Von Korff M, Katon W, et al. The role of the primary care physician in patients' adherence to antidepressant therapy. *Med Care.* 1995;33(1):67–74.

23. Maddox J, Levi M, Thompson C. The compliance with antidepressant in general practice. *J Psychopharmacol.* 1994;8:48–53.

24. Peveler R, George C, Kinmonth AL, Campbell M, Thompson C. Effect of antidepressant drug counseling and information leaflets on adherence to drug treatment in primary care: randomised controlled trial. *BMJ.* 1999;319:612–615.

25. Blackwell B. Compliance. *Psychother Psychosom.* 1992;58:161–169.

26. Berg JS, Dischler J, Wagner DJ, Raia JJ, Palmer-Shevlin N. Medication compliance: a healthcare problem. *Ann Pharmacother.* 1993;27(9 Suppl):S1–S24.

27. Schmaling KB, Afari N, Blume AW. Predictors of treatment adherence among asthma patients in the emergency department. *J Asthma.* 1998;35(8):631–636.

28. Fenton WS, Blyler CR, Heinssen RK. Determinants of medication compliance in schizophrenia: empirical and clinical findings. *Schizophr Bull.* 1997;23(4):637–651.

29. Daley DC, Salloum IM, Zuckoff A, Kirisci L, Thase ME. Increasing treatment adherence among outpatients with depression and cocaine dependence: results of a pilot study. *Am J Psychiatry.* 1998;155(11):1611–1613.

30. DeProspero T, Riffle WA. Improving patients' drug compliance. *Psychiatr Serv.* 1997;48(11):1468.

31. Melfi CA, Chawla AJ, Croghan TW, Hanna MP, Kennedy S, Sredl K. The effects of adherence to antidepressant treatment guidelines on relapse and recurrence of depression. *Arch Gen Psychiat.* 1998;55(12):1128–1132.

32. Melnikow J, Kiefe C. Patient compliance and medical research: issues in methodology. *J Gen Intern Med.* 1994;9(2):96–105.

33. Miller NH. Compliance with treatment regimens in chronic asymptomatic diseases. *Am J Med.* 1997;102(2A):43–49.

34. Rudd P. Clinicians and patients with hypertension: unsettled issues about compliance. *Am Heart J.* 1995;130(3 Pt 1):572–579.

35. Kruse W, Koch-Gwinner P, Nikolaus T, Oster P, Schlierf G, Weber E. Measurement of drug compliance by continuous electronic monitoring: a pilot study in elderly patients discharged from hospital. *J Am Geriatr Soc.* 1992;40(11):1151–1155.

36. Spagnoli A, Ostino G, Borga AD, et al. Drug compliance and unreported drugs in the elderly. *J Am Geriatr Soc.* 1989;37(7):619–624.

37. Nikolaus T, Kruse W, Bach M, Specht-Leible N, Oster P, Schlierf G. Elderly patients' problems with medication. An in-hospital and follow-up study. *Eur J Clin Pharmacol.* 1996;49(4):255–259.

38. Blenkiron P. The elderly and their medication: understanding and compliance in a family practice. *Postgrad Med J.* 1996;72(853):671–676.

39. Lowe CJ, Raynor DK, Courtney EA, Purvis J, Teale C. Effects of self medication programme on knowledge of drugs and compliance with treatment in elderly patients. *BMJ.* 1995;310(6989):1229–1231.

40. Esposito L. The effects of medication education on adherence to medication regimens in an elderly population. *J Adv Nurs.* 1995;21(5):935–943.

41. Lawrence J, Mayers DL, Hullsiek KH, et al. Structured treatment interruption in patients with multidrug-resistant human immunodeficiency virus. *N Engl J Med.* 2003;349(9):837–846.

42. Park D, Willis SL, Morrow D, Diehl M, Gaines CL. Cognitive function and medication usage in older adults. *J Appl Gerontology.* 1994;13:39–57.

43. Park D, Kidder DP. Prospective memory and medication adherence. In: Brandimonte MA, Einstein GO, McDaniel MA, eds. *Prospective Memory Theory and Application.* Hillsdale, NJ: Lawrence Erlbaum Associates; 1996:369–390.

44. Bosworth HB, Schaie KW. Medication knowledge and health status in the Seattle longitudinal study. *Gerontologist.* 1995;35:24.

45. Salthouse T. *Theoretical Perspectives in Cognitive Aging.* Hillsdale, NJ: Lawrence Erlbaum Associates; 1991.

46. Farmer ME, Kittner SJ, Abbott RD, Wolz MM, White LR. Longitudinally measured blood pressure, antihypertensive medication use, and cognitive performance: the Framingham Study. *J Clin Epidemiol.* 1990;43(5):475–480.

47. Wilson IB, Tchetgen E, Spiegelman D. Patterns of adherence with antiretroviral medications: an examination of between-medication differences. *J Acquir Immune Defic Syndr.* 2001;28(3):259–263.

48. Salzman C. Medication compliance in the elderly. *J Clin Psychiatry.* 1995;56 (Suppl 1):18–22.

49. Dunbar-Jacob J, Schlenk EA, Burke LE, et al. Predictors of patient adherence: patient characteristics. In: Schumaker S, McBee WL, Schron E, Ockene J, eds. *The Handbook of Health Behavior Change.* 2nd ed. New York: Springer; 1998.

50. Bosworth HB. Treatment adherence. In: Miller JR, Lerner RM, Schiamberg LB, Anderson PM, eds. *The Encyclopedia of Human Ecology.* Santa Barbara, CA: ABC-Clio; 2003:686–690.

51. Dunbar-Jacob J, Burkem LE, Pucyynski S, eds. *Clinical Assessment and Management of Adherence to Medical Regimens.* Washington, DC: American Psychological Association; 1995.

52. Weissberg-Benchell J, Glasgow AM, Tynan WD, et al. Adolescent diabetes management and mismanagement. *Diabetes Care.* 1995;18(1):77–82.

53. Steele RG, Grauer D. Adherence to antiretroviral therapy for pediatric HIV infection: review of the literature and recommendations for research. *Clin Child Fam Psychol Rev.* 2003;6(1):17–30.

54. Hanson CL, De Guire MJ, Schinkel AM, Kolterman OG. Empirical validation for a family-centered model of care. *Diabetes Care.* 1995;18(10):1347–1356.

55. Wamboldt FS, Wamboldt MZ, Gavin LA, Roesler TA, Brugman SM. Parental criticism and treatment outcome in adolescents hospitalized for severe, chronic asthma. *J Psychosom Res.* 1995;39(8):995–1005.

56. Shulman N, Cutter G, Daugherty R, Sexton M, et al. Correlates of attendance and compliance in hypertension detection and follow-up program. *Cont Clin Trials.* 1982;3:13–27.

57. Ahluwalia JS, McNagny SE, Rask KJ. Correlates of controlled hypertension in indigent, inner-city hypertensive patients. *J Gen Intern Med.* 1997;12(1):7–14.

58. Shea S, Misra D, Ehrlich MH, Field L, Francis CK. Predisposing factors for severe, uncontrolled hypertension in an inner-city minority population. *N Engl J Med.* 1992;327:776–781.

59. Moy E, Bartman BA, Weir MR. Access to hypertensive care: effects of income, insurance and source of care. *Arc Intern Med.* 1995;155:1497–1502.

60. Stason W. Cost and quality trade-offs in the treatment of hypertension. *Hypertension.* 1989;12:145–148.

61. Mojtabai R, Olfson M. Medication costs, adherence, and health outcomes among Medicare beneficiaries. *Health Aff (Millwood).* 2003;22(4):220–229.

62. Ley P. Memory for medical information. *Br J Soc Clin Psychol.* 1979;18:245–255.

63. Post K, Roter D. Predictors of recall of medication regimens and recommendations for lifestyle change in elderly patients. *Gerontologist.* 1988;27(4):510–515.

64. Ruscin JM, Semla TP. Assessment of medication management skills in older outpatients. *Ann Pharmacother.* 1996;30(10):1083–1088.

65. Ferrando SJ, Wall TL, Batki SL, Sorensen JL. Psychiatric morbidity, illicit drug use and adherence to zidovudine (AZT) among injection drug users with HIV disease. *Am J Drug Alcohol Abuse.* 1996;22(4):475–487.

66. Pablos-Mendez A, Knirsch CA, Barr RG, Lerner BH, Frieden TR. Nonadherence in tuberculosis treatment: predictors and consequences in New York City. *Am J Med.* 1997;102(2):164–170.

67. Chesney MA, Ickovics JR, Chambers DB, et al. Self-reported adherence to antiretroviral medications among participants in HIV clinical trials: the AACTG adherence instruments. Patient Care Committee & Adherence Working Group of the Outcomes Committee of the Adult AIDS Clinical Trials Group (AACTG). *AIDS Care.* 2000;12(3):255–266.

68. Malow RM, Baker SM, Klimas N, et al. Adherence to complex combination antiretroviral therapies by HIV-positive drug abusers. *Psychiatr Serv.* 1998;49(8): 1021–1022, 1024.

69. Singh RB, Suh IL, Singh VP, et al. Hypertension and stroke in Asia: prevalence, control and strategies in developing countries for prevention. *J Hum Hypertens.* 2000;14(10–11):749–763.

70. Bosworth HB, Bastian LA, Grambow SC, McBride CM, Skinner CS, Fish L, Rimer BK, Siegler IC. Initiation and discontinuation of hormone therapy for menopausal symptoms: results from a community sample. *J Behav Med.* In press.

71. Horne R, Weinman J, Hankins M. The beliefs about medicines questionnaire: the development and evaluation of a new method for assessing the cognitive representation of medication. *Psych Health.* 1999;14:1–24.

72. Horne R, Weinman J. Patients' beliefs about prescribed medicines and their role in adherence to treatment in chronic physical illness. *J Psychosom Res.* 1999;47(6):555–567.

73. Blessing-Moore J. Does asthma education change behavior? To know is not to do. *Chest.* 1996;109(1):9–11.

74. Becker M, Maiman L. Sociobehavioral determinants of compliance with health and medical care recommendations. *Med Care.* 1975;13:10–24.

75. Rosenstock I. Enhancing patient compliance with health recommendations. *Journal of Pediatric Health Care.* 1988;2:67–72.

76. Burroughs TE, Pontious SL, Santiago JV. The relationship among six psychosocial domains, age, health care adherence, and metabolic control in adolescents with IDDM. *Diabetes Educ.* 1993;19(5):396–402.

77. Eldred LJ, Wu AW, Chaisson RE, Moore RD. Adherence to antiretroviral and pneumocystis prophylaxis in HIV disease. *J Acquir Immune Defic Syndr Hum Retrovirol.* 1998;18(2):117–125.

78. Report of the NIH Panel to Define Principles of Therapy of HIV Infection. *Ann Intern Med.* 1998;128(12 Pt 2):1057–1078.

79. Casado JL, Sabido R, Perez-Elias MJ, et al. Percentage of adherence correlates with the risk of protease inhibitor (PI) treatment failure in HIV-infected patients. *Antivir Ther.* 1999;4(3):157–161.

80. Cramer JA. Practical issues in medication compliance. *Transplant Proc.* 1999;31 (4A):7S–9S.

81. Gatley MS. To be taken as directed. *J R Coll Gen Pract.* 1968;16(1):39–44.

82. Watts RW, McLennan G, Bassham I, el-Saadi O. Do patients with asthma fill their prescriptions? A primary compliance study. *Aust Fam Physician.* 1997;26 (Suppl 1):S4–S6.

83. Demyttenaere K. Compliance during treatment with antidepressants. *J Affect Disord.* 1997;43(1):27–39.

84. Kribbs N, Pack AI, Kline LR, et al. Objective measurement of patterns of nasal CPAP use by patients with obstructive sleep apnea. *Am Rev Respirat Dis.* 1993;147: 887–895.

85. Wadden T, Foster GD, Wang J, et al. Clinical correlates of short- and long-term weight loss. *Am J Clin Nutr.* 1992;56(Suppl 2):271S–274S.

86. Myers ED, Branthwaite A. Out-patient compliance with antidepressant medication. *Br J Psychiatry.* 1992;160:83–86.

87. Le Pen C, Levy F, Ravily V, Beuzen JN, Meurgey F. The cost of treatment dropout in depression. A cost–benefit analysis of fluoxetine vs. tricyclics. *J Affect Dis.* 1994;31:1–18.

88. Wannamaker BB, Morton WA Jr., Gross AJ, Saunders S. Improvement in antiepileptic drug levels following reduction of intervals between clinic visits. *Epilepsia.* 1980;21(2):155–162.

89. Cramer J, Scheyer RD, Mattson RH. Compliance declines between clinic visits. *Arch Intern Med.* 1990;150:1509–1510.

90. Donovan J, Blake DR. Patient non-compliance: deviance or reasoned decision-making? *Soc Sci Med.* 1992;34(5):507–513.

91. Sleath B, Roter D, Chewning B, Svarstad B. Asking questions about medication: analysis of physician–patient interactions and physician perceptions. *Med Care.* 1999;37(11):1169–1173.

92. Schwartz J. Clinical pharmacology. In: Hazzard WR, Blass JP, Halfer JB, Ouslander JO, eds. *Principles of Geriatric Medicine and Gerontology.* 3rd ed. New York: McGraw-Hill; 1994:259–276.

93. Black D, Brand RJ, Greenlick M, Hughes G, Smith J. Compliance to treatment for hypertension in elderly patients: the SHEP pilot study. *J Gerontol.* 1987;42: 552–557.

94. Neaton J, Grimm RH Jr., Prineas RJ, et al. For the Treatment of Mild Hypertension Study Research Group. Treatment of mild hypertension: final results. *JAMA.* 1993;270:713–724.

95. Benner JS, Glynn RJ, Mogun H, Neumann SD, Weinstein MC, Avorn J. Long-term persistence in use of statin therapy in elderly patients. *JAMA.* 2002; 288(4):455–461.

96. Jackevicius CA, Mamdani M, Tu JV. Adherence with statin therapy in elderly patients with and without acute coronary syndromes. *JAMA.* 2002;288(4): 462–467.

97. Juncos L. Patient compliance and angiotension converting enzyme inhibitors in hypertension. *J Cardiovasc Pharmaco.* 1990;15:S22–S25.

98. Clark L. Improving compliance and increasing control of hypertension needs of special hypertensive populations. *Am Heart J.* 1991;121:664–669.

99. Dunbar-Jacob J, Dwyer K, Dunning EJ. Compliance with antihypertensive regimen: a review of the research in the 1980s. *Ann Behav Med.* 1991;13(1):31–39.

100. Luscher T, Vetter W. Adherence to medication. *J Hum Hypertens.* 1990;4(Suppl 1):43–46.

101. Berlowitz D, Ash AS, Hickey EC, et al. Inadequate management of blood pressure in a hypertensive population. *N Engl J Med.* 1998;339(27):1957–1963.

102. Haynes R, Sackett DL, Gibson ES, et al. Improvement of medication compliance in uncontrolled hypertension. *Lancet.* 1976;1:1265–1268.

103. Berry SL, Hayford JR, Ross CK, Pachman LM, Lavigne JV. Conceptions of illness by children with juvenile rheumatoid arthritis: a cognitive developmental approach. *J Pediatr Psychol.* 1993;18(1):83–97.

104. Wechsler H, Levine S, Idelson RK, Rohman M, Taylor J. The physician's role in health promotion—a survey of primary-care practitioners. *N Engl J Med.* 1983; 308(2):97–100.

105. Working Group on Health Education and High Blood Pressure Control. The physician's guide: improving adherence among hypertensive patients. Bethesda, MD: U.S. Department of Health and Human Services, National Institutes of Health; 1987.

106. Hill MN, Bone LR, Kim MT, Miller DJ, Dennison CR, Levine DM. Barriers to hypertension care and control in young urban Black men. *Am J Hypertens.* 1999;12:951–958.

107. Burke L, Dunbar-Jacobs JM, Hill MN. Compliance with cardiovascular disease prevention strategies: a review of the research. *Ann Behav Med.* 1997;19:239–263.

108. Lemanek KL, Kamps J, Chung NB. Empirically supported treatments in pediatric psychology: regimen adherence. *J Pediatr Psychol.* 2001;26(5):253–275.

109. Belzer ME, Fuchs DN, Luftman GS, Tucker DJ. Antiretroviral adherence issues among HIV-positive adolescents and young adults. *J Adolesc Health.* 1999;25(5): 316–319.

110. Psaty B, Koepsel TD, Wagner EH, LoGerfo JP, Inui TS. The relative risk of incident coronary heart disease associated with recently stopping the use of beta-blockers. *JAMA*. 1990;263(12):1653–1657.

111. Mallion JM, Dutrey-Dupagne C, Vaur L, et al. Benefits of electronic pillboxes in evaluating treatment compliance of patients with mild to moderate hypertension. *J Hypertens*. 1996;14(1):137–144.

112. Dunbar-Jacob J, Burke LE, Rohay JM, et al. Comparability of self-report, pill count, and electronically monitored adherence data. *Control Clin Trials*. 1996;7(Suppl 2):805.

113. Namkoong K, Farren CK, O'Connor PG, O'Malley SS. Measurement of compliance with naltrexone in the treatment of alcohol dependence: research and clinical implications. *J Clin Psychiatry*. 1999;60(7):449–453.

114. Monane M, Bohn RL, Gurwitz JH, Glynn RJ, Avorn J. Noncompliance with congestive heart failure therapy in the elderly. *Arch Intern Med*. 1994;154: 433–437.

115. Monane M, Bohn RL, Gurwitz JH, Glynn RJ, Levin R, Avorn J. The effects of initial drug choice and comorbidity on antihypertensive therapy compliance: results from a population-based study in the elderly. *Am J Hypertension*. 1997;10(7 Pt 1):697–704.

116. Rudd P, Ahmed S, Zachary V, Barton C, Bonduelle D. Improved compliance measures: applications in an ambulatory hypertensive drug trial. *Clin Pharmacol Ther*. 1990;48(6):676–685.

117. Chesney MA. Factors affecting adherence to antiretroviral therapy. *Clin Infect Dis*. 2000;30(Suppl 2):S171–S176.

118. Kimmerling M, Wagner G, Ghosh-Dastidar B. Factors associated with accurate self-reported adherence to HIV antiretrovirals. *Int J STD AIDS*. 2003;14(4): 281–284.

119. Waltherhouse DM, Calzone KA, Mele C, Brenner DE. Adherence to oral tamoxifen: a comparison of patient self report, pill counts and microelectronic monitoring. *J Clin Oncol*. 1993;11:2547–2548.

120. Pullar T, Birtwell AJ, Wiles PG, Hay A, Feely MP. Use of a pharmacologic indicator to compare compliance with tablets prescribed to be taken once, twice, or three times daily. *Clin Pharmacol Ther*. 1988;44(5):540–545.

121. Maenpaa H, Javela K, Pikkarainen J, Malkonen M, Heinonen OP, Manninen V. Minimal doses of digoxin: a new marker for compliance to medication. *Eur Heart J*. 1987;8 Suppl I:31–37.

122. Gourevitch MN, Wasserman W, Panero MS, Selwyn PA. Successful adherence to observed prophylaxis and treatment of tuberculosis among drug users in a methadone program. *J Addict Dis*. 1996;15(1):93–104.

123. Volmink J, Garner P. Interventions for promoting adherence to tuberculosis management. *Cochrane Database Syst Rev*. 2000(4):CD000010.

124. Steiner JF, Koepsell TD, Fihn SD, Inui TS. A general method of compliance assessment using centralized pharmacy records. Description and validation. *Med Care*. 1988;26(8):814–823.

125. Paterson DL, Swindells S, Mohr J, et al. Adherence to protease inhibitor therapy and outcomes in patients with HIV infection. *Ann Intern Med.* 2000;133(1): 21–30.

126. Edelman R, Eitel P, Wadhwa NK, et al. Accuracy or bias in nurses' ratings of patient compliance: a comparison of treatment modality. *Perit Dial Int.* 1996; 16(3):321–325.

127. Morisky E, Green LW, Levine DM. Concurrent and predictive validity of a self-reported measure of medication adherence. *Med Care.* 1986;24:67–74.

128. Haynes R, Taylor DW, Sackett DL. Can simple clinical measurement detect patient noncompliance? *Hypertension.* 1980;2:759–782.

129. Fleece L, Summers MA, Schnaper H, et al. Adherence to pharmacotherapeutic regimen: assessment and intervention. *Alabama J Med Sciences.* 1988; 25(4):389–393.

130. Haubrich RH, Little SJ, Currier JS, et al. The value of patient-reported adherence to antiretroviral therapy in predicting virologic and immunologic response. California Collaborative Treatment Group. *AIDS.* 1999;13(9): 1099–1107.

131. Fong OW, Ho CF, Fung LY, et al. Determinants of adherence to highly active antiretroviral therapy (HAART) in Chinese HIV/AIDS patients. *HIV Med.* 2003;4(2):133–138.

132. George CF, Peveler RC, Heiliger S, Thompson C. Compliance with tricyclic antidepressants: the value of four different methods of assessment. *Br J Clin Pharmacol.* 2000;50(2):166–171.

133. Stephenson BJ, Rowe BH, Haynes RB, Macharia WM, Leon G. Is this patient taking the treatment as prescribed? *JAMA.* 1993;269(21):2779–2781.

134. Hays R, DiMatteo MR. Key issues and suggestions for patient compliance assessment: source of information, focus of measures, and nature of response options. *J Compliance Health Care.* 1987;2:37–53.

135. Inui TS, Carter WB, Pecoraro RE. Screening for noncompliance among patients with hypertension: is self-report the best available measure? *Med Care.* 1981;19(10):1061–1064.

136. Ley P. *Communicating With Patients.* London: Croom Helm; 1988.

137. Bosworth HB, Olsen MK, Dudley T, Goldstein MK, Orr M, Oddone EZ. *Antihypertensive medication adherence: Racial, clinical and psychosocial factors.* Paper presented at the 27th Annual VA Health Service Research and Development Meetings, March, 2004; Washington, DC.

138. Rand C, Wise RA. Measuring adherence to asthma medications. *Am J Respir Crit Care Med.* 1994;149:S69–S76.

139. Kravitz RL, Hays RD, Sherbourne CD, et al. Recall of recommendations and adherence to advice among patients with chronic medical conditions. *Arch Intern Med.* 1993;153(16):1869–1878.

140. Brooks CM, Richards JM, Kohler CL, et al. Assessing adherence to asthma medication and inhaler regimens: a psychometric analysis of adult self-report scales. *Med Care.* 1994;32(3):298–307.

141. Samet JH, Libman H, Steger KA, et al. Compliance with zidovudine therapy in patients infected with human immunodeficiency virus, type 1: a cross-sectional study in a municipal hospital clinic. *Am J Med.* 1992;92(5):495–502.

142. Knobel H, Alonso J, Casado JL, et al. Validation of a simplified medication adherence questionnaire in a large cohort of HIV-infected patients: the GEEMA Study. *AIDS.* 2002;16(4):605–613.

143. Kim MT, Hill MN, Bone LR, Levine DM. Development and testing of the Hill–Bone Compliance to High Blood Pressure Therapy Scale. *Prog Cardiovasc Nurs.* 2000;15(3):90–96.

144. McDonald HP, Garg AX, Haynes RB. Interventions to enhance patient adherence to medication prescriptions: scientific review. *JAMA.* 2002;288(22):2868–2879.

145. Haynes RB, McDonald H, Garg AX, Montague P. Interventions for helping patients to follow prescriptions for medications. *Cochrane Database Syst Rev.* 2002(2):CD000011.

146. Roter DH, Hall JA, Merisca R, Nordstrom B, Cretin D, Svarstad B. Effectiveness of interventions to improve patient compliance: a meta-analysis. *Med Care.* 1998;36(8):1138–1161.

147. Zygmunt A, Olfson M, Boyer CA, Mechanic D. Interventions to improve medication adherence in schizophrenia. *Am J Psychiatry.* 2002;159(10):1653–1664.

148. Swain MA, Steckel SB. Influencing adherence among hypertensives. *Res Nurs Health.* 1981;4(1):213–222.

149. Cummings KM, Becker MH, Kirscht JP, Levin NW. Intervention strategies to improve compliance with medical regimens by ambulatory hemodialysis patients. *J Behav Med.* 1981;4(1):111–127.

150. Morisky D. Five year blood pressure control and mortality following health education for hypertensive patients. *Am J Public Health.* 1983;73:153–162.

151. Nessman D, Carnahan JE, Nugent CA. Increasing compliance: patient-operated hypertension groups. *Arch Intern Med.* 1980;140:1427–1430.

152. Mullen PD, Green LW. Meta-analysis points way toward more effective medication teaching. *Promot Health.* 1985;6(6):6–8.

153. Levy M, Robb M, Allen J, Doherty C, Bland JM, Winter RJD. A randomized controlled evaluation of specialist nurse education following accident and emergency department attendance for acute asthma. *Resp Med.* 2000;94:900–908.

154. Bailey WC, Richards JM Jr., Brooks CM, Soong SJ, Windsor RA, Manzella BA. A randomized trial to improve self-management practices of adults with asthma. *Arch Intern Med.* 1990;150(8):1664–1668.

155. Tulda A, Fumaz CR, Ferrer MJ, et al. Prospective randomized two-arm controlled study to determine the efficacy of a specific intervention to improve long-term adherence to highly active antiretroviral therapy. *J Acquir Immune Defic Syndr.* 2000;25(3):221–228.

156. Owen PM, Johnson EM, Frost CD, Porter KA, O'Hare E. Reading, readability, and patient education materials. *Cardiovasc Nurs.* 1993;29:9–13.

157. Hussey LC. Minimizing effects of low literacy on medication knowledge and compliance among the elderly. *Clin Nurs Res.* 1994;3(2):132–145.

158. Kirsch I, Jungeblut A, Jenkins L, Kolstad A. *Adult Literacy in America: A First Look at the Results of the National Adult Literacy Survey.* Washington, DC: National Center for Education, U.S. Department of Education; 1993.

159. Williams M, Parker RM, Baker DW, et al. Inadequate functional health literacy among patients at two public hospitals. *JAMA.* 1995;274(21):1677–1682.

160. Parker R, Baker DW, Williams MV, Nurss JR. The test of functional health literacy in adults: a new instrument for measuring patients' literacy skills. *J Gen Intern Med.* 1995;10:537–541.

161. Baker D, Parker RM, Williams MV, Clark WS, Nurss J. The relationship of patient reading ability to self-reported health and use of services. *Am J Public Health.* 1997;87:1027–1030.

162. Weiss B, Har G, McGee DL, D'Estelle S. Health status of illiterate adults: relation between illiteracy and health status among persons with low literacy skills. *J Am Board Fam Pract.* 1992;5:254–257.

163. Health literacy: report of the Council on Scientific Affairs. Ad Hoc Committee on Health Literacy for the Council on Scientific Affairs, American Medical Association. *JAMA.* 1999;281(6):552–557.

164. Williams M, Baker DW, Parker RM, Nurss JR. Relationship of functional health literacy to patients' knowledge of their chronic disease: a study of patients with hypertension and diabetes. *Arch Intern Med.* 1998;158:166–172.

165. Morrow DG, Leirer VO, Andrassy JM, et al. The influence of list format and category headers on age differences in understanding medication instructions. *Exp Aging Res.* 1998;24(3):231–256.

166. Morrow D, Leirer V, Altieri PB. List formats improve medication instructions for older adults. *Educ Gerontology.* 1995;21(2):151–166.

167. Pratt J, Jones JJ. Noncompliance with therapy: an ongoing problem in treating hypertension. *Primary Cardiology.* 1995;21:34–38.

168. Urquhart J. Correlates of variable patient compliance in drug trials: relevance in the new health care environment. *Adv Drug Res.* 1995;26:237–257.

169. Sivarajan ES, Newton KM, Almes MJ, Kempf TM, Mansfield LW, Bruce RA. Limited effects of outpatient teaching and counseling after myocardial infarction: a controlled study. *Heart Lung.* 1983;12(1):65–73.

170. Chisholm MA, Vollenweider LJ, Mulloy LL, et al. Renal transplant patient compliance with free immunosuppressive medications. *Transplantation.* 2000; 70(8):1240–1244.

171. Giuffrida A, Torgerson DJ. Should we pay the patient? Review of financial incentives to enhance patient compliance. *BMJ.* 1997;315(7110):703–707.

172. Brody DA. The patient's role in clinical decision making. *Ann Intern Med.* 1980;93:718–722.

173. Piette JD, Weinberger M, McPhee SJ, Mah CA, Kraemer FB, Crapo LM. Do automated calls with nurse follow-up improve self-care and glycemic control among vulnerable patients with diabetes? *Am J Med.* 2000;108(1):20–27.

174. Burnier M, Schneider MP, Chiolero A, Stubi CL, Brunner HR. Electronic compliance monitoring in resistant hypertension: the basis for rational therapeutic decisions. *J Hypertens.* 2001;19(2):335–341.

175. Bosworth HB, Oddone EZ. A model of psychosocial and cultural antecedents of blood pressure control. *J Natl Med Assoc.* 2002;94(4):236–248.

176. Joint National Committee on Detection, Evaluation, and Treatment of High Blood Pressure. *The Sixth Report of the Joint National Committee on Detection, Evaluation, and Treatment of High Blood Pressure (JNC VI).* Bethesda, MD: U.S. Department of Health and Human Services, National Institutes of Health; 1997.

177. Bosworth HB, Oddone EZ. The role of patient and provider feedback and blood pressure control. *Am Heart J.* In press.

178. Kastrissios H, Flowers NT, Blaschke TF. Introducing medical students to medication noncompliance. *Clin Pharmacol Ther.* 1996;59(5):577–582.

179. Choo PW, Rand CS, Inui TS, et al. Validation of patient reports, automated pharmacy records, and pill counts with electronic monitoring of adherence to antihypertensive therapy. *Med Care.* 1999;37(9):846–857.

180. Haynes RB, McDonald HP, Garg AX. Helping patients follow prescribed treatment: clinical applications. *JAMA.* 2002;288(22):2880–2883.

181. Bender BG. Overcoming barriers to nonadherence in asthma treatment. *J Allergy Clin Immunol.* 2002;109(6 Suppl):S554–S559.

182. Horne R. Patients' beliefs about treatment: the hidden determinant of treatment outcome? *J Psychosom Res.* 1999;47(6):491–495.

183. Taggart AJ, Johnston GD, McDevitt DG. Does the frequency of daily dosage influence compliance with digoxin therapy? *Br J Clin Pharmacol.* 1981;11(1):31–34.

184. Heyscue BE, Levin GM, Merrick JP. Compliance with depot antipsychotic medication by patients attending outpatient clinics. *Psychiatr Serv.* 1998;49(9):1232–1234.

185. Levine RJ. Monitoring for adherence: ethical considerations. *Am J Respir Crit Care Med.* 1994;149(2 Pt 1):287–288.

186. Russel M. *Behavioral Counseling in Medicine: Strategies for Modifying At-Risk Behavior.* New York: Oxford University Press; 1986.

187. Taylor CB, Miller NH. The behavioral approach. In: Wenger NK, Weinstein HK, eds. *Rehabilitation of the Coronary Patient.* New York: Churchill Livingstone; 1992:461–471.

188. Lerman C, Hanjani P, Caputo C, et al. Telephone counseling improves adherence to colposcopy among lower-income minority women. *J Clin Oncol.* 1992;10(2):330–333.

189. DeBusk RF, West JA, Miller NH, Taylor CB. Chronic disease management: treating the patient with disease(s) vs treating disease(s) in the patient. *Arch Intern Med.* 1999;159(22):2739–2742.

190. DeBusk RF, Houston Miller N, West JA. Diabetes case management. *Ann Intern Med.* 1999;130(10):863.

191. Smith PM, Kraemer HC, Miller NH, DeBusk RF, Taylor CB. In-hospital smoking cessation programs: who responds, who doesn't? *J Consult Clin Psychol.* 1999;67(1):19–27.

192. DeBusk RF, Miller NH, Superko HR, et al. A case-management system for coronary risk factor modification after acute myocardial infarction. *Ann Intern Med.* 1994;120(9):721–729.

193. Szilagyi P, Bordley C, Vann JC, et al. Effect of patient reminder/recall interventions rates. *JAMA.* 2000;284(14):1820–1827.

194. Wasson J, Gaudette C, Whaley F, Sauvigne A, Baribeau P, Welch HG. Telephone care as a substitute for routine clinic follow-up. *JAMA.* 1992;267:1788–1793.

195. Weinberger M, Tierney WM, Cowpar PA, Katz BP, Booher PA. Cost-effectiveness of increased telephone contact for patients with osteoarthritis: a randomized controlled trial. *Arthritis Rheum.* 1993;26:243–246.

196. Yusuf S, Sleight P, Pogue J, Bosch J, Davies R, Dagenais G. Effects of an angiotensin-converting-enzyme inhibitor, ramipril, on cardiovascular events in high-risk patients. The Heart Outcomes Prevention Evaluation Study Investigators. *N Engl J Med.* 2000;342(3):145–153.

197. Dunbar-Jacob J, Sereika S, Burke LE, Starz T, Rohay JH, Kwoh CK. Can poor adherence be improved? *Ann Behav Med.* 1995;1995:17.

198. Peters AL, Davidson MB, Ossorio RC. Management of patients with diabetes by nurses with support of subspecialists. *HMO Pract.* 1995;9(1):8–13.

199. Curry S, Wagner EH, Gorthaus LC. Evaluation of intrinsic and extrinsic motivation interventions with a self help smoking cessation program. *J Consult Clin Psychol.* 1991;59:318–324.

200. Strecher VJ, Kreuter MW, DenBoer DJ, et al. The effects of tailored smoking cessation messages in family practice setting. *J Fam Pract.* 1994;39(3):262–270.

201. Rimer B, Orleans CT, Fleisher L, et al. Does tailoring matter? The impact of a tailored guide on ratings of short-term smoking-related outcomes for older smokers. *Health Education Research.* 1994;9:69–84.

202. Kreuter MW, Bull FC, Clark EM, Oswald DL. Understanding how people process health information: a comparison of tailored and nontailored weight-loss materials. *Health Psychol.* 1999;18(5):487–494.

203. Jameson JP, VanNoord GR. Pharmacotherapy consultation on polypharmacy patients in ambulatory care. *Ann Pharmacother.* 2001;35(7–8):835–840.

204. Tsuyuki RT, Johnson JA, Teo KK, et al. A randomized trial of the effect of community pharmacist intervention on cholesterol risk management: the Study of Cardiovascular Risk Intervention by Pharmacists (SCRIP). *Arch Intern Med.* 2002;162(10):1149–1155.

205. Grant RW, Devita NG, Singer DE, Meigs JB. Improving adherence and reducing medication discrepancies in patients with diabetes. *Ann Pharmacother.* 2003;37.

206. Miller N, Hill MN, Kottke T, Ockene IS. The multilevel compliance challenge: recommendations for a call to action. A statement for healthcare professionals. *Circulation.* 1997;95:1085–1090.

207. Haynes RB, Montague P, Oliver T, McKibbon KA, Brouwers MC, Kanani R. Interventions for helping patients to follow prescriptions for medications. *Cochrane Database Syst Rev.* 2000(2):CD000011.

208. Ockene IS, Hayman LL, Pasternak RC, Schron E, Dunbar-Jacob J. Task force #4—adherence issues and behavior changes: achieving a long-term solution. 33rd Bethesda Conference. *J Am Coll Cardiol.* 2002;40(4):630–640.

209. Williams AB. Adherence to HIV regimens: 10 vital lessons. *Am J Nursing.* 2001;101(6):37–43.

Chapter 7

Patient Adherence in Rehabilitation

Sandra Zinn

OVERVIEW

Rehabilitation is a descriptive term for a treatment process involving restoration of function or capacity, a process that is common to many medical disciplines. Indeed, the roots of the word *rehabilitation* translate as "to restore to a former rank or capacity." This restoration process can be applied to any damaged body organ, system, or function, from lung capacity to vocal flexibility, from cardiac muscle strength to athletic prowess. With rehabilitation thus broadly conceived, a cogent discussion of the issues surrounding patient adherence to rehabilitation would be nearly unmanageable. In this chapter, discussion is restricted to rehabilitation as practiced primarily by physiatrists and physical, occupational, and speech therapists. These practitioners seek to restore the physical functioning necessary for common activities of daily living such as walking, grooming, dialing a telephone number, or traveling to a medical appointment. Traditionally, physical medicine and allied rehabilitation disciplines have focused on treatment of musculoskeletal disorders, generally the result of orthopedic and/or neurological conditions that interfere with functioning in daily life. I follow that tradition here and consideration of adherence issues is focused on these types of disorders and diseases. However, some of these disorders—in particular, neurological disorders—often affect cognition, necessitating cognitive rehabilitation in addition to physical rehabilitation. Discussing adherence in rehabilitation without addressing cognitive impairment is akin to trying to diagnose a stalled automobile without referring to its electrical system. Therefore, cognitive impairment and its rehabilitation are reviewed throughout the chapter.

As one examines the issue of treatment adherence with respect to rehabilitation, it is immediately apparent that this is largely uncharted territory—at least if one searches the literature using the standard terms. Few studies address either the occurrence of, or promising interventions to, nonadherence to therapies. There are several reasons why this is the case. First, this is due, in part, to the relative youth of the discipline. Physical medicine and rehabilitation is one of the youngest medical disciplines. Muscle rehabilitation, for example, was not systematized as a treatment until the early 1900s. Physical medicine developed during World War I as a consequence of the need to treat disabilities inflicted by the war; the term *physiatrist* was first used in 1938. Although interventions for disabilities such as crutches and slings have doubtless been used since humans first began fashioning tools, the first reported controlled clinical trial in physical rehabilitation was conducted after World War II by Dr. Howard Rusk (1). Thus, research on the effectiveness of rehabilitation medicine is still relatively in the early stages of development and the literature has focused largely on the physical determinants of rehabilitation success. The field is still establishing the basic effectiveness of rehabilitation services (2). Once it is clear that treatment applications have been optimized to the extent that they can be without consideration of adherence issues, then obstacles to successful outcomes such as adherence will receive greater attention.

The relative dearth of literature relating to adherence issues may also arise from the unique challenges of rehabilitation medicine. The wide range of medical conditions producing a referral for rehabilitation—including stroke, multiple sclerosis (MS), traumatic brain injury (TBI), spinal cord injury (SCI), tumors, arthritis, muscular dystrophies, Parkinson's disease, and encephalitis—and the diversity of potential treatments—including such distinct therapies as prosthesis fitting, grooming adaptations, speech rehabilitation, remediation of spatial attention or disinhibition, and psychosocial adjustment to handicap—complicates the process of systematic investigation. Adding complexity to studies of adherence in rehabilitation are three considerations not found in chronic disease management more generally. First, for many diseases or conditions that include rehabilitation in the therapeutic armamentarium, there is a qualitatively different acute phase as well as a postacute or chronic phase. Second, the rehabilitation population includes a large proportion of patients with physical or cognitive impairments that are not readily accounted for in the normative-based theoretical models of adherence presented in chapter 2. Finally, the chronic handicaps experienced by many rehabilitation patients and the adaptive technology (such as wheelchairs or walkers) often required have an associated social stigma not found in diseases or treatments that do not significantly alter appearance.

However, though traditional adherence models have not found widespread application in this field, a careful sifting of studies on rehabilitation outcomes reveals a growing awareness of multiple factors that impact treatment success, especially those related to *patient motivation*. Anecdotally, physical, occupational, and speech therapists have repeatedly experienced the patient-centered barriers to successful involvement in therapy and can readily relate what they have observed. There is little evidence, however, that these observations have been systematically studied (3). Outcome studies for conditions that impact functional abilities such as joint replacement or stroke often report findings involving patient factors that are relevant to adherence difficulties, although typically these are not described as such. Furthermore, studies of rehabilitation success often acknowledge the importance of motivation, although it is rarely directly measured. Thus, despite little formal attention to patient adherence as an issue, there are numerous indicators in the existing literature suggesting that its role in rehabilitation outcomes is large indeed. This is not surprising. Adherence is fundamentally an issue of patient participation, and participation may be more crucial to successful rehabilitation than to other medical treatment regimes. Rehabilitative therapy cannot be "visited upon" the patient; the functioning to be restored can be remolded only through activity, especially purposeful activity versus repetitive or passive motion. It may be that the consideration of motivation and persistence is, of necessity, so central to the practice of rehabilitation that treatment efficacy and adherence may be inextricably intertwined (4).

In the sections that follow, I explore the current state of knowledge regarding patient adherence issues in rehabilitation, identify the gaps in knowledge and theory, and suggest a research agenda. As previously noted, the study of adherence in rehabilitation and physical medicine is a research frontier, and as such, it presents numerous opportunities to enterprising investigators to make substantive contributions. Accordingly, the application of existing theories and methodologies are reviewed; the emphasis is on the unique adherence issues in this field that suggest new conceptualizations and new methodological approaches for both epidemiological and interventional investigations. The goals of this chapter are to stimulate interest in these novel problems, to show how rehabilitation can serve as a paradigm for adherence, and to initiate the process of thinking through the methodological challenges that these novel problems create.

EPIDEMIOLOGY OF DISABILITY AND RISK FACTORS FOR NONADHERENCE

Magnitude of the Problem

On a number of counts, physical and rehabilitation medicine and, hence, patient adherence to rehabilitation therapies, is taking on increasing importance. For one, the aging of Western populations translates into a growing market for disability-related services. There is also improved survivorship for conditions, such as stroke or spinal cord injury, associated with residual deficits necessitating rehabilitation. Thus the incidence of disabled individuals is rising. Technological advances in materials and assistive devices expand the range of individuals who may benefit from them and may also spur greater interest in barriers to their use. In addition, the costs associated with rehabilitation are likely to motivate concerns for its effectiveness. A discussion of some of the specifics associated with each of these follows.

A brief consideration of the numbers involved in the expansion of the disabled population is telling. Stroke, for instance, is the leading cause of disability in North American adults (5); a single stroke is likely to result in disability in at least one activity of daily living (ADL; e.g., walking, dressing, toileting) (6). The incidence rate for stroke has been estimated at 700,000 annually (7) and may be increasing after a period of stabilization (8, 9). Estimates of the proportion of disablement among stroke survivors range from one to two thirds (10, 11). Surgical conditions requiring rehabilitation occur more frequently but are less likely to result in residual disability. The prevalence of hip replacement is 32 operations per 1,000 persons and for knee replacement, rates are 20 per 1,000 (12, 13). The incidence of first-time major amputation is approximately 32/100,000; rates are higher if second amputations are considered (14).

As the need for rehabilitation is chronic in some disorders, incidence rates convey neither the extent of the services needed, nor the protracted effects of nonadherence in these conditions. For example, traumatic brain injury or spinal cord injury patients are high-frequency, long-term users of rehabilitation because of the chronicity of the disability. Whereas the incidence of spinal cord injury is about 10,000 annually (15), the prevalence rate of 230,000, or 721 per million (16), is the more meaningful figure in assessing impact. In traumatic brain injury, the prevalence rate is similar (623 per million) (17), with 80,000 to 90,000 estimated to suffer long-term disability (18). Two thirds to four fifths of traumatic brain injury patients have one or more ADLs that require ongoing assistance (17, 19). Extrapolating from these estimates for the major disorders requiring rehabilitation, it is likely that there are at least 1 million potential users of rehabilitation therapies.

Technological advances also increase the focus on rehabilitation effectiveness. The development of new materials for synthetic joints, for example, has increased the number of arthroplasties performed in the United States. The imminent development of neural implants to stimulate nervous activity in paretic limbs will also call for the development or refinement of rehabilitative techniques.

Disability translates into increased costs, and less effective rehabilitation due to nonadherence worsens the fiscal impact. Functional rehabilitation is costly in terms of space, equipment, and personnel requirements. The cost of rehabilitation in stroke alone is estimated to be $7 billion per annum (20). Thus, optimizing its efficacy is crucial to increasing its cost-effectiveness. One might speculate that smaller facilities would be more likely to add rehabilitation units, thereby increasing the availability of these services, if these therapies were more cost-effective. Moreover, disability taxes multiple societal resources. Many disabled patients become high consumers of health care generally, further straining the resources of overburdened institutions. There are costs to society for untreated disability, not only in loss of productivity by the patients but also by those who must spend time caring for them.

Risk Factors for Nonadherence

Review of the literature for likely factors affecting adherence in rehabilitation is complicated by the fact that few articles in this field conceptualized their findings using adherence constructs. (The constructs of "participation," "motivation," and "alertness" or "cognitive impairment" that are assessed in various studies are likely related to several different aspects of adherence (4), but this research remains to be done.) Thus patient attributes and aspects of care that were judged likely to be relevant to rehabilitative treatment success form the bulk of this discussion. Evidence that these elements serve as barriers to treatment or treatment motivation is reviewed.

It is recognized that there are multiple disorders resulting in disability that requires rehabilitation, and these may each be associated with different adherence factors. However, as noted earlier there are several factors unique to rehabilitation users that are common to more than one disorder or condition within that population. These unique factors deserve an expanded consideration. Other factors appear to be common themes in adherence no matter what the condition or treatment. The lack of studies on adherence necessarily places our review at a broad anticipatory level for the most part, due to the lack of detailed information. The following discussion of adherence factors presents first the more unique and then the "typical" factors, with comments on their relevance in specific medical conditions referred for functional rehabilitation.

Unique Considerations for Adherence in Rehabilitation

Increasing effectiveness through addressing rehabilitation adherence will require understanding of issues not typically central to chronic disease that pertain to treatment of functional disabilities. As introduced earlier, there are three aspects of adherence in rehabilitation that make it unique: a qualitatively different acute phase as well as a chronic phase, high rates of physical or cognitive impairments, and the social stigma associated with handicap. Each of these is considered in this section.

Acute Care. The requirement for rehabilitation during the acute phase, in stroke or spinal cord injury, for example, presents adherence challenges that are different from those involved in the maintenance of prophylactic treatment. Physical medicine is not the only medical discipline to treat acute patients, but other acute treatment regimens typically require less active participation. Needed medications can be injected or dripped into an IV, for example; restraints can be used if the patient attempts to pull the IV out. When the therapeutic emphasis, however, is on functional abilities rather than disease, barriers to the patient's participation can effectively block treatment. (See Table 7.1 for a list of barriers.) This may occur in the acute stages following stroke, traumatic brain injury, spinal cord injury, or orthopedic surgery. These barriers may impact physical capacity, motivation, the patient–provider process, or all three.

Addressing these barriers is important, as rehabilitation during this time period may prove crucial for better recovery. For example, new evidence for poststroke brain plasticity from animal models suggests that rescue of perilesional tissue is more likely if functional use is initiated soon after the stroke (21). Such activity must be active, not passive. There is evidence that greater cortical reorganization, and thus greater functional recovery, is achieved with targeted, skill-oriented rehabilitative training than with unaided spontaneous recovery (22). Early induction of rehabilitation in stroke (23) and traumatic brain injury (24) has been associated with improved outcomes. In hip fracture patients, physical therapy in acute care reduced the total number of treatment days required compared to those receiving postacute therapy only (25), although another study of early treatment initiation in these patients found no outcome differences (26).

Chief among the factors affecting a patient's participation in rehabilitation in the acute phase is delirium. Acute confusion was identified in 20% of hip fracture patients (27); rates in patients with neurological conditions are likely higher (28). Attempting rehabilitative exercises in physical proximity to a patient who responds to his incomprehension of the situation by becoming violent is an adherence problem rarely encountered by the pri-

TABLE 7.1
Barriers to Participation in Acute Care

Delirium or transient confusion
Acute language impairment
Emotional lability
Reduced endurance
Postsurgical complications

mary-care physician seeking to get her patient to take his medications! Yet this appears to be an instance in which the patient needs to exhibit a different behavior in order to improve his health, and hence an adherence issue. In the acute setting, however, promoting adherence is better understood as a providing a facilitative external structure for the patient, rather than promoting individual responsibility. The provider must take a more active role in ensuring the outcome; this is addressed further in the section on treatment techniques. Although delirium affects the patient–provider process primarily, motivation in these patients is certainly derailed. One study reported that delirium persisting at 1 month was associated with poor rehabilitation outcome (29); however, another assessing orientation and alertness postsurgery found that these were not significantly associated with ambulation outcome in a multivariate model (30).

Confusion may also arise acutely in patients without delirium who require rehabilitation. Patients with central nervous system damage, or who are medically frail, may lapse into confusion when tired or excessively stimulated. Confusion and poor endurance are frequent in traumatic brain injury, stroke, and postsurgery (amputation or joint replacement) patients, especially if elderly.

Language impairments, or aphasias, are another major impediment to treatment. Aphasia is prevalent in stroke and acute traumatic brain injury patients. Although language capacity may return to a large extent later in recovery, the loss of this staple of human interaction can be devastating to the acute-care patient. Receptive aphasia, involving the comprehension of spoken or written language, impacts the capacity of the patient to understand and follow directions. Conveying a sequence of steps to be followed or communicating the purpose of a particular therapeutic technique becomes extremely difficult. The patient's frustration with incomprehension may become a direct barrier if complex activity is experienced as overwhelming. Expressive language deficits may present less of a barrier to rehabilitation, although clearly the patient's inability to describe goals or communicate their needs will affect the treatment process.

Emotional lability is another common sequela of stroke (31) and traumatic brain injury that is more often present in the acute phase with improvement over the days postinjury. Patients may respond to stress or effort with overwhelming emotions that interrupt their focus on rehabilitative exercises. More rare are the catastrophic emotional reactions, resulting in semiarbitrary outbursts of tears or laughter, that arise as a consequence of certain types of brain damage. As this is a behavioral response, typically not subjectively experienced as deep feeling (32), it is unlikely to impair the patient's response to treatment. It may nevertheless affect progress due to the response of the rehabilitation therapist, concerned by this unseemly behavior.

Chronic factors may also become greater barriers to participation in acute care. Factors such as poor resilience and medical comorbidity are known to influence long-term rehabilitation outcomes (23), but are also likely to affect acute-care performance. Both factors are associated with delayed initiation of postsurgery rehabilitation (33). Surgical complication has been identified as the primary reason for unanticipated transfer off of a rehabilitation unit (34). These chronic factors may also be associated with increased risk for the acute factors noted previously.

In summary, during the acute phase of disorders requiring rehabilitation, several factors with high prevalence in this population reduce the patient's ability to participate in rehabilitation therapy. Often, the barriers to participation cannot be overcome by the patient, so that greater responsibility for facilitating treatment falls to the provider. Optimization of the efficacy of physical medicine may require initiating treatment at the earliest opportunity. This will be dependent on the development of compensatory techniques to "bridge the gap" for extremely ill patients whenever possible. Research on such compensatory techniques is discussed in the section on interventions.

Cognitive Impairments. Another unique class of barriers to adherence arises from the high rates and wide range of cognitive impairments found in the rehabilitation population. If one asks physical and occupational therapists what factor most detracts from effective rehabilitation, the nearly universal first answer is "cognitive impairment." This is not surprising, as such impairments are an unfortunately common occurrence in the rehabilitation population. Stroke, traumatic brain injury, Parkinson's disease, multiple sclerosis, and cerebral neoplasms all have high rates of cognitive impairment. These impairments cover a full spectrum. Traumatic brain injury is nearly synonymous with cognitive impairment, with even mild cases demonstrating a constellation of behavioral problems despite apparently normal cognition on formal testing (35). Subtle executive function impairment, affecting attention, problem-solving, and planning behaviors needed for rehabilitation, is often present in early Parkinson's disease (36). Later in the disease course, Parkinson's patients often have impairment of visuoperceptual function (37). Among stroke patients especially, a broad spectrum of cognitive deficits may exist in varying combinations (38), challenging the provider's ingenuity in facilitating rehabilitation progress. In one report, more than 60% of the stroke patients had at least one higher cognitive deficit (39). Diabetes patients, with their high comorbidity of vascular disease, who are rehabilitating postamputation may also experience cognitive decline that affects their daily functioning (40, 41).

In addition to their prevalence, these impairments of communication, learning, and initiative are unique in that they create barriers to treatment at a more basic or profound level than those addressed by the usual adherence models. The social psychology theories on which many models of adherence are based operate at the level of beliefs and motivations but assume that basic cognition is intact. Mental processes that are assumed operational in typical adherence models may be altered or absent in patients with cognitive impairment. For example, how should one motivate a patient with anosognosia (lack of recognition of one's dysfunction as a result of brain damage) to engage in rehabilitation exercises? Such patients do not acknowledge their infirmities. To conceptualize these patients as being in the precontemplative stage (motivational interviewing theory) is not likely to be helpful. These impairments often become fundamental impediments to the treatment process. They may also be targets of the treatment process. Rehabilitation is first and foremost a process of relearning by the mind–body system. The altered configuration of body functioning must adjust to the demands of a patient's physical and psychosocial world. Even mild deficits in attention or memory can prove to be a barrier to this process and, hence, rehabilitation outcome (42). Patients with cognitive impairment typically require greater environmental support in order to effectively participate in treatment. Some of this support may involve assisting them in compensating for cognitive impairments. Improving their adherence requires techniques that minimize the effects of their barriers and maximize their strengths. Such techniques, which rely heavily on mechanisms used in behavioral treatment, are being developed primarily by providers working with traumatic brain injury patients and are discussed later in this chapter. The remainder of this section presents common categories of cognitive impairment (see Table 7.2) and discusses the effects of each on rehabilitation.

Awareness and Attention. Deficits of attention, learning, perception, language, persistence, initiation, and motivation have unique detrimental influences on treatment adherence; indeed, an entire chapter could be devoted to their effects and potential remediation techniques. Impairments of various kinds of awareness constitute a unique category of personal be-

TABLE 7.2
Cognitive Deficits Affecting Participation

Awareness and attention
Anosognosia
Language impairment (covered earlier)
Impulsivity
Executive functions
Memory
Apraxia

liefs that may interfere with treatment. Among these, perhaps the most frequently studied impairment of awareness is unilateral neglect, also known as attentional or spatial neglect, which is exemplified by inattention to one side of the body and its body space (43–45). In severe forms, patients may fail to dress or groom the body on the side opposite the cerebral lesion. The effect of inattention on training techniques for positioning and strengthening of extremities is obvious. Attentional neglect has a demonstrated association with increased disability (46) and reduced autonomy (42). Patients with neglect demonstrate lower mobility and reduced ADL functionality compared to patients without neglect, despite receipt of identical rehabilitation programs (47). The more "garden-variety" impairments of divided attention and flexible (switching) attention have also been associated with worse outcomes in stroke (48).

Anosognosia. The clearest direct threat to treatment adherence may come from anosognosia, in which the patient is unaware of their incapacity despite persistent effects of physical limitations (46, 49). Anosognosia is common early in recovery from traumatic brain injury (50) and occurs in approximately one quarter of both right- and left-hemisphere strokes (51). There appear to be different types of anosognosia, some due to a neurologically based incapacity for such perception, and some due to faulty reasoning or other executive dysfunction that may prove more amenable to direct intervention (52, 53). These different types of unawareness may have different effects on the rehabilitative process, but this is yet unknown. In that all types of anosognosias compromise patients' acceptance of the need for sustained rehabilitative effort, they represent a serious detraction from adherence. They also reduce adherence to safety precautions (51).

Impulsivity. Anterior circulation strokes and traumatic brain injury are often associated with impulsivity, which increases the risk of violating safety guidelines that are a cornerstone of disability education (54). Lesion-induced impulsivity is a significant risk factor for falls (54). Furthermore, impulsive patients who must learn to compensate for impaired balance or motor strength would seem to be at risk for slowed learning due to more frequent mistakes and potential for discouragement.

Executive Functions. Other executive-function impairments are also common in anterior circulation strokes and traumatic brain injury. Multiple sclerosis patients are vulnerable to executive-function deficits as well (55). These disorders of problem solving, planning, and abstract thinking can prevent the patient from being an effective collaborator in his or her treatment. Patients whose problem solving is compromised will have difficulty deriving compensatory solutions for physical impairments, and may be more likely to lapse into passive dependency. Impaired short-term memory and processing capacity often accompany problem-solving deficits, leading to a generalized cognitive impairment that saps the psychological resilience of the afflicted individual. Impairments of planning ability not only directly affect the capacity to implement ordered movement sequences (such as bed transfers) and anticipate consequences, but they likely affect an individual's ability to comprehend the rationale for rehabilitation and pursue an orderly course of treatment. Practitioners working with such patients may use their clinical acumen to adapt treatment processes for these deficits, but such adaptations need to be empirically tested and deliberately employed.

Memory. Memory disorders are also frequent in rehabilitation patients. Memory circuits are complex and distributed across many cortical and subcortical regions (56). Stroke (39), traumatic brain injury (57), and spinal cord injury (58) can produce lesions resulting in memory deficits. Memory deficits may be common in postsurgical patients as well (59); normal aging is also associated with mild retrieval losses that may be exacerbated by illness. Memory impairments in stroke patients have been related to rehabilitation progress (60). Premorbid learning disabilities have been associated with the occurrence of cognitive deficits in spinal cord injury patients (61); premorbid learning difficulties may have the same impact on treatment gains as injury-induced ones.

Apraxia. Apraxia, loss of skilled arm and hand movements, results from several types of cognitive impairment that can occur in either hemisphere (62). These different lesions are associated with different types of apraxia (63), each with its own threat to rehabilitation progress and presumably responding to different interventions. The incidence of apraxias in stroke is about 15% (39). Left-hemisphere prevalence may be as high as 28% (64) but may recover better than right-hemisphere apraxia (65). Apraxia clearly affects IADLs (independent activities of daily living) but it is not clear if it impacts adherence directly. Apraxia has been associated with worse outcome (66) but has also been shown to have little effect on functional outcome (67). Its frequent association with language or other higher level impairments may account for variations in its predictive strength (62, 68). Apraxia appears best rehabilitated by compensatory strategies (69).

Despite the fact that cognitive impairment is not directly related to disorders requiring joint replacement (i.e., osteoporosis or arthritis) and subsequent rehabilitation, its influence has been examined in a few studies. Dorra et al. found that hip fracture patients who showed poor functional gain during inpatient rehabilitation had a higher prevalence of behaviors indicating cognitive or participation problems documented in their charts than patients with good functional gains (70). Cognitive impairment has also been shown to predict ambulation (71) and independent living (72) 1 year postarthroplasty. However, another study found that presurgical mobility appeared to offset the negative effect of cognitive impairment (73). Establishing the prevalence of mild or moderate nondementing cognitive impairment in this population, which might otherwise go unaddressed, is merited.

Stigma-Related Barriers.   Finally, though treatments such as oral medication or change in diet are not obvious in casual encounters with treated patients, rehabilitation patients often require assistive devices such as wheelchairs or artificial limbs that identify them as disabled. Whereas patients treated for other conditions may have to internally address their loss of health, for rehabilitation patients, this loss is open to public scrutiny and reaction. The need for such obvious devices highlights the patient's deviance from the nearly universal cultural value of able-bodiedness. Social ostracism may accompany an infirmity that makes one visibly different. Although "disability rights" and an emphasis on fair access for disabled individuals in the United States has led to modifications of public edifices have probably reduced the stigma of disability, there is a societal contribution to its occurrence in a rehabilitation patient that is unlikely to be legislated away. The World Health Organization (WHO) model of disability uses the term *handicap* to label the barriers to a disabled individual that are of social origin. Patients who perceive such social barriers (whether accurately or not) may develop emotional responses that in turn become barriers to successful functional rehabilitation.

Patients whose prosthetics or orthotics are difficult to use and unsightly are more likely to discard them (74), unless doing so results in a significant restriction of activity. This creates a risk for nonuse of the stigmatized devices. More research is needed, however, to guide such treatment. Little information is available on who is at risk for sensitivity to stigma. Although older individuals' disability is more often viewed as socially acceptable (75), this does not necessarily mean that older persons would be less likely to experience stigma-related anxiety. There may be personality factors as well that influence one's susceptibility to stigma. Any contributor to social isolation, either currently or in the past, could sensitize a patient to potential sources of ostracism such as use of assistive devices.

The factors unique to rehabilitation that affect adherence arise from the fact that the loss of health in conditions necessitating rehabilitation create difficulties in real-world functioning; that is, the loss of health is by definition disabling. Rather than being "simply" a pathology of an organ system or physiological process, conditions requiring rehabilitation have impacted the interaction of the physique with its environment, and thus affect the individual in a dimension rarely considered in other medical domains. Assessment and treatment of these factors must expand the concept of adherence, then, in novel directions.

Factors Related to Adherence

In addition to these factors associated with disabling disorders, patient factors common to other disorders that may affect adherence are also found among those who present for rehabilitation. Common factors are discussed next (see Table 7.3).

Demographic Characteristics. Empirically, there is essentially no evidence that the patient's age, gender, or race, per se, puts him or her at higher risk for nonadherence to rehabilitative therapies. Theoretically, certain demographic populations may be more at-risk for nonadherence by virtue of being at higher risk for disorders requiring rehabilitation. Stroke, osteoporosis, arthritis, Parkinson's, and diabetes (due to risk of amputation) are clearly more prevalent among older individuals. As the relative proportion of persons over the age of 65 grows, the number of individuals with deconditioning (frailty), joint replacements, amputation, and stroke-related disability will increase. Decreased physical activity and increased obesity compound the problem. Similarly, African Americans are at greater risk for amputations and stroke. At the other end of the age continuum, younger persons are more likely to sustain traumatic injuries requiring rehabilitation, such as spinal cord injury and traumatic brain injury. Despite the better prognosis for survival and recovery that youth sometimes confers, severe traumatic injuries can create lifelong disability and the need for sustained treatment to prevent deterioration.

Patient demographic characteristics also may be associated—or confounded—with factors that are indicators of nonadherence to therapies and, hence, give the appearance of being risk factors. Some of these demographically defined groups may be more at-risk for nonadherence due to the same characteristics that place them at higher risk for disability. Impulsivity and substance abuse are risk factors for traumatic injury that also complicate adherence (76). Persons from lower socioeconomic groups may not

TABLE 7.3
Other Factors Affecting Participation

Demographic characteristics
Personality factors
Mood disorders
Frailty and other conditions affecting effort
Social support

only be more likely to experience greater disability from the same impairment as those of higher socioeconomic groups (77), but may experience problems in accessing rehabilitation services (78, 79) that might give the appearance of nonadherence. The decreased coping ability, the increased risk of cognitive impairment, frailty, and high comorbidity experienced by older individuals may also increase the risk of nonadherence, although this has not been definitively demonstrated. Though studies suggest that advanced age per se does not appear to be a factor in rehabilitation effectiveness in a postsurgical population (80, 81), it may be that age-related factors such as poor resilience and medical comorbidity influence these patients' adherence to exercises. For example, aging does seem to be associated with the success of rehabilitation after amputation. Several studies found that younger patients had better recovery (82, 83), but it is unclear whether this was related to adherence or more purely medical (healing and strength) factors. An examination of disability and handicap in amputees found that motivation, age, and comorbidity were highly correlated (84). Increased illness burden may reduce the coping resources of older patients, resulting in lower motivation for the arduous task of learning to walk with a prostheses.

Personality. Personality factors, such as an external locus of control (see chap. 2) or narcissistic traits, may prevent the patient from taking adequate responsibility for her or his participation (85). A cross-sectional study of knee surgery patients preoperatively indicated a relationship between locus of control and perceived functional limitations (86); however, the effect of these variables on rehabilitation effectiveness was not examined. Fortinsky et al.'s study of self-efficacy did examine outcomes and found that hip replacement patients with higher presurgical self-efficacy had a greater chance of ambulation recovery (87). A similar study found that hip replacement patients who had high self-efficacy prior to surgery showed better postsurgery functioning and less depression (88). Stroke patients who demonstrated self-efficacy for self-care showed better quality-of-life outcomes at 6 months (89). Dependency traits may actually produce resistance to improvement as there is secondary gain from the individual remaining disabled.

Psychological factors have received significant research attention in spinal cord injury. In spinal cord injury as in no other condition, there is a recognition that coping with disability is important to the overall health of the individual (90). Long-range goals include achievement of a stable medical condition without dependence on the medical establishment (91). In addition, there is an emphasis on psychological coping as an end in itself. The impact of psychological state on therapeutic effectiveness, which is often centered on continuing self-care, has been documented in several studies (92). Feeling "out of control" during admission is associated with worse long-term outcomes (93). Styles of coping have been studied in spinal cord injury patients and appear to be stable across the first year postinjury (85). Although these patients had a more external, fatalistic attributional style than controls, most spinal cord injury respondents endorsed adaptive coping styles. Those who had emotion-focused coping styles experienced more depression and rehospitalization than those using problem-focused coping (94).

Mood Disorders. Though depression and other psychiatric disorders can affect adherence in all medical conditions, mood disturbances are a neurological sequelae of stroke (95) and traumatic brain injury (96). Depression is prevalent in stroke patients (although Desmond et al., ref. 97, found much lower rates than others report) and has a demonstrated impact on rehabilitation outcomes (98–100). Depression in some patients is best understood as a reaction to the sudden, radical loss of physical function and capacity for independent living. In others, the mood disorder appears to be due to physiological alterations in brain function, particularly in patients in which the frontal-striatal or left frontotemporal circuits are damaged (101). Multiple risk factors for depression often coexist in rehabilitation patients. Clinical observations suggest very high rates of depression in spinal cord injury patients, but there appear to be discrepancies among observers, and between observers and psychometric instruments (102, 103). Minorities and women typically have higher rates of depression (98, 104). Those with chronic pain are more likely to experience depression (93, 105), and pain and depression become correlated over time in spinal cord injury patients (106). Depression in spinal cord injury patients has been associated with increased disability, both objective and subjective measures (107). Depression also reduces the activity level independently of disability (108). In stroke patients, depression is associated with slower progress in rehabilitation (98, 99), as well as poorer long-term outcomes (109). Patients with a history of mood disorder appear to use rehabilitation less effectively than their nondepressed counterparts (110).

Some of the effects of depression on rehabilitation may be due to its effect on locus of control or self-efficacy cognition. Patients who see themselves as inadequate due to their depressive syndrome are likely to view any impairment as more disabling. Depression in multiple sclerosis patients has been shown to increase their self-ratings of disablement (111), which in turn may reduce their motivation for pursuing healthy behaviors. Depression has been associated with lower self-efficacy in stroke patients (112). However, the relationship of depression and psychological responses to disability appear complex (113); further investigation is needed.

The course of depression is typically not static, and further exploration of this phenomenon is merited. Rates of depression in spinal cord injury patients during their initial inpatient stay range from 14% to 33%

(114–117), irrespective of whether the injury was of traumatic etiology or not (118). This rate peaks near the end of lengthy inpatient admissions (117), and appears to drop to 15% or less in community-dwelling patients (108). Various models of depression, such as a diathesis stress model combining neurobiological bases with social triggers, have been proposed to explain the trajectory of depressive symptoms (117, 119). In stroke patients, Zinn et al. reported that the 12-month trajectory of depression was associated with stroke subtype (120). Depression in arthroplasty patients appears to peak at 3 months postsurgery but dwindles by 9 months (121). Unfortunately, rates of depression are often highest soon after onset of the condition requiring rehabilitation.

Other mood or emotional disorders can effect rehabilitation, although these are less well studied than depression (122). Irritability is common early in recovery and may or may not be associated with confusion, exacerbating uncooperativeness. Lesion-induced mania can also occur after right-hemisphere strokes affecting the frontal or temporal lobes or limbic connections thereof (122, 123), resulting in disinhibition that interferes with rehabilitative processes. As many spinal cord injuries are from traumatic causes, the incidence of posttraumatic stress disorder (PTSD) has also been examined and affects one fifth of spinal cord injury patients (124). There is also evidence that concomitant cognitive impairment affects not only psychosocial adaptation but also medical stability (61).

Frailty.   Frailty and fatigue may reduce effort during rehabilitation, through either physical incapacity or beliefs and fears about one's incapacity, or both. Frailty seems likely to impact self-efficacy for mobility and other physical activities. Cognitions related to the frailty that necessitated arthroplasty, for example, would likely affect one's motivation during rehabilitation. Many hip replacement patients required surgery due to fractures caused by falls; amputation patients also fear falls (125). Fear of falling, if not addressed in rehabilitation, may reduce self-efficacy and attenuate rehabilitation progress (126). Older persons who have perceived themselves as brittle due to osteoporosis may be physically timid and lack self-efficacy for rehabilitation, yet we can find no consideration of this in the literature.

Distinguishing between medically related frailty, psychologically induced poor effort, and lesion-induced impairments such as fatigue, apathy, or impaired motor initiation can be a significant problem for the rehabilitation team. Fatigue and lethargy are common sequelae of stroke and can affect the patient's ability to persist in rehabilitative exercises even when motivation is unaffected (127). Some evidence suggests that persistent fatigue may be a physiological sequela of stroke (127). Apathy is one of the neurological consequences of traumatic brain injury (127) that seems likely to impact effort.

Pain also affects the amount of effort a patient exerts in the rehabilitation process. The amount of pain experienced also affects residual disability (128) and may affect, and be affected by, coping and adherence issues. Stump pain or phantom limb pain has been documented in up to 50% of amputation patients (129). Phantom limb pain has been associated with poorer postamputation adjustment (130), and one study of correlates of phantom pain and its change over time found that catastrophizing cognitions were associated with less improvement in perceived pain (131). Models of pain in amputation, such as the biopsychosocial model, may lead to further understanding of the role of pain in adherence, and thus potential treatments, but need further development (132).

Both depression and cognitive impairment are more prevalent in older rehabilitation patients, who may therefore be at risk for poor treatment adherence. Premorbid deconditioning can reduce physical endurance and patients' abilities to participate with adequate frequency and intensity in rehabilitative exercises (34). Older patients tolerated an intense physical therapy regime well in one study (133), but another found significant attrition that was thought to be related to motivation as well as medical burden (134).

Social Support.   The role of families and other sources of social support are crucially important factors in the adherence equation for rehabilitation treatment. Family perceptions can influence patient satisfaction with rehabilitation outcome (135). Recovery from stroke and other disabling conditions often requires extended outpatient treatment. The family or significant others must often become the facilitators of continued participation in rehabilitation exercises (136). Loss of gains achieved during inpatient rehabilitation once the patient is discharged are common (137). Higher levels of social support increase long-term outcome for moderate to severe stroke patients discharged to home (138). Social support at home appears to be as important for postsurgical functional recovery as it is for stroke (139). In fact, arthroplasty patients appear to increase their levels of social support postoperatively, despite improved functioning (140).

Family support also seems to relate to abnormal illness behavior (AIB), in which patients adopt the sick role (141). AIB has been associated with functional progress postdischarge (141). If a family member encourages a patient, however subtly, to remain in a victim role (131), or becomes resentful due to misunderstanding of the changes caused by the stroke in the patient, then the support that is often needed to sustain rehabilitation may be compromised. Characteristics of families associated with poststroke treatment adherence include high levels of communication and problem-solving efficacy (142).

For amputation patients, there are more frequent investigations of psychosocial factors related to treatment adherence and recovery in the literature. This may be due to the recognition of amputation's impact on body image (143) and self-esteem, clearly psychological issues. Furthermore, patients with amputations as a result of trauma may be younger; for them an emphasis on living as full a life as possible requires a more global approach to rehabilitation (144). Outcomes relevant to patient satisfaction and adjustment, in themselves clinically useful, have been investigated. One study of return to work after amputation did not examine psychological factors directly but concluded that they might account for their finding of frequent failure to return to work (145). The utility of providing psychological support and treatment of any tendency for social withdrawal in amputees has been documented (146). Having a partner increases life satisfaction for amputees and presumably improves their adjustment to wearing a prostheses (147). The perception of social support also led to reductions in phantom limb pain in amputees 5 months postsurgery (131). However, even in this literature, an examination of the impact of these psychosocial constructs on the process and effectiveness of rehabilitation itself has not been conducted.

The need for social support, or the type of support needed, may change over time. Support in the form of information may be important initially, but emotional support becomes more crucial as the rehabilitating individual contemplates returning to society (148). The relationship between social support and coping may also be complex, and warrants further investigation (148).

Not only the family, but the larger sociological institutions that the patient is a part of, can impact the effectiveness of rehabilitation. The standards and expectations of a rehabilitation therapist or unit can influence outcome (149). A highly motivated patient who is considered a poor candidate may have difficulty overcoming staff perceptions (150). Once in the community, a patient who has adapted his self-view of disability may find that further adaptation to the responses of others is necessary, especially if his disability is stigmatized. Iatrogenic causes of poor adherence due to polypharmacy are common in the elderly (151). Other instances of the social environment affecting patient participation in rehabilitation are likely to arise from the multiple combinations of disabilities, individuals, and social situations.

INTERVENTIONS TO IMPROVE ADHERENCE
IN REHABILITATION

Interventions are guided by the conceptualization of the desired state. Interventions to improve adherence, then, would be guided by one's conceptualization of adherence to rehabilitation treatment. As I have argued, however, treatment in rehabilitation occurs in multiple modalities across a wide range of pathological conditions that necessitate a reconceptualization of adherence. This enhancement of the concept unfolds along two primary dimensions: our understanding of patient responsibility/participation, and our understanding of healthy functioning as being primarily an interactive process, an adaptation of the individual to the environment.

The first reconceptualization involves a recognition that participation varies not only across individuals, but within individuals and across treatment demands. The typical model of adherence implies that the patient bears responsibility for participating in and contributing to the success of treatment. Indeed, this emphasis on the patient's autonomous participation is precisely why the term *compliance* has fallen into disfavor. However, because rehabilitation therapies span a broad range of conditions, the need for a spectrum in the degree of appropriate responsibility required must be recognized. Patient responsibility should be viewed as existing on a continuum from minimal to total, with care providers taking more responsibility when the patient is less able (152). During recovery, providers facilitate the assumption of increasing responsibility by the patient. As noted previously, during acute care when the rehabilitation patient may be minimally able to act in her own behalf, the practitioners may need to ensure participation using external structure. On the other hand, maximizing the recovery possible through long-term rehabilitation may demand not just adherence but an extraordinary commitment on the part of many patients. Physiatrists and other rehabilitation providers can optimize the patient's return to functioning by promoting high levels of dedication to the task of recovery.

Interventions to Maximize Commitment

The phenomenal advances in physical and rehabilitative medicine that have or will yield new, more effective therapies are likely to push consideration of adherence as optimized participation to the forefront. Recent studies of neural plasticity show that neural circuits undergo adaptive changes throughout life, particularly in response to acute demands such as learning and recovery from injury (153). Neuroplasticity drugs, once developed, will still not replace the need for the patient to learn to function with their altered physique (154). Neural plasticity serves the individual by enabling adaptation to new conditions, but novel neural connections are established only through practice (155, 156). This is why current therapies relying on neural plasticity, such as constraint-induced therapy, require persistent practice and effort to obtain results. Effective rehabilitation demands the patient's thorough participation, yet interventions promoting the patient's engagement are nonexistent.

Developing these interventions will require a conceptualization of rehabilitation as an process of radical adaptation. One's gross physiology is altered, in movement, sensation, or composition. The rehabilitation patient must learn to perform the same ADLs with a body and/or brain that may be radically altered. The retuning required must occur at the mental, psychological, and social levels as well as the physical. This is very unlikely to occur in 1 hour per day of scheduled treatment. The moderately to severely disabled patient must be dynamically engaged in this process that is essentially a reconfiguring of her life. Intense or multidisciplinary approaches to rehabilitative treatment demonstrate great promise (133, 157, 158). Treating the whole person can generate a synthesizing effect that improves outcomes, but only if the patient who is the target of the multimodal treatments can participate at all levels.

The amounts of energy and attention needed to realign one's body, mind, and environment are similar to that of the original learning process that occurred in childhood. Grasp, reach, balance, and stride develop through the persistent zeal of the young child, who repeats an action again and again in an apparently tireless effort to achieve mastery. Remastery of functional skills requires a similar investment of time and energy on the part of the patient. One occupational therapist wryly observed that farmers, being used to hard work, tended to do well in rehabilitation, but that salesmen, used to talking their way to success, often had more difficulty. Rehabilitation often demands a supranormal effort for fullest success, so characteristics that are associated with high achievement, such as those of outstanding athletes, are likely to predict successful outcomes. Those factors that sports psychologists must consider in optimizing performance should be considered by rehabilitation practitioners in optimizing adherence.

In summary, the potential for recovery from existing as well as new techniques may not be realized unless we conceptualize adherence as the nearly full-time job of a rehabilitation patient, and facilitate their engagement in this task. However, the extent to which high levels of recovery, and thus maximal effort, are required for an individual are determined by that individual's functional adaptation needs. This introduces the second reconceptualization of adherence: that functional health is always situational, and the patient's adaptational success depends on the environment to which it is adapting.

For example, it makes very little sense for a demented individual who has been living in a nursing home to be considered nonadherent if they do not exert heroic efforts to recover from a stroke. In disabled individuals, optimal functioning may be achieved by compensating and adapting to a new health state. Some of this compensation and adaptation occurs within the patient; some of it occurs in the patient's environment. Appropriate functioning, which is the goal of rehabilitation, is determined by the interaction of patient and environment. Thus a failure of rehabilitation can be due to a failure of the environment to adapt to or compensate for the individual's irremediable disability. Better outcomes from rehabilitation involve enabling a patient to function in a wider variety of environments; this suggests that teaching the patient how to solicit the proper compensation from her or his environment is an important part of rehabilitation. This concept is addressed further in the discussion of adjustment to disability later in this section; both of these extensions of the adherence concept are integral to interventions for the unique factors affecting adherence in rehabilitation.

Interventions for the Acute Phase of Care

In the acute phase when disease sequelae may impair the patient's ability to be a willing and able partner in rehabilitative therapy, facilitation is achieved by providing a fairly concrete supportive scaffolding for the patient. Early in the course of treatment, responsibility for participation may reside largely with the provider, whose goal is to enable the patient to take increasing responsibility for participation. Intervention techniques, then, must construct a bridge from the patient's current incapacity to the next step forward in self-management.

Rehabilitation-related research on patient adherence that is conducted according to this conceptualization of patient responsibility may yield techniques for facilitating adherence earlier in the acute phase especially for patients who are currently considered poor candidates for treatment. Examples may be found from the literature on treating traumatic brain injury patients, in which practitioners have developed treatment protocols for dependent, severely impaired individuals (159). Analyses of which incapacities are barriers and identification of the natural *zone of proximal improvement* (where recovery is next likely to proceed, to modify Vygotsky's phrase) are a necessary first step in this research.

Other patients require far more structure from the environment to succeed. Often these patients have significant brain damage that results in persistent maladaptive, treatment-interfering behaviors. Practitioners working with traumatic brain injury patients have developed treatment protocols for dependent, severely impaired individuals (159). Strict behavioral systems that are implemented systematically across staff must be employed, and staff must be trained to respond consistently to target behaviors. Such intensive programs are clearly costly, but principles derived from them may be useful on a smaller scale to assist acute patients.

Interventions for Cognitive Impairment

Although cognitive impairment itself may be the target of remediation, we restrict our description to those techniques designed to prevent or minimize the impairment from interfering with the rehabilitation process. Because there are few data on applying these techniques to rehabilitation tasks, this discussion targets those areas of greatest promise for such application. It should be noted that the treatment effects of cognitive rehabilitation tend to wash out over time without continued intervention. Continued outpatient utilization of learned strategies is thus crucial to the maintenance of functional gains.

Aphasia. Patients who can no longer verbally organize their understanding or responses often have difficulty learning. These patients have to learn how to plan, communicate, and conduct their lives without language. Proprioceptive or biofeedback methods of training, which increase the patients' sensitivity to their body states through visual feedback, may be effective with these patients (160). Such patients are highly dependent on social support and the rehabilitation team can improve outcomes by assisting these patients in developing and integrating their social networks.

Anosognosia. Remediation of impaired awareness can be facilitated in some cases by gradually pointing to the effects of disabilities that the patient cannot apprehend (161). Having patients predict performance then evaluate their predictions, for example, can improve realistic anticipation (162). For other patients, however, confrontational approaches only exacerbate the difficulty, and bypassing the cognitive disbelief by focusing on behavioral implementation may meet with more success (163). At times, the threat to the patient's integrity is sufficiently disruptive as to prevent treatment (164). In severe cases, the practitioner may have to decide whether to win over the patient to perform compensatory techniques that the patient is still unable to perceive the need for. Maintaining rapport and mutual respect in this situation is difficult but necessary to provide needed care.

Disinhibition. For this threat to adherence, behavioral approaches, based on techniques that selectively increase or decrease the frequency of specific responses, may be "best practices." Some behavioral control may return naturally in the course of recovery, but instituting a behavioral plan makes it possible for rehabilitation to proceed in the interim. Such approaches work best when they are explicit, detailed, and reinforced by both team and family members. These can be applied to safety procedures, the learning of transfers (165), or other treatment-interfering impulsive behaviors.

Executive-Function Disorders.   For these cognitive impediments to rehabilitation, creative techniques must be developed to recover or compensate
for any of several component functions that may be impaired. Attentional
deficits are one of these components that interfere with therapy but prove
resistant to rehabilitation. Interventions typically involve computer-based
training (166, 167) and may show gains after treatment, but attentional
control does not readily generalize to real-life tasks. Wilson and colleagues
reported success with external cuing systems for a patient with deficits in
planning and executing activities (168). Organizational skills are also frequently impaired in executive dysfunction; external support in the form of
an organized environment can be effective (169). During rehabilitation,
multiple opportunities for organizing the patient's therapeutic environment usually exist and may provide the repetitive opportunities for learning that these patients require. In some patients, frontal damage may reduce the patient's sensitivity to reward, so alternative training incentives
such as response cost are required (112). Virtual-reality programs may also
provide new rehabilitation techniques that focus on real-world behavioral
sequences for attention and other executive function disorders (170).

Memory Disorders.   Mild deficits in traumatic brain injury may show a response to intervention but moderate deficits appear to show little benefit
(171). In a small-group controlled trial, stroke patients receiving a memory-
training intervention showed improvement on the training task but little
generalization to other memory tasks (172). These studies suggest that
compensatory strategies may be more effective in improving functioning
and quality of life. The use of calendars and notebooks are the most familiar compensatory aids. Memory compensations that are spontaneously developed by patients are likely to be less effective than those developed
systematically (57). Errorless learning techniques involve training the individual to rely on written manuals and notebooks set up for the patient's
needs (173). Memory uncertainty is sidestepped with the rote use of these
materials, and reduces frustration on the part of the patient. The use of mi-
crocomputers and handheld electronic devices shows promise (174), and
seems a natural avenue for treatment in a discipline that has already developed interventions for the incorporation of devices into a daily regime. To
date, compensatory strategies and learning techniques for rehabilitation
material (i.e., step sequence in bed transfers, exercise regimens) have
rarely been empirically tested. Wilson, however, has provided a review of
techniques that are applicable to rehabilitation settings (175).

Interventions for Mood and Anxiety Disorders

Interventions for mood disorders that affect rehabilitation are usually
based on pharmacological or cognitive-behavioral therapy. These methods
appear to work with the same effectiveness in a rehabilitation population as

they do in other patient groups. To the extent that depression is a response to disability onset, group therapy may be effective (176). Cognitive behavioral interventions for distressed geriatric rehabilitation patients enable participants to achieve similar rehabilitation outcomes as their nondistressed peers (177). Developing methods to increase the rates of detection and treatment of mood and anxiety disorders in rehabilitation candidates is perhaps the most crucial issue here.

Interventions for Adjustment to Visible Disability

One important source of adherence difficulties with physical disabilities and prostheses, as previously mentioned, is the associated stigma (74). Medical professionals, who may be inured to the presence of impairment, may fail realize the full effect of stigma on their patients, and thus aggravate its impact by failing to address it directly. Emphasis in rehabilitation may be on how to properly use an orthotic device, without assisting the patient in considering the cost–benefit ratio of such use.

The solution may be not to "fix" the person, but to adapt the treatment (the prosthesis). Improving the appearance and skin verisimilitude of prostheses increase patients' adaptation to them and their willingness to participate in more normal activities (178). The factors to be considered are likely a combination of prosthetic type, patient concerns, and available technology for adapting the device to minimize concerns about appearance. Pursuing this comedogenic category of intervention would initially require an elaboration of which concerns are associated with which devices. Such a detailed natural history may drive the development of technology to respond to the highlighted issues.

There are other patient-centered psychological issues that are best addressed with psychotherapeutic interventions. When the very need for, or act of engaging in, the healthy behavior is a threat to one's self-image, assisting the individual in negotiating self- and social acceptance may need to come first. Studies are needed to determine whether standard interventions for adjustment to illness are sufficient, or whether modules specifically addressing social or body image aspects of disability are warranted. A recent review of adaptation to disability in spinal cord injury noted that empirical definition of the problem has only begun (179).

Existing evidence suggests that blanket treatment approaches will not suffice. Coping style, associated in other disorders with adherence, has been associated with adjustment to wearing prostheses (130); yet it appears that there are different coping styles used by wheelchair patients with different disorders (180)! Different age groups may also require different interventions. Distressing levels of concern about one's altered appearance may be more likely in young persons (130), perhaps because infirmity is more acceptable in older persons. Different treatments may be efficacious for adjustment to disability at different points in the disability process. Although advance preparation is not always possible, facilitating adjustment by openly discussing likely outcomes with patients prior to surgery or prosthetic provision has been found beneficial (143). For patients who already have prostheses, emotional disclosure may be more effective in promoting self-acceptance and thus adaptation (181).

Treatment modalities that have proven beneficial for adjustment to illness in other medical conditions may be adapted for adjustment to the stigma of disability. Cognitive therapy can provide a structured means of reviewing and updating beliefs about the usefulness and impact of prosthetics in verbally oriented patients. For some patients, behavioral interventions such as exposure therapy techniques, used to treat anxieties or phobias, may speed the reduction in self-consciousness that appears to develop gradually in the natural course of adaptation to orthoses (182). In some cases, the negative impact of stigma may respond to the cognitive-behavioral interventions used to support dietary or lifestyle changes in the face of contravening social pressure. Rehabilitation scientists may also want to draw on the body image literature from breast cancer studies, translating those concepts and methodologies to a new population. These studies have yet to be done, but the benefits to patients faced with an altered self-image are likely to be significant.

Adjustment to Disability in General

In large part, the issue of adjustment to disability involves shifting the patient from being "disabled" to being "re-abled" (183). Amputation patients themselves have noted that psychological factors, including expectations, influence their ambulation success after their amputation (184). Individuals can cope better with their alteration in functioning if they perceive themselves as having control over their future through their capacity to improve their condition and its ramifications. Clearly, Bandura's concept of self-efficacy applies here, and several studies have investigated this or related approaches to adjustment issues impacting rehabilitation. Older rehabilitation patients who received a self-efficacy-boosting intervention demonstrated higher participation and reported less pain at discharge (185). Marks has reviewed the application of self-efficacy theory in arthritis (186), and parallel investigations in other rehabilitation disorders would seem likely to produce similar results. Interventions to build confidence and increase self-efficacy may be reflected in improved functioning at discharge (126).

Coping style shows promise as a point of intervention. In a study of coping in prosthetics patients, denial was found to be more common in those who lost a limb due to trauma, suggesting that interventions directed at this maladaptive avoidance of disability awareness in trauma patients may improve prosthetics fit and use (130). Fostering problem-oriented coping rather than emotion-oriented coping may improve mood and reduce rehospitalization (94). A stress appraisal and coping (SAC) model, and its related intervention of coping effectiveness training, has been applied with good results to spinal cord injury patients (187, 188). The SAC model posits that health and mood are moderated by a person's appraisal of events as stressful and their confidence in their ability to cope with perceived stressors. Coping effectiveness is achieved by matching coping mechanisms to problems. Problems that cannot be resolved (such as the loss of limb function due to injury) respond best to coping that focuses on acceptance and adaptation of internal expectations. Relaxation may promote this type of coping in spinal cord injury patients (189). Active problem solving (i.e., problem-oriented as opposed to a passive, feeling-oriented style) has been associated with better adaptation to amputation (190), so development of active coping responses in patients who do not self-generate them would seem to be a fruitful avenue of treatment. This may also promote an orientation toward the future rather than the past, which has been implicated as conducive to adjustment to prosthesis (130). Hypnosis has even been used to reduce negativity and increase motivation for rehabilitative exercises (191).

Family and friends also affect the patient's sense of self-efficacy. Families who directly or inadvertently encourage a disabled person's self-perception as a victim can influence rehabilitation outcomes (131). Families who encourage problem solving can contribute to a patient's self-efficacy (192). Community group exercise-and-support programs (193) can be used to help older or disabled patients stay active. Empowering traumatic brain injury patients to draw on their societal networks beyond the family (194) for support and practical assistance has proven helpful. As noted previously, effective rehabilitation likely requires enabling patients to elicit necessary support, structure, and adaptation from their social environments.

IMPLICATIONS FOR RESEARCH AND CLINICAL PRACTICE

Completing the Epidemiology of Adherence in Rehabilitation

The epidemiology of adherence or nonadherence to rehabilitation therapies is at a rudimentary stage of development. An understanding of the magnitude of problem and associated risk factors are lacking. Thus, we need estimates of the occurrence of specific adherence problems in rehabilitation for specific disorders, and within disorders, for specific therapies; a nosology identifying likely syndromes of disability requiring greater environmental support is also required.

Initial Steps

A consistent terminology to denote the problem with treatment adherence is necessary to achieve the scientific rigor that is especially crucial. Use of the term *motivation* is common among rehabilitation practitioners, but is ill-defined and possibly prejudicial (4). Rehabilitation-specific measures of treatment readiness, expectancies, and self-efficacy for exercises and training are likely needed. Some instruments of this type exist (195–197), but lack an overarching conceptual framework or consistency of approaches.

Establishing Baseline Efficacy

One reason that adherence lacks attention in rehabilitation is that the basic effectiveness of rehabilitation services has not been established. Rehabilitation has been referred to as a "black box" for that reason (2). Multiple disease- and physiology-related factors influence outcomes after rehabilitation, and these have not been well characterized. Some functional recovery will spontaneously occur after stroke without rehabilitation, for example, whereas others may be so frail and deconditioned that even intense, targeted rehabilitation may fail to restore much functionality (133). Identification of patient factors influencing selection for participation in treatment studies is needed to measure and analyze the effect of treatment confounds. Identification of groups excluded from studies would assist in highlighting patient groups for whom traditional treatment must be supplemented or replaced by targeted techniques. Although this type of research is proceeding apace, the need for further evaluation of key treatment parameters and targeted, meaningful outcomes can scarcely be overemphasized.

The effectiveness of specific rehabilitative treatment techniques needs to be established to provide a sound basis for adherence research. There is considerable variability in the results of controlled trials for specific rehabilitative therapies, with little evidence of reduced mortality or long-term disability (198). However, use of specific outcomes such as earlier return-to-home or patient satisfaction has indicated improved outcomes for sophisticated rehabilitation programs. These studies would not only yield data on the current efficacy of particular techniques, but would distinguish more promising techniques from those with a weaker empirical basis. Adaptations in applications of treatment by therapists are often ignored, and yet such adaptations often constitute an alteration of the basic treatment package in response to patient factors that may affect outcome. Both preventive (i.e., for bedsores and contractures) and restorative therapies may need to be investigated.

Targeting Interventions

Better understanding of barriers is needed to improve the efficacy of rehabilitation interventions. Multiple questions need to be answered. How do patients view their own participation in the rehabilitation process? How do their expectations for recovery change over time? What factors impact acceptance of disability? How does acceptance of disability affect motivation? What attributes enable patients to persist in therapy in the face of miniscule functional gains? Though studies addressing these issues are limited in the physical medicine literature, there is a body of clinical knowledge that can be used to direct investigations in the interim. Investigating those factors associated with successful rehabilitation and adaptation to disability can generate a model of the attributes of effective patients (199). Patient characteristics contradictory to these become the focus of epidemiological investigations and development of interventions.

Promoting Adherence After Discharge

A key element in the issue of adherence in rehabilitation is the postdischarge need for ongoing training, exercise and generalization of techniques. This necessitates continued therapeutic activity by patients who are typically facing multiple life challenges. Creating a "portable rehabilitation system" to provide a therapeutic environment and increase the likelihood of sustained rehabilitative effort is a challenging but necessary goal for physical medicine (200, 201). The disciplines of rehabilitation must develop new routes of administration and delivery techniques. Early, supported discharge may be effective (202), but attrition in home-based, independent exercise programs is high (203). Home visits by therapists, however, appear to be as effective as clinic- or inpatient-based programs (204). Home visits may also increase effectiveness of rehabilitation by acting as boosters to motivation and by bringing a "hospital context" to the home environment. Alternately, interventions that boost supportive family characteristics may improve adherence long-term (142). Recovery from hip surgery at 1 year postsurgery was better for patients who received home visits spaced over time than those with an inpatient 1-month rehabilitation stay (205). Maintaining functionality gains from inpatient treatment in a cost-effective manner may require the development of local outpatient centers (206), community services (198) or lay therapists to facilitate ongoing treatment.

SUMMARY

In rehabilitation, a fundamental issue of adherence is the issue of adjustment to disability. One has to be able to begin living in accordance with new health facts, whether these involve the need for medication, exercise, diet change, or an artificial limb. Encouraging participation in rehabilitation may be best conceptualized as a coaching process. Selecting a goal, developing a game plan, and encouraging the patient when the pursuit of success becomes daunting would thus be an important model of intervention. The primary goal would be to adapt oneself and one's environment to enable a positive, rewarding life to continue beyond rehabilitation.

This focus on adherence can stimulate approaches to rehabilitation research that will not just identify the "human factors" that are important in recovery, but will also provide a road map for the process from program entry to beyond discharge. An integral part of the rehabilitation process would be assessment of those patient attributes that may prevent the goal from being reached. Means of transferring "ownership" of the therapeutic process and empowering patients to alter old habits and foster new ones, both in themselves and in their familiar environments, would be central to the practitioner's tool kit. Characterization of successful rehabilitation patients beyond their physical attributes can facilitate the identification of higher-risk patients. New techniques will need to be developed for patients at-risk for failure. Cognitive impairment is a huge issue, due to its prevalence and its manifold effects on rehabilitation efficacy. Psychiatric disorders and maladaptive coping styles represent another large area of concern. Maintenance of therapeutic exercise postdischarge may translate into a powerful source of outcome gains. Development of interventions for these and for those adherence issues unique to rehabilitation such as acute-care demands and issues with prostheses are best undertaken by partnerships among those who have the relevant knowledge: rehabilitation scientists, physical-medicine clinicians, and investigators in the mental-health and behavioral-medicine fields.

REFERENCES

1. Association of Academic Physiatrists. History of Physiatry. *www.physiatry.org.* Available at: http://www.physiatry.org. 2003.

2. Pomeroy VM, Tallis RC. Need to focus research in stroke rehabilitation. *Lancet.* 2000;355(9206):836–837.

3. Bajo A, Fleminger S. Brain injury rehabilitation: what works for whom and when? *Brain Injury.* 2002;16(5):385–395.

4. Maclean N, Pound P, Wolfe C, Rudd A. The concept of patient motivation: a qualitative analysis of stroke professionals' attitudes. *Stroke.* 2002;33(2):444–448.

5. Truelsen T, Mahonen M, Tolonen H, et al. Trends in stroke and coronary heart disease in the WHO MONICA Project. *Stroke.* 2003;34(6):1346–1352.

6. Di Carlo A, Baldereschi M, Gandolfo C, et al. Stroke in an elderly population: incidence and impact on survival and daily function. The Italian Longitudinal Study on Aging. *Cerebrovascular Diseases.* 2003;16(2):141–150.

7. Williams GR, Jiang JG, Matchar DB, Samsa GP. Incidence and occurrence of total (first-ever and recurrent) stroke. *Stroke.* 1999;30(12):2523–2528.

8. Feigin VL, Lawes CM, Bennett DA, Anderson CS. Stroke epidemiology: a review of population-based studies of incidence, prevalence, and case-fatality in the late 20th century. [comment]. *Lancet. Neurology.* 2003;2(1):43–53.

9. Wolfe CD. The impact of stroke. *Br Med Bull.* 2000;56(2):275–286.

10. Hankey GJ, Jamrozik K, Broadhurst RJ, Forbes S, Anderson CS. Long-term disability after first-ever stroke and related prognostic factors in the Perth Community Stroke Study, 1989–1990. *Stroke.* 2002;33(4):1034–1040.

11. Prencipe M, Ferretti C, Casini AR, Santini M, Giubilei F, Culasso F. Stroke, disability, and dementia: results of a population survey. *Stroke.* 1997;28(3):531–536.

12. Fear J, Hillman M, Chamberlain MA, Tennant A. Prevalence of hip problems in the population aged 55 years and over: access to specialist care and future demand for hip arthroplasty. *Br J Rheumatol.* 1997;36(1):74–76.

13. Tennant A, Fear J, Pickering A, Hillman M, Cutts A, Chamberlain MA. Prevalence of knee problems in the population aged 55 years and over: identifying the need for knee arthroplasty. *BMJ.* 1995;310(6990):1291–1293.

14. Group TG. Epidemiology of lower extremity amputation in centres in Europe, North America and East Asia. The global lower extremity amputation study group. *Br J Surg.* 2000;87(3):328–337.

15. Ergas Z. Spinal cord injury in the United States: a statistical update. *Central Nervous System Trauma.* 1985;2(1):19–32.

16. Berkowitz M. Assessing the socioeconomic impact of improved treatment of head and spinal cord injuries. *J Emerg Med.* 1993;11(Suppl 1):63–67.

17. Moscato BS, Trevisan M, Willer BS. The prevalence of traumatic brain injury and co-occurring disabilities in a national household survey of adults. *J Neuropsychiatry Clin Neurosci.* 1994;6(2):134–142.

18. Thurman DJ, Alverson C, Dunn KA, Guerrero J, Sniezek JE. Traumatic brain injury in the United States: a public health perspective. *J Head Trauma Rehabil.* 1999;14(6):602–615.

19. Dawson DR, Chipman M. The disablement experienced by traumatically brain-injured adults living in the community. *Brain Inj.* 1995;9(4):339–353.

20. Duncan P. Evaluating the outcomes of stroke. *Monitor.* 1998;3(3A).

21. Levin HS, Grafman J, eds. *Cerebral Reorganization of Function After Brain Damage.* New York: Oxford University Press; 2000:xvi.

22. Nudo RJ, Barbay S, Kleim JA. Role of neuroplasticity in functional recovery after stroke. In: Levin HS, Grafman J, eds. *Cerebral Reorganization of Function After Brain Damage.* New York: Oxford University Press; 2000:168–200.

23. Musicco M, Emberti L, Nappi G, Caltagirone C, Italian Multicenter Study on Outcomes of Rehabilitation of Neurological P. Early and long-term outcome of rehabilitation in stroke patients: the role of patient characteristics, time of initiation, and duration of interventions. *Arch Phys Med Rehabil.* 2003;84(4):551–558.

24. Wagner AK, Fabio T, Zafonte RD, Goldberg G, Marion DW, Peitzman AB. Physical medicine and rehabilitation consultation: relationships with acute functional outcome, length of stay, and discharge planning after traumatic brain injury. *Am J Phys Med Rehabil.* 2003;82(7):526–536.

25. Harada ND, Chun A, Chiu V, Pakalniskis A. Patterns of rehabilitation utilization after hip fracture in acute hospitals and skilled nursing facilities. *Med Care.* 2000;38(11):1119–1130.

26. Koval KJ, Aharonoff GB, Su ET, Zuckerman JD. Effect of acute inpatient rehabilitation on outcome after fracture of the femoral neck or intertrochanteric fracture. *J Bone Joint Surg Am.* 1998;80(3):357–364.

27. Duppils GS, Wikblad K. Acute confusional states in patients undergoing hip surgery: a prospective observation study. *Gerontology.* 2000;46(1):36–43.

28. Brust JCM, Caplan LR. Agitation and delirium. In: Bogousslavsky J, Caplan LR, eds. *Stroke Syndromes.* 2nd ed. Cambridge: Cambridge University Press; 2001: 222–231.

29. Marcantonio ER, Flacker JM, Michaels M, Resnick NM. Delirium is independently associated with poor functional recovery after hip fracture. *J Am Geriatr Soc.* 2000;48(6):618–624.

30. Barnes B. Ambulation outcomes after hip fracture. *Phys Ther.* 1984;64(3): 317–323.

31. Caplan B, Moelter S. Stroke. In: Frank RG, Elliott TR, eds. *Handbook of Rehabilitation Psychology.* Washington, DC: American Psychological Association; 2000: 75–108.

32. Feinstein A, Feinstein K, Gray T, O'Connor P. Prevalence and neurobehavioral correlates of pathological laughing and crying in multiple sclerosis. *Arch Neurol.* 1997;54(9):1116–1121.

33. Kehlet H. Multimodal approach to control postoperative pathophysiology and rehabilitation. *Br J Anaesth.* 1997;78(5):606–617.

34. Siegler EL, Stineman MG, Maislin G. Development of complications during rehabilitation. *Arch Intern Med.* 1994;154(19):2185–2190.

35. Varney NR, Menefee L. Psychosocial and executive deficits following closed head injury: implications for orbital frontal cortex. *J Head Trauma Rehabil.* 1993;8(1):32–44.

36. Owen AM, Sahakian BJ, Hodges JR, Summers BA, al. e. Dopamine-dependent frontostriatal planning deficits in early Parkinson's disease. *Neuropsychology.* 1995;9(1):126–140.

37. Troster AI. Movement and demyelinating disorders. In: Nussbaum PJSPD, ed. *Clinical Neuropsychology: A Pocket Handbook for Assessment.* Washington, DC: American Psychological Association; 1998:266–303.

38. Boettger S, Prosiegel M, Steiger H-J, Yassouridis A. Neurobehavioural disturbances, rehabilitation outcome, and lesion site in patients after rupture and re-

pair of anterior communicating artery aneurysm. *J Neurol Neurosurg Psychiatry.* 1998;65(1):93–102.

39. Hoffmann M. Higher cortical function deficits after stroke: an analysis of 1,000 patients from a dedicated cognitive stroke registry. *Neurorehabil Neural Repair.* 2001;15(2):113–127.

40. Sinclair AJ, Girling AJ, Bayer AJ. Cognitive dysfunction in older subjects with diabetes mellitus: impact on diabetes self-management and use of care services. All Wales Research into Elderly (AWARE) Study. *Diabetes Res Clin Pract.* 2000; 50(3):203–212.

41. Gregg EW, Yaffe K, Cauley JA, et al. Is diabetes associated with cognitive impairment and cognitive decline among older women? Study of Osteoporotic Fractures Research Group [see comments]. *Arch Intern Med.* 2000;160(2):174–180.

42. Paolucci S, Antonucci G, Gialloreti LE, et al. Predicting stroke inpatient rehabilitation outcome: the prominent role of neuropsychological disorders. *Eur Neurol.* 1996;36(6):385–390.

43. Cherney LR, Halper AS, Kwasnica CM, Harvey RL, Zhang M. Recovery of functional status after right hemisphere stroke: relationship with unilateral neglect. *Arch Phys Med Rehabil.* 2001;82(3):322–328.

44. Pizzamiglio L, Antonucci G, Judica A, Montenero P, Razzano C, Zoccolotti P. Cognitive rehabilitation of the hemineglect disorder in chronic patients with unilateral right brain damage. *J Clin Exp Neuropsychol.* 1992;14(6):901–923.

45. Robertson IH, Tegner R, Tham K, Lo A, Nimmo-Smith I. Sustained attention training for unilateral neglect: theoretical and rehabilitation implications. *J Clin Exp Neuropsychol.* 1995;17(3):416–430.

46. Appelros P, Karlsson GM, Seiger A, Nydevik I. Neglect and anosognosia after first-ever stroke: incidence and relationship to disability. *J Rehabil Med.* 2002; 34(5):215–220.

47. Paolucci S, Antonucci G, Grasso MG, Pizzamiglio L. The role of unilateral spatial neglect in rehabilitation of right brain-damaged ischemic stroke patients: a matched comparison. *Arch Phys Med Rehabil.* 2001;82(6):743–749.

48. McDowd JM, Filion DL, Pohl PS, Richards LG, Stiers W. Attentional abilities and functional outcomes following stroke. *J Geront B Psychol Sci Soc Sci.* 2003;58(1): P45–P53.

49. Katz N, Fleming J, Keren N, Lightbody S, Hartman-Maeir A. Unawareness and/ or denial of disability: implications for occupational therapy intervention. *Can J Occup Ther.* 2002;69(5):281–292.

50. Ranseen JD, Bohaska LA, Schmitt FA. An investigation of anosognosia following traumatic head injury. *International Journal of Clinical Neuropsychology.* 1990;12 (1):29–36.

51. Hartman-Maeir A, Soroker N, Katz N. Anosognosia for hemiplegia in stroke rehabilitation. *Neurorehabil Neural Repair.* 2001;15(3):213–222.

52. Jehkonen M, Ahonen JP, Dastidar P, Laippala P, Vilkki J. Unawareness of deficits after right hemisphere stroke: double-dissociations of anosognosias. *Acta Neurol Scand.* 2000;102(6):378–384.

53. Giacino JT, Cicerone KD. Varieties of deficit unawareness after brain injury. *J Head Trauma Rehabil.* 1998;13(5):1–15.

54. Rapport LJ, Webster JS, Flemming KL, et al. Predictors of falls among right-hemisphere stroke patients in the rehabilitation setting. *Arch Phys Med Rehabil.* 1993;74(6):621–626.

55. Grigsby J, Kravcisin N, Ayarbe SD, Busenbark D. Prediction of deficits in behavioral self-regulation among persons with multiple sclerosis. *Arch Phys Med Rehabil.* 1993;74(12):1350–1353.

56. Leon-Carrion J. Rehabilitation of memory. In: Leon-Carrion J, ed. *Neuropsychological Rehabilitation: Fundamentals, Innovations and Directions.* Delray Beach, FL: GR/St. Lucie Press; 1997:371–398.

57. Tate RL. Beyond one-bun, two-shoe: Recent advances in the psychological rehabilitation of memory disorders after acquired brain injury. *Brain Inj.* 1997; 11(12):351–356.

58. Morris J, Roth E, Davidoff G. Mild closed head injury and cognitive deficits in spinal-cord-injured patients: Incidence and impact. *J Head Trauma Rehabil.* 1986; 1(2):31–42.

59. Milisen K, Abraham IL, Broos PL. Postoperative variation in neurocognitive and functional status in elderly hip fracture patients. *J Adv Nurs.* 1998;27(1):59–67.

60. Mysiw WJ, Beegan JG, Gatens PF. Prospective cognitive assessment of stroke patients before inpatient rehabilitation. The relationship of the Neurobehavioral Cognitive Status Examination to functional improvement. *Am J Phys Med Rehabil.* 1989;68(4):168–171.

61. Davidoff GN, Roth EJ, Richards JS. Cognitive deficits in spinal cord injury: epidemiology and outcome. *Arch Phys Med Rehabil.* 1992;73(3):275–284.

62. Heilman KM, Rothi LJG. Apraxia. In: Heilman KM, Valenstein E, eds. *Clinical Neuropsychology.* 3rd ed. New York: Oxford University Press; 1993:141–163.

63. Gonzalez Rothi LJ, Raade AS, Heilman KM. Localization of lesions in limb and buccofacial apraxia. In: Kertesz A, ed. *Localization and Neuroimaging in Neuropsychology. Foundations of Neuropsychology.* San Diego: Academic Press, Inc; 1994: 407–427.

64. Donkervoort M, Dekker J, van den Ende E, Stehmann-Saris JC, Deelman BG. Prevalence of apraxia among patients with a first left hemisphere stroke in rehabilitation centres and nursing homes. *Clin Rehabil.* 2000;14(2):130–136.

65. Sunderland A, Tinson D, Bradley L. Differences in recovery from constructional apraxia after right and left hemisphere stroke? *J Clin Exp Neuropsychol.* 1994; 16(6):916–920.

66. Giaquinto S, Buzzelli S, Di Francesco L, et al. On the prognosis of outcome after stroke. *Acta Neurol Scand.* 1999;100(3):202–208.

67. Pedersen PM, Jorgensen HS, Kammersgaard LP, Nakayama H, Raaschou HO, Olsen TS. Manual and oral apraxia in acute stroke, frequency and influence on functional outcome: The Copenhagen Stroke Study. *Am J Phys Med Rehabil.* 2001;80(9):685–692.

68. van Heugten CM, Dekker J, Deelman BG, Stehmann-Saris JC, Kinebanian A. Rehabilitation of stroke patients with apraxia: the role of additional cognitive and motor impairments. *Disabil Rehabil.* 2000;22(12):547–554.

69. van Heugten CM. Rehabilitation and management of apraxia after stroke. *Rev Clin Gerontol.* 2001;11(2):177–184.

70. Dorra HH, Lenze EJ, Kim Y, et al. Clinically relevant behaviors in elderly hip fracture inpatients. *Int J Psychiatry Med.* 2002;32(3):249–259.

71. Chiu CC, Chen CE, Wang TG, Lin MC, Lien IN. Influencing factors and ambulation outcome in patients with dual disabilities of hemiplegia and amputation. *Arch Phys Med Rehabil.* 2000;81(1):14–17.

72. Svensson O, Stromberg L, Ohlen G, Lindgren U. Prediction of the outcome after hip fracture in elderly patients. *J Bone Joint Surg Brit.* 1996;78(1):115–118.

73. Beloosesky Y, Grinblat J, Epelboym B, Weiss A, Grosman B, Hendel D. Functional gain of hip fracture patients in different cognitive and functional groups. *Clin Rehabil.* 2002;16(3):321–328.

74. Basford JR, Johnson SJ. Form may be as important as function in orthotic acceptance: a case report. *Arch Phys Med Rehabil.* 2002;83(3):433–435.

75. Menec VH, Perry RP. Reactions to stigmas. The effect of targets' age and controllability of stigmas. *J Aging Health.* 1995;7(3):365–383.

76. Hanks RA, Wood DL, Millis S, et al. Violent traumatic brain injury: occurrence, patient characteristics, and risk factors from the Traumatic Brain Injury Model Systems project. *Arch Phys Med Rehabil.* 2003;84(2):249–254.

77. Lawrence ES, Coshall C, Dundas R, et al. Estimates of the prevalence of acute stroke impairments and disability in a multiethnic population. *Stroke.* 2001; 32(6):1279–1284.

78. Gerszten PC, Witham TF, Clyde BL, Welch WC. Relationship between type of health insurance and time to inpatient rehabilitation placement for surgical subspecialty patients. *Am J Med Qual.* 2001;16(6):212–215.

79. Horner RD, Swanson JW, Bosworth HB, Matchar DB, Team VAASS. Effects of race and poverty on the process and outcome of inpatient rehabilitation services among stroke patients. *Stroke.* 2003;34(4):1027–1031.

80. Jones CA, Voaklander DC, Johnston DW, Suarez-Almazor ME. The effect of age on pain, function, and quality of life after total hip and knee arthroplasty. *Arch Int Med.* 2001;161(3):454–460.

81. Duke RG, Keating JL. An investigation of factors predictive of independence in transfers and ambulation after hip fracture. *Arch Phys Med Rehabil.* 2002;83(2): 158–164.

82. Traballesi M, Brunelli S, Pratesi L, Pulcini M, Angioni C, Paolucci S. Prognostic factors in rehabilitation of above knee amputees for vascular diseases. *Disabil Rehabil.* 1998;20(10):380–384.

83. Munin MC, Espejo-De Guzman MC, Boninger ML, Fitzgerald SG, Penrod LE, Singh J. Predictive factors for successful early prosthetic ambulation among lower-limb amputees. *J Rehabil Res Dev.* 2001;38(4):379–384.

84. Greive AC, Lankhorst GJ. Functional outcome of lower-limb amputees: a prospective descriptive study in a general hospital. *Prosthet Orthot Int.* 1996;20(2): 79–87.

85. Hancock K, Craig A, Tennant C, Chang E. The influence of spinal cord injury on coping styles and self-perceptions: a controlled study. *Aust NZ J Psychiatry.* 1993;27(3):450–456.

86. Nyland J, Johnson DL, Caborn DN, Brindle T. Internal health status belief and lower perceived functional deficit are related among anterior cruciate ligament-deficient patients. *Arthroscopy.* 2002;18(5):515–518.

87. Fortinsky RH, Bohannon RW, Litt MD, et al. Rehabilitation therapy self-efficacy and functional recovery after hip fracture. *Int J Rehabil Res.* 2002;25(3): 241–246.

88. Kurlowicz L. Perceived self-efficacy, functional ability, and depressive symptoms in older elective surgery patients. *Nurs Res.* 1998;47(4):219–226.

89. Robinson-Smith G, Johnston MV, Allen J. Self-care self-efficacy, quality of life, and depression after stroke. *Arch Phys Med Rehabil.* 2000;81(4):460–464.

90. Bracken MB, Shepard MJ, Webb SB Jr. Psychological response to acute spinal cord injury: an epidemiological study. *Paraplegia.* 1981;19(5):271–283.

91. Frost FS. Role of rehabilitation after spinal cord injury. *Urol Clin North Am.* 1993;20(3):549–559.

92. Malec J, Neimeyer R. Psychologic prediction of duration of inpatient spinal cord injury rehabilitation and performance of self-care. *Arch Phys Med Rehabil.* 1983;64(8):359–363.

93. Craig AR, Hancock KM, Dickson HG. Spinal cord injury: a search for determinants of depression two years after the event. *Br J Clin Psychol.* 1994;33(Pt 2): 221–230.

94. Moore AD, Bombardier CH, Brown PB, Patterson DR. Coping and emotional attributions following spinal cord injury. *Int J Rehabil Res.* 1994;17(1):39–48.

95. Rao R. Cerebrovascular disease and late life depression: an age old association revisited. *Int J Geriatr Psychiatry.* 2000;15(5):419–433.

96. Busch CR, Alpern HP. Depression after mild traumatic brain injury: a review of current research. *Neuropsychol Rev.* 1998;8(2):95–108.

97. Desmond DW, Remien RH, Moroney JT, Stern Y, Sano M, Williams JB. Ischemic stroke and depression. *J Int Neuropsychol Soc.* 2003;9(3):429–439.

98. Paolucci S, Antonucci G, Pratesi L, Traballesi M, Grasso MG, Lubich S. Post-stroke depression and its role in rehabilitation of inpatients. *Arch Phys Med Rehabil.* 1999;80(9):985–990.

99. Schubert DS, Taylor C, Lee S, Mentari A, Tamaklo W. Physical consequences of depression in the stroke patient. *Gen Hosp Psychiatry.* 1992;14(1):69–76.

100. Pohjasvaara T, Leskela M, Vataja R, et al. Post-stroke depression, executive dysfunction and functional outcome. *Eur J Neurol.* 2002;9(3):269–275.

101. Beblo T, Wallesch CW, Herrmann M. The crucial role of frontostriatal circuits for depressive disorders in the postacute stage after stroke. *Neuropsychiatry Neuropsychol Behav Neurol.* 1999;12(4):236–246.

102. Dijkers M, Cushman LA. Differences between rehabilitation disciplines in views of depression in spinal cord injury patients. *Paraplegia.* 1990;28(6):380–391.

103. Elliott TR, Frank RG. Depression following spinal cord injury. *Arch Phys Med Rehabil.* 1996;77(8):816–823.

104. Krause JS, Kemp B, Coker J. Depression after spinal cord injury: relation to gender, ethnicity, aging, and socioeconomic indicators. *Arch Phys Med Rehabil.* 2000;81(8):1099–1109.

105. Rintala DH, Loubser PG, Castro J, Hart KA, Fuhrer MJ. Chronic pain in a community-based sample of men with spinal cord injury: prevalence, severity, and relationship with impairment, disability, handicap, and subjective well-being. *Arch Phys Med Rehabil.* 1998;79(6):604–614.

106. Cairns DM, Adkins RH, Scott MD. Pain and depression in acute traumatic spinal cord injury: origins of chronic problematic pain? *Arch Phys Med Rehabil.* 1996;77(4):329–335.

107. Tate D, Forchheimer M, Maynard F, Dijkers M. Predicting depression and psychological distress in persons with spinal cord injury based on indicators of handicap. *Am J Phys Med Rehabil.* 1994;73(3):175–183.

108. MacDonald MR, Nielson WR, Cameron MG. Depression and activity patterns of spinal cord injured persons living in the community. *Arch Phys Med Rehabil.* 1987;68(6):339–343.

109. Paolucci S, Antonucci G, Grasso MG, et al. Post-stroke depression, antidepressant treatment and rehabilitation results. A case-control study. *Cerebrovasc Dis.* 2001;12(3):264–271.

110. Gillen R, Tennen H, McKee TE, Gernert-Dott P, Affleck G. Depressive symptoms and history of depression predict rehabilitation efficiency in stroke patients. *Arch Phys Med Rehabil.* 2001;82(12):1645–1649.

111. Smith SJ, Young CA. The role of affect on the perception of disability in multiple sclerosis. *Clin Rehabil.* 2000;14(1):50–54.

112. Alderman N, Ward A. Behavioural treatment of the dysexecutive syndrome: reduction of repetitive speech using response cost and cognitive overlearning. *Neuropsychological Rehabilitation.* 1991;1(1):65–80.

113. Clark MS, Smith DS. The effects of depression and abnormal illness behaviour on outcome following rehabilitation from stroke. *Clin Rehabil.* 1998;12(1): 73–80.

114. Judd FK, Burrows GD, Brown DJ. Depression following acute spinal cord injury. *Paraplegia.* 1986;24(6):358–363.

115. Judd FK, Stone J, Webber JE, Brown DJ, Burrows GD. Depression following spinal cord injury. A prospective in-patient study. *Br J Psychiatry.* 1989;154: 668–671.

116. Kishi Y, Robinson RG, Forrester AW. Prospective longitudinal study of depression following spinal cord injury. *J Neuropsychiatry Clin Neurosci.* 1994;6(3): 237–244.

117. Kennedy P, Rogers BA. Anxiety and depression after spinal cord injury: a longitudinal analysis. *Arch Phys Med Rehabil.* 2000;81(7):932–937.

118. McKinley WO, Tewksbury MA, Godbout CJ. Comparison of medical complications following nontraumatic and traumatic spinal cord injury. *J Spinal Cord Med.* 2002;25(2):88–93.

119. Boekamp JR, Overholser JC, Schubert DS. Depression following a spinal cord injury. *Int J Psychiatry Med.* 1996;26(3):329–349.

120. Zinn S, Bosworth HB, Horner RD. *Stroke characteristics as factors in post-stroke depression.* Paper presented at meeting of American Association of Geriatric Psychiatry, 2003; Honolulu, HI.

121. Orbell S, Johnston M, Rowley D, Espley A, Davey P. Cognitive representations of illness and functional and affective adjustment following surgery for osteoarthritis. *Soc Sci Med.* 1998;47(1):93–102.

122. Robinson RG. Neuropsychiatric consequences of stroke. *Annu Rev Med.* 1997; 48:217–229.

123. Starkstein SE, Robinson RG. The role of the frontal lobes in affective disorder following stroke. In: Levin HS, Eisenberg HM, Benton AL, eds. *Frontal Lobe Function and Dysfunction.* New York: Oxford University Press; 1991:288–303.

124. Nielsen MS. Post-traumatic stress disorder and emotional distress in persons with spinal cord lesion. *Spinal Cord.* 2003;41(5):296–302.

125. Miller WC, Speechley M, Deathe B. The prevalence and risk factors of falling and fear of falling among lower extremity amputees. *Arch Phys Med Rehabil.* 2001;82(8):1031–1037.

126. Petrella RJ, Payne M, Myers A, Overend T, Chesworth B. Physical function and fear of falling after hip fracture rehabilitation in the elderly. *Am J Phys Med Rehabil.* 2000;79(2):154–160.

127. Andersson S, Krogstad JM, Finset A. Apathy and depressed mood in acquired brain damage: relationship to lesion localization and psychophysiological reactivity. *Psychol Med.* 1999;29(2):447–456.

128. Marshall M, Helmes E, Deathe AB. A comparison of psychosocial functioning and personality in amputee and chronic pain populations. *Clin J Pain.* 1992; 8(4):351–357.

129. Hagberg K, Branemark R. Consequences of non-vascular trans-femoral amputation: a survey of quality of life, prosthetic use and problems. *Prosthet Orthot Int.* 2001;25(3):186–194.

130. Gallagher P, MacLachlan M. Psychological adjustment and coping in adults with prosthetic limbs. *Behav Med.* 1999;25(3):117–124.

131. Jensen MP, Ehde DM, Hoffman AJ, Patterson DR, Czerniecki JM, Robinson LR. Cognitions, coping and social environment predict adjustment to phantom limb pain. *Pain.* 2002;95(1–2):133–142.

132. Hill A. Phantom limb pain: a review of the literature on attributes and potential mechanisms. *J Pain Symptom Manage.* 1999;17(2):125–142.

133. Hauer K, Specht N, Schuler M, Bartsch P, Oster P. Intensive physical training in geriatric patients after severe falls and hip surgery. *Age & Ageing.* 2002; 31(1):49–57.

134. Lauridsen UB, de la Cour BB, Gottschalck L, Svensson BH. Intensive physical therapy after hip fracture. A randomised clinical trial. *Dan Med Bull.* 2002; 49(1):70–72.

135. Clark MS, Smith DS. Factors contributing to patient satisfaction with rehabilitation following stroke. *Int J Rehabil Res.* 1998;21(2):143–154.

136. Burton CR. Re-thinking stroke rehabilitation: the Corbin and Strauss chronic illness trajectory framework. *J Adv Nurs.* 2000;32(3):595–602.

137. Werner RA, Kessler S. Effectiveness of an intensive outpatient rehabilitation program for postacute stroke patients. *Am J Phys Med Rehabil.* 1996;75(2): 114–120.

138. Tsouna-Hadjis E, Vemmos KN, Zakopoulos N, Stamatelopoulos S. First-stroke recovery process: the role of family social support. *Arch Phys Med Rehabil.* 2000;81(7):881–887.

139. Ceder L, Thorngren KG, Wallden B. Prognostic indicators and early home rehabilitation in elderly patients with hip fractures. *Clin Orthop.* 1980(152): 173–184.

140. Orbell S, Espley A, Johnston M, Rowley D. Health benefits of joint replacement surgery for patients with osteoarthritis: prospective evaluation using independent assessments in Scotland. *J Epidemiol Community Health.* 1998;52(9):564–570.

141. Clark MS, Smith DS. Psychological correlates of outcome following rehabilitation from stroke. *Clin Rehabil.* 1999;13(2):129–140.

142. Evans RL, Halar EM, Bishop DS. Family function and treatment compliance after stroke. *Int J Rehabil Res.* 1986;9(1):70–72.

143. Butler DJ, Turkal NW, Seidl JJ. Amputation: preoperative psychological preparation. *J Am Board Fam Pract.* 1992;5(1):69–73.

144. Kent R, Fyfe N. Effectiveness of rehabilitation following amputation. *Clin Rehabil.* 1999;13(Suppl 1):43–50.

145. Fisher K, Hanspal RS, Marks L. Return to work after lower limb amputation. *Int J Rehabil Res.* 2003;26(1):51–56.

146. Gerhards F, Florin I, Knapp T. The impact of medical, reeducational, and psychological variables on rehabilitation outcome in amputees. *Int J Rehabil Res.* 1984;7(4):379–388.

147. Ide M, Watanabe T, Toyonaga T. Sexuality in persons with limb amputation. *Prosthet Orthot Int.* 2002;26(3):189–194.

148. McColl MA, Lei H, Skinner H. Structural relationships between social support and coping. *Soc Sci Med.* 1995;41(3):395–407.

149. Durance JP, Warren WK, Kerbel DB, Stroud TW. Rehabilitation of below-knee amputees: factors influencing outcome and costs in three programmes. *Int Disabil Stud.* 1989;11(3):127–132.

150. Heim M, Wershavski M, Arazi-Margalit D, Azaria M. The will to walk—a partnership involving dual dynamics. *Disabil Rehabil.* 1998;20(2):74–77.

151. Williams LS, Lowenthal DT. Clinical problem-solving in geriatric medicine: obstacles to rehabilitation. *J Am Geriatr Soc.* 1995;43(2):179–183.

152. Judd T. *Neuropsychotherapy and Community Integration: Brain Illness, Emotions, and Behavior.* London: Kluwer Academic; 1999.

153. Johansson BB. Brain plasticity and stroke rehabilitation. The Willis lecture. *Stroke.* 2000;31(1):223–230.

154. Gaillard F. Recovery as a mind-brain paradigm. *Int J Rehabil Res.* 1983;6(3): 331–338.

155. Liepert J, Miltner WH, Bauder H, et al. Motor cortex plasticity during constraint-induced movement therapy in stroke patients. *Neurosci Lett.* 1998;250 (1):5–8.

156. Kopp B, Kunkel A, Muhlnickel W, Villringer K, Taub E, Flor H. Plasticity in the motor system related to therapy-induced improvement of movement after stroke. *Neuroreport.* 1999;10(4):807–810.

157. Collaboration SUT. Collaborative systematic review of the randomised trials of organised inpatient (stroke unit) care after stroke. *BMJ.* 1997;314(7088): 1151–1159.

158. Naglie G, Tansey C, Kirkland JL, et al. Interdisciplinary inpatient care for elderly people with hip fracture: a randomized controlled trial. *Can Med Assoc J.* 2002;167(1):25–32.

159. Peters MD, Gluck M, McCormick M. Behaviour rehabilitation of the challenging client in less restrictive settings. *Brain Inj.* 1992;6(4):299–314.

160. Balliet R, Levy B, Blood KM. Upper extremity sensory feedback therapy in chronic cerebrovascular accident patients with impaired expressive aphasia and auditory comprehension. *Arch Phys Med Rehabil.* 1986;67(5):304–310.

161. Prigatano GP. Motivation and awareness in cognitive neurorehabilitation. In: Stuss DT, Winocur G, et al., eds. *Cognitive Neurorehabilitation.* New York: Cambridge University Press; 1999:240–251.

162. Youngjohn JR, Altman IM. A performance-based group approach to the treatment of anosognosia and denial. *Rehabil Psychol.* 1989;34(3):217–222.

163. Bieman-Copland S, Dywan J. Achieving rehabilitative gains in anosognosia after TBI. *Brain Cogn.* 2000;44(1):1–5.

164. Langer KG, Padrone FJ. Psychotherapeutic treatment of awareness in acute rehabilitation of traumatic brain injury. *Neuropsychological Rehabilitation.* 1992; 2(1):59–70.

165. Stanton KM, Pepping M, Brockway JA, Bliss L, Frankel D, Waggener S. Wheelchair transfer training for right cerebral dysfunctions: an interdisciplinary approach. *Arch Phys Med Rehabil.* 1983;64(6):276–280.

166. Sohlberg MM, McLaughlin KA, Pavese A, Heidrich A, Posner MI. Evaluation of attention process training and brain injury education in persons with acquired brain injury. *J Clin Exp Neuropsychol.* 2000;22(5):656–676.

167. Podd MH, Seelig DP. Computer-assisted cognitive remediation of attention disorders following mild closed head injuries. In: Long CJ, Ross LK, eds. *Handbook of Head Trauma: Acute Care to Recovery. Critical Issues in Neuropsychology.* New York: Plenum Press; 1992:231–244.

168. Evans JJ, Emslie H, Wilson BA. External cueing systems in the rehabilitation of executive impairments of action. *J Int Neuropsychol Soc.* 1998;4(4):399–408.

169. Ylvisaker M, Szekeres SF, Haarbauer-Krupa J. Cognitive rehabilitation: organization, memory, and language. In: Ylvisaker M, ed. *Traumatic Brain Injury Rehabilitation: Children and Adolescents.* 2nd ed. Woburn, MA: Butterworth-Heinemann; 1998:181–220.

170. Trepagnier CG. Virtual environments for the investigation and rehabilitation of cognitive and perceptual impairments. *Neurorehabilitation.* 1999;12(1): 63–72.

171. Ryan TV, Ruff RM. The efficacy of structured memory retraining in a group comparison of head trauma patients. *Arch Clin Neuropsychol.* 1988;3(2): 165–179.

172. Doornhein K, De Haan EHF. Cognitive training for memory deficits in stroke patients. *Neuropsychological Rehabilitation.* 1998;8(4):393–400.

173. Squires EJ, Hunkin NM, Parkin AJ. Take note: using errorless learning to promote memory notebook training. In: Parkin AJ, ed. *Case Studies in the Neuropsychology of Memory.* Hove, England: Psychology Press; 1997:191–203.

174. Kim HJ, Burke DT, Dowds MM, George J. Utility of a microcomputer as an external memory aid for a memory-impaired head injury patient during inpatient rehabilitation. *Brain Inj.* 1999;13(2):147–150.

175. Wilson BA. Dealing with memory problems in rehabilitation. *Rev Clin Gerontol.* 1995;5(4):457–463.

176. Craig AR, Hancock K, Chang E, Dickson H. Immunizing against depression and anxiety after spinal cord injury. *Arch Phys Med Rehabil.* 1998;79(4):375–377.

177. Lopez MA, Mermelstein RJ. A cognitive-behavioral program to improve geriatric rehabilitation outcome. *Gerontologist.* 1995;35(5):696–700.

178. Donovan-Hall MK, Yardley L, Watts RJ. Engagement in activities revealing the body and psychosocial adjustment in adults with a trans-tibial prosthesis. *Prosthet Orthot Int.* 2002;26(1):15–22.

179. Woodbury B. Psychological adjustment to spinal cord injury: a literature review, 1950–1977. *Rehabil Psychol.* 1978;25(3):119–163.

180. Wheeler G, Krausher K, Cumming C, Jung V, Steadward R, Cumming D. Personal styles and ways of coping in individuals who use wheelchairs. *Spinal Cord.* 1996;34(6):351–357.

181. Gallagher P, Maclachlan M. Evaluating a written emotional disclosure homework intervention for lower-limb amputees. *Arch Phys Med Rehabil.* 2002;83 (10):1464–1466.

182. Richards JS. Psychologic adjustment to spinal cord injury during first postdischarge year. *Arch Phys Med Rehabil.* 1986;67(6):362–365.

183. O'Hara CC, Harrell M. The empowerment rehabilitation model: meeting the unmet needs of survivors, families, and treatment providers. *Cognitive Rehabilitation.* 1991;9(1):14–21.

184. Chan KM, Tan ES. Use of lower limb prosthesis among elderly amputees. *Ann Acad Med Singapore.* 1990;19(6):811–816.

185. Resnick B. Efficacy beliefs in geriatric rehabilitation. *J Gerontol Nurs.* 1998; 24(7):34–44.

186. Marks R. Efficacy theory and its utility in arthritis rehabilitation: review and recommendations. *Disabil Rehabil.* 2001;23(7):271–280.

187. Galvin LR, Godfrey HP. The impact of coping on emotional adjustment to spinal cord injury (SCI): review of the literature and application of a stress appraisal and coping formulation. *Spinal Cord.* 2001;39(12):615–627.

188. King C, Kennedy P. Coping effectiveness training for people with spinal cord injury: preliminary results of a controlled trial. *Br J Clin Psychol.* 1999;38(Pt 1): 5–14.

189. Curcoll ML. Psychological approach to the rehabilitation of the spinal cord injured: the contribution of relaxation techniques. *Paraplegia.* 1992;30(6): 425–427.

190. Livneh H, Antonak RF, Gerhardt J. Psychosocial adaptation to amputation: the role of sociodemographic variables, disability-related factors and coping strategies. *Int J Rehabil Res.* 1999;22(1):21–31.
191. Crasilneck HB, Hall JA. The use of hypnosis in the rehabilitation of complicated vascular and post-traumatic neurological patients. *Int J Clin Exp Hypn.* 1970;18(3):145–159.
192. Evans RL, Bishop DS, Matlock AL, Stranahan S, Smith GG, Halar EM. Family interaction and treatment adherence after stroke. *Arch Phys Med Rehabil.* 1987;68(8):513–517.
193. Brown-Watson AV. *Still Kicking: Restorative Groups for Frail Older Adults.* Baltimore: Health Professions Press; 1999.
194. Man DW. A preliminary study to investigate the empowerment factors of survivors who have experienced brain damage in rehabilitation. *Brain Inj.* 2001;15(11):961–973.
195. Chervinsky AB, Ommaya AK, deJonge M, Spector J, Schwab K, Salazar AM. Motivation for traumatic brain injury rehabilitation questionnaire (MOT-Q): Reliability, factor analysis, and relationship to MMPI-2 variables. *Arch Clin Neuropsychol.* 1998;13(5):433–446.
196. Fleury J. The Index of Readiness: development and psychometric analysis. *J Nurs Meas.* 1994;2(2):143–154.
197. Bombardier CH, Heinemann AW. The construct validity of the readiness to change questionnaire for persons with TBI. *J Head Trauma Rehabil.* 2000;15(1):696–709.
198. Evans RL, Connis RT, Hendricks RD, Haselkorn JK. Multidisciplinary rehabilitation versus medical care: a meta-analysis. *Soc Sci Med.* 1995;40(12):1699–1706.
199. Brillhart B, Johnson K. Motivation and the coping process of adults with disabilities: a qualitative study. *Rehabil Nurs.* 1997;22(5):249–252, 255–256.
200. Hoffmann B, Duwecke C, von Wild KR. Neurological and social long-term outcome after early rehabilitation following traumatic brain injury. 5-year report on 240 TBI patients. *Acta Neurochir Suppl.* 2002;79:33–35.
201. Martin BJ, Yip B, Hearty M, Marletta S, Hill R. Outcome, functional recovery and unmet needs following acute stroke. Experience of patient follow up at 6 to 9 months in a newly established stroke service. *Scott Med J.* 2002;47(6):136–137.
202. von Koch L, de Pedro-Cuesta J, Kostulas V, Almazan J, Widen Holmqvist L. Randomized controlled trial of rehabilitation at home after stroke: one-year follow-up of patient outcome, resource use and cost. *Cerebrovasc Dis.* 2001;12(2):131–138.
203. Frost H, Lamb SE, Robertson S. A randomized controlled trial of exercise to improve mobility and function after elective knee arthroplasty. Feasibility, results and methodological difficulties. *Clin Rehabil.* 2002;16(2):200–209.
204. Baskett JJ, Broad JB, Reekie G, Hocking C, Green G. Shared responsibility for ongoing rehabilitation: a new approach to home-based therapy after stroke. *Clin Rehabil.* 1999;13(1):23–33.

205. Kuisma R. A randomized, controlled comparison of home versus institutional rehabilitation of patients with hip fracture. *Clin Rehabil.* 2002;16(5):553–561.

206. Roderick P, Low J, Day R, et al. Stroke rehabilitation after hospital discharge: a randomized trial comparing domiciliary and day-hospital care. *Age & Ageing.* 2001;30(4):303–310.

Part III

TREATMENT ADHERENCE
IN SPECIAL POPULATIONS

Chapter 8

Nonadherence in Pediatrics

Jennifer Cheng
Emmanuel Chip Walter

Nonadherence to prescribed treatments is prevalent in pediatric practice (1–6). Medical nonadherence has far-reaching implications for both the future health of children as well as our health care establishment. Pediatric medical nonadherence results in poor health outcomes, unreliable treatment efficacy assessments, unnecessary clinical interventions, and enormous costs to American taxpayers (7). Recent studies indicate that 30% to 60% of all patients do not optimally adhere to prescribed medical regimens (6).

Nonadherence in pediatrics is associated with unique causative factors. For example, practitioners must be aware of the additional dimension of complexity introduced by the interests of the parent or caregiver (8). In today's society, nontraditional families are increasingly commonplace, and adherence becomes a challenge in environments where different and perhaps unreliable adults may participate in the parental caregiver role. As children become adolescents and young adults, complex psychosocial and developmental issues, including the establishment of self-identity and conforming to peer norms, further complicate adherence (9, 10).

Yet whereas some issues are unique, pediatric patients are subject to the same difficulties faced by adults in today's health care environment. Technological advancements in disease management have resulted in increasing numbers of patients who must live with and manage their own chronic health conditions (11, 12). With the advent of managed care, there is a shift in the responsibilities of disease management from physicians to patients.

This is evidenced by increased use of physician extenders in patient treatment, shorter hospitalization stays, and increased utilization of outpatient versus inpatient treatment settings (8, 13). Children with complex diseases and their families are often saddled with multiple medical appointments and complicated medication, dietary, and lifestyle regimens that compete with their desire to lead a normal life at home.

Nonadherence in the pediatrics population is a clear concern for the entire health care establishment. The physiological bases for changes seen in many chronic diseases of adulthood are established during childhood and adolescence. Furthermore, adherence has been shown to be a reliable predictor of future adherence (10, 14–16). Nonadherence in children results in increased numbers of nonadherent adults. Lifestyle and behavior choices that become refractory to modification in adulthood also contribute to many chronic illnesses. Any discussion of nonadherence in medicine, therefore, must start with a thorough examination of nonadherence in children.

This chapter reviews the factors that affect adherence in children and adolescents and examines the extent of treatment nonadherence. Our goal is to present evidence-based recommendations to help improve adherence in the pediatric population for the practitioner.

PREVALENCE OF NONADHERENCE IN PEDIATRICS

Prevalence of Nonadherence to Medical Regimens in Children and Adolescents

Estimates of the prevalence of nonadherence with medical treatment in the pediatric literature vary tremendously. These estimates depend on a number of variables, including the specific criteria used for classifying acceptable adherence and nonadherence, the method of assessment, the behavior assessed, the disease studied, the population examined, and the setting in which the study takes place (7, 13). What constitutes an "acceptable" level of medical adherence in children is unclear, as the threshold level of adherence or nonadherence that will result in a therapeutic or deleterious effect is not well established for most pediatric medical conditions (17).

Nevertheless, in general terms, the average adherence rate to medical regimens in children and adolescents approximates 50% (10, 18) and ranges from 43% to 100% (19). Approximately 50%–60% of children underuse medication and less than 10% overuse medication (13). In the few studies that examine adherence exclusively in children, the average adherence rate reported was 54% (20). Several studies have shown that children are less likely to adhere to medical regimens when compared to adults

(9, 21). This is, at least in part, due to higher cognitive functioning in adults, who may be more motivated to adhere to treatment regimens in order to achieve a desired outcome (8). In children, different developmental stages can have a profound impact on adherence behavior (8). For younger children, future health benefits are less compelling than the immediacy of pain or unpalatability (8, 22). In situations where the child and the caregiver share responsibility for medical regimens, factors related to both parties interact and impact adherence rates.

During adolescence, developmental tasks such as the need to establish greater autonomy while conforming to peer norms complicate medical adherence (9, 10). Adolescents have been found to be less adherent than young children to regimens for diabetes (23), renal disease (20, 24), asthma (5), and HIV (15, 25). Although adolescents have a better cognitive understanding of the importance of medical adherence than younger children (26), they deviate from regimen recommendations if these conflict with peer-accepted behavior (27, 28) or produce unacceptable effects such as weight gain (29, 30). For example, in a study of juvenile rheumatoid arthritis, adolescents were found to be less likely to adhere to splint use and other regimens that made them feel or look different than their peers (31). In another study, youth discontinued their steroid regimen following renal transplantation as a result of perceived changes in physical appearance (20). Poor adherence in adolescents may reflect rebellion against the regimen's control over their lives (10, 19) or denial of their susceptibility to disease (9, 10, 15, 25, 32). Adolescents with higher denial had significantly poorer adherence to anticancer agents (33). Privacy concerns may also be a significant barrier to medical adherence in adolescence (34). Adolescents with HIV who had undisclosed disease status reported missing more doses of antiretroviral therapy due to concerns about privacy than those with disclosed HIV status (15). Adolescents on oral contraceptives also reported hesitation about returning for medical appointments due to confidentiality concerns (35). High-risk behaviors such as substance use and unsafe sexual practices are associated with poor adherence to medical regimens (36, 37) whereas positive behaviors such as high educational goals predict improved adherence (10, 38).

Prevalence of Nonadherence to Regimens for Acute Illness

Approximately 33%–50% of children inadequately adhere to regimens for acute illness (8, 39, 40). Adherence rates tend to decline over the course of therapy with the onset of symptomatic relief (6, 8, 17) or with poor improvement despite treatment (30). Most of the literature on pediatric nonadherence to acute disease regimens has focused on otitis media and streptococcal pharyngitis.

Otitis media is the most frequently reported illness among children seen in the acute-care setting, accounting for more than 20 million clinical encounters per year and a total treatment cost of >$3.5 billion annually (40). Streptococcal pharyngitis is also an important pediatric clinical entity, accounting for an average of 3.3 ambulatory care visits per 100 children per year for youth less than 15 years (41). In a study of oral penicillin prescribed for streptococcal pharyngitis or otitis media, 56% of children had stopped therapy by the third day, 71% by the sixth day, and 82% by the ninth day (1, 7). In another study of 300 children taking antibiotics for otitis media, full adherence was observed in only 7.3% of patients, and 53% took less than half of the prescribed medicine (42). Nonadherence to regimens for these two illnesses has been linked to treatment failures and adverse sequelae including acute rheumatic fever and chronic serous otitis media with related hearing loss and speech delay, while contributing to antibiotic resistance (4, 39, 43–46).

Prevalence of Nonadherence to Regimens for Chronic Illness

Nonadherence is a greater problem with chronic regimens than acute ones (7, 13, 17, 30). Children with chronic illness and their families are often asked to make significant behavioral and lifestyle changes in order to adhere to long-term, if not lifelong, regimens to control disease symptoms and prevent complications (13, 47). Such changes can be difficult to integrate into everyday life, particularly if they significantly alter previous behavior patterns (19). It is estimated that approximately 50% (11%–83%) of patients inadequately adhere to chronic disease protocols (7, 17). Adherence to chronic regimens is dynamic, generally increasing during times of high disease activity and decreasing as symptoms abate (13, 15, 17, 48).

For chronic-disease prophylaxis, nonadherence is higher than for nonprophylaxis treatment (7, 9). Among children receiving isoniazid for tuberculosis prophylaxis, for example, 30% were nonadherent during the 6-month course (49). Almost a third (32%) of children on oral penicillin for rheumatic fever prophylaxis were nonadherent (50). Only 47% of parents of children taking antibiotics for otitis media prophylaxis claimed to be adherent (51). In this case, actual adherence rates may be even lower because self-reports have consistently been found to overestimate true adherence (1, 6, 52). In a study of adolescents who had undergone renal transplantation, 14% were nonadherent to chronic medications, 23% did not follow recommendations for blood testing, and 58% did not return for clinic appointments as requested (53).

Each chronic disease presents its own constellation of adherence problems (18). A study of youth with acute lymphocytic leukemia or Hodgkin's disease found 52% to be nonadherent with prednisone regimens, and 48% to be nonadherent with penicillin for postsplenectomy prophylaxis (removal of the spleen) (54). Adherence to highly active antiretroviral therapy (HAART) limits viral replication in HIV-infected children (55, 56); however, adherence is difficult due to high regimen complexity, unpalatability, toxicity, and frequency of drug interactions (15, 55–59). In one study, only 58% of children were adherent to HAART during the first 180 days, and that figure declined further after 200 days of therapy (55). Pediatric studies on asthma and diabetes mellitus best illustrate specific disease-related issues.

Asthma. Asthma, the most common chronic disease of childhood, affects 5 million American children and is the third leading cause of hospitalization in the pediatric population, representing more than 200,000 hospitalizations a year at a cost in excess of $12.7 billion (60). The mean medical expenditure of American families for children who have asthma has been estimated to range between 5.5% and 14.5% of family income (61). In families where caretakers overestimated the level of adolescent involvement in asthma self-care, higher levels of nonadherence and functional morbidity have been found (62).

Adherence is difficult in the management of asthma. Long periods of quiescence alternate with acute exacerbations, so many asthmatics treat exacerbations while ignoring their persistent chronic illness (5). Nonadherence rates for asthma have been reported to vary from 3% to 88% regardless of age, race, or gender (63). Less than 50% of pediatric patients (5) and as few as 30% of adolescents (19) with asthma adequately adhere to recommended inhalation medication regimens. Adherence to asthma medications is sporadic, with inhalers used in only 5 out of 45 treatment days with inappropriately low inhaled doses, in one study (5). Inability to use the inhaler properly and inappropriate timing of treatment are the primary reasons for nonadherence with inhalation regimens (8, 64–67). Proper technique education is essential for adherence to asthma regimens (68, 69).

Diabetes Mellitus. Diabetes mellitus is a growing pediatric public health concern. Chronic poor glycemic control leads to a host of multisystemic end-organ disorders. Medical adherence to diabetic regimens is poor in all age groups. Only 7% of patients adhere fully to all aspects of their diabetes regimens (70). A significant proportion (30%–70%) of patients do not adequately monitor blood glucose, 20%–80% do not correctly administer insulin, 70%–80% do not adhere to exercise guidelines, and 35%–75% do not follow dietary recommendations (70, 71).

Parental supervision (71) and warmth (72), family cohesion (73), and support from friends (74) have been consistently associated with improved adherence and metabolic control in children and adolescents. In contrast, parent–child conflict (75), high stress levels (76), and confusion over who has primary responsibility for regimen tasks (77) negatively impact adherence. Youth who were given "excessive self-care autonomy" over their diabetes regimens had poorer adherence, less knowledge, and higher hospitalization rates than those who had active parental participation (78, 79). As the disease progresses, the pancreas makes less insulin and metabolic control becomes more difficult (13). Thus, adherence in children with diabetes worsens with longer duration of illness (80).

Prevalence of Nonadherence to Nonmedication Lifestyle Regimens

Long-term adherence to lifestyle modification such as diet or exercise is lower than adherence to medication regimens (13, 79). Diabetic patients, for instance, cite greater barriers to dietary and exercise adherence than insulin injections (81).

Diet. Nonadherence to dietary guidelines can result in adverse health consequences for children with diabetes, renal disease, cystic fibrosis, and metabolic disorders (82–86). However, long-term dietary modification is difficult. Skill and knowledge deficits (17, 87) contribute to the 34%–50% of children with diabetes mellitus (87–89), and 43%–80% of those with cystic fibrosis (89, 90) who inadequately adhere to dietary aspects of their regimens. Unpalatability of low-protein diets has been implicated in nonadherence to regimens for phenylketonuria (91). In adolescents with phenylketonuria, time constraints, social pressures, financial limitations, and growing independence from the family combine to further interfere with dietary control (83). Better coping with dietary temptations has resulted in better dietary adherence in adolescents with hyperlipidemia (92). A brief motivational intervention has been shown to improve short-term dietary adherence in adolescents with diabetes (93). Other evidence suggests that nutritional education in combination with behavioral strategies is important to effect meaningful, lasting dietary change (94).

Exercise. Exercise training is an important aspect in the treatment of many conditions including juvenile rheumatoid arthritis, cerebral palsy, diabetes mellitus, obesity, cystic fibrosis, and asthma (12, 88, 95–98). Lifestyle exercise programs produce the best long-term health benefits (97, 99). Unfortunately, long-term adherence to exercise programs is universally poor. A majority (60%) of children with juvenile rheumatoid arthritis have difficulty adhering to exercise programs (96). In children with hemophilia, adherence to a therapeutic exercise program was 55% (100). Parents of children with juvenile rheumatoid arthritis reported more difficulty adhering to a range of motion exercises and splint use than to medications due to their children's resistance (101). In children with cystic fibrosis, fatigue and time required for other treatments hindered exercise adherence (102). Factors that have been associated with better adherence to exercise in children include enjoyment, variety, social support, and perceptions of competency and self-esteem (102). Family-centered behavioral strategies can enhance exercise adherence (99, 103, 104). Future research should determine the type, intensity, and duration of exercise that will produce acceptable adherence and ascertain the reinforcing factors that determine youth behavior choice (99).

UNINTENTIONAL AND INTENTIONAL NONADHERENCE

Unintentional nonadherence, the most common form of medical nonadherence in pediatrics, results from human error (105). Examples include forgetting to take medicines as prescribed, misunderstanding instructions, and running out of medication. It has been estimated that 40%–60% of patients forget physician instructions within 10–80 minutes of having heard them, and that over 60% of patients misinterpret them (6). Patients are also more likely to remember the diagnosis than the treatment prescribed (6, 106). Poor knowledge and communication contribute to unintentional nonadherence.

Intentional nonadherence is less commonly reported than unintentional nonadherence, because it is more difficult to detect. Examples of intentional nonadherent behavior include stopping medications because of perceived symptomatic improvement, perceived ineffectiveness, perceived low susceptibility to disease, concerns about safety, or resistance of the child. Cultural, ethnic, and religious health beliefs have an important impact on intentional nonadherence and should be considered in designing interventions.

RISK FACTORS/DETERMINANTS OF NONADHERENCE

Over the past several years, researchers have examined adherence risk factors in an attempt to derive a "risk profile" for targeting by future interventions. Unfortunately, adherence prediction is an imperfect science because no single or group of factors has been shown to accurately predict adherence behavior (7, 10). The most frequently studied correlates of adherence can be organized into demographic, disease, regimen, and provider factors.

Demographic

Age.   Several studies have shown that age is a significant determinant of adherence behavior. Young children often lack the skills needed to perform regimen tasks and must rely on adult supervision and assistance to adequately adhere to medical treatments (9). Successful adherence in this age group depends on the adherence of both the adult and the child (9). Palatability and pain play a large role in the adherence of young children (22, 107), and may be counteracted with parental warmth and support (18). As children enter school, they spend less time at home with their parents and are increasingly influenced by their peers and social environment (19). Adherence rates in adolescence are lower than those found in both adults (9, 10) and children (9, 19, 20, 29, 108). Although adolescents are capable of greater autonomy in carrying out regimen tasks, their struggle with self-esteem, body image, and social role definition in peer groups affects medical adherence (7, 9, 19).

Socioeconomic Status (SES).   Socioeconomic factors have been found to be important determinants of medical nonadherence in a number of studies (19, 109–112). Until an individual's basic needs are met, adherence to a medical regimen is unlikely to become a high priority (10). Families from low socioeconomic groups may encounter a multitude of barriers including lack of reliable transportation, limited social support networks, and few financial resources that make it difficult for them to adhere to prescribed regimens and medical follow-up (107, 113). For adolescents with HIV, adherence to antiretroviral medication has been linked to housing stability (114) and availability of child care and transportation (15, 115). Several studies have found lower SES and lower parental education levels to be associated with nonadherence to regimens for acute otitis media, diabetes, asthma, cystic fibrosis, familial hypercholesterolemia, phenylketonuria, and renal disease (17, 42, 112, 116). However, other studies have failed to establish an association between socioeconomic variables and medical adherence (117, 118).

Parental marital status has also been studied, with lone parenthood, separation, and divorce being associated with poorer adherence to asthma (108), diabetes mellitus (119, 120), renal disease (121), otitis media (42), contraceptive regimens (122), and liver transplantation (123). Large family size has been associated with lower adherence to regimens for malignancy (124), asthma (60, 125), diabetes (125), cystic fibrosis (17), and antibiotic prophylaxis for rheumatic fever (126).

Gender.   Studies examining patient gender have yielded conflicting results. Some found that boys were less likely than girls to adhere to diabetes (127) and cystic fibrosis (128) regimens. Others found boys more likely to adhere to diabetes (129, 130) and weight control (131) programs. Many found no relationship between gender and medical adherence (32, 33, 90, 108, 132, 133). One study found adolescent girls diagnosed with chlamydial infection to be more adherent with doxycycline treatment than boys (134); in the latter study, is has been theorized that girls may have recognized their higher susceptibility to more severe disease and perceived a greater benefit of therapy as compared to their male counterparts (10), who more often may be asymptomatic or mildly symptomatic.

Race. Several studies examining race as a correlate of adherence have also produced varying results. In studies that find a difference, culture or social inequalities may play a role (19). One study found that glycemic control of African American adolescents was significantly better than that of White youths when controlled for age, parent marital, socioeconomic, and insurance status (110). Christiansee et al. found that White patients were less likely than Black patients to adhere to asthma regimens (108) whereas Bender found the opposite (135). Other groups found adolescent teens from minority groups less likely than White teens to adhere to oral contraceptives (122) and antituberculous medications (136).

Other Demographic Factors. Additional factors that have been correlated with poor medical adherence include medical-insurance type, language barrier, and inner-city geographic location (10). Children with cystic fibrosis who had Medicaid coverage were found to have worse lung function and more pulmonary exacerbations than more advantaged counterparts (137). Inadequate access to specialty care, greater exposure to pollutants, and poorer regimen adherence among Medicaid patients may have contributed to these findings (137). Adolescents treated in a suburban clinic have demonstrated better adherence to oral contraceptives than matched controls treated in an inner-city setting (122). Hispanic patients whose providers demonstrated some understanding of Hispanic culture were more likely to adhere to medication recommendations (6, 138). Patients who communicated with their doctors through a translator were less likely to be informed about medication side effects, and more likely to have decreased satisfaction with medical care and poorer adherence (139).

Psychosocial

Family Dynamics and Social Support. Social support has been consistently associated with better medical adherence in children (19, 27, 116, 140–144). Children whose parents are supportive, flexible, good problem solvers, and not overly critical have better medical adherence (5, 7, 9, 73, 107, 145–147) than those whose parents are restrictive, hostile, disengaged, or stressed (10, 146, 148). In children with phenylketonuria (PKU), a positive correlation was found among family cohesion, dietary adherence, and child IQ (112). Adequate parental oversight and participation is important (30, 149, 150). Shifting too much responsibility to children and adolescents results in higher nonadherence and functional morbidity (10, 19, 62, 72, 77, 78). Youth whose parents accompanied them to appointments or supervised treatments had better adherence to regimens for renal transplantation (149) and contraception (150). Diabetic children stating that they were primarily responsible for glucose monitoring and insulin administration had poorer metabolic control than those with more active parental participation (71).

Unfortunately, what parents view as support, older children and adolescents may perceive as a threat to their autonomy (9, 10). In a study of youth requiring seizure prophylaxis, poorer adherence was associated with perceived lower personal freedom (27). Among teenage patients who had undergone renal transplantation, autonomy conflicts were cited as a primary reason for nonadherence (151). Families should strive to provide ongoing support while respecting the evolving autonomy of adolescents (10).

Peer support can facilitate disease adjustment, improve adherence, and reduce the time devoted by health care providers to the management of medical conditions (19, 27, 152). Teenagers who received contraceptive counseling from peers have demonstrated better adherence than those counseled by nurses (153). A combined family/peer intervention that paired HIV-positive adolescents with "treatment buddies" reported improved adherence to medications, reduced viral loads, and improvements in other health parameters including rates of medical and dental visits, hepatitis B and influenza immunizations, and referrals to mental health and dental appointments (154). Additional research is needed to develop strategies for incorporating peers and friends into the management of youth with medical illness.

Factual Knowledge. Improved knowledge has not been consistently linked to better medical adherence. Knowledge gaps have been associated with poorer adherence to regimens for cystic fibrosis, cancer, and diabetes, but improved knowledge has not been consistently linked to better adherence in renal disease (17, 124, 149, 155). In one study of renal transplantation, 44% of nonadherent children did not improve adherence despite receiving extensive education about medications (149). Another intensive educational intervention for diabetic teenagers improved disease-related knowledge but had no effect on adherence behavior or metabolic control (156).

Parental knowledge has been shown to significantly influence medical adherence by young children (17). In a study of children with cystic fibrosis in which only 16% of children adhered to dietary recommendations, maternal nutritional knowledge specific to cystic fibrosis predicted children's dietary adherence patterns and adherence scores (157). Another study showed that children whose caregivers were unable to describe the medication regimen or who failed to keep appointments were not likely to adhere to medication regimens (52).

Cognitive delays or psychiatric illness may affect information processing and retention and subsequently affect adherence (158, 159).

Adjustment and Coping to Disease. Patients and families with maladaptive reactions to diagnosis or treatment have poorer medical adherence (17, 160). Excessive anger, denial, rebellion, and anxiety have been linked with worse adherence to regimens for renal transplantation, cancer, scoliosis, and diabetes (5, 33, 53, 160–162). Depression or a history of previous psychiatric diagnosis also predict nonadherence (5, 33, 159, 163, 164). Clinically depressed patients are three times more likely to be nonadherent to diabetes regimens than nondepressed ones (159).

Parental worry is associated with restrictive behavior, and predicts poor adherence (165). Parental self-confidence affects adherence. In a study of children with HIV, parental self-perception of their ability to successfully administer their child's medication was positively correlated with adherence; parents of nonadherent children were more likely to agree with the statement that full adherence to antiretroviral medications was "almost impossible" (58).

Disease

Disease symptomatology, severity, duration, and course impact adherence. Asymptomatic and mild disease are associated with low patient motivation to follow treatment recommendations (9). Paradoxically, high symptomatology, high severity, and more functional impairment are also linked with increased nonadherence, perhaps due to pessimism about the ability of therapies to alter the course or outcome of serious illness (5). Poorer adherence has been observed in children with refractory epilepsy (165), aggressive malignancy (113), severe asthma (5), and end-stage renal disease (121). Adherence deteriorates over time in regimens for acute disease as symptoms abate or fail to improve despite treatment (7, 42, 153). Adherence to regimens for chronic disease fluctuates with overall decline over the course of illness (28, 107, 114, 121, 166, 167). Further characterization of vulnerable periods would allow providers to intervene more effectively.

Regimen

The administration of medical therapies to children can be difficult (42). Young children often resist the administration of eye, nose, or eardrops (42). Fear of needles is an obstacle for children receiving injected medications (168). Several studies examining adherence to pediatric liquid medications have found clear taste preferences (22, 169, 170) and marked variations in acceptance and adherence (170). Tablets and capsules are usually more palatable than liquids or suspensions but are not preferred for younger children secondary to choking risks (7). Adolescents with asthma have also voiced concerns about the taste of inhaled medications as an important problem in their regimen adherence (171). Adolescents with asthma object to having to carry inhalers and spacers to school and do not like to take medication in front of their peers (171).

Regimen characteristics play a critical role in pediatric adherence. Regimens that are aversive (9, 172), complex (5, 7, 10, 96, 107), protracted (7, 9), costly (5, 9, 173, 174), and preventive rather than curative (5–7, 9) are associated with poor adherence in children. Regimens requiring frequent dosing and/or food restrictions are harder to take as directed (5, 7, 15). Medical adherence has been shown to be improved with simplified regimens (7, 17, 107), fewer medications prescribed (7, 42, 175, 176), less frequent medication dosing (6, 8, 126, 175, 177), less expensive treatment options (6, 174), and nocturnal dosing of medications (7, 10, 28, 167, 178). The latter may be the result of fewer competing tasks or increased parental supervision at night.

Provider/Health System

Physician and health system attributes are also important factors in medical adherence (6, 9). Poor patient–doctor communication is one of the most frequently cited reasons for nonadherence to medical regimens (6, 7, 9, 17, 107, 179). In today's busy clinical setting, encounters are brief and communication may be inadequate, resulting in decreased patient education for disease management. Adequate support from physicians, nurses, and pharmacists has been shown to positively impact adherence in the pediatric population (28, 30, 143). Adolescents with epilepsy who had physician support had a 10-fold higher likelihood of adherence compared with teens without such support (28). Specific provider communication skills associated with better adherence include avoidance of jargon and increased attention to patients' concerns (10, 17, 63). Providers who are familiar with their patients or described as warm, empathetic, attentive, or friendly are associated with higher patient satisfaction and adherence (2, 5–7, 9, 165, 180, 181).

More frequent and longer clinical encounters also result in improved adherence to regimens (10, 30, 105).

An environment supportive of confidentiality is important to adolescents (10, 35). Attributes linked to poor medical adherence include distant or inconvenient facility locations, unfriendly staff, difficulty scheduling appointments, long waiting times, and medication dispensing difficulties (5, 6, 182). One study found that 43% of families had trouble filling prescriptions after clinic hours, but only 3% of providers gave patients either sample medications or parental antibiotics to provide medication until the morning (42). Table 8.1 summarizes the factors associated with medical adherence (5–7, 17, 18, 30, 105, 152, 159, 163, 183, 184).

CONSEQUENCES OF NONADHERENCE

Evidence supporting the relationship between medical nonadherence and poor clinical outcomes in children is plentiful. Suboptimal adherence has been associated with therapeutic failure in group A streptococci infections, otitis media, recurrent urinary tract infections, congenital heart disease, and asthma (4, 17, 39, 43, 185, 186). It has also been linked with increased antimicrobial resistance in tuberculosis, otitis media, recurrent urinary tract infection, and HIV (7, 19, 47, 136, 187). In addition, nonadherence has been implicated in the rates of unplanned pregnancy among adolescents (30), relapse of childhood cancer (188, 189), and graft failure in kidney, liver, and heart transplantation (109, 123, 132, 151, 184, 190). One study found 50% of children and 64% of adolescents to be nonadherent to their regimens for renal transplantation, resulting in subsequent graft rejection in 13% (17, 191). Nonadherence affects the quality of life for children and their families in the form of increased time, money, and energy spent in the clinic or hospital setting. Ultimately, nonadherence leads to unfavorable health outcomes directly as a result of therapeutic failure or lack of desired effect, or indirectly due to iatrogenic effects of unnecessary clinical interventions (7, 10).

INTERVENTIONS TO IMPROVE MEDICAL ADHERENCE

Over the past few years, a significant number of strategies have been designed and implemented with the aim to improve medical adherence in children and adolescents. Interventions to improve adherence fall into four main categories: educational, behavioral, affective, or organizational.

TABLE 8.1
Factors Associated With Non-Adherence

Patient and Family Factors	Associated With Better Adherence	Associated With Poorer Adherence	Inconsistent Association
DEMOGRAPHICS Patient Characteristics Socioeconomic status (SES)		• Adolescent age • Lower SES • Lower educational level • Language barrier • Single parenthood • Inner-city location	• Gender • Race
PSYCHOSOCIAL Parental/Caregiver traits	• Supportive • Flexible • Warm • Problem solver • Not overly critical	• Disengaged • Hostile • Stressed • Poor coping skills • Low health motivation	
Family traits Parental supervision	• Cohesion • Active	• Discord • Inadequate • Restrictive	
Peer group	• Peer support • Peer counseling		
Factual knowledge	• Better parental knowledge	• Knowledge deficits	• Patient knowledge
Adjustment to disease/ coping skills Psychological Developmental	• Good coping skills	• Maladaptive (anger, denial, anxiety) • Depression • Mental illness • Cognitive impairment • Developmental delay	
DISEASE FACTORS		• Long duration • Asymptomatic disease • Severe symptoms causing functional impairment	
REGIMEN FACTORS	• Simplified • Non-aversive • Non-intrusive • Nocturnal dosing • Curative	• Prolonged • Complex • Aversive • Intrusive • Costly • Preventive	
PROVIDER FACTORS	• Familiar • Empathetic • Good communicator • Friendly	• Impersonal • Apathetic • Poor communication skills	
HEALTH SYSTEM FACTORS	• Convenient location • Good accessibility • Supportive staff	• Distant location • Poor accessibility • Long waiting times • Unfriendly staff	

Educational Interventions. These strategies focus on providing patients and their families factual information about disease and treatment (107). Children and parents often make mistakes following complex protocols (6, 107, 192), especially when the rationale is unclear. Children formulate health beliefs and expectations about medications early in their development (193). Children and adolescents want to learn about their medicines, but providers rarely discuss medical regimens with them (194). Evidence suggests that children who are taught to use medication wisely and given some responsibility for their own care become more discerning about medical information, and less likely to engage in high-risk behaviors (18). Successful educational interventions are focused, organized, personalized, and age-appropriate (107). Information should be presented gradually and in a variety of formats to improve information retention and to accommodate different learning styles (6). For younger children, materials should be brief, interactive, and fun. Animated books, videos, and interactive computer games are favored by older children and adolescents (18). Because parents can strongly influence children's beliefs and attitudes, well-designed strategies must be family centered and include caregivers (195).

How should this education be provided by the provider? Crucial regimen components should be reiterated by the provider and repeated by the patient to ensure understanding. Scare tactics do not result in improved adherence and may be counterproductive (18, 30, 196). Teaching patients ways to integrate regimens into their daily routine is important (18). Peer teaching has been found to be an effective educational tool among adolescents (30, 153). Group education is generally more effective than individual education because of the social support and practical advice that is shared (15, 197). Nurses, pharmacists, case managers, and other staff members can also serve as educational resources (10, 15, 30).

Interventions to improve patient knowledge, however, have not always translated into better medical adherence or clinical outcome (7, 107). One intervention that educated caretakers about the physical findings of acute otitis media did not affect adherence to medication, appointment keeping, or clinical outcome (198). An intensive educational intervention for diabetic teenagers and their families improved disease-related knowledge but had no effect on adherence behavior or metabolic control (156). Because the effects of education may not be long lasting (7, 29, 199), additional strategies may be needed to maintain optimal medical adherence over time (107).

Behavioral Interventions. Behavioral approaches, focused on shaping or reinforcing specific behaviors, are among the most widely used adherence interventions (107). The underlying assumption is that "established behaviors are difficult to alter and that lasting change is only possible by breaking down habitual patterns and building up new behavior patterns" (107). Simple behavioral techniques that are easily incorporated into patient lifestyles have improved adherence in asthma and diabetes (107, 172, 200). Such methods include reward or token economies, mnemonic devices, cues, contracts, and goal setting (6, 7). For example, cueing techniques such as refrigerator notes or an association with teeth brushing, postcards, or telephone reminders can be successful (6, 10). In one study, stickers and medication labels imprinted with a clock reminding patients to take medicine improved adherence to antibiotics twofold over controls (201). Verbal or written contracts have improved adherence to regimens for otitis media (202), asthma (8), and diabetes mellitus (203). Token economies have improved adherence to regimens for pediatric asthma, diabetes mellitus, thalassemia (form of anemia), allergic rhinitis, juvenile rheumatoid arthritis, and renal disease (96, 204–207). Cognitive behavioral approaches such as distraction, imagery, or hypnosis have been effective in the management of pain and anxiety in children (208–213). Behavioral interventions seem to be effective in the short term, but further studies are needed to examine their long-term effects (107, 214).

Affective Strategies. Affective strategies focus on mediating patients' emotional responses to illness and treatment. These strategies typically involve individual and family psychosocial counseling. Adolescents who were counseled by trained peers have demonstrated better adherence to oral contraceptives than those who received counseling by an adult nurse (153). However, with the exception of peer counseling, affective strategies have had limited success in altering adherence behavior (197). Affective interventions are most commonly employed in conjunction with behavioral or other strategies (10).

Organizational Strategies. Organizational strategies focus on improving the quality and accessibility of health care services. Examples of such strategies include simplifying regimens, increasing appointment availability, improving provider supervision, or widening outreach efforts (17). A sound organizational infrastructure is crucial to optimizing health care delivery. Whether organizational efforts improve medical adherence and health outcomes requires further study.

Analysis of Successful Strategies. Evidence suggests that educational and organizational strategies (e.g., extended patient education or automated phone reminders) can positively impact adherence to regimens for acute disease (17, 174). For chronic illness, however, behavior strategies that result in enduring change are needed to improve adherence (17). A meta-analysis of interventions to improve adherence to chronic disease regimens found that those that used a multifaceted approach were more effective than those that relied on single strategies. Educational and behavioral interventions were found to be equally effective individually, and most effective when used jointly; each was found to work better than affective strategies alone (7, 10, 176, 197).

METHODOLOGICAL ISSUES
AND RECOMMENDATIONS

Choice of Informants. Adherence measures are generally obtained from patients or their parents whereas diagnostic laboratory procedures usually require that the information be provided by a properly trained health care professional (17). Because patients, parents, and providers may have equally valid but strikingly different views regarding the same subject matter *(cross-informant variance)*, the choice of informants should be carefully considered depending on the specific disease entity under evaluation, the adherence measure chosen, the individual with primary responsibility for regimen tasks, and the setting in which the study is to take place (17). For instance, physical education teachers or sports coaches are convenient informants in a study of pediatric adherence to inhaled medication for exercise-induced asthma whereas parents may be more appropriate informants in a study of pediatric adherence to nightly growth hormone injections. A study of adolescents' adherence to fluid restriction would ideally utilize informants in both home and school environments. In order for clinicians and researchers to attain an accurate depiction of adherence in pediatrics, efforts should be made to utilize multiple informants (patients, parents, teachers, etc.) whenever possible (17).

Representativeness. Most current adherence measures represent only a "snapshot" view of true adherence behavior. How closely this snapshot approaches the real picture depends on the frequency of assessment, the quality of adherence measures used, and duration of disease. In acute disease regimens, a single adherence measurement is likely to be more representative of true adherence than a single measurement in chronic illness. However, frequent health assessments are impractical unless patients are hospitalized or seen frequently in outpatient clinics (17). This can create a "severity bias" in which those patients who have more poorly controlled disease are assessed most frequently (17). Frequent health assessments, however, would facilitate access to adherence interventions (17).

To ensure accurate depiction of disease and health status, assessments should be frequent and sensitive enough to detect incremental changes over time. In addition, it is important that validated measures incorporate both subjective and objective data from multiple sources and perspectives including those of the child, the family, the teacher, and the health care provider (17).

CLINICAL IMPLICATIONS

Through recent research efforts, significant insight has been gained about the factors that contribute to medical nonadherence in children. Developmentally appropriate, family-centered interventions are critical in improving adherence in the pediatric population. Interventions that fail to address the particular needs of children and their families are short-lived and ineffective. The following is a compendium of clinical, research, and policy implications that follow from observed adherence trends in the pediatric literature. It is important to remark, however, that these observed associations do not imply causality. More rigorous research is needed to establish such claims.

Patient and Family Correlates. Human error contributes significantly to nonadherence. Parents forget 50% of medical information imparted verbally in 15 minutes, recall best the first third of the discussion, and remember more about diagnosis than therapy (6, 9, 106, 215). Clear and concise verbal and written information with repetition of important points can improve recall and enhance adherence (8). Behavioral strategies including memory cues such as "refrigerator notes" and taking medication in association with a daily habit such as teeth brushing improve adherence (34). Ongoing support is critical to ensure adherence. Because peers assume increasing importance as children mature, strategies that incorporate the peer group have shown benefit in improving adherence among adolescents (30, 153). Interventions that promote self-reliance in children and adolescents empower them to become informed medication consumers (193, 194). As children assume greater responsibility for their care, parental supervision and support can be eased but not discontinued.

Disease-Related Correlates. Patient adherence decreases with increasing length of illness, and when patients are either asymptomatic or highly symptomatic. Ideally, adherence interventions should be timed to coincide with these vulnerable periods. Messages about severity and risks of disease should be communicated in a positive manner, as children and adolescents often react negatively to such messages (17). The benefits of performing specific and manageable tasks to prevent or minimize disease severity or risk should be emphasized (17).

Regimen Correlates.   Adherence is inversely related to regimen complexity, duration, intensity, inconvenience, aversiveness, and intrusiveness (9, 118, 172). Whenever two or more equally effective regimens are available, the simplest, least intrusive, best-tasting, most economical regimen with the shortest treatment duration and fewest side effects should be selected to ensure optimal adherence (17, 173, 202). When multiple medications must be taken, they should ideally be organized to minimize confusion, and synchronized to the patient's daily routine. Medication packaging and measuring aids can also be specified to minimize dosing errors (46). Complex regimens should be implemented in a stepwise manner to enhance self-reliance and mastery (34). Critical aspects of the treatment plan such as completing the full course of antibiotics should be emphasized by the physician and reiterated by the patient.

Provider and Health System Correlates.   Poor provider–patient communication has been found to be one of the most important determinants of medical nonadherence. Providers cite time constraints and reimbursement limitations as important barriers to optimal adherence management (19). In addition, medical adherence can be significantly impaired by poorly developed health services and poor accessibility to providers due to lack of appointment availability, poor communication networks, inconvenient facility location, transportation problems, or long waiting times. Systemwide strategies include improving communication and access to health care, improving adherence counseling reimbursement, and allowing adequate time during clinical encounters for effective communication. Ancillary medical staff, pharmacists, and other community-based affiliates can offer continuing support and assistance. Timely follow-up via office visits or phone calls may allow earlier intervention (10). Evidence suggests that ongoing communication efforts to keep the patient engaged in health care may be the simplest and most cost-effective strategy for improving adherence (19).

Length of treatment and frequency of dosing impact medical adherence. Choosing medications with daily or twice dosing improves adherence in comparison to medications requiring greater dosing frequencies (6, 7, 96, 126, 170, 216). Several studies investigating shorter regimens of newer antibiotics for both otitis media and streptococcal pharyngitis have shown similar efficacy and safety profiles and better adherence as compared to traditional 10-day courses (217–219). Choosing lower cost medication options may be important with the increasing prevalence of medical copayments for pharmaceutical benefits. Successful strategies to improve medical adherence to acute-disease regimens would decrease problems associated with treatment failure and have a substantial impact on overall health costs.

TECHNOLOGICAL ADVANCES AND FUTURE DIRECTIONS

Electronic devices that measure dispensed medications represent incremental improvements from pill counting. There is greater difficulty with the measurement of dispensed liquid suspensions. Furthermore, the relative expense of such devices prohibits widespread use. Current efforts are under way to develop cost-effective pediatric adherence measures that can be incorporated into routine clinical practice.

Recent technological advances such as computerized medication databases, automated physician order entry, and preprinted medication information will likely reduce the frequency of medication errors in both inpatient and outpatient settings (220). This is expected to result in lower rates of adverse events and hopefully, higher rates of medical adherence. An innovative Internet-based intervention that included a video assessment of children's adherence to asthma regimens improved inhaler technique and reduced rescue medication use, emergency department visits, and hospitalizations. In addition, caregivers in the virtual-education group reported an increase in their children's quality-of-life scores (221). Another intervention that integrated video technology with qualitative research methods to assess asthmatic children's perspectives on illness found risk factors, barriers, and beliefs that were not identified by standard clinical tools (222).

Computerized applications now exist that create self-care plans with individualized medication, procedure, and condition-specific instructions. These applications allow patients and their caregivers to track completion of regimen tasks online and can also generate reminders to bolster adherence. However, further research is needed to assess whether these innovations will result in lasting behavior change or improved health outcomes.

LIMITATIONS OF CURRENT ADHERENCE RESEARCH IN CHILDREN

Global methodological limitations of adherence research are well described elsewhere in this book. They include the lack of standardized adherence measures (7) and of consistent definitions of adherence (7, 17). Pediatric adherence research suffers from a lack of longitudinal randomized controlled studies (13, 17). Many studies examine a single aspect of a complex regimen, and fail to control for multiple variables. The narrow focus of these studies tend to leave unstudied nonmedication aspects of medical regimens such as adherence to exercise recommendations, dietary guidelines, or medical follow-up (9). Many studies rely on indirect adherence measures with questionable validity. Unfortunately, direct adherence measures are invasive, expensive, and inconvenient for children and their families. Few studies examine pediatric adherence from ethnic, religious, or cultural, psychosocial perspectives (223), or study patients who live in isolated rural areas, whose lifestyles are outside of the mainstream, and have special needs and disabilities (224).

AN ADHERENCE RESEARCH AGENDA

A research agenda for future investigators of pediatric adherence includes the following:

- To explore strategies to improve the patient–doctor relationship and the patient and provider health care experience.
- To further explore the relationship between responsibility for regimens tasks and adherence.
- To develop improved health outcome measures that incorporate quality of life.
- To examine the multifactorial causation of adherence behavior from the different perspectives of caregivers, children, and health care workers via longitudinal trials.
- To further study the link between treatment adherence and health outcomes in children.
- To analyze the cost and effectiveness of different adherence measures and interventions.

Such an agenda demands a relatively large commitment in terms of time, money, and other resources. However, investments in adherence improvement have consistently yielded significant systemwide cost savings. Indeed, experts suggest that improving adherence might have a greater impact on public health than any improvement in specific disease treatments (19).

SUMMARY

Medical nonadherence is prevalent in pediatrics, with only about 50% of children adhering to prescribed treatments, and only 30% adhering to regimens for chronic illness. Long-term adherence to lifestyle modification such as diet or exercise is lower than adherence to medication regimens. Nonadherence does not indicate that patients and their caregivers do not give primacy to health and welfare. Rather, medical nonadherence results from a complex interplay of factors that affect children's and families' willingness or ability to adhere to treatment recommendations.

These factors may be related to the patient, family, disease, regimen, or health care provider. The different interests of the parent and the child complicate pediatric nonadherence. Factors such as patient age, SES, and psychosocial support also affect adherence. In adolescence, peers play an increasing role in behaviors affecting adherence. Medical adherence declines over the course of chronic illnesses and is low in asymptomatic conditions and in severe illnesses. Complex, unpleasant, protracted, or costly regimens are associated with lower adherence.

The doctor–patient relationship is of critical importance to medical adherence. Good physician communication fosters frank exchange with patients regarding treatment regimens, and the ability to tailor regimens to optimize adherence. Health care services that are efficient and convenient while allowing physicians to perform adequate teaching and counseling can improve adherence.

Specific interventions to improve adherence fall into educational, behavioral, affective, and organizational categories. Educational and organizational strategies improve adherence to regimens for acute disease. The addition of behavioral strategies helps to create long-term adherence to regimens for chronic disease.

Adherence strategies should be personalized, developmentally appropriate, family centered, and multifaceted. Physicians should work with children and their families to construct an acceptable treatment regimen that will cause the least disruption to the lives of children and their families. Health workers should inquire about difficulties with medical regimens to continuously improve adherence by removing barriers to prescribed treatments. By identifying and eliminating such barriers while maintaining communication and support, health care providers can create the optimal environment to help children and their families achieve their therapeutic goals and thus attain the highest potential quality of life despite their illness.

REFERENCES

1. Bergman AB, Werner RJ. Failure of children to receive penicillin by mouth. *N Engl J Med.* 1963;268:1334–1338.

2. Charney E, Bynum R, Eldredge D, et al. How well do patients take oral penicillin? A collaborative study in private practice. *Pediatrics.* 1967;40(2):188–195.

3. Mohler DN, Wallin DG, Dreyfus EG. Studies in the home treatment of streptococcal disease. I. Failure of patients to take penicillin by mouth as prescribed. *N Engl J Med.* 1955;252(26):1116–1118.

4. Green JL, Ray SP, Charney E. Recurrence rate of streptococcal pharyngitis related to oral penicillin. *J Pediatr.* 1969;75(2):292–294.

5. Bender BG. Overcoming barriers to nonadherence in asthma treatment. *J Allergy Clin Immunol.* 2002;109(6 Suppl):S554–S559.

6. Gottlieb H. Medication nonadherence: finding solutions to a costly medical problem. *Drug Benefit Trends.* 2002;12(6):57–62.

7. Matsui D. Drug compliance in pediatrics: clinical and research issues. *Pediatr Clin of North America.* 1997;44(1):1–14.

8. Buck M. Improving compliance with medication regimens. *Pediatr Pharmacotherapy.* 1997;3(8):1–3.

9. Fotheringham MJ, Sawyer MG. Adherence to recommended medical regimens in childhood and adolescence. *J Paediatr Child Health.* 1995;31(2):72–78.

10. Staples B, Bravender T. Drug compliance in adolescents. *Pediatr Drugs.* 2002;8 (8):503–513.

11. Pidgeon V. Compliance with chronic illness regimens: school-aged children and adolescents. *J Pediatr Nurs.* 1989;4(1):36–47.

12. Ayyangar R. Health maintenance and management in childhood disability. *Phys Med Rehabil Clin N Am.* 2002;13(4):793–821.

13. Riekert K. Adherence to medical treatment in pediatric chronic illness: critical issues and answered questions. In: Drotar D, ed. *Promoting Adherence to Medical Treatment in Chronic Childhood Illness.* Mahwah, NJ: Lawrence Erlbaum Associates; 2000:3–33.

14. Litt IF. Know thyself—adolescents' self-assessment of compliance behavior. *Pediatrics.* 1985;75(4):693–696.

15. Cheever L. Adherence to HIV therapies. Available at: http://hab.hrsa.gov/publications/chapter5/chapter5.htm.

16. Norman P, Searle A, Harrad R, Vedhara K. Predicting adherence to eye patching in children with amblyopia: an application of protection motivation theory. *Br J Health Psychol.* 2003;8(Pt 1):67–82.

17. Rapoff M. Medical nonadherence. In: *Adherence to Pediatric Medical Regimens.* New York: Kluwer Academic/Plenum Publishers; 1999:1–21.

18. Nichols-English G, Poirier S. Optimizing adherence to pharmaceutical care plans. *J Am Pharm Assoc (Wash).* 2000;40(4):475–485.

19. Burkhart PV, Sabate E. Adherence to long-term therapies: evidence for action. *J Nurs Scholarsh.* 2003;35(3):207.

20. Korsch BM, Fine RN, Negrete VF. Noncompliance in children with renal transplants. *Pediatrics.* 1978;61:872–876.

21. Blackwell B. Drug therapy: patient compliance. *N Engl J Med.* 1973;289(5): 249–252.

22. Powers JL, Gooch WM 3rd, Oddo LP. Comparison of the palatability of the oral suspension of cefdinir vs. amoxicillin/clavulanate potassium, cefprozil and azithromycin in pediatric patients. *Pediatr Infect Dis J.* 2000;19(12 Suppl):S174–S180.

23. Johnson S, Silverstein J, Rosebloom A, et al. Assessing daily management in childhood diabetes. *Health Psychol.* 1986;5:545–564.

24. Bond GG, Aitken LS, Somerville SC. The health belief model and adolescents with insulin dependent diabetes mellitus. *Health Psychol.* 1992;11:190–198.

25. Cheever LW, Wu AW. Medication adherence among HIV infected patients: understanding the complex behavior of taking complex therapy. *Curr Infect Dis Rep.* 1999;1:401–407.

26. Thomas AM, Peterson L, Goldstein D. Problem solving and diabetes regimen adherence by children and adolescents with IDDM in social pressure situations: a reflection of normal development. *J Pediatr Psychol.* 1997;22(4):541–561.

27. Friedman IM, Litt IF, King DR, et al. Compliance with anticonvulsant therapy by epileptic youth. Relationships to psychosocial aspects of adolescent development. *J Adolesc Health Care.* 1986;7(1):12–17.

28. Kyngas H. Predictors of good compliance in adolescents with epilepsy. *Seizure.* 2001;10(8):549–553.

29. Litt IF, Cuskey WR. Compliance with medical regimens during adolescence. *Pediatr Clin North Am.* 1980;27(1):3–15.

30. Jay S, Litt IF, Durant RH. Compliance with therapeutic regimens. *J Adol Health Care.* 1984;5:124.

31. Kroll T, Barlow JH, Shaw K. Treatment adherence in juvenile rheumatoid arthritis—a review. *Scand J Rheumatol.* 1999;28(1):10–18.

32. Buston KM, Wood SF. Non-compliance amongst adolescents with asthma: listening to what they tell us about self-management. *Fam Pract.* 2000;17(2):134–138.

33. Tamaroff MH, Festa RS, Adesman AR, Walco GA. Therapeutic adherence to oral medication regimens by adolescents with cancer. II. Clinical and psychologic correlates. *J Pediatr.* 1992;120(5):812–817.

34. Friedman IM, Litt IF. Adolescents' compliance with therapeutic regimens. *J Adolesc Health Care.* 1986;8:52–67.

35. Peremans L, Hermann I, Avonts D, Van Royen P, Denekens J. Contraceptive knowledge and expectations by adolescents: an explanation by focus groups. *Patient Educ Couns.* 2000;40(2):133–141.

36. Lloyd A, Horan W, Borgaro SR, Stokes JM, Pogge DL, Harvey PD. Predictors of medication compliance after hospital discharge in adolescent psychiatric patients. *J Child Adolesc Psychopharmacol.* 1998;8(2):133–141.

37. Durant RH, Jay MS, Linder CW, Shoffitt T, Litt I. Influence of psychosocial factors on adolescent compliance with oral contraceptives. *J Adolesc Health Care.* 1984;5(1):1–6.

38. Chacko MR, Kozinetz CA, Smith PB. Assessment of oral contraceptive pill continuation in young women. *J Pediatr Adolesc Gynecol.* 1999;12(3):143–148.

39. Wandstrat TL, Kaplan B. Pharmacoeconomic impact of factors affecting compliance with antibiotic regimens in the treatment of acute otitis media. *Pediatr Infect Dis J.* 1997;16S:27–29.

40. Stool SE, Field MJ. The impact of otitis media. *Pediatr Infect Dis J.* 1989;8(1 Suppl):S11–S14.

41. Freid VM, Makuc DM, Rooks RN. Ambulatory health care visits by children: principal diagnosis and place of visit. *Vital Health Stat.* 1998;13:1–23.

42. Mattar ME, Markello J, Yaffe SJ. Inadequacies in the pharmacologic management of ambulatory children. *J Pediatr.* 1975;87(1):137–141.

43. Harrison CJ, Belhorn TH. Antibiotic treatment failures in acute otitis media. *Pediatr Ann.* 1991;20(11):600–601, 603–608.

44. Dillon HC Jr. Streptococcal pharyngitis in the 1980s. *Pediatr Infect Dis J.* 1987;6 (1):123–130.

45. Gottlieb MI, Zinkus PW, Thompson A. Chronic middle ear disease and auditory perceptual deficits: is there a link? *Clin Pediatr (Phila).* 1979;18(12):725–732.

46. Shulman ST. Acute streptococcal pharyngitis in pediatric medicine: current issues in diagnosis and management. *Paediatr Drugs.* 2003;5 Suppl 1:13–23.

47. Seel K, Grosch-Worner I. [HIV infection in childhood]. *MMW Fortschr Med.* 2000;142 Suppl 1:54–57.

48. Sawyer SM, Aroni RA. Sticky issue of adherence. *J Paediatr Child Health.* 2003; 39(1):2–5.

49. Alperstein G, Morgan KR, Mills K, Daniels L. Compliance with anti-tuberculosis preventive therapy among 6-year-old children. *Aust NZ J Public Health.* 1998; 22(2):210–213.

50. Gordis L, Markowitz M, Lilienfeld AM. Why patients don't follow medical advice: a study of children on long-term anti-streptococcal prophylaxis. *J Pediatr.* 1969;75:957.

51. Goldstein NA, Sculerati N. Compliance with prophylactic antibiotics for otitis media in a New York City clinic. *Int J Pediatr Otorhinolaryngol.* 1994;28:129.

52. Katko E, Johnson GM, Fowler SL, Turner RB. Assessment of adherence with medications in human immunodeficiency virus-infected children. *Pediatr Infect Dis J.* 2001;20(12):1174–1176.

53. Penkower L, Dew MA, Ellis D, et al. Psychological distress and adherence to the medical regimen among renal transplant recipients. *Am J Transplantation.* 2003; 3(11):1418.

54. Festa RS, Tamaroff MH, Chasalow F, Lanzkowsky P. Therapeutic adherence to oral medication regimens by adolescents with cancer. I. Laboratory assessment. *J Pediatr.* 1992;120(5):807–811.

55. Watson DC, Farley JJ. Efficacy of and adherence to highly active antiretroviral therapy in children infected with human immunodeficiency virus type 1. *Pediatr Infect Dis J.* 1999;18(8):682–689.

56. Chesney M. Adherence to HAART regimens. *AIDS Patient Care STDS.* 2003; 17(4):169–177.

57. Chesney MA. Factors affecting adherence to antiretroviral therapy. *Clin Infect Dis.* 2000;30 Suppl 2:S171–S176.

58. Reddington C, Cohen J, Baldillo A, et al. Adherence to medication regimens among children with human immunodeficiency virus infection. *Pediatr Infect Dis J.* 2000;19(12):1148–1153.

59. Havens PL. Principles of antiretroviral treatment of children and adolescents with human immunodeficiency virus infection. *Semin Pediatr Infect Dis.* 2003; 14(4):269–285.

60. Redd SC. Asthma in the United States: burden and current theories. *Environ Health Perspect.* 2002;110(Suppl 4):557–560.

61. Marion RJ, Creer TL, Reynolds RV. Direct and indirect costs associated with the management of childhood asthma. *Ann Allergy.* 1985;54(1):31–34.

62. Walders N, Drotar D, Kercsmar C. The allocation of family responsibility for asthma management tasks in African-American adolescents. *J Asthma*. 2000; 37(1):89–99.

63. Bauman LJ, Wright E, Leickly FE, et al. Relationship of adherence to pediatric asthma morbidity among inner-city children. *Pediatrics*. 2002;110:e6.

64. Rand CS, Wise RA. Measuring adherence to asthma medication regimens. *Am J Respir Crit Care Med*. 1994;149(2 Pt 2):S69–S76; discussion S77–S78.

65. Kelloway JS, Wyatt RA, Adlis SA. Comparison of patients' compliance with prescribed oral and inhaled asthma medications. *Arch Intern Med*. 1994;154(12): 1349–1352.

66. Weinstein AG. Clinical management strategies to maintain drug compliance in asthmatic children. *Ann Allergy Asthma Immunol*. 1995;74(4):304–310.

67. Farber HJ, Capra AM, Finkelstein JA, et al. Misunderstanding of asthma controller medications: association with nonadherence. *J Asthma*. 2003;40(1):17–25.

68. Fish L, Lung CL. Adherence to asthma therapy. *Ann Allergy Asthma Immunol*. 2001;86(6 Suppl 1):24–30.

69. Celano M, Geller RJ, Phillips KM, Ziman R. Treatment adherence among low-income children with asthma. *J Pediatr Psychol*. 1998;23(6):345–349.

70. McNabb W. Adherence in diabetes: can we define it and can we measure it? *Diabetes Care*. 1997;20:215–218.

71. Diabetes, your child, your family. In: Diabetic Lifestyle. www.diabetic-lifestyle. com. Accessed 11/20/03.

72. Davis CL, Delamater AM, Shaw KH, et al. Parenting styles, regimen adherence, and glycemic control in 4- to 10-year-old children with diabetes. *J Pediatr Psychol*. 2001;26(2):123–129.

73. Hauser ST, Jacobson AM, Lavori P, et al. Adherence among children and adolescents with insulin-dependent diabetes mellitus over a four-year longitudinal follow-up: II. Immediate and long-term linkages with the family milieu. *J Pediatr Psychol*. 1990;15(4):527–542.

74. La Greca AM, Auslander WF, Greco P, Spetter D, Fisher EB Jr., Santiago JV. I get by with a little help from my family and friends: adolescents' support for diabetes care. *J Pediatr Psychol*. 1995;20(4):449–476.

75. Miller-Johnson S, Emery RE, Marvin RS, Clarke W, Lovinger R, Martin M. Parent–child relationships and the management of insulin-dependent diabetes mellitus. *J Consult Clin Psychol*. 1994;62(3):603–610.

76. Hanson CL, De Guire MJ, Schinkel AM, Kolterman OG. Empirical validation for a family-centered model of care. *Diabetes Care*. 1995;18(10):1347–1356.

77. Anderson BJ, Auslander WF, Jung KC, Miller JP, Santiago JV. Assessing family sharing of diabetes responsibilities. *J Pediatr Psychol*. 1990;15(4):477–492.

78. Anderson B, Ho J, Brackett J, Finkelstein D, Laffel L. Parental involvement in diabetes management tasks: relationships to blood glucose monitoring adherence and metabolic control in young adolescents with insulin-dependent diabetes mellitus. *J Pediatr*. 1997;130(2):257–265.

79. Glasgow RE, McCaul KD, Schafer LC. Self-care behaviors and glycemic control in type I diabetes. *J Chronic Dis*. 1987;40(5):399–412.

80. Kovacs M, Goldston D, Obrosky DS, Iyengar S. Prevalence and predictors of pervasive noncompliance with medical treatment among youths with insulin-dependent diabetes mellitus. *J Am Acad Child Adolesc Psychiatry.* 1992;31(6): 1112–1119.

81. Glasgow RE, McCaul KD, Schafer LC. Barriers to regimen adherence among persons with insulin-dependent diabetes. *J Behav Med.* 1986;9(1):65–77.

82. Huijbregts SC, de Sonneville LM, Licht R, van Spronsen FJ, Verkerk PH, Sergeant JA. Sustained attention and inhibition of cognitive interference in treated phenylketonuria: associations with concurrent and lifetime phenylalanine concentrations. *Neuropsychologia.* 2002;40(1):7–15.

83. Levy HL, Waisbren SE. PKU in adolescents: rationale and psychosocial factors in diet continuation. *Acta Paediatr Suppl.* 1994;407:92–97.

84. Anthony H, Bines J, Phelan P, Paxton S. Relation between dietary intake and nutritional status in cystic fibrosis. *Arch Dis Child.* 1998;78(5):443–447.

85. Levin ME. Understanding your diabetic patient. *Clin Podiatr Med Surg.* 1987; 4(2):315–330.

86. Raymond NG, Dwyer JT, Nevins P, Kurtin P. An approach to protein restriction in children with renal insufficiency. *Pediatr Nephrol.* 1990;4(2):145–151.

87. Lorenz RA, Christensen NK, Pichert JW. Diet-related knowledge, skill, and adherence among children with insulin-dependent diabetes mellitus. *Pediatrics.* 1985;75(5):872–876.

88. Assuncao MC, Santos Ida S, Costa JS. [Process assessment of health care: adequacy of the diabetes mellitus treatment in Pelotas, Southern Brazil]. *Cad Saude Publica.* 2002;18(1):205–211.

89. Passero MA, Remor B, Salomon J. Patient-reported compliance with cystic fibrosis therapy. *Clin Pediatr (Phila).* 1981;20(4):264–268.

90. Borowitz D, Wegman T, Harris M. Preventive care for patients with chronic illness. Multivitamin use in patients with cystic fibrosis. *Clin Pediatr (Phila).* 1994; 33(12):720–725.

91. MacDonald A. Diet and compliance in phenylketonuria. *Eur J Pediatr.* 2000; 159(Suppl 2):S136–S141.

92. Hanna KJ, Ewart CK, Kwiterovich PO Jr. Child problem solving competence, behavioral adjustment and adherence to lipid-lowering diet. *Patient Educ Couns.* 1990;16(2):119–131.

93. Berg-Smith SM, Stevens VJ, Brown KM, et al. A brief motivational intervention to improve dietary adherence in adolescents. The Dietary Intervention Study in Children (DISC) Research Group. *Health Educ Res.* 1999;14(3):399–410.

94. Brownell KD, Cohen LR. Adherence to dietary regimens. 2: components of effective interventions. *Behav Med.* 1995;20(4):155–164.

95. Robertson E. [Exercise therapy for children with cerebral palsy]. *Sven Lakartidn.* 1955;52(49):3038–3042.

96. Rapoff MA, Lindsley CB, Christophersen ER. Improving compliance with medical regimens: case study with juvenile rheumatoid arthritis. *Arch Phys Med Rehabil.* 1984;65(5):267–269.

97. Epstein LH, Coleman KJ, Myers MD. Exercise in treating obesity in children and adolescents. *Med Sci Sports Exerc.* 1996;28(4):428–435.

98. Gulmans VA, de Meer K, Brackel HJ, Faber JA, Berger R, Helders PJ. Outpatient exercise training in children with cystic fibrosis: physiological effects, perceived competence, and acceptability. *Pediatr Pulmonol.* 1999;28(1):39–46.

99. Fulton JE, McGuire MT, Caspersen CJ, Dietz WH. Interventions for weight loss and weight gain prevention among youth: current issues. *Sports Med.* 2001; 31(3):153–165.

100. Greenan-Fowler E, Powell C, Varni JW. Behavioral treatment of adherence to therapeutic exercise by children with hemophilia. *Arch Phys Med Rehabil.* 1987; 68(12):846–849.

101. Rapoff MA, Lindsley CB, Christophersen ER. Parent perceptions of problems experienced by their children in complying with treatments for juvenile rheumatoid arthritis. *Arch Phys Med Rehabil.* 1985;66(7):427–429.

102. Prasad SA, Cerny FJ. Factors that influence adherence to exercise and their effectiveness: application to cystic fibrosis. *Pediatr Pulmonol.* 2002;34(1):66–72.

103. De Bourdeaudhuij I, Crombez G, Deforche B, Vinaimont F, Debode P, Bouckaert J. Effects of distraction on treadmill running time in severely obese children and adolescents. *Int J Obes Relat Metab Disord.* 2002;26(8):1023–1029.

104. Coates TJ, Thoresen CE. Treating obesity in children and adolescents: a review. *Am J Public Health.* 1978;68(2):143–151.

105. Tebbi C. Treatment compliance in childhood and adolescence. *Cancer.* 1993; 71:3441.

106. Ley P, Bradshaw PW, Eaves D, Walker CM. A method for increasing patients' recall of information presented by doctors. *Psychol Med.* 1973;3(2):217–220.

107. Fielding D, Duff A. Compliance with treatment protocols: interventions for children with chronic illness. *Arch Dis Child.* 1999;80:196–200.

108. Christiaanse ME, Lavigne JV, Lerner CV. Psychosocial aspects of compliance in children and adolescents with asthma. *J Dev Behav Pediatr.* 1989;12(4):75–80.

109. Meyers KE, Thomson PD, Weiland H. Noncompliance in children and adolescents after renal transplantation. *Transplantation.* 1996;62(2):186–189.

110. Auslander WF, Thompson S, Dreitzer D, White NH, Santiago JV. Disparity in glycemic control and adherence between African American and Caucasian youths with diabetes: family and community contexts. *Diabetes Care.* 1997; 20(10):1569–1575.

111. Smith LK, Thompson JR, Woodruff G, Hiscox F. Factors affecting treatment compliance in amblyopia. *J Pediatr Ophthalmol Strabismus.* 1995;32(2):98–101.

112. Shulman S, Fisch RO, Zempel CE, Gadish O, Chang PN. Children with phenylketonuria: the interface of family and child functioning. *J Dev Behav Pediatr.* 1991;12(5):315–321.

113. Manne SL, Jacobsen PB, Gorfinkle K, Gerstein F, Redd WH. Treatment adherence difficulties among children with cancer: the role of parenting style. *J Pediatr Psychol.* 1993;18:47–62.

114. Martinez J, Bell D, Camacho R, et al. Adherence to antiviral drug regimens in HIV-infected adolescent patients engaged in care in a comprehensive adolescent and young adult clinic. *J Natl Med Assoc.* 2000;92(2):55–61.

115. Johnson RL, Botwinick G, Sell RL, et al. The utilization of treatment and case management services by HIV-infected youth. *J Adolesc Health.* 2003;33(2 Suppl):31–38.

116. Tonstad S, Sivertsen M. Dietary adherence in children with familial hypercholesterolemia. *Am J Clin Nutr.* 1997;65(4):1018–1026.

117. Becker MH, Maiman LA. Sociobehavioral determinants of compliance with health and medical care recommendations. *Med Care.* 1975;13(1):10–24.

118. Becker MH, Drachman RH, Kirscht JP. Predicting mothers' compliance with pediatric medical regimens. *J Pediatr.* 1972;81(4):843–854.

119. Overstreet S, Goins J, Cheng RS, et al. Family environment and the interrelation of family structure, child behavior, and metabolic control for children with diabetes. *J Pediatr Psychol.* 1995;20:435–447.

120. Thompson SJ, Auslander WF, White NH. Influence of family structure on health among youths with diabetes. *Health Soc Work.* 2001;26(1):7–14.

121. Brownbridge G, Fielding DM. Psychological adjustment and adherence to dialysis treatment regimens. *Pediatr Nephrol.* 1994;8:744–749.

122. Emans SJ, Grace E, Wood ER, et al. Adolescents' compliance with the use of oral contraceptives. *JAMA.* 1987;257:3377–3381.

123. Lurie S, Shemesh E, Sheiner PA, et al. Non-adherence in pediatric liver transplant recipients—an assessment of risk factors and natural history. *Pediatr Transplant.* 2000;4(3):200–206.

124. Tebbi CK, Cummings KM, Zevon MA, Smith L, Richards M, Mallon J. Compliance of pediatric and adolescent cancer patients. *Cancer.* 1986;58(5):1179–1184.

125. Daviss WB, Coon H, Whitehead P, Ryan K, Burkley M, McMahon W. Predicting diabetic control from competence, adherence, adjustment, and psychopathology. *J Am Acad Child Adolesc Psychiatry.* 1995;34(12):1629–1636.

126. Dajani AS. Adherence to physicians' instructions as a factor in managing streptococcal pharyngitis. *Pediatrics.* 1996;97(6 Pt 2):976–980.

127. Williams C. Gender, adolescence, and the management of diabetes. *J Adv Nurs.* 1999;30(5):1160–1166.

128. Patterson J. Critical factors affecting family compliance with home treatment for children with cystic fibrosis. *Family Relations.* 1985;34:79–89.

129. Johnson SB, Freund A, Silverstein J, Hansen CA, Malone J. Adherence-health status relationships in childhood diabetes. *Health Psychol.* 1990;9(5):606–631.

130. Kaar ML, Akerblom HK, Huttunen NP, Knip M, Sakkinen K. Metabolic control in children and adolescents with insulin-dependent diabetes mellitus. *Acta Paediatr Scand.* 1984;73(1):102–108.

131. Epstein LH, Paluch RA, Raynor HA. Sex differences in obese children and siblings in family-based obesity treatment. *Obes Res.* 2001;9(12):746–753.

132. Blowey DL, Hebert D, Arbus GS, Pool R, Korus M, Koren G. Compliance with cyclosporine in adolescent renal transplant recipients. *Pediatr Nephrol.* 1997; 11(5):547–551.

133. Cromer BA, Steinberg K, Gardner L, Thornton D, Shannon B. Psychosocial determinants of compliance in adolescents with iron deficiency. *Am J Dis Child.* 1989;143(1):55–58.

134. Bachmann LH, Stephens J, Richey CM, et al. Measured vs self-reported compliance with doxycycline therapy for chlamydia-associated syndromes: high therapeutic success rates despite poor compliance. *Sex Transm Dis.* 1999;26(5): 272–278.

135. Bender B, Wamboldt FS, O'Connor SL, et al. Measurement of children's asthma medication adherence by self report, mother report, canister weight, and Doser CT. *Ann Allergy Asthma Immunol.* 2000;85(5):416–421.

136. Pablos-Mendez A, Knirsch CA, Barr RG, Lerner BH, Frieden TR. Nonadherence in tuberculosis treatment: predictors and consequences in New York City. *Am J Med.* 1997;102(2):164–170.

137. Schechter MS, Margolis PA. Relationship between socioeconomic status and disease severity in cystic fibrosis. *J Pediatr.* 1998;132(2):260–264.

138. Ruiz P. The role of culture in psychiatric care. *Am J Psychiatry.* 1998;155(12): 1763–1765.

139. David RA, Rhee M. The impact of language as a barrier to effective health care in an underserved urban Hispanic community. *Mt Sinai J Med.* 1998;65(5–6): 393–397.

140. Schlenk EA, Hart LK. Relationship between health locus of control, health value, and social support and compliance of persons with diabetes mellitus. *Diabetes Care.* 1984;7:566–574.

141. Christiansen AJ, Smith TW, Turner CW, Holman JM Jr., Gregory MC, Rich MA. Family support, physical impairment, and adherence in hemodialysis: an investigation of main and buffering effects. *J Behav Med.* 1992;15:313–325.

142. Byrne M, Honig J, Jurgrau A, Heffernan SM, Donahue MC. Achieving adherence with antiretroviral medications for pediatric HIV disease. *AIDS Read.* 2002;12(4):151–154, 161–164.

143. Kyngas H, Rissanen M. Support as a crucial predictor of good compliance of adolescents with a chronic disease. *J Clin Nurs.* 2001;10(6):767–774.

144. DuRant RH, Jay MS. A social psychologic model of female adolescents' compliance with contraceptives. *Semin Adolesc Med.* 1987;3(2):135–144.

145. Wamboldt MZ, Wamboldt FS. Role of the family in the onset and outcome of childhood disorders: selected research findings. *J Am Acad Child Adolesc Psychiatry.* 2000;39(10):1212–1219.

146. Davis MD, Eichern RL. Compliance with medical regimens: a panel study. *J Health Hum Behav.* 1963;4:240.

147. Salabarria-Pena Y, Trout PT, Gill JK, Morisky DE, Muralles AA, Ebin VJ. Effects of acculturation and psychosocial factors in Latino adolescents' TB-related behaviors. *Ethn Dis.* 2001;11(4):661–675.

148. Lansky SB, Smith SD, Cairns NU, Cairns GF Jr. Psychological correlates of compliance. *Am J Pediatr Hematol Oncol.* 1983;5(1):87–92.

149. Beck DE, Fennell RS, Yost RL, Robinson JD, Geary D, Richards GA. Evaluation of an educational program on compliance with medication regimens in pediatric patients with renal transplants. *J Pediatr.* 1980;96(6):1094–1097.

150. Scher PW, Emans SJ, Grace EM. Factors associated with compliance to oral contraceptive use in an adolescent population. *J Adolesc Health Care.* 1982;3(2):120–123.

151. Wolff G, Strecker K, Vester U, Latta K, Ehrich JH. Non-compliance following renal transplantation in children and adolescents. *Pediatr Nephrol.* 1998;12(9):703–708.

152. La Greca AM, Bearman KJ, Moore H. Peer relations of youth with pediatric conditions and health risks: promoting social support and healthy lifestyles. *J Dev Behav Pediatr.* 2002;23(4):271–280.

153. Jay MS, DuRant RH, Shoffitt T, Linder CW, Litt IF. Effect of peer counselors on adolescent compliance in use of oral contraceptives. *Pediatrics.* 1984;73(2):126–131.

154. Lyon ME, Trexler C, Akpan-Townsend C, et al. A family group approach to increasing adherence to therapy in HIV-infected youths: results of a pilot project. *AIDS Patient Care STDS.* 2003;17(6):299–308.

155. Gudas LJ, Koocher GP, Wypij D. Perceptions of medical compliance in children and adolescents with cystic fibrosis. *J Dev Behav Pediatr.* 1991;12(4):236–242.

156. Mendez FJ, Belendez M. Effects of a behavioral intervention on treatment adherence and stress management in adolescents with IDDM. *Diabetes Care.* 1997;20(9):1370–1375.

157. Anthony H, Paxton S, Bines J, Phelan P. Psychosocial predictors of adherence to nutritional recommendations and growth outcomes in children with cystic fibrosis. *J Psychosom Res.* 1999;47(6):623–634.

158. Sunder TR. Meeting the challenge of epilepsy in persons with multiple handicaps. *J Child Neurol.* 1997;12(Suppl 1):S38–S43.

159. Martinez Chamorro MJ, Lastra Martinez I, Luzuriaga Tomas C. [Psychopathology and child and adolescent type 1 diabetes mellitus outcome]. *Actas Esp Psiquiatr.* 2002;30(3):175–181.

160. Brownbridge G, Fielding DM. Psychosocial adjustment and adherence to dialysis treatment regimes. *Pediatr Nephrol.* 1994;8(6):744–749.

161. Knowles HC, Guest GM, Lampe J, et al. The course of diabetes mellitus treated with unmeasured diet. *Diabetes.* 1965;14:239–270.

162. Wickers FC, Bunch WH, Barnett PM. Psychological factors in failure to wear the Milwaukee brace for treatment of idiopathic scoliosis. *Clin Orthop.* 1977;(126):62–66.

163. Thiruchelvam D, Charach A, Schachar RJ. Moderators and mediators of long-term adherence to stimulant treatment in children with ADHD. *J Am Acad Child Adolesc Psychiatry.* 2001;40(8):922–928.

164. Simoni JM, Asarnow JR, Munford PR, Koprowski CM, Belin TR, Salusky IB. Psychological distress and treatment adherence among children on dialysis. *Pediatr Nephrol.* 1997;11(5):604–606.

165. Hazzard A, Hutchinson SJ, Krawiecki N. Factors related to adherence to medication regimens in pediatric seizure patients. *J Pediatr Psychol.* 1990;15(4): 543–555.

166. Hudson J, Fielding D, Jones S, McKendrick T. Adherence to medical regime and related factors in youngsters on dialysis. *Br J Clin Psychol.* 1987;26(Pt 1): 61–62.

167. Jonasson G, Carlsen KH, Mowinckel P. Asthma drug adherence in a long term clinical trial. *Arch Dis Child.* 2000;83(4):330–333.

168. Sandberg DE, Mazur TA, Alliger DA, et al. Promoting adherence to growth hormone therapy among children with growth failure. In: Drotar D, ed. *Promoting Adherence to Medical Treatment in Chronic Childhood Illness.* Mahwah, NJ: Lawrence Erlbaum Associates; 2000:429–451.

169. Bagger-Sjoback D, Bondesson G. Taste evaluation and compliance of two paediatric formulations of phenoxymethylpenicillin in children. *Scand J Prim Health Care.* 1989;7(2):87–92.

170. Dagan R, Shvartzman P, Liss Z. Variation in acceptance of common oral antibiotic suspensions. *Pediatr Infect Dis J.* 1994;13(8):686–690.

171. Slack MK, Brooks AJ. Medication management issues for adolescents with asthma. *Am J Health Syst Pharm.* 1995;52(13):1417–1421.

172. Creer TL, Burns KL. Self-management training for children with bronchial asthma. *Psychother Psychosomatics.* 1979;32:270–278.

173. Brand FN, Smith RT, Brand PA. Effect of economic barriers to medical care on patients' noncompliance. *Public Health Rep.* 1977;92(1):72–78.

174. Haynes RB, McKibbon KA, Kanani R. Systematic review of randomised trials of interventions to assist patients to follow prescriptions for medications. *Lancet.* 1996;348(9024):383–386.

175. Hussar DA. Importance of patient compliance in effective antimicrobial therapy. *Pediatr Infect Dis J.* 1987;6(10):971–975.

176. Thatcher S. Medication compliance. *Pediatr Clin North Am.* 1981;28:5.

177. Richter A, Anton SE, Koch P, Dennett SL. The impact of reducing dose frequency on health outcomes. *Clin Ther.* 2003;25(8):2307–2335; discussion 2306.

178. Moncica I, Oh PI, ul Qamar I, et al. A crossover comparison of extended release felodipine with prolonged action nifedipine in hypertension. *Arch Dis Child.* 1995;73(2):154–156.

179. Kessler D. Communicating with patients about their medications. *N Engl J Med.* 1991;325:1650–1652.

180. Korsch BM, Gozzi EK, Francis V. Gaps in doctor–patient communication. Doctor–patient interaction and patient satisfaction. *Pediatrics.* 1968;42:855.

181. Ley P. Satisfaction, compliance and communication. *Br J Clin Psychol.* 1982; 21(Pt 4):241–254.

182. Davidson PO, Schrag AR. Factors affecting the outcome of child psychiatric consultations. *Am J Orthopsychiatry.* 1969;39(5):774–778.

183. Home R. One to be taken as directed: reflections on non-adherence (non-compliance). *J Soc Admin Pharm.* 1993;10(4):150–156.
184. Zerwic JJ, Sherry DC, Simmons B, Wung SF. Noncompliance in heart transplantation: a role for the advanced practice nurse. *Prog Cardiovasc Nurs.* 2003; 18(3):141–146.
185. Matsui D, Hermann C, Braudo M, et al. Clinical use of the medication event monitoring system: a new window into pediatric compliance. *Clin Pharmacol Ther.* 1992;52:102.
186. Daschner F, Maget W. Treatment of recurrent urinary tract infection in children. *Acta Paediatr Scand.* 1975;64:105.
187. Bangsberg D. Adherence to protease inhibitors, HIV-1 viral load, and development of drug resistance in an indigent population. *AIDS.* 2000;14:357–366.
188. Smith SD, Cairns NU, Sturgeon JK, et al. Poor drug compliance in an adolescent with leukemia. *Am J Hematol Oncol.* 1981;3:297.
189. Snodgrass W, Smith S, Trueworthy R, Vats TS, Klopovich P, Kisker S. Pediatric clinical pharmacology of 6-mercaptopurine; lack of compliance as a factor in leukemia relapse. *Am Soc Clin Oncol.* 1984;3:204.
190. Tuchman M, Freese DK, Sharp HL, et al. Persistent succinylacetone excretion after liver transplantation in a patient with hereditary tyrosinaemia type I. *J Inherit Metab Dis.* 1985;8(1):21–24.
191. Ettenger RB, Rosenthal JT, Marik JL, et al. Improved cadaveric renal transplant outcome in children. *Pediatr Nephrol.* 1991;5(1):137–142.
192. Johnson S, Pollak RT, Silverstein J, et al. Cognitive and behavioral knowledge about insulin dependent diabetes among children and parents. *Pediatrics.* 1982;69:708–713.
193. Bush PJ, Iannotti RJ. A children's health belief model. *Med Care.* 1990;28(1): 69–86.
194. Menacker F, Aramburuzabala P, Minian N, Bush P, Bibace R. Children and medicines: what they want to know and how they want to learn. *J Soc Adm Pharm.* 1999;16(1):38–51.
195. Bush PJ, Iannotti RJ. Origins and stability of children's health beliefs relative to medicine use. *Soc Sci Med.* 1988;27(4):345–352.
196. Evans RI, Rozelle RM, Lasater TM, Dembroski TM, Allen BP. Fear arousal, persuasion, and actual versus implied behavioral change: new perspective utilizing a real-life dental hygiene program. *J Pers Soc Psychol.* 1970;16(2):220–227.
197. Roter DL, Hall JA, Merisca R, Nordstrom B, Cretin D, Svarstad B. Effectiveness of interventions to improve patient compliance: a meta-analysis. *Med Care.* 1998;36(8):1138–1161.
198. Williams R. Illness visualization and therapeutic adherence. *J Fam Pract.* 1989;28(2):185–192.
199. Rapoff MA, Purviance MR, Lindsley CB. Educational and behavioral strategies for improving medication compliance in juvenile rheumatoid arthritis. *Arch Phys Med Rehabil.* 1988;69(6):439–441.
200. Delamater AM, Smith JA, Kurtz SM, White NH. Dietary skills and adherence in children with type I diabetes mellitus. *Diabetes Educ.* 1988;14(1):33–36.

201. Lima J, Nazarian L, Charney E, Lahti C. Compliance with short-term antimicrobial therapy: some techniques that help. *Pediatrics.* 1976;57(3):383–386.

202. Kulik JA, Carlino P. The effect of verbal commitment and treatment choice on medication compliance in a pediatric setting. *J Behav Med.* 1987;10(4): 367–376.

203. Weinstein A. Clinical management strategies to maintain compliance in asthmatic children. *Ann Allergy Asthma Immunol.* 1995;74:304–310.

204. da Costa IG, Rapoff MA, Lemanek K, Goldstein GL. Improving adherence to medication regimens for children with asthma and its effect on clinical outcome. *J Appl Behav Anal.* 1997;30(4):687–691.

205. Magrab PR, Papadopoulou ZL. The effect of a token economy on dietary compliance for children on hemodialysis. *J Appl Behav Anal.* 1977;10(4):573–578.

206. Finney JW, Lemanek KL, Brophy CJ, Cataldo MF. Pediatric appointment keeping: improving adherence in a primary care allergy clinic. *J Pediatr Psychol.* 1990;15(4):571–579.

207. Koch DA, Giardina PJ, Ryan M, MacQueen M, Hilgartner MW. Behavioral contracting to improve adherence in patients with thalassemia. *J Pediatr Nurs.* 1993;8(2):106–111.

208. Jay SM, Elliott CH, Woody PD, Siegel S. An investigation of cognitive-behavior therapy combined with oral valium for children undergoing painful medical procedures. *Health Psychol.* 1991;10(5):317–322.

209. Ellis JA, Spanos NP. Cognitive-behavioral interventions for children's distress during bone marrow aspirations and lumbar punctures: a critical review. *J Pain Symptom Manage.* 1994;9(2):96–108.

210. Moore KE, Geffken GR, Royal GP. Behavioral intervention to reduce child distress during self-injection. *Clin Pediatr (Phila).* 1995;34(10):530–534.

211. McCarthy AM, Cool VA, Petersen M, Bruene DA. Cognitive behavioral pain and anxiety interventions in pediatric oncology centers and bone marrow transplant units. *J Pediatr Oncol Nurs.* 1996;13(1):3–12; discussion 13–14.

212. Mazur J, Mierzejewska E. [Health-related quality of life (HRQL) in children and adolescents—concepts, study methods and selected applications]. *Med Wieku Rozwoj.* 2003;VII(1 Pt 2):35–48.

213. Vessey JA, Carlson KL. Nonpharmacological interventions to use with children in pain. *Issues Compr Pediatr Nurs.* 1996;19(3):169–182.

214. Miller DL, Stark LJ. Contingency contracting for improving adherence in pediatric populations. *JAMA.* 1994;271(1):81, 83.

215. Liptak GS. Enhancing patient compliance in pediatrics. *Pediatr Rev.* 1996; 17(4):128–134.

216. Greenberg RN. Overview of patient compliance with medication dosing: a literature review. *Clin Ther.* 1984;6(5):592–599.

217. Esposito S, Marchisio P, Bosis S, et al. Comparative efficacy and safety of 5-day cefaclor and 10-day amoxicillin treatment of group A streptococcal pharyngitis in children. *Int J Antimicrobial Agents.* 2002;20(1):28–33.

218. Powers JL. Properties of azithromycin that enhance the potential for compliance in children with upper respiratory tract infections. *Pediatr Infect Dis J.* 1996;15(9 Suppl):S30–S37.

219. Gerber MA. A comparison of cefadroxil and penicillin V in the treatment of streptococcal pharyngitis in children. *Drugs.* 1986;32(Suppl 3):29–32.

220. Kaushal R, Barker KN, Bates DW. How can information technology improve patient safety and reduce medication errors in children's health care? *Arch Pediatr Adolesc Med.* 2001;155(9):1002–1007.

221. Chan DS, Callahan CW, Sheets SJ, Moreno CN, Malone FJ. An Internet-based store-and-forward video home telehealth system for improving asthma outcomes in children. *Am J Health Syst Pharm.* 2003;60(19):1976–1981.

222. Rich M, Lamola S, Gordon J, Chalfen R. Video intervention/prevention assessment: a patient-centered methodology for understanding the adolescent illness experience. *J Adolesc Health.* 2000;27(3):155–165.

223. Matza LS, Swensen AR, Flood EM, Secnik K, Leidy NK. Assessment of health-related quality of life in children: a review of conceptual, methodological, and regulatory issues. *Value Health.* 2004;7(1):79–92.

224. Bender B, Milgrom H, Apter A. Adherence intervention research: what have we learned and what do we do next? *J Allergy Clin Immunol.* 2003;112(3):489–494.

Chapter 9

The Effects of Clinical Depression and Depressive Symptoms on Treatment Adherence

Jodi M. Gonzalez
John W. Williams, Jr.

PREVALENCE AND IMPACT OF DEPRESSION

Depressive disorders are prevalent, cause marked personal suffering, and are associated with increased mortality. In primary care settings, the prevalence of major depression ranges from 4.8% to 8.6%, and dysthymia ranges from 2.1% to 3.7% (1). Less severe depressive disorders, such as minor depression and adjustment disorders, are even more common. Depressive episodes are about twice as common in women as in men, peak in middle age, and are strongly associated with adverse social and economic circumstances such as unemployment, divorce or separation, inadequate housing, and lower socioeconomic status. Ethnic minority status can affect depression rates. The most recent U.S. epidemiologic study reported that non-Hispanic Blacks had lower odds of lifetime depression than non-Hispanic Whites, whereas Hispanics did not differ from Whites in lifetime or 12-month depression (2). Depression increases when a family history of depression is present (3).

The World Health Organization estimates that major depression alone was the fourth leading cause of disability worldwide in 1990, and will soon be second only to heart disease as a cause of disability (4). In a longitudinal study of over 2,500 older adults with one of eight chronic medical conditions, depressive symptoms were associated with a marked reduction in quality of life. After adjusting for potential confounders, only arthritis and heart disease were more strongly associated with decreases in quality-adjusted life years when compared to depression (5).

Depressive disorders are at least 2 to 3 times more common in hospitalized patients, nursing home residents, or outpatients with chronic medical disorders. In particular, the "3 C's—cardiovascular disease (CVD), central nervous system disorders (e.g., strokes, dementia, Parkinsons disease), and cancer"—are medical conditions prevalent in older adults and associated with a high risk for coexisting depression (6). Comorbid medical illness is a marker for poor outcomes in patients with depression. Conversely, depression adversely affects the course of coexisting medical illness, contributing to increased symptom burden, functional impairment, and mortality (7, 8). Patients who have suffered a recent myocardial infarction (MI) and have concurrent depression are approximately 3 times more likely to die within 6 months than those who are not depressed (7–9). For patients with diabetes mellitus, depression is associated with worse glycemic control and higher risk of heart disease (10, 11). Depression is also associated with an increased risk of mortality in elderly patients following hospital discharge, and in nursing home residents (12). (See Table 9.1 for a breakdown of the prevalence of depression in patients with chronic medical illness.)

TABLE 9.1
Prevalence of Depression in Patients With Chronic Medical Illness

Medical Illness	Depressive Disorder	Prevalence (%)
Alzheimer's disease (1)	Major depression	5–15
Arthritis (7)	Major depression, dysthymia, or mania	11
Cardiovascular disease (2):		
Angina	Major depression	15–23
Congestive heart failure	Major depression	17–37
Post–myocardial infarction	Major depression	16–27
Post–coronary artery bypass	Major depression	20
Cancer (1)		
Hospitalized patients	Depressive symptoms	25–50
Hospitalized patients	Major depression	6–13
Chronic lung disease (7)	Major depression, dysthymia, or mania	14
Diabetes mellitus (5–8)	Major depression	10–14
Human immunodeficiency virus infection (3)	Major depression	3–36
Hypertension (7)	Major depression, dysthymia, or mania	11
Parkinson's disease (1)	Major depression	15–20
Poststroke (4)		
Acute and rehabilitation hospitals	Major depression	19
Outpatients	Major depression	23

Clinical depression is a final common pathway resulting from the interaction of biological, psychological, and social factors. It is a syndrome characterized by persistent depressed mood or anhedonia, additional psychological (e.g., feeling worthless) and somatic symptoms (e.g., appetite change, motor retardation), and significant functional impairment. Interpersonal withdrawal and decreased social support are also common features of depression. Various theories exist as to why depression is often comorbid with medical illness. One leading hypothesis is that structures of the brain may be impaired as a cause, or result, of depression (13–15). These impaired structures may make the brain more vulnerable to not only depression but other medical illnesses. For example, Krishnan (15) reported that in poststroke patients with depression, there were more structural abnormalities in the brain than poststroke patients without depression. A second set of hypotheses involve the functioning of neuroendocrine systems, which are often dysregulated in depression (16). This dysregulation may be the resultant effect of stress and depression on the brain, increasing the likelihood of neuroendocrine-related medical illness such as cardiovascular disease or impaired immune or metabolic systems (17). Or, biological predisposition to dysregulation of neuroendocrine systems may cause patients to be more vulnerable to both depression and related medical illnesses.

Neurotransmitter and neuroendocrine system malfunctions may also affect medical illness via decreased adherence to medical treatment. Serotonin, dopamine, and other neurotransmitters are implicated in depression and contribute to sad mood and diminished interest in social contact. Neuroendocrine changes may also cause disturbances in sleep, appetite, and energy levels. Medical treatments requiring significant motivation level, cognitive skills, and daily physical and mental effort are more difficult to follow in the face of pessimistic mood, decreased ability to concentrate, and low energy. Furthermore, social isolation may decrease the emotional and material social support needed to foster treatment adherence.

The goals of this chapter are to identify the independent effects of depression on adherence to medical treatments, mental health treatments, and preventive care. As suggested by the theoretical models described in chapter 3 (of this volume), adherence to medical treatment is a multi-determined pathway. There are without doubt other mechanisms affecting adherence other than depression. However, in this chapter we discuss the impact of depression on adherence.

We summarize the extant literature, limited to publications in English conducted since 1980. Although a considerable amount of literature correlates depression with medical and psychiatric morbidity, we hone the discussion to studies where adherence is included as a specific variable, in the form of failure to initiate treatment, limited adherence to treatment, or discontinuing treatment. We discuss the clinical implications of our findings and directions for future research.

IMPACT OF DEPRESSION ON ADHERENCE TO GENERAL MEDICAL TREATMENT

Adherence to Treatments for Chronic Medical Illness

Chronic illnesses such as CVD, diabetes, and asthma often involve multifaceted, complex treatments. Treatment regimens may include (a) attending office visits, (b) collaborating with physicians, (c) altering one's diet, (d) increasing or adding exercise, (e) taking medications regularly, (f) self-monitoring activities, such as checking blood glucose or blood pressure, (g) decreasing potentially harmful behaviors such as drinking alcohol or smoking, and (h) tolerating the physical or psychological discomfort and financial costs of these treatments (13). It is logical to hypothesize that adherence suffers when highly demanding treatment plans intersect with clinical depression. In a meta-analysis of the effects of depression and anxiety on adherence to various medical treatments, Di Matteo (18) reported adherence was 3 times lower in depressed patients as compared to nondepressed patients. We selected highly prevalent, chronic medical conditions where sufficient evidence is available for detailed review to evaluate this association.

Cardiovascular Disease. Depression increases the risk of heart disease morbidity and mortality, even after adjusting for other established risk factors. Biological, behavioral, and treatment disparities are hypothesized as explanatory mechanisms. One likely mechanism is reduced adherence to medical treatments demonstrated to improve cardiac outcomes (18–23). Another possibility is the provision of less aggressive treatment for depressed patients. Recent evidence shows that post-MI, depressed patients may be less likely to be prescribed medications (24) or have important cardiovascular procedures performed (22). In a Medline review, we searched for articles that empirically address the effects of depression on adherence to medical and related treatments for CVD.

The majority of studies show a reciprocal relationship between increasing depressive symptoms and short-term adherence. Ziegelstein (23) followed 204 patients for 4 months following an MI. Depressed patients reported lower adherence to recommended changes in diet, regular exercise, reducing stress, and increasing social support. A subset analysis confirmed these results in patients 65 years and older (24). Blumenthal (19) prospectively evaluated 35 patients with recent MIs who were prescribed an exercise rehabilitation program. Depression, significant in univariate analyses, did not remain significantly associated with dropout in multivariate analyses, but the small sample size limited power to detect a significant association. Carney (20) studied 55 patients over 64 years old with coronary artery disease who were prescribed daily aspirin. Over 3 weeks, depressed patients adhered to the regimen significantly less often than nondepressed patients. The effects of depression on longer-term adherence have not been well studied, but two studies evaluating effects on exercise and medication have not shown an effect. Dorn (25) studied 308 men from the 1976–1979 National Exercise and Heart Disease Project, and did not find a relationship between depressive symptoms and adherence to a 3-year exercise treatment regimen. Irvine (26) prospectively evaluated 2-year medication adherence via pill counts in 671 patients post-MI, and did not find a relationship of depression to adherence.

For patients with hypertension, several studies have shown an association with adherence and depression. Ford (27) analyzed 31 hypertensive adults, and found that depression negatively affected adherence to medication treatments. In a 1-year prospective study, Wang (28) studied 248 VA (Veterans Affairs) patients and 248 HMO patients with hypertension. After adjusting for potential confounders, depressive symptoms were significantly associated with decreased adherence to antihypertensive medications. Davies (29) studied 233 hypertensive patients, and found that reported intolerance to hypertensive drugs was significantly associated with depression and anxiety. The authors hypothesized that depressed patients may focus on and amplify negative aspects of treatment, or may misinterpret symptoms of psychiatric illness as drug side effects.

Diabetes Mellitus.   Diabetes mellitus is a psychologically and behaviorally demanding illness. For optimal clinical outcomes, patients are asked to monitor glucose, exercise, inspect their feet, follow a restrictive diet, and adhere to medication regimens. Treatment plans are increasingly complex as greater emphasis is placed on achieving normal blood pressures and near normal fasting and average blood glucose. Because patients implement the majority of diabetes disease management and treatment, depression has significant potential to adversely affect adherence. In a recent retrospective study of patients with predominantly type 2 diabetes (30), depressive symptom severity was associated with poorer diet and medication adherence, functional impairment, and higher health care costs. In their follow-up study of type 1 and 2 diabetic patients, depressive symptoms were associated with decreased adherence to exercise regimens and diet, increased diabetes symptoms, and poor physical functioning. Poorer glycemic control was associated with depressive symptoms in type 1 but not type 2 diabetes (31).

Van Tilburg (32) also investigated the association of mild depression on adherence. In their study of patients with type 1 diabetes, depression was associated with decreased adherence, including less blood glucose monitoring and higher hemoglobin levels. This study replicated a similar finding with type 1 patients and glycemic control, where symptoms of mild depression were associated with poorer glycemic control (33).

Kidney Disease and Hemodialysis.   End-stage kidney disease requires dialysis, most commonly hemodialysis three times weekly, and careful adherence to complex medical and dietary regimens. Depression is highly prevalent in kidney disease, affecting an estimated 20%–25% of patients (34–36). Previous studies investigating the effects of depression on mortality have shown conflicting findings. However, several recent large-scale studies have reported a detrimental effect of depression in kidney disease; adherence rates were reported in only two of the studies.

DeOreo (34) followed 1,000 hemodialysis patients at three sites over 2 years. Mental-health status was measured with a component of the medical outcomes study short-form-36 (SF-36). Patients with poorer self-reported mental health status (mood, emotional and social functioning) were more likely to skip two or more treatments per month and had more days of hospitalization. However, mortality rates and albumin level were not affected by self-reported mental health.

Kimmel (37) prospectively studied 295 patients across several U.S. sites and reported depression as a predictor of mortality in chronic hemodialysis patients. The Dialysis Outcomes and Practice Patterns Study (DOPPS) is an observational, cross-national study of approximately 5,000 patients on hemodialysis (36). The authors found that self-reported depression was associated with an increased risk of hospitalization and mortality. Depression-related adherence as a mediator of mortality was not assessed in their study; however, depressed patients had significantly higher rates of withdrawal from dialysis. Knight (38) studied 14,815 patients receiving hemodialysis at the facilities of a national medical-care company. The authors assessed mental health using a component of the SF-36. Poorer mental-health status (mood, social and emotional functioning) at baseline was independently associated with increased 1- and 2-year mortality. In addition, a decline in mental-health function from baseline to 6 months was associated with additional increased risk of mortality (38); those with poorer mental-health status did *not* withdraw from dialysis at a significantly higher rate.

AIDS-HIV Infection.   Individuals who are HIV positive are required to take large numbers of pills daily, at complex intervals, typically indefinitely. High adherence rates of greater than 90% are essential to successful drug therapy (39–41). One recent study found that only 22% of the HIV-infected drug users were highly adherent to combination antiretroviral therapy (41). Poor adherence affects the illness acutely and also has long-term implications due to increased viral resistance.

Affective disorders are the most common mental-health problems in individuals with HIV infection (42). Prevalence rates of depression range from 17% to 36% (43–45). Depression in HIV-affected individuals tends to affect women more than men, with 30%–60% of women and 20%–30% of men reporting significant depressive symptoms (41). HIV-infected women are more likely than men to be depressed and less likely to enter into care or adhere to antiretroviral regimens (41). In a longitudinal analysis of 765 women in the HIV Epidemiology Research Study, depressive symptoms were associated with disease progression and mortality; adherence per se was not evaluated as a mediating factor of progression or mortality (46). Although some investigators have proposed socioeconomic factors or disease etiology (e.g., IV drug use) as potential confounders to the observed relationship between female gender and poor adherence (47, 48), the high rates of depression in HIV-infected women is a plausible alternative.

In a population of over 5,000 Medicaid recipients who were also current illicit-drug users, Turner (41) used claims data to study the correlates of adherence to HIV therapies. In their study, an administrative code for depression was associated with *increased* adherence to HIV treatment. However, most individuals diagnosed with depression were being treated in mental health–specialty settings, which also was associated with the greater adherence levels. Women with a diagnosis of depression who received psychiatric and antidepressant treatment, as compared to depressed women without either form of care, had nearly twofold greater adjusted odds of adherence. For men and women, counseling sessions were associated with 50% greater odds of adherence, where antidepressant treatment alone showed a nonsignificant association (41). Although a clear relationship was demonstrated for depression and adherence, the authors were not able to determine causality. That is, whether depression treatment produced improved adherence, or those individuals seeking treatment were a priori more adherent to medical and psychiatric treatments.

We found one prospective study that investigated predictors of adherence to antiretroviral therapy in 445 HIV patients; one independent variable was depression (49). Depressive symptoms at baseline did not predict later adherence, but an increase in depression scores during the study was significantly related to nonadherence at 4-month follow-up.

Summary. In adults with chronic medical illness, depressive symptoms are consistently associated with disease progression or mortality. For most conditions, depressive symptoms are associated with lower short-term adherence. Given the limited number of studies conducted in this area and confounding or latent variables affecting adherence, it is very challenging to demonstrate evidence that depression causes nonadherence.

Few studies have evaluated longer-term adherence. An important methodological issue identified by several authors was mistimed depression assessments, which may obscure an association between depression and short- or especially long-term outcomes. Depressive symptoms may be transiently increased after a chronic medical illness is diagnosed or after hospitalization for an acute event. It may be more meaningful to measure depressive symptoms after a wait period of several weeks in order to identify individuals with persistent depressive symptoms. These individuals are more likely to be clinically depressed and experience adverse effects on adherence.

Adherence to Preventive Care (e.g., Mammography, Pap Smear)

Health promotion and prevention are big topics in health care settings and national-awareness days for screening/examinations are proliferating. For women, pap smears and mammography in adulthood are considered essential screenings for early identification of cancer. In older men, some organizations recommend prostate cancer screening. For all of us, blood pressure checks, appropriate immunizations, alcohol use history, dental care, and colorectal cancer screening in later life are recommended. How does depression affect the choice to engage in preventive-care practices? Does depression produce less involvement in preventive care and screening? Our search identified cancer screening as the area where most of the research on depression and its relationship to preventive care has been published.

Lerman, Kash, and Stefanek (50) investigated adherence to mammography in 780 women age 20–75 at risk for breast cancer. They found that general psychological distress was associated with nonadherence to mammography. Siegler, Feaganes, and Rimer (51) prospectively studied women under age 50 in the University of North Carolina Alumni Heart Study, and found that depression predicted lower adherence to mammography; when adherence was adjusted for various factors, depression no longer predicted adherence. Banks (52) retrospectively inquired about reasons for not attending a cancer screening, and found no differences in depression among 1,064 women invited for cancer screening. These few studies provide equivocal evidence about the effects of depression on an act of screening. Given the national priority on cancer prevention, further studies are needed to determine if, and to what degree, depression is associated with nonadherence to preventive screening and other prevention behaviors.

Adherence to Antidepressants in General Medical Settings

Primary-care physicians provide the majority of depression treatment in the United States. When depression is treated in primary care, the treatment of choice is antidepressant medication. Patient nonadherence to treatment in the form of not taking an antidepressant or discontinuing prior to an adequate trial is common. Reported nonadherence rates average 50% among primary-care patients (53, 54). For this section, we focus on primary-care studies. In our search of Medline articles that included primary, general, or family practice and adherence to depression treatment as an outcome, those articles that included an intervention to increase adherence are discussed in the section Interventions of this chapter. Here we discuss the articles where variables predictive of nonadherence were investigated.

A retrospective study that was one of the first to examine primary-care patients' reasons for nonadherence to antidepressant medications identified several contributing factors. Side effects, negative attitudes toward medication, and poor doctor–patient communication were the most common reasons for nonadherence (55). Lin (56) sought to identify specific educational messages, side effects, and features of the doctor–patient collaboration that influenced adherence to antidepressant treatments in 155 primary-care patients initiating antidepressant medication. When specific educational messages about the medication were given, there was improved adherence to antidepressant treatment in the 1st month. The messages were: Take the medication daily, it will take 2–4 weeks to see effect, mild side effects are common but usually resolve with time, keep taking medication even when you begin to feel better, and check with your physician before stopping the medication. Severe side effects were associated with early discontinuation. At the 4th month of treatment, the only significant predictor of adherence was whether the patient had used antidepressants previously, which demonstrated a positive effect on adherence.

A large-scale study (57) of over 15,000 general-practice patients found that 33% of patients stopped antidepressant treatment with fluoxetine over a 6-week period. Of those, 64% stopped because of marked or complete improvement in symptoms, 11% of patients terminated therapy because of insufficient response, 14% for worsening, adverse events, and side effects, and 11% for a variety of other reasons. Maidment, Livingston, and Katona (58) studied 67 primary-care patients ≥65 years old. Nonadherence was associated with more severe psychological distress and depression, less education about antidepressants, worse side effects, more negative attitudes about the necessity of taking antidepressants, and more concerns about doing so. Cognitive functioning was also assessed and the authors found that *lower* cognitive functioning predicted higher adherence (these patients were hypothesized to have greater support from a significant other).

Demyttenaere (59) studied 272 patients receiving antidepressant therapy over 6 months; 53% discontinued antidepressant therapy at 6 months. Of those, 55% did so because they were feeling better, 23% for adverse events, 10% reported a fear of drug dependence, 10% cited lack of efficacy, 9% stated they wanted to solve their problems without drugs, and 9% reported their generalist physician told them to stop the medication. Sleath (60) studied 81 primary- and specialty-care patients obtaining antidepressant prescriptions at a pharmacy. Patients reported information about their medication adherence over the previous week. Adherence decreased as the number of side effects experienced increased; adherence increased in parallel with greater numbers of information sources on antidepressant treatment. Dietrich (61) asked patients about barriers to taking antidepressants. Of the 50% of patients who reported barriers to taking medication, 50% reported medication side effects as a barrier and 23% reported ambivalence about medication as a barrier.

Because adverse effects are clearly related to adherence, it was hoped that antidepressants with fewer adverse effects would be associated with greater adherence. Selective serotonin reuptake inhibitors (SSRIs) have a number of potential advantages over older antidepressants, including fewer adverse effects, less dose titration, and less frequent dosing (1, 62). The SSRI's impact on adherence, although positive, has been less than anticipated (63–66). Two meta-analyses have provided useful information. A meta-analysis of randomized controlled trials comparing SSRIs to older tricyclic antidepressants (TCAs) found that SSRIs were associated with 5% fewer dropouts due to adverse effects (67). A more recent meta-analysis focused specifically on primary-care settings. MacGillivray (65) included a total of 11 studies that compared SSRIs to tricyclics. They found that SSRIs were equally efficacious, and confirmed a greater dropout rate for tricyclics, specifically due to adverse effects. Tai-Seale, Croghan, and Obenchain (68) retrospectively studied 2,012 claims (primary and specialty) and found that when controlling for other potential variables, individuals taking fluoxetine were more likely to continue their treatment, as compared to those on TCAs.

Summary. Several consistent themes are evident in studies of antidepressant medication treatment in primary care. A central theme is the importance of negative side effects in early medication discontinuation. A second consistent factor is the importance of patient attitudes toward psychotropic medications and their knowledge about expected benefits and risks (e.g., side effects) of treatment with antidepressants. This includes early termination due to improvement, which likely include individuals at low and high risk for future episodes, so for at least a subset early discontinuation because of improvement remains a concern. Adherence appears to improve when physicians address the timing of clinical benefit, common adverse effects, and duration of treatment. In our experience, we have found it important to reassure patients that antidepressant medications are not addicting. A third theme, highly related to the first two, is the quality of doctor–patient communication and how this interacts with attitudes, knowledge, and willingness to engage in treatment. Basco and Rush (69) reach similar conclusions in their review of medication adherence for mood disorders in specialty and primary care. They reported that the most consistently cited reasons for poor adherence were poor-quality patient–clinician relationship, medication side effects, and resistance to taking psychotropic medication.

Adherence to Mental-Health Referrals From Generalist Physicians

Generalist physicians (GPs) refer to mental-health specialists for specialized care due to physician or patient preference, in response to high-risk patient characteristics, or when initial treatments have not been successful. When patients are recognized as depressed, primary-care physicians refer 5% to 40% of the time (70, 71). One survey found that when depression is moderate to severe, referrals to mental-health specialty occur more than 50% of the time (72). Referral rates might be even higher, except for physicians' reports that patient reluctance is a considerable problem (71). Nonadherence to mental-health referral appointments occurs in 10% to 70% of referrals (73–79), rates that exceed those seen for referrals to medical specialists (80, 81). Numerous factors may contribute to nonacceptance/nonadherence of a referral to a mental-health specialist. These include demographic and illness characteristics, negative attitudes about mental health, and provider and organizational barriers. We summarize studies from a MedLine and PsychInfo review that report on variables affecting adherence to referrals from a GP to a mental-health provider. In most studies the reason for referral (i.e., depression, anxiety) was not a variable assessed.

Olfson (82) conducted a case-control study of 65 primary-care patients referred for mental-health care. Adherent patients were more likely to be married, had met with their GP in person (as opposed to on the phone), and attended fewer medical visits the 2 years preceding and the 2 years following the referral. Adherent patients' general medical visits *more* often had a discussion of mental-health concerns; nonadherent patients tended to report symptoms that were either somatically focused or not identified by the patient as psychological in nature. The nonadherent group had a higher proportion of medical visits with unexplained physical complaints the 2 years preceding the referral, and was more likely to have been nonadherent to other referrals. Finally, there was significant variability between physicians, with some achieving very high follow-through on referrals, suggesting that physician factors were also important.

Farid and Alapont (83) studied referral letters for 130 new psychiatric appointments. They found that younger age men, those of a "lower social class," and those living *nearer* the hospital were less likely to attend (the hospital may have been located in a poorer neighborhood). The worse the quality of the referral letter, the more likely patients were to be nonadherent. Nonadherent patients had a history of not attending previous psychiatric or medical appointments. Killaspy et al. (84) were primarily interested in how communication between referral parties affected adherence. They investigated the quality of referral letters in 224 patients, and did not find a difference in adherence based on the quality and content of letters from the GP. In a subsequent report (85) of those 224 patients, nonattendees were less likely to have agreed with the referral. Nonattendees also waited longer for their appointment.

Grunebaum (74) was one of the few studies we found that included ethnicity as a variable. They found that Anglos, African Americans, and Hispanics attended initial appointments at similar rates. In their sample of 270 patients, those with cognitive impairment were significantly *less* likely to miss appointments, perhaps due to assistance from family members or friends. Patients who expressed less distress to their GP were more likely to be nonadherent, as well as those who had expressed greater resistance to the seeing a psychiatrist and who had a longer wait time before the referral appointment.

Neeleman and Mikhail (86) studied 50 adherent and 46 nonadherent patients referred from their GP to psychiatry. Fewer social and relationship problems and a diagnosis of depression or anxiety (as opposed to psychosis or something else) were independently associated with higher adherence. Livianos-Aldana (87) investigated adherence among 1,311 individuals referred from their GP to a Spanish Community Mental Health Center. Patients with early-morning appointments, without a contacting telephone number, a longer time lapse to appointment, or a substance-related referral were less likely to attend. Attendance rates also varied by season.

Peeters and Bayer (77) investigated adherence to 1,713 initial referrals to psychiatry, the majority of which were GP referred; only 9.6% were nonadherent to the referral. Nonadherence occurred more often with self-initiated appointments and referrals by other medical specialties, as opposed to their GP. Of the 94 who were nonadherent and responded to the questionnaire, the most common reasons for nonattendance were longer wait time or another clinic had appointed them earlier (31.9%), persistent problem but lack of motivation for treatment at that clinic (29.8%), and resolution of the problem (21.3%).

Summary. Demographic characteristics such as age, ethnicity, and gender were not consistently related to follow-through on mental-health referrals. Variables that consistently predicted nonadherence were longer wait times, confusing or difficult-to-define symptoms, negative attitudes about seeking mental health, and a history of nonattendance. The doctor–patient relationship also is likely a factor in that primary-care-generated referrals improved attendance in some cases, whereas poor-quality referral letters and lack of agreement about treatment negatively impacted adherence.

ADHERENCE TO PSYCHOLOGICAL TREATMENT

Correlates and predictors of adherence to specific psychological treatments, or psychotherapy, is covered in chapter 10 of this book. We focus our review by briefly summarizing the literature on adherence to psychological treatments for unipolar depression. Compared to medication treatments, there is considerably less literature on adherence to psychological interventions for depression. In general and specialty settings, a Medline search for research studies that included either compliance or adherence and depression as key terms, found 15 articles (empirical and theoretical) for psychotherapy depression, whereas 104 articles were found for antidepressant treatment. We duplicated this search in PsychInfo and found 17 studies for psychotherapy and 105 for antidepressant treatment.

One reason why adherence is not as well addressed in the psychological literature is the different approach that psychological treatments take toward the issue of adherence. That is, adherence tends to be characterized more in terms of dropouts, rather than number of visits attended or treatment adherence (e.g., integration of feedback or homework completion). Discontinuation of therapy is often the operational definition of whether a patient adhered to a treatment. For example, in the most recent (fifth) edition of the *Handbook of Psychotherapy and Behavior Change* (88), an 800-page comprehensive review of psychotherapy research, the subject index does not include the terms adherence or compliance. Attrition is included, in 11 pages of the book.

Treatment studies report that a participant "completed" a 16-week trial of cognitive behavioral therapy, but rarely detail how many sessions were missed and how well the patient adhered to in-therapy treatment suggestions. This may be due to the qualitative differences of psychological interventions. Dropout rates for psychosocial depression treatments in clinical trials are typically 20%–40%. However, if adherence to weekly treatments and "homework" were included, a more comprehensive view of adherence, adherence would likely be closer to the 50% adherence rates we reported for antidepressants and mental-health referrals.

In psychotherapy, there is an increased level of patient–provider collaboration. In this paradigm, the professional is held more accountable for intreatment success, and the patient is understandably held to a "lower" standard of adherence. For example, it is highly unusual for patients to attend 100% of sessions and comply with most or all suggestions/homework over a 16-week trial of therapy. This paradigm is of value, in that there is not an expectation that a depressed person can or should adhere to the demands of a weekly therapy intervention and related outcomes. The clinician's role is more partner-like than has been traditionally defined for medication treatment. The patient would have to ask him or herself, "Is it me or the doctor?", whereas changing a medication can occur with some ease, whether or not one is particularly pleased with their provider. If a treatment fails, it is much easier to switch medications than psychotherapists. Moreover, there is a considerable amount of literature showing that the "treatment alliance," as it is called, is predictive of outcomes in psychotherapy, and experienced therapists are more adept at reducing the likelihood of dropout to a treatment (89).

This is not to downplay the importance of the physician in successful treatment, which has already been established. An issue that arises that is very similar to medication management is fitting the particular treatment to the particular patient. In trials where psychological treatments are compared to antidepressants, or psychotherapies are compared head to head (e.g., the National Institute of Mental Health Collaborative Depression Study) new insights are gained. For example, the accumulated evidence shows that although severely depressed patients may respond equally as well to psychological treatments, a greater length of time is required in comparison to antidepressant treatments. Milder depressions may respond more positively to a psychological intervention, where minimal improvements may be seen with antidepressant treatments (90).

INTERVENTIONS

Does Treatment of Depression Improve Adherence to Medical Treatments?

Is there evidence that effective treatment for depression improves patient's adherence to their medical treatments? If this phenomenon is true, it would most likely be shown in the treatment of CVD. In cardiovascular studies, however, the answer is not clear. Linden (91) performed a meta-analysis of 23 randomized controlled trials that evaluated the additional impact of psychosocial treatment in cardiac rehabilitation programs. Psychosocial treatments were not specifically targeted for depression, and any resultant effects on adherence to treatments were not studied. Psychosocial interventions yielded greater reductions in systolic blood pressure, heart rate, and cholesterol level; overall mortality and recurrent cardiac events were also decreased at 2-year follow-up. Two recent large-scale randomized clinical trials have investigated the effects of treating depression in patients following an MI. The SADHART study found that sertraline was safe and superior to placebo for depression outcomes (92). The study did not have a sufficient number of patients to demonstrate an effect on cardiovascular or mortality outcomes but showed a promising trend toward fewer cardiovascular events. The ENRICHD trial (93), which evaluated cognitive behavioral therapy in 2,481 patients, also did not show an effect on mortality among post-MI patients with clinical depression and/or low perceived social support. Neither trial reported effects on adherence to medical treatments. Our Medline search found no studies that directly examined the effects of depression treatments on adherence to cardiovascular treatments. Thus, we are still sorely lacking evidence that treatment of depression improves adherence to treatments for CVD.

Diabetes mellitus is another behaviorally complex illness where there is evidence that depression is associated with poor outcomes and low adherence to recommended treatments. Three short-duration efficacy trials evaluated the effects of depression treatment in patients with coexisting depression and diabetes. All showed positive effects on depression symptoms but effects on diabetes outcomes varied, and the one reported effect on adherence was negative. In a study of 51 patients with major depression and poorly controlled type 2 diabetes (mean glycohemoglobin >10%), cognitive behavioral therapy plus diabetes education improved glycohemoglobin by more than 1% compared to education alone; however, adherence to glucose monitoring was adversely affected (94). The positive effects on glycemic control persisted at 6 months for individuals whose depression improved. A trial of nortriptyline for 28 patients with major depression and diabetes showed no effect on glycemic control or glucose monitoring, but path analysis showed a negative effect of nortriptyline on glucose control; power to detect clinically significant differences was limited (95). The third study evaluated fluoxetine in 60 patients with type 1 or 2 diabetes and major depression (96). Glycohemoglobin improved by a nonstatistically significant degree; self-care behaviors were not measured.

A recent 12-month effectiveness trial evaluated the effects of depression care management on depression outcomes, diabetes self-care behaviors, and glycemic control in 417 older adults with major depression or dysthymia and type 2 diabetes mellitus. This trial differed from previous studies in that patients were age 60 and older, had relatively good glycemic control at baseline (mean Hemoglobin A1c = 7.3), and the intervention was a process change that allowed for flexible approaches to depression treatment rather than a specific antidepressant or psychological treatment. At 12 months, intervention subjects experienced lower depression severity, and greater improvement in mental and physical functioning than participants assigned to usual care. Intervention subjects were more likely to adhere to antidepressant medications and increased their weekly exercise days by 0.59 days compared to usual-care subjects. Other self-care behaviors for diabetes, such as foot inspections, adherence to hypoglycemics, and dietary adherence, were not affected. Glycemic control as measured by Hemoglobin A1c at 6 and 12 months was unaffected by the intervention but the investigators could not exclude a clinically important effect in patients with poor glycemic control at baseline.

Collectively, these diabetes trials provide mixed support for the hypothesis that effective depression treatments may improve glycemic control in patients with poorly controlled diabetes. Although likely related to adherence, effects on self-care behaviors and adherence to hypoglycemic medications have not been adequately evaluated. However, given the mixed data, we think it is likely that adherence to diabetes treatments will need to be targeted directly, either concurrently with depression treatments or sequentially, to show important changes in adherence.

Summary. The hypothesis that effective treatment for depression would indirectly improve adherence to other chronic medical treatments is both intriguing and logical. Individuals freed from the burden of pessimistic thoughts, low energy, and difficulty concentrating should be able to participate more actively in medical care. In cardiovascular illness, psychosocial interventions appear to benefit physiological measures and mortality but it remains unclear whether improved adherence is an explanatory mechanism. Although the research may be lagging, experienced clinicians believe that treatment of depression is essential. Angelino and Treisman (97) noted the effect of psychiatric disorders, including major depression, on HIV adherence at the Johns Hopkins Moore (HIV) clinic. They note: "treatment of these disorders [psychiatric illnesses] greatly improves patient adherence to treatment and outcomes of HIV infections."

One important methodological issue when interpreting these studies is a matter of dose response. That is, is the intervention applied in a particular study of a great enough "dose" to affect adherence or disease outcomes? Linden (91) noted that as follow-up was extended from months to years, treatment effects weakened. Thus, for these interventions, we need to be certain that psychosocial and medical interventions are potent enough to show an effect on adherence and outcome. As for other medical illnesses, we did not identify any depression treatment studies reporting effects on adherence for patients with depression and coexisting HIV infection or chronic kidney disease.

How Effective Are Interventions Aimed at Improving Adherence to Depression Treatment?

General-Care Settings. A number of patient-centered interventions to improve adherence to depression treatments have been tested including patient education and multimodal interventions. Peveler (98) investigated adherence to antidepressant medication in a primary-care setting, using two interventions: a printed brochure or a two-session nurse intervention focused on the treatment of depression. Counseling sessions were lead by experienced nurses at 2 and 8 weeks following treatment initiation. The nurses assessed the patient's daily routine, attitudes toward treatment, and understanding of the reasons for treatment. Education was given about depressive illness, self-help behaviors, local resources, management of medication side effects, and the importance of antidepressant drug treatment. Nurses emphasized the need to continue treatment for up to 6 months and offered advice about using reminders and cues to enhance adherence. The brochure contained information about the antidepressant medication, unwanted effects, and what to do if a dose was missed. At 12 weeks, counseling significantly improved adherence (OR = 2.6, 95% CI 1.6 to 4.8), but the educational leaflet had no effect.

In the mid-1990s, new models of care, called Collaborative Care, began to be tested in randomized controlled trials. In these studies, depressed patients in primary-care settings received enhanced treatment, which resulted in better treatment adherence and depression outcomes for up to 12 months later (99). These improvements were observed consistently for patients with major depression or dysthymia, but not for patients with subsyndromal depression.

Early studies (100) colocated a mental-health professional in the primary-care setting and depression management was shared between this specialist and the primary-care clinician, often by alternating visits. Brief, didactic sessions on guideline concordant depression care were offered for the primary-care clinicians. Although effective, this model was not sustained in study practices, in part, because of the high cost. Subsequent studies (101–104) used nurses or other non-mental-health paraprofessionals, and importantly, augmented the primary-care physician visits with telephone follow-up. These telephone follow-ups focused on treatment adherence, and objective assessments of depression symptoms. In most studies a psychiatrist supervised the telephone care manager and provided written or verbal treatment recommendations to the primary-care physician. The

Antidepressant adherence*

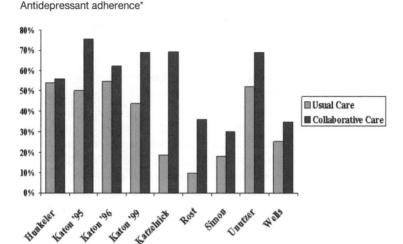

FIG. 9.1. Effects of care management for depression on antidepressant medication adherence. Time intervals for assessment of medication adherence
varied from 2 to 7 months. Studies assessed for adequate dose based on
Agency for Health Care Policy and Research guidelines or taking any antidepressant dose (5, 100–104, 122–125).

change to telephone follow-up and non-mental-health professionals increased the feasibility of the approach. These models have continued to
evolve and now contain many elements of the chronic-care model (105).
Using the chronic-care model as the conceptual framework, a recent literature synthesis identified key components of enhanced care as: patient education and support, monitoring depressive symptoms and treatment adherence, support for self-care behaviors, and the option of psychological
treatments offered in the primary-care setting. Absolute improvements in
antidepressant medication adherence ranged from 2% to almost 51% (Fig.
9.1). The absolute increases in the proportion of patients achieving clinically significant improvement ranged from 16% to 30.6%.

Pharmacist interventions also hold promise (106). In an observational
study, Bultman and Svarstad (107) reported better adherence to depression medication therapy when pharmacist-monitoring services were included as routine care. Finley (108) reported on a similar study involving
two to three brief visits with pharmacists and several phone contacts over a
period of 6 months. The intervention group adhered significantly more to
antidepressant therapy at 6 months (51% vs. 76%). These encouraging observational findings are being tested in a randomized controlled trial that
utilizes frequent telephone-based contacts by a clinical pharmacist (109).
Pharmacist-based interventions are promising because they fit within the
context of current primary-care delivery models.

Specialty-Care Settings. Combining antidepressant treatment with psychotherapy is the most potent method to increase adherence and improve outcome in specialty-care settings. Adding rapidly acting medications to ameliorate specific symptoms, such as anxiety, may also be beneficial. Furukawa (110) performed a meta-analysis of nine randomized controlled trials, conducted primarily in psychiatric outpatient clinics, comparing antidepressant monotherapy to antidepressant plus benzodiazepine therapy. They found that those on combination treatment were 37% less likely to drop out of treatment in the initial 4 to 8 weeks. It is unclear whether this short-term benefit would be sustained with longer-term treatment and whether the potential benefits offset the potential harms of dependence, increased fall risk, and increased medication costs.

Larsen (111) attempted to reduce no-shows at a community mental-health clinic. When time to appointment was decreased to below 5 days and therapists made verbal contact prior to the appointment, no-show rates were significantly reduced by 10%. The authors also attempted to reduce early dropout by randomly assigning 52 patients to either a 15-minute pretherapy orientation or no orientation. The oriented patients were significantly less likely to drop out or miss appointments in the 1st month. The oriented group reported fewer symptoms at 1 month, and were more likely to have terminated services and have a better global functioning score at 22 months. Clinical benefits were not explained by differences in service use; continuity and missed appointments did not differ between groups (111).

Daley (112) looked at the effects of a motivational interviewing intervention on treatment adherence among depressed cocaine-dependent patients recently discharged from inpatient care. Motivational interviewing was targeted at depression and drug dependence concurrently. Although this was a preliminary study ($n = 23$), they found that the patients who received the motivational interviewing intervention attended more treatment sessions during the 1st month, and completed 30 and 90 days of patient care at higher rates. For these patients, adherence was correlated with fewer psychiatric rehospitalizations and days in the hospital in the 1st year of their outpatient treatment.

Summary. In general and specialty care, providing higher quality, patient-centered, and more comprehensive treatments increase adherence. As Chen (113) and Tinsley (114) noted more than a decade ago, decreasing wait times, verbal or written contact prior to appointments, education about the nature of treatment, and an invested, involved referral source can decrease missed appointments and early dropout. Again, the most robust finding from randomized controlled trials and other studies is that a combination of medication and psychotherapy improves adherence rates to medication treatments more than medication alone.

CLINICAL IMPLICATIONS

Changing Practice

Clinical depression is highly prevalent in primary-care settings. In patients with chronic medical illness, the prevalence increases about twofold. Depression causes significant disability, and in patients with coexisting medical illness, is associated with worse treatment adherence and medical outcomes. Effective treatments for depression are available, including antidepressant medications and psychological treatments. We recommend systematic screening for depression in patients with chronic medical illness. Treatments are most effective when a systematic approach to treatment is used, including efforts to promote adherence. Although not proven to improve depression-related adherence, assessing treatment preferences for antidepressant medication, psychological treatments, or both is consistent with patient-centered care. Because nonadherence to depression treatments is common, we recommend routine assessment of treatment adherence. A review of specific clinical and systems strategies to promote adherence to depression treatments are listed in Table 9.2.

In specialty mental-health care, evidence supports the combination of medicine and psychological treatments to improve adherence to antidepressant medication. The American Psychiatric Association recommends a combination of antidepressant medication and psychological treatments for nonadherent patients with major depression (115). Short-term combination medication treatments for depressed patients with prominent anxiety may improve adherence and depressive symptoms.

Because of the link between clinical depression and worse medical outcomes, it is hoped that effective depression treatment will improve adherence to treatments for chronic medical conditions. To date, evidence supporting this hypothesis is inconclusive. Clinicians should implement adherence-enhancing strategies for depression treatments based on expected benefits for depression and functional outcomes, not indirect benefits on adherence to other medical treatments.

RESEARCH IMPLICATIONS/FUTURE DIRECTIONS

Theoretical Underpinnings for Depression's Effect on Adherence

Conceptual models of the link between depression and adherence are informed by a detailed understanding of the clinical syndrome. Initially proposed by Radloff (116), numerous cross-cultural research studies with thou-

TABLE 9.2

Strategies to Improve Adherence to Depression Treatments

Antidepressant medication

Choose medications with fewer adverse effects.

Assess patient attitudes toward taking medications; address reluctance or resistance prior to prescription.

Tell patients:

- Take the medication daily.
- It will take 2–4 weeks to see effect.
- Mild side effects are common but usually resolve with time.
- Keep taking medication even when you begin to feel better.
- Check with your physician before stopping the medication.

Offer collaborative care or its key elements, which should include an interactive experience where the following are addressed: symptom and adherence monitoring, patient education, support for self-care.

- Additional psychological treatment in the primary-care setting may be required for those at risk of nonadherence (history of nonadherence, high medical-treatment users, minimal social support, or continuing resistance despite education/collaborative care).

Assess adherence routinely, including early response and initial side effects.

- Change or add medication if adherence is affected by side effects or lack of response.
- Support a change of provider, if necessary to improve the doctor–patient relationship.

Referrals to Mental Health Specialists

From referring end:

- Assess if patient agrees with the need for a mental-health referral and address reluctance or resistance prior to completion of the referral.
- Educate patients about mental-health specialty care (benefits, risks, what to expect).
- Inform patient of potential for excessive wait time and offer more than one referral choice.
- Colocate mental-health specialist in primary care.
- Physician or nurse follow-up with patients regarding referral when at risk of nonadherence (history of nonadherence, high medical-treatment users, minimal social support, continued resistance despite education/collaborative care).

From specialty end:

- Reduce wait times for mental-health specialty appointment.
- Make verbal contact prior to the appointment, address concerns/questions regarding upcoming appointment.
- Provide in-person orientation regarding expectations about psychosocial treatment.

---

sands of individuals have replicated a general-factor structure underlying depression. The most widely accepted, four-factor structure, includes somatic symptoms, negative affect, positive affect, and interpersonal symptoms (116–119).

Biological/Somatic Symptoms. Depression impairs physical functioning. Somatic symptoms of depression are: being bothered by things that don't usually bother someone, not feeling like eating, restless sleep, decreased concentration, feeling that everything is an effort, talking less than usual, and not being able to "get going." Diminished physical well-being makes one less likely to engage in life's activities, responsibilities, and social roles; decreased involvement in medical treatments is no exception.

Negative Affect and Thought.   Depression also increases negativity of thought and mood. Characteristic symptoms are: not being able to shake off the blues, feeling one's life has been a failure, pessimism, feeling fearful, lonely, sad, and having crying spells. Depressed individuals are often negative. It is difficult for a person to be proactive, motivated, and positive about treatment, when their view of self, others, and the world is negative.

Positive Affect and Thought.   Depressed individuals lack positive affect such as: feeling just as good as other people, feeling hopeful about the future, and feeling happy and enjoying life. Hopelessness is a significant factor in depression. Anhedonia, or lack of pleasure in life, negatively impacts the desire to engage in potentially mundane activities such as treatment for chronic medical illness.

Interpersonal Factors.   The interpersonal component of depression includes believing that people are unfriendly and feeling that people dislike them. The provider–patient relationship is an important determinant of adherence. In addition, interactions with treatment team members including administrative staff and nurses may influence adherence. From our clinical experience, even calling the clinic staff for treatment-related reasons can feel overwhelming in depressed individuals. Individuals who feel that others do not like them or that people are unfriendly are less likely to seek social support, professional or personal. Understanding this factor provides theoretical support for studies that improve adherence through increased social involvement of professionals and paraprofessionals.

In summary, clinical dimensions of depression may inform explanatory models linking depression to adherence and interventions to improve adherence. Decreased adherence to effective medical treatments may explain the association between depression and worse chronic-illness outcomes. Many of the commonly used depression scales, such as the Center for Epidemiological Studies Depression Scale, measure the four factors of clinical depression. Investigators conducting natural-history studies or treatment interventions that require a good deal of patient participation should consider measuring depression as a mediating variable.

Gaps in Knowledge for Further Study

Available evidence shows a consistent, and relatively strong negative effect of depression on chronic medical illness. Behavioral mechanisms such as decreased adherence and biological mechanisms have been proposed as etiologic. Depending on the illness and possibly the complexity of the medical regimen, we think that current evidence supports decreased adherence as a mechanism. As investigators seek to determine the strength of this association with greater certainty, they will need to pay attention to the measurement of depression. Measurement issues include the timing of the assessment in relation to acute illness, care to measure the different factors or domains of depression, and careful consideration of whether to measure depressive symptoms only or to make a criterion-standard diagnosis of the full clinical syndrome.

For observational studies, it will be important to control for potential confounding variables such as coping factors, coping styles (120), and personality factors or traits. Prior studies have identified personality types and adherence, such as accepters, deniers, and pragmatists (121). Ford (27) found that a measure of interpersonal sensitivity affected adherence to medication and lifestyle changes in asthmatics. Given the observation that depressed patients post-MI are offered less aggressive treatment, issues of access and medical appropriateness will also need to be considered.

When considering the relationship between depression and chronic medical illness, a number of lines of investigation seem appropriate. Are the effects of depression magnified by more complex medical treatments or treatments requiring more self-care such as home monitoring? Does depression adversely affect patient–physician communication and if so, would these negative effects be overcome by printed materials to reinforce key messages or communication training? Another exciting area for future research will be interventions designed to relieve depression and concurrently address another chronic medical illness. Depression, coexisting with cardiovascular disease, is a promising target given its high prevalence, high patient impact, and studies showing benefits from nonspecific psychosocial interventions.

We also reviewed the evidence on adherence to antidepressant medications, psychological treatments, and specialty referrals for patients with depression. Poor adherence to antidepressant medications has been well documented and does not require further study. Multimodal care management programs are demonstrated to improve medication adherence and depression outcomes. Interventions should be of adequate dose. However, investigators have not determined the essential elements or methods to disseminate the programs beyond the research setting. Understanding these elements is key to promoting dissemination and developing the most cost-effective approaches to enhancing adherence. Even if care management programs were widely implemented, there remains an urgent need to develop approaches promoting adherence, either through medications with fewer adverse effects, or innovative uses of technology such as e-mail reminders, or monitoring of medication refills. The dose or intensity of interventions should be carefully considered when endeavoring to improve long-term outcome of morbidity and mortality. In addition to developing more efficacious interventions, we believe the most pressing need for depressed patients is to develop cost-effective adherence-enhancing strategies, and invite readers to take up this charge.

REFERENCES

1. Katon W, Von Korff M, Lin E, Bush T, Ormel J. Adequacy and duration of antidepressant treatment in primary care. *Medi Care.* 1992;30(1):67–76.
2. Kessler RC, Berglund P, Demler O, et al. The epidemiology of major depressive disorder; results from the National Comorbidity Survey Replication (NCS-R). *JAMA.* 2003;289(23):3095–3105.
3. Doebbling CC. Epidemiology, risk factors, and prevention. In: Levinson JL, ed. *Depression.* Philadelphia, PA; American College of Physicians; 2000:23–45.
4. Murray CJ, Lopez AD. *The Global Burden of Disease,* ed. H.U. Press. 1996, Cambridge, MA.
5. Unutzer J, Patrick DL, Diehr P, Simon G, Grembowski D, Katon w. Quality adjusted life years in older adults with depressive symptoms and chronic medical disorders. *Int Psychogeriatr.* 2000;12(1):15–33.
6. Kroenke K. A 75-year-old man with depression. *JAMA.* 2002;287(12):1568–1576.
7. Sullivan MD, LaCroix AZ, Baum C, Grothaus LC, Katon WJ. Functional status in coronary artery disease; a one-year prospective study of the role of anxiety and depression. *Am J Med.* 1997;103:348–356.
8. Barefoot JC, Helms MJ, Mark DB, et al. Depression and long-term mortality risk in patients with coronary artery disease. *Am J Cardiol.* 1996;78(6):613–617.
9. Frasure-Smith N, Lesperance F, Talajic M. Depression and 18-month prognosis after myocardial infarction. *Circulation.* 1995;91(4):999–1005.
10. deGroot M, Anderson R, Freedland KE, Clouse RE, Lustman PJ. Association of depression and diabetes complications: a meta-analysis. *Psychosom Med.* 2001;63: 619–630.
11. Lustman PJ, Anderson RJ, Freedland KE, et al. Depression and poor glycemic control: a meta-analytic review of the literature. *Diabetes Care.* 2000;23:934–942.
12. Covinsky KE, Kahana E, Chin MH, Palmer RM, Fortinsky RH, Landefeld CS. Depressive symptoms and 3-year mortality in older hospitalized medical patients. *Ann Intern Med.* 1999;130(7):563–569.
13. Katon W. Clinical and health services relationships between major depression, depressive symptoms, and general medical illness. *Biol Psychiatry.* 2003;54: 216–226.
14. Sheline Y. Neuroimaging studies of mood disorder effects on the brain. *Biol Psychiatry.* 2003;54:338–352.
15. Krishnan KR. *Vascular Disease and Depression.* Paper presented at Psychiatry Grand Rounds of the University of Texas Health Science Center, San Antonio, Texas (November 4, 2003).

16. Nemeroff CB. The neurobiology of depression. *Sci Am.* 1998;278:42–49.

17. McEwen B. Mood disorders and allostatic load. *Biol Psychiatry.* 2003;54:200–207.

18. Di Matteo R, Lepper H, Croghan T. Depression is a risk factor for noncompliance with medical treatment: Meta analysis of the effects of anxiety and depression on patient adherence. *Arch Int Med.* 2000;160:2101–2107.

19. Blumenthal JA, Williams RS, Wallace AG, Williams RB, Needles TL. Physiological and psychological variables predict compliance to prescribed exercise therapy in patients recovering from myocardial infarction. *Psychosom Med.* 1982; 44(6):519–527.

20. Carney R, Freedland K, Eisen S, Rich MW, Jaffe AS. Major depression and medication adherence in elderly patients with coronary artery disease. *Health Psychol.* 1995;14(1):88–90.

21. Carney R, Freedland K, Miller G, et al. Depression as a risk factor for cardiac mortality and morbidity: A review of potential mechanisms. *J Psychosom Res.* 2002;53:897–902.

22. Druss BG, Bradford DW, Rosenheck RA, Radford MJ, Krumholz HM. Mental disorders and use of cardiovascular procedures after myocardial infarction. *JAMA.* 2000;283:506–511.

23. Ziegelstein R, Fauerbach J, Stevens S, Romanelli J, Richter DP, Bush DE. Patients with depression are less likely to follow recommendations to reduce cardiac risk during recovery from a myocardial infarction. *Arch Int Med.* 2000;160: 1818–1823.

24. Romanelli J, Fauerbach J, Bush D, Ziegelstein RC. The significance of depression in older patients after myocardial infarction. *J Am Geriatr Soc.* 2002;50: 817–822.

25. Dorn J, Naughton J, Imamura D, et al. Correlates of compliance in randomized exercise trial in myocardial infarction patients. *Med Sci Sports Exercise.* 2001; 33(7):1081–1089.

26. Irvine J, Baker B, Smith J, et al. Poor adherence to placebo or amiodarone therapy predicts mortality: results from the CAMIAT study. *Psychosom Med.* 1999;61: 566–575.

27. Ford F, Hunter M, Hensley M, et al. Hypertension and asthma: psychological aspects. *Soc Sci Med.* 1989;29(1):79–84.

28. Wang P, Bohn R, Knight E, Glynn RJ, Mogun H, Avorn J. Noncompliance with antihypertensive medications: the impact of depressive symptoms and psychosocial factors. *J Gen Intern Med.* 2002;17:504–511.

29. Davies S, Jackson P, Ramsay L, Ghahramani P. Drug intolerance due to nonspecific adverse effects related to psychiatric morbidity in hypertensive patients. *Arch Intern Med.* 2003;163:592–600.

30. Ciechanowski P, Katon W, Russon J. Depression and diabetes: Impact of depressive symptoms on adherence, function and costs. *Arch Intern Med.* 2000;160(21): 3278–3285.

31. Ciechanowski P, Katon WJ, Russo JE, Hirsch IB. The relationship of depressive symptoms to symptom reporting, self-care and glucose control in diabetes. *Gen Hosp Psychiatry.* 2003;25(4):246–252.

32. Van Tilburg M, McCaskill C, Lane J, et al. Depressed mood is a factor in glycemic control in type 1 diabetes. *Psychosom Med.* 2001;63:551–555.

33. Mazze RS, Lucido D, Shamoon H. Psychological and social correlates of glycemic control. *Diabetes Care.* 1984;7(4):360–366.

34. DeOreo P. Hemodialysis patient-assessed functional health status predicts continued survival, hospitalization, and dialysis-attendance compliance. *Am J Kidney Dis.* 1997;30(2):204–212.

35. Kimmel PL, Peterson RA, Weihs KL, et al. Behavioral compliance with dialysis prescriptions in hemodialysis patients. *J Am Soc Nephrol.* 1995;5:1826–1834.

36. Lopes A, Bragg J, Young E, et al. Depression as a predictor of mortality and hospitalization among hemodialysis patients in the United States and Europe. *Kidney Int.* 2002;62:199–207.

37. Kimmel P, Peterson R, Weihs K, et al. Multiple measurements of depression predict mortality in a longitudinal study of chronic hemodialysis outpatients. *Kidney Int.* 2000;57:2093–2098.

38. Knight E, Ofsthun N, Teng M, Lazarus JM, Curhan GC. The association between mental health, physical function and hemodialysis mortality. *Kidney Int.* 2003;63:1843–1851.

39. Singh N, Squier C, Sivek C, Wagener M, Nguyen MH, Yu VL. Determinants of compliance with antiretroviral therapy in patients with immunodeficiency virus: prospective assessment with implications for enhancing compliance. *AIDS Care.* 1996;8(3):261–269.

40. Bogart L, Kelly J, Catz S, Sosman JM. Impact of medical and nonmedical factors on physician decision making for HIV/AIDS antiretroviral treatment. *J Acquir Immune Defic Syndr.* 2000;23(5):396–404.

41. Turner B, Laine C, Cosler L, Hauck WW. Relationship of gender, depression, and health care delivery with antiretroviral adherence in HIV-infected drug users. *J Gen Int Med.* 2003;18:248–257.

42. Starace F, Ammassari A, Trotta M, et al. Depression is a risk factor for suboptimal adherence to highly active antiretroviral therapy. *J Acquir Immune Defic Syndr.* 2002;31:S136–S139.

43. Bing E, Burnam A, Longshore D, et al. Psychiatric disorders and drug use among human immunodeficiency virus-infected adults in the United States. *Arch Gen Psychiatry.* 2001;58:721–728.

44. Fernando S, Evans S, Goggin K, Sewell M, Fishman B, Rabkin J. Fatigue in HIV illness: Relationship to depression, physical limitations and disability. *Psychosom Med.* 1998;60:759–764.

45. Rabkin J, Wagner G, Rabkin R. Fluoxetine treatment for depression in patients with HIV and AIDS. *Am J Psychiatry.* 1999;156:101–107.

46. Ickovics J, Hamburger M, Vlahov D, et al. Mortality, CD4 cell count decline, and depressive symptoms among HIV-seropositive women: Longitudinal analysis from the HIV epidemiology research study. *JAMA.* 2001;285(11):1466–1474.

47. Powell-Cope GM, White J, Henkelman EJ, Turner BJ. Qualitative and quantitative assessments of HAART adherence of substance-abusing women. *AIDS Care.* 2003;15(2):239–249.

48. Moore J, Schuman P, Schoenbaum E, Solomon L, Smith D. Severe adverse life events and depressive symptoms among women with, or at risk for, HIV infection in four cities in the United States of America. *AIDS.* 1999;13:2459–2468.

49. Spire B, Duran S, Souville M, et al. Adherence to highly active antiretroviral therapies (HAART) in HIV-infected patients: from a predictive to a dynamic approach. *Soc Sci Med.* 2002;54:1481–1496.

50. Lerman C, Kash K, Stefanek M. Younger women at increased risk for breast cancer: perceived risk, psychological well-being, and surveillance behavior. *J Natl Cancer Inst Monogr.* 1994;16:171–176.

51. Siegler I, Feaganes J, Rimer B. Predictors of adoption of mammography in women under age 50. *Health Psychol.* 1995;14(3):274–278.

52. Banks E, Beral V, Cameron R, et al. Comparison of various characteristics of women who do and do not attend for breast cancer screening. *Breast Cancer Res.* 2002;4(1):R1.

53. Haynes RB, Montague P, Oliver T, McKibbon KA, Brouwers MC, Kanani R. Interventions for helping patients to follow prescriptions for medications. *Cochrane Database Syst Rev.* 2000;(2):CD000011.

54. Ruscher SM, de Wit R, Mazmanian D. Psychiatric patients' attitudes about medication and factors affecting noncompliance. *Psychiatr Serv.* 1997;48(1):82–85.

55. Johnson D. Depression: treatment compliance in general practice. *Acta Psychiatr Scand.* 1981;290:447–453.

56. Lin EHB, Von Korff M, Katon W, et al. The role of the primary care physician in patients' adherence to antidepressant therapy. *Med Care.* 1995;33(1):67–74.

57. Linden M, Gothe H, Dittman R, Schaaf B. Early termination of antidepressant drug treatment. *J Clin Psychopharmacol.* 2000;20(5):523–530.

58. Maidment R, Livingston G, Katona C. Just keep taking the tablets: Adherence to antidepressant treatment in older people in primary care. *Int J Geriatr Psychiatry.* 2002;17:752–757.

59. Demyttenaere K, Enzlin P, Dewe W, et al. Compliance with antidepressants in a primary care setting, 1: beyond lack of efficacy and adverse events. *J Clin Psychiatry.* 2001;62(S22):30–33.

60. Sleath B, Wurst K, Lowery T. Drug information sources and antidepressant adherence. *Community Ment Health J.* 2003;39(4):359–368.

61. Dietrich A, Oxman T, Burns M, Winchell CW, Chin T. Application of a depression management office system in community practice: a demonstration. *J Am Board Fam Pract.* 2003;16:107–114.

62. Keller M, Hirschfeld R, Demyttenaere K, Baldwin DS. Optimizing outcomes in depression: focus on antidepressant compliance. *Int Clin Psychopharmacol.* 2002; 17:265–271.

63. Demyttenaere K, Haddad P, Compliance with antidepressant therapy and antidepressant medications. *Acta Psychiatr Scand.* 2000;S403:50–56.

64. Hotopf M, Hardy R, Lewis G. Discontinuation rates of SSRIs and tricyclic antidepressants: a meta-analysis and investigation of heterogeneity. *Br J Psychiatry.* 1997;170:120–127.

65. MacGillivray S, Arroll B, Hatcher S, et al. Efficacy and tolerability of selective serotonin reuptake inhibitors compared with tricyclic antidepressants in depression treated in primary care: a systematic review and meta-analysis. *BMJ.* 2003;326(7397):1014.

66. Thompson C, Peveler R, Stephenson D, McKendrick J. Compliance with antidepressant medication in the treatment of major depressive disorder in primary care: a randomized, comparison of fluoxetine and a tricyclic antidepressant. *Am J Psychiatry.* 2000;157(3):338–343.

67. Williams JW Jr., Mulrow CD, Chiquette E, Noel PH, Aguilar C, Cornell J. A systematic review of newer pharmacotherapies for depression in adults: evidence report summary. *Ann Intern Med.* 2000;132(9):743–756.

68. Tai-Seale M, Croghan T, Obenchain R. Determinants of antidepressant treatment compliance: implications for policy. *Med Care Res Rev.* 2000;57(4): 491–512.

69. Basco M, Rush J. Compliance with pharmacotherapy in mood disorders. *Psychiatr Ann.* 1995;25(5):269–279.

70. Orleans C, George L, Houpt J, Brodie HK. How primary care physicians treat psychiatric disorders: a national survey of family practitioners. *Am J Psychiatry.* 1985;142(1):52–57.

71. Williams J, Rost K, Dietrich AJ, Ciotti MC, Zyzanski SJ, Cornell J. Primary care physicians' approach to depressive disorders. Effects of physician specialty and practice structure. *Arch Fam Med.* 1999;8(1):57–67.

72. Gallo J, Meredith L, Gonzales J, et al. Do family physicians and internists differ in knowledge, attitudes and self-reported approaches for depression? *Int J Psychiatry Med.* 2002;32(1):1–20.

73. Dobscha S, Delucchi K, Young M. Adherence with referrals for outpatient follow-up from a VA psychiatric emergency room. *Community Ment Health J.* 1999;35(5):451–458.

74. Grunebaum M, Luber P, Callahan M, Leon AC, Olfson M, Portera L. Predictors of missed appointments for psychiatric consultations in a primary care clinic. *Psychiatr Serv.* 1996;47(8):848–852.

75. Koshes R, Rothberg J. Compliance with consultations in a military psychiatry clinic. *Mil Med.* 1994;159(4):310–313.

76. Minoletti A, Perez E, Blouin A. Compliance with referrals from psychiatric emergency services to ambulatory facilities: a 20-year literature review. *Am J Soc Psychiatry.* 1984;4(2):57–61.

77. Peeters F, Bayer H. No-show for initial screening at a community mental health centre: rate, reasons and further help-seeking. *Soc Psychiatry Psychiatr Epidemiol.* 1999;34:323–327.

78. Sparr L, Moffitt B, Ward M. Missed psychiatric appointments: who returns and who stays away. *Am J Psychiatry.* 1992;150(5):801–805.

79. Solomon P, Gordon B. Outpatient compliance of psychiatric emergency room patients by presenting problems. *Psychiatr Q.* 1988;59(4):271–283.

80. McGlade K, Bradley T, Murphy G, Lundy GP. Referrals to hospital by general practitioners: A study of compliance and communication. *BMJ.* 1988;297: 1246–1248.

81. Reuben D, Maly R, Hirsch S, et al. Physician implementation of and the patient adherence to recommendations from comprehensive geriatric assessment. *Am J Med.* 1996;100:444–451.

82. Olfson M. Primary care patients who refuse specialized mental health services. *Arch Intern Med.* 1991;151:129–132.

83. Farid B, Alapont E. Patients who fail to attend their first psychiatric outpatient appointment: non-attendance or inappropriate referral? *J Ment Health.* 1993;2: 81–83.

84. Killaspy H, Banerjee S, King M, Lloyd M. Non-attendance at psychiatric outpatient clinics: communication and implications for primary care. *Br J Gen Pract.* 1999;49:880–883.

85. Killaspy H, Banerjee S, King M, Lloyd M. Prospective controlled study of psychiatric outpatient non-attendance. *Br J Psychiatry.* 2000;176:160–165.

86. Neeleman J, Mikhail W. A case-control study of GP and patient-related variables associated with non-attendance at new psychiatric out-patient appointments. *J Ment Health.* 1997;6(3):301–306.

87. Livianos-Aldana L, Vila-Gomez M, Rojo-Moreno L, Luengo-Lopez MA. Patients who miss initial appointments in community psychiatry? A Spanish community analysis. *Int J Soc Psychiatry.* 1999;45(3):198–206.

88. Lambert M. *Bergin and Garfield's Handbook of Psychotherapy and Behavior Change.* New York: John Wiley and Sons; 2004.

89. Garland A, Scott J. Cognitive therapy for depression in women. *Psychiatr Ann.* 2002;32(8):465–476.

90. Paykel E. Psychotherapy, medication combinations, and compliance. *J Clin Psychiatry.* 1995;56(S1):24–30.

91. Linden W, Stossel C, Maurice J. Psychosocial interventions for patients with coronary artery disease. A meta-analysis. *Arch Intern Med.* 1996;156:745–752.

92. Glassman A, O'Connor C, Califf R, et al. Sertraline treatment of major depression in patients with acute MI or unstable angina. *JAMA.* 2002;288(6):701–709.

93. Writing Committee for the ENRICHD Investigators. Effects of treating depression and low perceived social support on clinical events after myocardial infarction. The Enhancing Recovery in Coronary Heart Disease Patients (ENRICHD) Randomized Trial. *JAMA.* 2003;289(23):3106–3116.

94. Lustman PJ, Griffith LS, Freedland KE, Kissel SS, Clouse RE. Cognitive behavior therapy for depression in type 2 diabetes mellitus: a randomized, controlled trial. *Ann Intern Med.* 1998;129(8):613–621.

95. Lustman PJ, Griffith LS, Clouse RE, et al. Effects of nortriptyline on depression and glycemic control in diabetes: results of a double-blind, placebo-controlled trial. *Psychosom Med.* 1997;59:241–250.

96. Lustman PJ, Freedland KE, Griffith LS, Clouse RE. Fluoxetine for depression in diabetes: a randomized double-blind placebo-controlled trial. *Diabetes Care.* 2000;23:618–623.

97. Angelino A, Treisman G. Management of psychiatric disorders in patients infected with human immunodeficiency virus. *HIV/AIDS.* 2001;33:847–856.

98. Peveler R, George C, Kinmonth AL, Campbell M, Thompson C. Effect of antidepressant drug counseling and information leaflets on adherence to drug treatment in primary care: randomized controlled trial. *BMJ.* 1999;319: 612–615.

99. Badamgarav E, Weingarten S, Henning J, et al. Effectiveness of disease management programs in depression: a systematic review. *Am J Psychiatry.* 2003; 160(12):2080–2090.

100. Katon W, Von Korff M, Lin E, et al. Collaborative management to achieve treatment guidelines: impact on depression in primary care. *JAMA.* 1995;273: 1026–1031.

101. Simon G, Von Korff M, Rutter C, Wagner E. Randomised trial of monitoring, feedback, and management of care by telephone to improve treatment of depression in primary care. *BMJ.* 2000;320:550–554.

102. Hunkeler E, Meresman J, Hargreaves W, et al. Efficacy of nurse telehealth care and peer support in augmenting treatment of depression in primary care. *Arch Fam Med.* 2000;9:700–708.

103. Katzelnick D, Simon G, Pearson S, et al. Randomized trial of a depression management program in high utilizers of medical care. *Arch Fam Med.* 2000;9: 345–351.

104. Rost K, Nutting P, Smith J, Werner J, Duan N. Improving depression outcomes in community primary care practice. *J Gen Intern Med.* 2001;16(3):143–149.

105. Wagner EH, Austin BT, Davis C, Hindmarsh M, Schaefer J, Bonomi A. Improving chronic illness care: translating evidence into action. *Health Aff (Millwood).* 2001;20(6):64–78.

106. Kehoe W. Pharmacists and the treatment of depression. *Am J Health Syst Pharm.* 2002;59(16):1509.

107. Bultman D, Svarstad B. Effects of physician communication style on client medication beliefs and adherence with antidepressant treatment. *Patient Educ Couns.* 2000;40:173–185.

108. Finley P, Rens H, Pont J, et al. Impact of a collaborative pharmacy practice model on the treatment of depression in primary care. *Am J Health Syst Pharm.* 2002;59(16):1518–1526.

109. Boudreau D, Capoccia K, Sullivan S, et al. Collaborative care model to improve outcomes in major depression. *Ann Pharmacother.* 2002;36:585–591.

110. Furukawa T, Streiner D, Young T. Is antidepressant-benzodiazepine combination therapy clinically more useful? A meta-analytic study. *J Affect Disord.* 2001; 65:173–177.

111. Larsen D, Nguyen T, Green R, et al. Enhancing the utilization of outpatient mental health services. *Community Ment Health J.* 1983;19(4):305–320.

112. Daley D, Salloum I, Zuckoff A, Kirisci L, Thase ME. Increasing treatment adherence among outpatients with depression and cocaine dependence: results of a pilot study. *Am J Psychiatry.* 1998;155(11):1611–1613.

113. Chen A. Noncompliance in community psychiatry: a review of clinical interventions. *Hosp Commun Psychiatry.* 1991;42(3):282–287.

114. Tinsley H, Bowman S, Ray S. Manipulation of expectancies about counseling and psychotherapy: Review and analysis of expectancy manipulation strategies and results. *Journal of Counseling Psychology*. 1988;35(1):99–108.
115. Karasu TB, Gelenberg A, Merriam AE, Wang P. American Psychiatric Association practice guideline for the treatment of patients with major depressive disorder. *Am J Psychiatry*. 2000 Apr;157(4 Suppl):1–45.
116. Radloff S. The CES-D Scale: a self-report depression scale in the general population. *Appl Psychol Meas*. 1977;1:385–401.
117. Gatz M, Johansson B, Pedersen N, Berg S, Reynolds C. A cross-national self-report measure of depressive symptomatology. *Int Psychogeriatr*. 1993;5:147–156.
118. Hertzog C, Van Alstine J, Usasl P, Hultsch DF, Dixon R. Measurement properties of the center for epidemiological studies depression scale (CES-D) in older populations. *J Consult Clin Psychol*. 1990;2:64–72.
119. Sheehan T, Fifield J, Reisine S, et al. The measurement structure of the center for epidemiological studies depression scale. *J Pers Assess*. 1995;64:507–521.
120. Felton B, Revenson T, Hinrichsen G. Stress and coping in the explanation of psychological adjustment among chronically ill adults. *Soc Sci Med*. 1984;18(10):889–898.
121. Adams S, Pill R, Jones A. Medication, chronic illness and identity: the perspective of people with asthma. *Soc Sci Med*. 1997;45(2):189–201.
122. Katon W, Robinson P, Von Korff M, et al. A multifaceted intervention to improve treatment of depression in primary care. *Arch Gen Psychiatry*. 1996;53:924–932.
123. Katon W, Von Korff M, Lin E, et al. Stepped collaborative care for primary care patients with persistent symptoms of depression: a randomized trial. *Arch Gen Psychiatry*. 1999;56:1109–1115.
124. Wells KB, Sherbourne C, Schoenbaum M, et al. Impact of disseminating quality improvement programs for depression in managed primary care. *JAMA*. 2000;283:212–220.
125. Unutzer J, Katon W, Callahan CM, et al. Collaborative care management of late-life depression in primary care: a randomized controlled trial. *JAMA*. 2002;288:2836–2845.

Treatment Adherence Among Individuals With Severe Mental Illness

Patrick S. Calhoun
Marian I. Butterfield

A major challenge in medicine is ensuring that patients adhere to their schedules for treatment and clinical appointments. The estimated yearly cost of nonadherence to treatment for all medical disorders in the United States is $100 billion (1). As described in earlier chapters of this volume, mental illness has been identified as a risk factor for poor adherence. In chapter 9, Gonzalez and Williams outline the deleterious effects of clinical depression on adherence to general medical care. In this chapter, we focus on issues surrounding adherence to psychiatric treatment among individuals with severe mental illness (SMI). Improving treatment adherence of patients with SMI is one of the biggest challenges facing psychiatry today. Among patients with SMI, nonadherence with psychiatric treatment is associated with increased social, economic, and clinical costs and is closely related to relapse, rehospitalization, and poor outcomes (2).

People with SMI represent about 2.6% of the population in the United States (3). Although there are widespread inconsistencies in the definitions of SMI (4, 5), common criteria include the presence of a major mental illness, chronicity, and pervasive social and occupational impairment (4–7). Although major mental illness may include major depression, bipolar disorder, and severe anxiety disorders, including obsessive-compulsive disorder and posttraumatic stress disorder, the overwhelming majority of research examining adherence among patients with SMI focuses on studies of patients with schizophrenia or other psychotic illnesses.

Schizophrenia is an often devastating, chronic mental illness that has severe social and economic effects. Approximately 1% to 2% of adults in the general population will suffer from the disorder during their lifetime (8). The usual onset for schizophrenia is late adolescence or early adulthood, and it typically follows a recurrent and chronic course (8). Studies suggest that 1.5% to 3% of health expenditures in developed countries and 22% of the costs of mental illness are related to schizophrenia and associated psychotic illness (9). For example, in the United States, where about 2 million patients have schizophrenia, the estimated yearly cost of this disorder is about $33 billion to $65 billion (9–11). In comparison, for depression, diagnosed in around 19 million Americans, the estimated yearly cost is $30 billion (11).

The goals of this chapter are to summarize the prevalence, costs, risks, and clinical interventions for poor adherence among patients with SMI. Although severe mental illness includes a wide variety of mental disorders, we focus the majority of attention on adherence among patients with psychotic disorders. We conclude with a discussion of the research and clinical implications of our findings, and offer several directions for future research.

PREVALENCE AND COST OF NONADHERENCE

Nonadherence is responsible for much of the high costs associated with medical treatment for schizophrenia and related SMIs (11). Nonadherence with medical appointments and medication regimens is very prevalent both among patients with psychiatric disorders in general and among patients with SMI in particular. Disturbingly, research suggests that fewer than half of all patients diagnosed with a mental disorder initiate treatment (12, 13). Among those who do initiate treatment, missed outpatient appointments are a significant problem. Rates of missed outpatient psychiatric appointments range from 9% to 60% (2, 14–17) and tend to be higher for patients with SMI (14). In community-based clinic settings, patients with SMI miss about 25% of their outpatient psychiatric appointments (16).

Adherence rates with medication regimens are similarly problematic. Although rates of adherence differ among studies, which use various methods of estimating medication compliance, including patient report, clinician's judgment, or pill counts, those studies uniformly find troubling rates of adherence. Adherence rates to antipsychotic medications among patients with schizophrenia range from 20% to 90% (18–22).

The wide range, or inconsistency, in the incidence of nonadherence, that is, 10%–80%, is likely due, in part, to the problem of accurately measuring adherence. For example, one study suggesting that only 10% of patients were nonadherent relied on clinician judgment (23). In contrast, studies showing much higher rates of nonadherence relied on patient reports. Reviews of the literature, however, consistently estimate that the average rate of nonadherence to psychiatric medications among patients with SMI is around 50% (18, 19).

The rate of nonadherence among patients with SMI is thus disturbingly high. It is unclear, however, whether adherence rates actually differ between patients with mental disorders and those with physical disorders (24). In a review of almost 12,000 articles, half of which were review articles and half papers reporting original data, Blackwell concluded that there are few data to suggest that the rates differ (24). His review, however, pooled patients with SMI and patients with other, less chronic mental illnesses. In a more recent review, Cramer and Rosenheck (19) found that patients requiring antipsychotic medication had a much wider range of nonadherence than did both patients with depression and patients with physical disorders: They found that patients receiving antipsychotic medication take an average of 58% of the recommended amount of medications; patients receiving antidepressant medication take an average rate of 65%, and patients with physical disorders take 76% of the recommended amount.

It is also unclear as to whether patients with SMI take nonpsychiatric medications as prescribed. Almost no attention is paid to this issue. The overwhelming number of studies examining adherence among patients with SMI focus solely on adherence to neuroleptic medications (19), possibly because of the severe implications that nonadherence has on relapse and course of the illness. One study did find that adherence to antihypertensive, antihyperlipidemic, and antidiabetic medications were poor, ranging from 64% to 52%, among middle-aged and older patients with psychotic disorders followed at a Veterans Affairs medical center (25).

There are high social, economic, and clinical costs associated with nonadherence among patients with SMI. The majority of the direct health costs associated with the treatment of schizophrenia is attributable to hospitalizations for both initial and later relapses (11). Nonadherence is closely related to relapse, rehospitalization, and increased emergency room visits among patients with SMI (26, 27). In fact, medication nonadherence is the best predictor of relapse after a psychotic episode (28) and is responsible for over half of all relapses (27). A review of the literature suggests that approximately 75% of patients with poor adherence will relapse, compared with about 35% of patients with good adherence (11, 24, 28–31).

In one of the most cited studies in the field, Weiden and Olfson (27) estimate that upwards of 40% of rehospitalization costs among persons with schizophrenia are attributable to nonadherence. They estimate that, in terms of actual dollars, $2.3 billion of U.S. hospitalization annual costs are due to relapse associated with nonadherence (27). Subsequent studies suggest that the Weiden and Olfson estimate is likely to be an underestimate of the true burden associated with nonadherence, because their model includes the costs associated with only the first rehospitalization when, in practice, 30% of patients are rehospitalized more than once a year (32, 33).

Whereas the direct medical costs of nonadherence to medication use among patients with psychotic illness receives significant attention, relatively little research examines the indirect costs associated with the resultant loss of productivity and decreased quality of life. For patients with chronic mental illness, antipsychotic medications and, more recently, the introduction of atypical antipsychotics open new possibilities for reintegration into the community through meaningful work and independent living. The likelihood of their sustaining work and community living is likely dependent on their potentially lifelong adherence to psychiatric medications in an unsupervised setting (34).

Treatment guidelines published by the American Psychiatric Association (APA) recommend at least 1 year of antipsychotic therapy for individuals experiencing a first psychotic episode. For patients with multiple psychotic episodes, a minimum of 5 years of maintenance therapy is suggested, and, in practice, indefinite therapy is often prescribed (35). There is a paucity of research, however, examining the long-term adherence of patients with psychotic illness to antipsychotic medications under conditions of routine care (11, 34). The overwhelming majority of studies examining treatment adherence to neuroleptic medication among patients with SMI examine adherence only for a year or less (11, 19). Almost none examine adherence for a period as long as 5 years, the period recommended by the APA's treatment guidelines for patients with multiple psychotic episodes (36). More research is needed to examine adherence to long-term neuroleptic medication regimens. Nonadherence to maintenance medication use is likely to reduce quality of life and lead to decreased community living and unemployment among patients with SMI.

Another high cost of nonadherence among patients with SMI is increased mortality. In epidemiological studies, excess mortality among persons with schizophrenia is one of the most consistent and accepted findings (37). The relative mortality rate is more than twice that of the general population and is poorly understood (38). One factor attributed to the increase risk of mortality is the increased rate of suicide, which is as high as 10% among patients with SMI (39). A number of variables predict suicide in patients with SMI. These include hopelessness, high stress, being young, single, male, having high socioeconomic background, high intelligence, poor social support, and being recently discharged from the hospital. Another key variable associated with an increased risk of completed suicide among persons with schizophrenia is treatment nonadherence (40, 41). For example, in one case-control study of 63 young patients who had committed suicide and 63 controls, a negative attitude toward treatment and treatment nonadherence significantly increased the odds of death (OR = 7.0) (40).

Although suicide is a factor in increased mortality, the high rate of suicide does not fully account for the excess premature death (37, 38). Patients with SMI appear at greater risk for dying prematurely from natural causes as well (37, 38). The mechanisms are unclear and may be associated with factors that affect mortality in the general population, including socioeconomic status, unhealthy diet, substance abuse, smoking, and possible medication side effects (38, 42). One identified mechanism, however, is nonadherence or refusal of treatment for medical disease (43).

RISK FACTORS FOR NONADHERENCE

Given the high cost associated with nonadherence in patients with SMI, clinicians and researchers attempt to define the factors that are associated with it. A number of methodological problems flaw much of the research, to some degree limiting our understanding of the critical factors associated with adherence. Furthermore, many studies were conducted 20 to 30 years ago, before the advent of atypical antipsychotic medications and significant changes in the context of health service delivery (44).

The problem of reliably measuring adherence continues to plague studies attempting to identify factors associated with nonadherence. Many studies classify patients into two groups, compliant or noncompliant, despite adherence's often being partial rather than all-or-none (19). Other common flaws of research in this area are problems associated with reactivity and generalizability. There is a risk that the assessment procedures themselves are an important intervention. Poor adherence tends to diminish when patients know that their behaviors are under scrutiny (24). Also, it is difficult to ensure that study participants are representative of the population of interest. Nonadherent patients may be more likely to refuse to participate in research studies than adherent patients are, potentially leading to a source of bias and limiting the generalizability of results.

Despite these limitations, a number of factors appear to be important predictors of nonadherence among patients with SMI (see Table 10.1). A number of studies suggest that psychotic symptoms and psychotic symptom severity may be important factors (18). In an interview study of 40 patients who refused antipsychotic medication, Appelbaum and Gutheil (45) identify paranoia, grandiosity, and delusional beliefs about medicine as important factors. Subsequent cross-sectional research finds similar results (18); however, longitudinal studies are more ambiguous. Only one of four longitudinal studies examining symptom severity at hospital discharge and subsequent adherence support the link between severity and adherence (46).

TABLE 10.1
Factors Associated With Adherence
to Treatment Among Persons With SMI

Factor	Influence on Adherence
Patient-related factors	
Psychotic symptoms (paranoia, grandiosity, delusions)	–
Symptom severity	–
Neurobehavioral cognitive status	?
Lack of insight	–
Comorbid substance abuse	–
Medication factors	
Adverse effects	–
Suboptimal dosing	–
Use of atypical antipsychotic medications	+
Clinician factors	
Therapeutic alliance	+
Forced treatment	–
Social and environmental factors	
Adequate social support	+
Economic barriers	–

Another patient factor that appears very important to adherence is insight. Among patients with SMI, insight is defined as an understanding that one has an illness, an ability to recognize symptoms as part of the disease, and acceptance of the need for treatment. Consistent with the health belief model, which postulates that persons reach decisions on health actions on the basis of their perception of the seriousness of the illness, their susceptibility to it, and the benefits of adherence, patients with physical disorders who accept that they have an illness and perceive it as serious tend to be more adherent compared with persons without these perceptions (47) (see chap. 2).

Despite significant differences in the way insight is defined across studies, the majority of research examining the relationship between insight and adherence provides consistent results (18, 44). Although there are some negative findings (48), most studies find that greater insight is associated with increased adherence (18). Patients who deny having a mental illness have higher rates of medication nonadherence than do patients who have more insight into their illness.

A number of authors theorize that the deleterious effects of chronic psychotic illness on cognition and motivation may underlie the high rates of nonadherence in this population (18). Schizophrenia has been associated with neuropsychological deficits and deficits in motivation. A thorough review of the literature in this area, however, suggests no clear association between adherence and neurobehavioral cognitive status (18).

Among patients with SMI, there appears to be a strong relationship between substance abuse and adherence (18, 46, 49). The majority of studies examining the impact of comorbid substance abuse on adherence show a strong relationship between substance abuse and poor adherence (46, 50–52), although a few studies find no relationship (53). Active substance abuse may lead to a chaotic and disorganized lifestyle that makes adherence difficult (49). Intoxication may impair judgment about health-related behaviors (49, 54) and lead to a devaluation of the benefits of antipsychotic medications, which may be perceived as less effective than they are, slow to act, and having more side effects than they do (55).

Medication side effects are commonly cited as the main reason patients fail to take psychotropic medications. The side effects of neuroleptic medication can be severe. Extrapyramidal side effects (EPSs) are among the most common. Acute EPSs, including parkinsonism, akinesia, and dystonia, create discomfort and physical disability related to movement disorder. The effects of long-term use, including tardive dyskinesia and akathisia, are extremely debilitating and contribute to both the stigma and the social isolation associated with SMI (56).

The evidence that the severe side effects associated with antipsychotic medication are a significant factor in nonadherence is not as clear-cut as one might imagine. Several studies show that when patients are asked why they did not take medication, they report side effects as a significant factor (57–59). Prospective studies document a relationship between nonadherence and EPSs, including bradykinesia, dystonia, and akathisia (56, 60, 61). Other research, however, fails to find an association between side effects and nonadherence in retrospective (62), cross-sectional (63), or prospective studies (64, 65). Although adverse effects are clearly one possible reason that patients with SMI do not take their medication, more research is needed to clarify the strength of relationship between side effects and nonadherence among patients with SMI.

Atypical antipsychotic medications have an improved side-effect profile, including a lower incidence of EPSs and tardive dyskinesia, compared with older typical antipsychotics (22). Many speculate that as a result of reduced side effects, adherence will be better among patients on these newer medications. Although showing a trend toward improved adherence with atypical antipsychotic medications, the evidence indicates that adherence tends to remain poor overall. For example, in a study examining haloperidol, perphenazine, risperidone, olanzapine, and quetiapine, Dolder and colleagues (22) found that patients on the atypical agents were moderately more adherent. Patients on typical antipsychotics were without medication for an average of 7 days per month compared with 4 days per month for those patients on atypical agents. At 12 months, patients taking atypical agents filled prescriptions at a higher rate than did patients on typical antipsychotics (55% vs. 50%); however, this difference was not statistically significant (22). In a double-blind, randomized trial of haloperidol or clozapine, Rosenheck and colleagues (66) found that although there was no difference in the proportion of pills returned each week between treatment conditions, patients receiving clozapine did take their medication significantly longer.

A number of other factors are linked with adherence among patients with SMI. Perhaps one of the most important factors is the patient–provider relationship. Outpatients who develop a strong therapeutic alliance with their provider are more likely to adhere to medications and treatment recommendations than are patients with a less strong relationship (67). Inpatients who are adherent with medication suggestions are more satisfied with their care and trusting of staff (63). Through building a trusting and collaborative clinical relationship, patients may perceive the practical advantages of continuing medications (46).

Conversely, there is some evidence that coercion may deter adherence. Patients who receive forced treatment or are detained against their will may be less adherent (68). Although there are strongly held views for and against coerced treatment, there is relatively little empirical evidence about its effectiveness or harmful effects (69, 70). Several studies found that patients who feel more coerced at hospital admission are less likely to take medications or use mental-health services upon discharge (70, 71). Other studies, however, found no relationship between perceived coercion at hospital admission and adherence to outpatient treatment (69, 72). More research is needed to examine the suggestion that coercive treatment reduces future treatment adherence (73).

Other factors empirically related to treatment adherence among patients with SMI include social support and economic barriers. Not surprisingly, adherence appears to be higher among patients with family members who are available to supervise medication regimens (46, 48). In contrast, patients with family members who have ambivalent attitudes about antipsychotic medications appear at increased risk of nonadherence (46). Economic barriers, including poverty and homelessness, are also associated with poorer adherence. Sociocultural background may be a factor but has received little empirical support (44).

INTERVENTIONS DESIGNED TO IMPROVE ADHERENCE AMONG PATIENTS WITH SMI

Given that the most effective treatment for SMI is symptomatic and typically involves the use of neuroleptic or other psychotropic medications, perhaps it is not surprising that the majority of interventions aimed at improving adherence among this population focus on improving the rate at which patients take their psychotropic medication as prescribed. We group these interventions into three broad categories (education, psychotherapy, or service delivery; see Table 10.2) reflecting the focus or target of the intervention. Education, or *psychoeducation* as it is commonly called, reflects interventions with a knowledge-based emphasis (74). Most psychoeducational interventions provide information in both written and verbal formats about SMI, treatment, and medications (75). In contrast, psychotherapeutic interventions focus on attitudinal and behavioral changes needed to achieve medication adherence. Finally, interventions focused on service de-

TABLE 10.2
Interventions Designed to Improve
Adherence Among Patients With SMI

Type of Intervention	*Description—Orientation*	*Impact on Adherence*
Psychoeducation	Focus on the dissemination of knowledge about mental illness, treatment, and medications.	Ineffective
Psychotherapy		
Cognitive-behavioral	Target patient's attitudes and beliefs about treatment and medications. Behavioral modification techniques employed to target, shape, or reinforce specific behaviors.	Effective
Group	Stresses importance of peer support and shared identification.	Modest support for behavioral interventions
Family	Focuses on the family as a critical component of treatment.	Modest support for behavioral interventions
Service Delivery		
Open-access clinics and prompts	Policies that allow patients to be seen on a walk-in basis or employ telephone calls to remind patients of appointments.	Effective
Assertive community treatment models	Include provision of a supportive social network; close monitoring of clinical status, and provision of stable housing. Often include multiservice treatment teams, small caseloads, 24-hour services, and assertive outreach and rehabilitation.	Modest support of effectiveness
Case management models	Involve a support person or "case manager" who monitors patient, performs needs assessment, gains access to services, and helps with advocacy.	Modest support of effectiveness

livery investigate the impact of prompts or telephone calls on adherence. Service delivery interventions also have investigated the efficacy of newer community-based models of care that involve a variety of supportive and rehabilitative services (75).

A consistent finding among reviews and meta-analyses of interventions aimed at improving adherence among patients with SMI, is the failure of educational interventions to produce significant change (74–77). Both broad-based psychoeducation programs, in which education about mental illness, symptoms, and treatment is provided, and medication-focused programs, characterized by the provision of information about the benefits and side effects of medications, appear to increase participants' knowledge about mental illness and their medication. There is little evidence, however, that educational strategies improve the rate at which patients take their medication as prescribed (74, 75, 77).

In contrast, there is good support for psychotherapeutic interventions, particularly cognitive-behavioral interventions aimed at improving adherence. Cognitive treatments target patients attitudes and beliefs about medications, whereas behavioral interventions target and shape specific behavioral patterns (74, 75). Kemp and colleagues (78, 79) demonstrated sustained gains in adherence over 18 months among patients who received "compliance therapy," which combined cognitive approaches and motivational interviewing techniques (see chap. 2 for more details on motivation interviewing). Similarly, there is consistent support for interventions that include a form of behavioral tailoring (75, 77). Behavioral tailoring involves helping patients develop strategies to include medication into their daily routine. Examples include simplifying the medication regimen such as taking medications once or twice per day instead of many times, and pairing medications with other routine activities of daily living such as brushing one's teeth (77).

Interventions with groups of patients with mental illness stress the importance of peer support and shared identification in an effort to increase adherence. Group interventions are also thought to be cheaper because more patients can be seen with fewer resources. The majority of group interventions, however, were psychoeducational in nature and did not demonstrate efficacy (75). One group intervention that was a combination of psychoeducation and a behavioral intervention did show some promise (80). Seltzer and colleagues (80) provided nine sessions of psychoeducation, group discussion of fears and beliefs that interfere with adherence, and positive reinforcement for advantageous medication-taking regimens. They found increased adherence among the intervention group at a 5-month follow-up. Results of this study are limited, however, by significant dropouts in both the intervention and comparison group, raising concerns of attrition bias (75, 80).

Owing to the evidence that patients with families who have ambivalent attitudes about antipsychotic medications are at increased risk of non-adherence (46), families are a focus for intervention. Family-focused interventions include a variety of psychoeducational and behavioral strategies to facilitate better outcomes for patients (75). In a thorough review of interventions from 1980 to 2000, Zygmunt and colleagues found that only 3 of 12 family interventions reported a significant difference in adherence. Two of the three successful interventions included a strong behavioral therapy component (75).

Although the intervention literature shows some promise for psychotherapeutic interventions, it is unclear to what extent patients with SMI are actually adherent with this form of treatment. For example, although Kemp and colleagues (78) reported the success of their cognitive-behavioral intervention, they administered four to six sessions of compliance therapy to patients who were hospitalized on an inpatient unit. It is unknown how many patients would complete similar treatment on an outpatient basis. Increasingly, investigators in Great Britain are conducting cognitive-behavioral treatment for improved medication adherence and for the actual treatment of persistent psychotic symptoms. Several controlled trials were published regarding the use of cognitive-behavioral therapy for schizophrenia and the results were reported as promising in a recent review (81). In general, however, the literature examining the efficacy of cognitive-behavioral therapy and other psychotherapies for treatment of psychoses is in its infancy. Few studies report adherence with specific psychotherapy appointments, and fewer report adherence with specific components of treatment, for example, homework assignments. More research is needed to examine patient and therapist factors that affect adherence to psychotherapy and clinical outcomes (82).

Increasingly investigators are examining service policies and new models of treatment provision in an effort to increase adherence. These interventions range from relatively straightforward ones using telephone prompts to much more complex community-based models of care. Two large studies investigated the use of telephone prompts to remind patients of their upcoming mental-health appointment (83, 84). Patients who were reminded of their appointment via a telephone call were more likely to attend than were. patients enrolled in usual care (76). Results from a recent meta-analysis examining clinical interventions for nonadherence provide support for interventions that provide patients with predischarge outpatient clinician contact (76). Patients with SMI who are provided contact with an outpatient provider before they are discharged from an inpatient psychiatric unit are more likely to attend their first postdischarge appointment.

More complex service delivery interventions involving community-based care are becoming increasingly popular. Only a relatively small proportion of studies examining community care, most notably, those involving assertive community treatment and intensive case management models, have included assessment of medication adherence as an outcome (75). Assertive community treatment, or the program for assertive community treatment (PACT) model, is a comprehensive team-based psychosocial intervention that provides treatment and rehabilitation services to persons with SMI. Much of the service delivery takes place outside of the outpatient clinic setting. PACT programs target those most underserved by the traditional treatment system. The six basic elements of the PACT model are: (a) multiservice teams, which may include case managers, a psychiatrist, and additional clinicians and supervisor, (b) 24-hour service availability, (c) small caseloads, usually 10–20 patients per team, (d) ongoing and continuous services, (e) assertive outreach as most service takes place outside the clinic setting, and (f) a rehabilitation component—social, educational, vocational, housing, financial (85).

Case management has become an increasingly important component of mental-health services in both the public and private sector. Case management interventions are need-based services that enlist a "case manager" to help persons with SMI in pragmatic ways to enhance functioning. The overall goals of case management are twofold: to achieve continuity of care and to improve clinical outcomes. Case management services have at least six recognized functions: identification and outreach, assessment of needs, planning services, linkage to services, monitoring and evaluation of progress, and advocacy (86). Case managers may provide assistance to persons with SMI in procuring housing and employment, or with tasks such as grocery shopping or supportive counseling. They may also support the patient's treatment plan through transportation to appointments and ensuring medication availability.

In a review of assertive community-based treatment and intensive case management programs, Zygmunt and colleagues (75) found that 4 of 10 studies examining these interventions reported that the intervention was associated with greater medication adherence. These positive studies were limited, however, by a nonrigorous assessment of adherence. Despite the variability in the quality of research examining the impact of community-based interventions on adherence, these programs tend to closely monitor patients with a history of nonadherence and view medication adherence as an important goal (75, 87). As a result, many suggest that the reduction in hospitalization that has been widely associated with these models of care is likely due to increased medication adherence.

Treatment adherence is a perplexing issue for clinicians and researchers working with SMI cohorts. Reviews of the effectiveness of mental-health services interventions on treatment adherence and clinical outcomes in this population report limited efficacy in general. Psychoeducational interventions are largely unsuccessful. Similarly, group and family psychotherapeutic interventions do not have large effects on adherence (75). Conversely, cognitive and behavioral interventions show promise and appear to be superior in promoting adherence. Emerging evidence demonstrates that assertive community treatment and case management models are effective in promoting adherence to medication treatment.

RESEARCH IMPLICATIONS AND NEW DIRECTIONS

As outlined in the first chapter of this volume, defining and measuring adherence is a problem that has limited much of the work is this area. This certainly continues to be a problem for research examining adherence among patients with SMI. There is no generally accepted definition of adherence among patients with SMI. The majority of studies examining medication adherence among patients with SMI rely on subjective reports of medication taking. This approach tends to overestimate adherence and reduces the likelihood of detecting intervention effects (18, 75). Objective measures of adherence may provide greater accuracy, but have the drawbacks associated with increased cost.

Some have suggested that complete cessation of oral medications for at least 1 week should be the definition of nonadherence of neuroleptic medications (75, 88). The majority of patients (91%) who fail to take medication for 1 week continue not to take their medication until they relapse (89). Until a gold standard for defining and measuring adherence exists, however, multiple measures, for example, subjective reports, pill counts, electronic measuring, and so on, should be used. Improved measurement would allow researchers to define various subtypes of nonadherence. For example, intentional versus accidental mistakes in dosing could be defined and used to develop more specific interventions. Interventions that target motivation such as compliance therapy (78) may be more useful for patients who intentionally stop medications, whereas behavioral interventions may be more appropriate for those patients with cognitive deficits (75).

Research in this area focuses predominantly on younger adult patients with schizophrenia. More research with a wider variety of patients is needed. The success of an intervention may vary depending on the population. For example, Nose and colleagues (76) reported that results from their meta-analysis indicated that studies that enrolled only homogeneous samples of people with schizophrenia were associated with a more favorable treatment effect, suggesting that the tested interventions may be less effective for patients with different diagnoses. It is possible that interventions designed for patients with schizophrenia are not easily transferable to patients with other SMI.

There is clearly a need for more research that investigates adherence in other SMI. Although the prevalence of nonadherence among patients with bipolar disorder is thought to be high (ranging from 18% to 52%), fewer than a dozen controlled studies examine adherence interventions in this group of patients (90, 91). Even less is known about adherence among patients with severe anxiety disorders, such as obsessive-compulsive disorder and posttraumatic stress disorder (PTSD).

PTSD is a highly prevalent disorder that can have serious affective, behavioral, and social consequences. There is clear evidence that patients with PTSD experience both significant intrapersonal and interpersonal difficulties, including problems with communication, self-disclosure, sexual intimacy, family cohesion, substance abuse, hostility, aggression, and interpersonal violence (92–94). Furthermore, there is increasing evidence that PTSD is associated with poor physical health, increased medical utilization, and mortality (95, 96). Yet, almost nothing is known to what extent poor adherence limits the effectiveness of PTSD treatment and how it may affect the course of illness.

Recently, researchers began to investigate whether PTSD may be a risk factor for poor adherence among patients with medical illness (97, 98). For example, Shemesh and colleagues (98) hypothesized that patients who are traumatized by their medical illness and develop PTSD symptoms, may avoid taking medication as prescribed because it is a reminder of their illness. In a sample of patients with myocardial infarction (MI), they found that PTSD was associated with medication nonadherence 1 year following MI. We recently have found that comorbid PTSD is highly prevalent and unrecognized in patients with primary psychotic illness (99). Comorbid PTSD may be a risk factor for poor adherence in this population. Given that PTSD leads to increased irritability and estrangement from others, PTSD symptoms may increase the difficulty of developing good therapeutic relationships. More research investigating the impact of comorbid PTSD is warranted as are studies examining the prevalence and impact of nonadherence among patients with primary PTSD.

The literature examining adherence among patients with SMI is also limited by a lack of studies examining the long-term effects of interventions. Only a small minority of studies examining intervention outcomes examine adherence for as long as 1 year, and fewer examine adherence for a period as long as 5 years, the period recommended by the American Psychiatric Association's treatment guidelines for patients with multiple psychotic episodes (36). Trials of adequate duration are needed to measure both the immediate effects on adherence and the long-term effects of the intervention.

In summary, differences between study designs, interventions, and measures of adherence make it difficult to categorize studies and thus to make generalizable conclusions (74). The differences in the definition of adherence and adherence measures make it difficult to compare studies and success of outcomes directly. Collectively, this literature supports the need for more research using standardized interventions, defined adherence outcome measures, diverse cohorts as most studies focus on schizophrenia, and longitudinal follow-up of adherence effects.

The development of interventions to improve adherence would benefit from the use of conceptual models. Much of the work examining adherence in patients with SMI is atheoretical and problem focused. Building on psychological principles and theoretical foundations of behavior change is preferable to an approach that is only empirically driven.

Much of the development of interventions to reduce adherence overlooks the risk factors associated with nonadherence. For example, a poor therapeutic alliance is frequently linked to nonadherence, but only recently was applied to interventions that seek to improve the therapeutic relationship (75). Other factors such as the negative impact of repeated involuntary commitment or forced treatment have not received much attention.

We are currently investigating the effectiveness of psychiatric advance directives (PADs), which are designed to increase therapeutic alliance and decrease the distress associated with forced treatment by giving patients an opportunity to direct their care even under conditions when they are no longer able to make rational decisions. PADs are legal documents that allow competent persons to declare their treatment preferences in advance of a mental-health crisis, when they may lose capacity to make reliable health care decisions. Fifteen states have now adopted PAD legislation. Federal mandates, and the actions of 15 state legislatures that have approved these documents, suggest that PADs are supported in both policy and theory.

Although the goals of PADs are to improve the working alliance between patients and clinicians, enhance treatment engagement, and provide a potential shift in patterns of service use from inpatient to outpatient services, little is known on the downstream effects of PADs. We are currently investigating the impact of PADs on patient care, service use, and clinical outcomes in a randomized trial of a PAD intervention in a sample of 400 veterans with SMI. The study specifically will describe veteran preferences for PAD content and completion, determine the effects of PADs on patients' willingness to engage in treatment, examine the effectiveness of PADs in guiding treatment during a mental-health crisis, and evaluate the effects of PADS on mental-health service use and clinical outcomes.

CLINICAL IMPLICATIONS AND CONCLUSIONS

Ensuring adherence among patients with SMI is clearly challenging and involves a variety of factors that can influence adherence. The sheer rate of medication nonadherence among patients with SMI underscores the importance of consistent multimodal monitoring of patients' medication adherence. In addition to patients' self-report, data from family members or caregivers and objective measures, including pill counts and refill records, should be gathered.

When a patient appears nonadherent with treatment, conceptualizing adherence in the context of one of the many behavioral change models described in chapter 1 of this volume may help clinicians formulate treatment plans. Perkins (100) modified the health belief model in the context of schizophrenia to include perceived susceptibility to illness, perceived severity of illness, perceived benefits of taking health action, perceived barriers of taking action, and various cues to action. Modifying a patient's perceptions of the relative costs and benefits of treatment may require targeting a variety of risk factors for nonadherence, including poor insight, substance abuse, therapist alliance, and negative attitudes about medication (74).

When faced with any of these issues, clinicians need to implement strategies to address them. Changing service policies to include preappointment telephone prompts should be implemented. This is a relatively low-cost intervention that has been shown to be effective in increasing adherence with scheduled appointments. The use of medications with fewer side effects such as the newer atypical antipsychotic medications should be used, although nonadherence with these medications can still be substantial (75).

Cognitive-behavioral interventions that target negative attitudes and shape behavior to increase adherence have the most empirical support and should be offered to patients who demonstrate poor adherence. Although these could be easily incorporated into routine care by the prescribing clinician, there is substantial evidence that the involvement of other health care professionals, for example, clinical psychologists or social workers, increases adherence (101). Patients who demonstrate repeated nonadherence and have multiple psychiatric admissions may be best served by community-based treatment such as PACTs or intensive case management models.

Medication management remains the treatment of choice for patients with psychotic disorders and many other severe mental illnesses. Ensuring that patients with mental illness adhere to treatment is one of the biggest challenges faced today by the mental-health sector. Our understanding of ways to improve adherence lags well behind the advances in psychopharmacology (75). There is a continued need for the development of effective interventions to enhance adherence to psychotropic medication therapy.

REFERENCES

1. Breen R, Thornhill JT. Noncompliance with medication for psychiatric disorders. *CNS Drugs.* 1998;9:457–471.

2. Delaney C. Reducing recidivism: medication versus psychosocial rehabilitation. *J Psychosocial Nurs.* 1998;36:28–34.

3. *United States Mental Health.* Washington, DC: U.S. Department of Health and Human Services; 1996.

4. Schinnar A, Rothbard A, Kanter R, Yung YS. An empirical literature review of definitions of severe and persistent mental illness. *Am J Psychiatry.* 1990;147: 1602–1608.

5. Slade M, Powell R, Strathdee G. Current approaches to identifying the severely mentally ill. *Soc Psychiatry Psychiatr Epidemiol.* 1996;32:177–184.

6. Goldman H, Gattozzii A, Taube C. Defining and counting the chronically mentally ill. *Hospital and Community Psychiatry.* 1981;32:21–27.

7. National Institute of Mental Health. *Announcement of community support system strategy development and implementation.* Rockville, MD: Author; 1994.

8. Warner R, de Girolamo G. *Epidemiology of Mental Disorders and Psychosocial Problems: Schizophrenia.* Geneva: World Health Organization; 1995.

9. Rice DP. The economic impact of schizophrenia. *J Clin Psychiatry.* 1999;60 (Suppl 1):4–6.

10. Wyatt RJ, Henter I, Leary MC, Taylor E. An economic evaluation of schizophrenia—1991. *Soc Psychiatry Psychiatr Epidemiol.* 1995;30(5):196–205.

11. Thieda P, Beard S, Richter A, Kane J. An economic review of compliance with medication therapy in the treatment of schizophrenia. *Psychiatr Serv.* 2003;54: 508–516.

12. Wells KB, Katon W, Rogers B, Camp P. Use of minor tranquilizers and antidepressant medications by depressed outpatients: results from the Medical Outcomes Study. *Am J Psychiatry.* 1994;151:694–700.

13. Wang PS, Gilman SE, Guardino M, et al. Initiation of and adherence to treatment for mental disorders: examination of patient advocate group members in 11 countries. *Med Care.* 2000;38(9):926–936.

14. Solomon P, Davis J, Goson B. Discharged state hospital patient's characteristics and use of aftercare. *Am J Psychiatry.* 1984;141:1566–1570.

15. Sparr LF, Moffitt MC, Ward MF. Missed psychiatric appointments: who returns and who stays away. *Am J Psychiatry.* 1993;150:801–805.

16. Centorrino F, Hernan MA, Drago-Ferrante G, et al. Factors associated with noncompliance with psychiatric outpatient visits. *Psychiatr Serv.* 2001;52(3):378–380.

17. Cruz M, Cruz RF, McEldoon W. Best practices for managing noncompliance with psychiatric appointments in community-based care. *Psychiatr Serv.* 2001;52: 1443–1445.

18. Fenton WS, Blyer CR, Heinssen RK. Determinants of medication compliance in schizophrenia: empirical and clinical findings. *Schizophr Bull.* 1997;23:637–651.

19. Cramer JA, Rosenheck R. Compliance with medication regimens for psychiatric and medical disorders. *Psychiatr Serv.* 1998;49:196–210.

20. Cramer JA, Rosenheck R. Enhancing medication compliance for people with serious mental illnesses. *J Nerv Ment Dis.* 1999;187:53–55.

21. McCombs JS, Nichol MB, Stimmel GL, Shi J, Smith RR. Use patterns for antipsychotic medications in Medicaid patients with schizophrenia. *J Clin Psychiatry.* 1999;60:5–11.

22. Dolder CR, Lacro J, Dunn L, Jeste DV. Antipsychotic medication adherence: is there a difference between typical and atypical agents? *Am J Psychiatry.* 2002;159: 103–108.

23. Quitkin F, Rifkin A, Kane J, Ramos Lorenzi JR, Klein DF. Long-acting oral vs injectable antipsychotic drugs in scizophrenia: a one-year double-blind comparison in multiple episode schizophrenics. *Arch Gen Psychiatry.* 1978;35(7): 889–892.

24. Blackwell B. From compliance to alliance: a quarter century of research. *Arch Gen Psychiatry.* 1996;48:140–149.

25. Dolder CR, Lacro JP, Jeste DV. Adherence to antipsychotic and nonpsychiatric medications in middle-age and older patients with psychotic disorders. *Psychosom Med.* 2003;65:156–162.

26. Terkelsen KG, Menifoff A. Measuring the costs of schizophrenia: implications for post-institutional era in the US. *Pharmacoeconomics.* 1995;8(3):199–222.

27. Weiden PJ, Olfson M. Cost of relapse in schizophrenia. *Schizophr Bull.* 1995;21: 419–429.

28. Ayuso-Gutierrez JL, del Rio Vega JM. Factors influencing relapse in the long-term course of schizophrenia. *Schizophr Bull.* 1997;28:199–206.

29. Weiden P, Aquila R, Standard J. Atypical antipsychotic drugs and long-term outcome in schizophrenia. *J Clin Psychiatry.* 1996;57:53–60.

30. Kane JM. What can we achieve by implementing a compliance improvement program? *Int Clin Psychopharmacology.* 1997;12:S43–S97.

31. Rabinowitz J, Lichtenberg P, Kaplan Z, Mark M, Nahon D, Davidson M. Rehospitalization rates of chronically ill schizophrenic patients discharged on a regimen of risperidone, olanzapine, or conventional antipsychotics. *Am J Psychiatry.* 2001;158:266–269.

32. Dickey B, Normand SLT, Norton E, Azeni H, Fisher W, Altaffer F. Managing the care of schizophrenia: lessons from a 4-year Massachusetts Medicaid study. *Arch Gen Psychiatry.* 1996;53(10):945–952.

33. Svarstad BL. Using drug claims data to assess the relationship of medication adherence with hospitalization and costs. *Psychiatr Serv.* 2001;52:805–811.

34. Vanelli M, Burstein P, Cramer J. Refill patterns of atypical and conventional antipsychotic medications at a national retail pharmacy chain. *Psychiatr Serv.* 2001;52:1248–1250.

35. American Psychiatric Association. Practice guidelines for the treatment of patients with schizophrenia. *Am J Psychiatry.* 1997;154(APR Suppl):1–63.

36. Palmer CS, Revicki DA, Genduso LA, Hamilton SH, Brown RE. A cost-effectiveness clinical decision analysis model for schizophrenia. *Am J Managed Care.* 1998;4(3):345–355.

37. Jablensky A. Schizophrenia: the epidemiological horizon. In: Weinberger DR, ed. *Schizophrenia.* Oxford: Blackwell; 1995:206–252.

38. Brown S. Excess mortality of schizophrenia. A meta-analysis. *Br J Psychiatry.* 1997;171:502–508.

39. Caldwell CB, Gottesman II. Schizophrenics kill themselves too; a review of risk factors for suicide. *Schizophr Bull.* 1990;16:571–589.

40. DeHert M, McKenzie K, Peuskens J. Risk factors for suicide in young people suffering from schizophrenia: a long-term follow-up study. *Schizophr Res.* 2001;47: 127–134.

41. Siris SG. Suicide and schizophrenia. *J Psychopharmacology.* 2001;15:127–135.

42. Mortensen PB, Juel K. Mortality and causes of death in schizophrenic patients in Denmark. *Acta Psychiatr Scand.* 1990;81:372–377.

43. Jeste DV, Gladsjo JA, Lindamer LA, Lacro JP. Medical co-morbidity in schizophrenia. *Schizophr Bull.* 1996;22(3):413–430.

44. Gray R, Wykes T, Gournay K. From compliance to concordance: a review of the literature on interventions to enhance compliance with antipsychotic medication. *J Psychiatr Ment Health Nurs.* 2002;9(3):277–284.

45. Appelbaum PS, Gutheil TG. Drug refusal: a study of psychiatric inpatients. *Am J Psychiatry.* 1980;137:340–346.

46. Olfson M, Mechanic D, Hansell S, Boyer CA, Walkup J, Weiden PJ. Predicting medication noncompliance after hospital discharge among patients with schizophrenia. *Psychiatr Serv.* 2000;51:216–222.

47. Meichenbaum D, Tusk DC. *Facilitating Treatment Adherence: A Practitioner's Guidebook.* New York: Plenum Press; 1987.

48. McEvoy JP, Apperson LJ, Appelbaum PS, et al. Insight in schizophrenia: its relationship to acute psychopathology. *J Nerv Mental Dis.* 1989;177:43–47.

49. Magura S, Laudet A, Mahmood D, Rosenblum A, Knight E. Adherence to medication regimens and participation in dual-focus self-help groups. *Psychiatr Serv.* 2002;53:310–316.

50. Drake RE, Osher FC, Wallach MA. Alcohol use and abuse in schizophrenia: a prospective community study. *J Nerv Mental Dis.* 1989;177:408–414.

51. Kashner TM, Radr LE, Rodell DE. Family characteristics substance abuse, and hospitalization patterns of patients with schizophrenia. *Hospital Community Psychiatry.* 1991;42:195–197.

52. Owen RR, Fischer EP, Booth BM, Cuffel BJ. Medication noncompliance and substance abuse among patients with schizophrenia. *Psychiatr Serv.* 1996;47: 853–858.

53. Kovasznay B, Fleischer J, Tanenberg-Karant M, Jandorf L, Miller AD, Bromet E. Substance use disorder and the early course of illness in schizophrenia and affective psychosis. *Schizophr Bull.* 1997;23(2):195–201.

54. Sowers W. Treatment of persons with severe mental illness and substance use disorders in addiction programs. *Drug Alcohol Forum.* 1997;191:15–21.

55. Sowers W, Golden S. Psychotropic medication management in persons with co-occurring psychiatric and substance abuse disorders. *J Psychoactive Drugs.* 1999; 31:59–70.

56. Kane JM. Extrapyramidal side effects are unacceptable. *Eur Neuropsychopharmacol.* 2001;11:397–403.

57. Weiden PJ, Shaw E, Mann JJ. Causes of neuroleptic noncompliance. *Psychiatric Ann.* 1986;16:571–575.

58. Hodge SK, Appelbaum PS, Lawlor T, et al. A prospective, multicenter study of patients' refusal of antipsychotic medication. *Arch Gen Psychiatry.* 1990;47: 949–956.

59. Ruscher SM, de Wit R, Mazmanian D. Psychiatric patients attitudes about medication and factors affecting noncompliance. *Psychiatr Serv.* 1997;48:82–85.

60. Van Putten T. Why do schizophrenic patients refuse to take their drugs? *Arch Gen Psychiatry.* 1974;31:67–72.

61. Van Putten T, May P, Marder S. Responses to antipsychotic medication: the doctors and consumers view. *Am J Psychiatry.* 1984;141:116–119.

62. Renton CA, Affleck JW, Carstairs GM, et al. A follow-up of schizophrenic patients in Edinburgh. *Acta Psychiatr Scand.* 1963;39:548–600.

63. Pan PC, Tantam D. Clinical characteristics, health beliefs, and compliance with maintenance treatment: a comparison between regular and irregular attenders at a depot clinic. *Psychiatr Serv.* 1989;79:564–570.

64. Buchanan A. A 2-year prospective study of treatment compliance in patients with schizophrenia. *Psychological Med.* 1992;22:787–797.

65. Fleischhacker WW, Meise U, Gunther V, Kurz M. Compliance with antipsychotic drug treatment: influence of side-effects. *Acta Psychiatr Scand Suppl.* 1994;382:11–15.

66. Rosenheck R, Chang S, Choe Y, et al. Medication continuation and compliance: a comparison of patients treated with clozapine and haloperidol. *J Clin Psychiatry.* 2000;61:382–386.

67. Frank AF, Gunderson JG. The role of the therapeutic alliance in the treatment of schizophrenia. *Arch Gen Psychiatry.* 1990;47:228–236.

68. Kemp R, David A. Psychological factors of insight and compliance in psychotic patients. *Br J Psychiatry.* 1996;169:444–450.

69. Rain S, Williams V, Robbins P, Monahan J, Steadman HJ, Vesselinov R. Perceived coercion at hospital admission and adherence to mental health treatment after discharge. *Psychiatr Serv.* 2003;54:103–105.

70. Blanch A, Parrish J. Reports of three roundtable discussions on involuntary interventions. In: *Psychiatric Rehabilitation and Community Support Monograph 1.* Rockville, MD: National Institute of Mental Health, Division of Applied and Services Research; 1990.

71. Kaltiala-Heino R, Laippala P, Salokangas RKR. Impact of coercion on treatment outcome. *Int J Law Psychiatry.* 1997;20:311–322.

72. Rain S, Steadman H, Robbins P. Perceived coercion and treatment adherence in an outpatient commitment program. *Psychiatr Serv.* 2003;54:399–401.

73. Parrish J. Involuntary use of interventions: pros and cons. *Innovations and Research.* 1993;2:15–22.

74. Dolder CR, Lacro JP, Leckband S, Jeste DV. Interventions to improve antipsychotic medication adherence: review of recent literature. *J Clin Psychopharmacol.* 2003;23:389–399.

75. Zygmunt A, Olfson M, Boyer CA, et al. Interventions to improve medication adherence in schizophrenia. *Am J Psychiatry.* 2002;159:1653–1664.

76. Nose M, Barbui C, Gray R, Tansella M. Clinical interventions for treatment nonadherence in psychosis: meta analysis. *Br J Psychiatry.* 2003;183:197–206.

77. Mueser KT, Corrigan PW, Hilton DW, et al. Illness management and recovery: a review of the research. *Psychiatr Serv.* 2002;53:1271–1284.

78. Kemp R, Hayward P, Applewhaite G, Everitt B, David A. Compliance therapy in psychotic patients; randomised controlled trial. *Br J Psychiatry.* 1996;372:345–349.

79. Kemp R, Krov G, Hayward P, Haywood P, David A. Randomized controlled trial of compliance therapy; 18 month follow-up. *Br J Psychiatry.* 1998;172:413–419.

80. Seltzer A, Roncari I, Garfinkel P. Effect of patient education on medication compliance. *Can J Psychiatry.* 1980;25:638–645.

81. Jones C, Cormac I, Mota J, Campbell C. *Cognitive Behavior Therapy for Schizophrenia.* Oxford, England: U.S. Cochrane Library; 1999.

82. Sensky T, Turkington D, Kingdon D, et al. A randomized controlled trial of cognitive-behavioral therapy for persistent symptoms in schizophrenia resistant to medication. *Arch Gen Psychiatry.* 2000;57:165–172.

83. Shivack IM, Sullivan CW. Use of telephone prompts at an inner-city outpatient clinic. *Hospital Community Psychiatry.* 1989;40(8):851–853.

84. Boswell PC, Brauzer B, Postlethwaite N, et al. Improving aftercare patient's compliance with appointments through phone calls and letters. *Hospital Community Psychiatry.* 1983;34(4):358–360.

85. Lachance KR, Santos AB. Modifying the PACT model; preserving critical elements. *Psychiatr Serv.* 1995;46(6):601–604.

86. Joint Commission on Accreditation of Hospitals. *Principles for Accreditation of Community Mental Health Service Programs.* 1979.

87. Dixon L, Weiden P, Torres M, Lehman A. Assertive community treatment and medication compliance in the homeless mentally ill. *Am J Psychiatry.* 1997;154:1302–1304.

88. Kelly GR, Scott JA. Medication compliance and health education among outpatients with chronic mental disorders. *Med Care.* 1990;28:1181–1197.

89. Weiden PJ, Dixon L, Frances A, Appelbaum P, Haas G, Rapkin B. Neuroleptic noncompliance in schizophrenia. In: Tamminga CA, Schulz SC, eds. *Advances in Neuropsychiatry and Psychopharmacology.* Vol. 1. New York: Raven Press; 1991:285–296.

90. Sajatovic M, Davies M, Hrouda DR. Enhancement of treatment adherence among patients with bipolar disorder. *Psychiatr Serv.* 2004;55(3):264–269.

91. Scott J, Pope M. Self-reported adherence to treatment with mood stabilizers, plasma levels, and psychiatric hospitalization. *Am J Psychiatry.* 2002;159:1927–1929.

92. Calhoun PS, Beckham JC, Bosworth HB. Caregiver burden and psychological distress in partners of veterans with chronic posttraumatic stress disorder. *J Trauma Stress*. 2002;15:205–212.
93. Calhoun PS, Beckham JC, Feldman ME, et al. Partners' ratings of combat veteran's anger. *J Trauma Stress*. 2002;15:133–136.
94. Calhoun PS, Sampson WS, Bosworth HB, et al. Drug use and validity of substance use self-reports in veterans seeking help for posttraumatic stress disorder. *J Consult Clin Psychology*. 2000;68:923–927.
95. Calhoun PS, Bosworth HB, Beckham JC, Grambow SC, Dudley TK. Medical service utilization of veterans seeking help for posttraumatic stress disorder. *Am J Psychiatry*. 2002;159:2081–2086.
96. Beckham JC, Calhoun PS, Glenn DM, Barefoot JC. Posttraumatic stress disorder, hostility, and health in women. *Ann Behav Med*. 2002;24:219–228.
97. Cohen MA, Alfonso CA, Hoffman RG, Milan V, Carrera G. The impact of PTSD on treatment adherence in persons with HIV infection. *Gen Hosp Psychiatry*. 2001;23:294–296.
98. Shemesh E, Rudnick A, Kaluski E, et al. A prospective study of posttraumatic stress symptoms and nonadherence in survivors of a myocardial infaction (MI). *Gen Hosp Psychiatry*. 2001;23(4):215–222.
99. Calhoun PS, Stechuchak KM, Bosworth HB, et al. Medical morbidity and self-rated health in veterans with SMI and PTSD. Poster presented at the annual meeting of the American Psychiatric Association, San Francisco, 2003.
100. Perkins DO. Adherence to antipsychotic medications. *J Clin Psychiatry*. 1999;60(Suppl 21):25–30.
101. Ockene IS, Hayman LL, Pasternak RC, Schron E, Dunbar-Jacob J. Task force #4—adherence issues and behavior changes: achieving a long-term solution. *J Am Coll Cardiol*. 2002;40(4):630–640.

Provider–Patient Communication and Treatment Adherence

Stewart C. Alexander
Betsy Sleath
Carol E. Golin
Carolyn T. Kalinowski

Provider–patient communication has been identified as one of the most important factor for improving patient adherence (1–12). However, to be able to use patient–provider communication to increase adherence, a detailed understanding of the mechanisms by which provider–patient communication influences treatment adherence is required. Many of the questions, and perhaps many of the insights, regarding adherence and provider–patient communication are not new. In spite of this, only recently have researchers begun to look at the underlining mechanisms that mediate how provider–patient communication affects treatment adherence.

This chapter begins with a discussion of the theoretical mechanisms by which provider–patient communication influences treatment adherence. Observational research on specific aspects of provider–patient communication associated with patient adherence in four common chronic conditions is then reviewed. A discussion of the unique communication challenges encountered when providers work with diverse patient populations follows, specifically covering issues related to cultural competency, health literacy, and working with elderly patients with complex treatment regimens. Then, interventions to improve provider–patient communication and patient adherence to treatment regimens are reviewed. The chapter then closes with a discussion of the limitations of existing research on provider–patient communication and treatment adherence and directions for future research.

MECHANISMS BY WHICH PROVIDER–PATIENT COMMUNICATION INFLUENCES TREATMENT ADHERENCE

A number of researchers have examined the theoretical mechanisms by which provider–patient communication influences adherence. Researchers have argued that there are a number of ways that improved provider–patient communication can help increase treatment adherence. Effective communication can improve adherence by (a) increasing patient knowledge and understanding, (b) changing patient beliefs and attitudes, and (c) increasing patient motivation by encouraging patients to actively participate in their health care.

Patient Knowledge and Understanding

For some patients, nonadherence is the result of lack of knowledge concerning their illness and what specifically needs to be done in order to adhere to their treatment regimen. Although providers believe that they give adequate information to patients, observational studies show that providers spend little to no time during an office visit giving patients information (5, 13, 14). In one observational study, providers estimated that during a typical 20-minute office visit, approximately 10 to 15 minutes of that time was devoted to providing patients with medical information about their illness and its treatment; however, when actually observed they spent less than 1 minute per visit discussing these issues with their patients (14). Furthermore, when providers were observed during another study, three fourths of all providers failed to give clear instructions to their patients on how to adhere to their prescribed treatments (15).

In addition to providers spending little to no time with patients discussing how to adhere to treatment regimens, when providers do give information about illness and its treatment to patients, patients often report that the information they receive is confusing or inadequate (16–18). In one observational study, patients were able to recall very little information about their treatments because their providers either did not tell them or assumed that the patient was already aware of the information for adherence (5). Furthermore, when patients are asked by researchers whether they mention these topics to their providers, patients overwhelmingly agreed that they do not know how to tell their provider that they are uninformed and need information on how to adhere to their treatment regimen (9). Because patients often do not express their confusion or lack of knowledge on how to adhere to treatment regimens, the transfer of information between providers and patients is an essential component to help patient adherence to treatment regimens (14–16, 19–28).

TABLE 11.1
Commonly Recommended Strategies for Increasing
Patient Knowledge and Understanding

- Start visit by asking patient to identify and address problems with current adherence to treatment (19).
- Assess patient recall and comprehension of treatment regimen (20, 21, 169).
- Clear up misunderstanding patient has about treatment (10).
- Try to avoid medical terminology (16, 22, 23).
- Provide additional information about patient's illness and treatment (10, 14, 15, 21, 24, 25, 28).
- Elicit further questions and/or concerns patient has with treatment (19, 21).
- Provide complete information in easy-to-understand language on what a patient needs to do to adhere to treatment (16, 20, 23, 26, 27).
- Have patient summarize treatment regimen at end of visit (19).
- Incorporate other health care providers, such as nurses and pharmacists, in patient education (174, 175, 178–180).
- Provide written instructions (8, 16, 22).

There is a dearth of research on provider–patient communication that provides a number of useful recommendations providers can use to help improve a patients' knowledge and understanding of their illness and treatment (see Table 11.1). Although information giving is important to help improve treatment adherence, providers do not necessarily need to increase the time the provider spends with a patient to transfer this information to their patients. Within office visits, incorporating other health care providers (16, 20, 23, 26, 27) can be used to provide patients with information as well as giving patients written instructions (8, 16, 22) to take home to review at a later time.

Although providing patients with adequate information to understand the medical regimen that is recommended is a necessary first step to improving adherence, providing more information alone is not sufficient to ensure patient adherence. In addition, it may be that different types of information have more influence on adherence than others, however, this has not been well studied. For example, some studies have shown that when patients are more knowledgeable about the regimen, they are more adherent (29). This type of knowledge may be more important than simply general knowledge of the disease.

Patient Beliefs and Attitudes

Although nonadherence is often mentioned as a result of patients having a lack of information on their illness and its treatment, not all nonadherence is because of a lack of knowledge. For some patients, they are fully aware of the causes of their illness and what they need to do in order to comply; however, they believe that this information does not pertain to their specific situation. For example, there is an abundant amount of information available to our society that smoking is detrimental to a person's health, yet there are many people who continue to smoke regardless of this information. For these type of patients, adherence is not necessarily a matter of giving the patient more information; rather, it is about changing the patients' health beliefs and attitudes associated with their situation. In these situations, providers are in a position to not only influence a patient's behavior but also to change the patient's awareness of their health status (2, 30).

It is important to get an understanding of patients' health beliefs and attitudes when communicating with them about medication, diet, exercise, and other treatments, because these beliefs can impact whether they will adhere to prescribed therapies (10, 15, 25, 31–36). Patients may not share their health beliefs until a safe environment has been created and a trusting relationship has been established. For example, there is evidence that approximately one out of three Americans uses alternative therapies yet very few patients tell their health care providers about this use (37). Therefore, providers need to be open to different ways of thinking about health and illness. The research on provider–patient communication provides a number of useful recommendations providers can use to help improve a patients' beliefs and attitudes of their illness and treatment (see Table 11.2).

Patient Motivation

One of the most common reasons why a patient does not adhere to their treatment regimen is due to a lack of motivation. Perhaps one of the more difficult tasks a provider can encounter is how to get a patient committed to a treatment regimen; however, prior research has shown that actively involving patients in treatment regimen decisions can positively influence ad-

TABLE 11.2
Commonly Recommended Strategies for Influencing
Patients' Health Beliefs and Attitudes.

- Elicit patient's concerns and beliefs about their illness and its treatments (10, 14, 15, 22, 30).
- Assess patients' perception of whether they believe they can change or change their lifestyle (31–34).
- Provide patients with information regarding benefits of various treatment regimens.
- Work with patient to develop a treatment regimen that has highest probability of success based on patients' beliefs and lifestyle (35).
- Do not manipulate the perceived threat of illness or its treatment (35).
- Provide clear and specific instructions on various ways patient can adhere to treatment (30, 35).
- Provide additional resources (30, 35).

herence and health outcomes (2, 7, 8, 38–48). By actively participating, patients are able to communicate their concerns, lifestyle, and their priorities to the provider and tailor their treatment regimen to maximize the likelihood of adherence (36).

There is an abundant literature that discusses how providers can involve patients in their health care by incorporating a "patient-centered" style of communication (7, 36, 42, 49–54). In general, patient-centered style of communication involves four parts: (a) establishing a encouraging environment, (b) determining patients' goals and concerns, (c) providing patients information, and (d) negotiating a treatment regimen (43). The research on provider–patient communication provides a number of useful recommendations providers can use to help improve a patients' motivation through patient participation (see Table 11.3).

In order for a patient-centered interaction to occur, a provider needs to provide an environment where a patient feels comfortable expressing their concerns and emotions, raise questions, and disclose personal information. For some providers, dealing with expressed concerns and emotions is an uncomfortable or difficult activity, especially concerning a patient's expressed emotion. However, in order to help negotiate a treatment regimen that motivates a patient, a patient needs to be able to feel they can express their emotions concerning their illness and treatment (42).

A person's emotional expression is often fundamental to learning more about a patient and how they are handling their illness (45). Therefore, a provider needs to be able to respond to a patients' expressed "emotions with empathy, respect, humility, and sensitivity a provider is able to develop a stronger relationship with the patient" (45). Through empathic communication, a provider gains a better understanding of their patient's health problems and allows for more open communication and self-disclosure to occur by patients. It is through open communication and self-disclosure that a provider gains a greater understanding about the patient, their illness, and its effect on the patient. In addition, empathic communication al-

TABLE 11.3
Commonly Recommended Strategies for Improving
Patient Motivation in Their Treatment Regimens

- Engage in nondirective, open-ended questions or statements to elicit patient information about their concerns (2, 42, 48).
- Elicit and explore patient's life context (2, 43).
- Negotiate agenda with patient to determine what issues to address during medical visit and which issues to address at future time (44, 45, 48).
- Provide patient with options concerning various treatments (36, 42).
- Allow patient to express preference for specific treatment regimens (36, 42).
- Make recommendation for treatment based on what the best fit for the patient's life circumstances (40, 46, 47).

lows for the sharing of emotional concerns a patient has about their illness, which helps increase a patient's motivation and emotional commitment to their treatment. It is through both the provider's greater understanding about a patient's illness and the patient's increased motivation to the treatment that allows for stronger adherence to a treatment regimen.

Although enhancing patient motivation through a patient-centered approach to medical care, it is important to point out that not all patients prefer the same level of participation in their care (17, 24, 28, 55–58). In general, younger patients prefer a more active level of participation in their health care compared to older patients (28, 36). As for preferences based on race, ethnicity, and gender, there seems to be no correlation with preferred level of particpation (17, 24, 26, 28, 55–58). Therefore, providers should be cautious in assuming how active they believe a patient wishes to be involved in their health care.

OBSERVATIONAL RESEARCH ON PROVIDER–PATIENT COMMUNICATION AND DISEASE-SPECIFIC ADHERENCE

The next section of this chapter reviews observational studies on provider–patient communication about patient adherence and diabetes, hypertension, HIV/AIDS, and asthma. These four illnesses were selected because the majority of nonintervention work in the field has focused on these areas and these are some of the disease states most commonly seen in practice. A review of the work done in these areas will hopefully give providers insight on how to optimally communicate with patients who have diabetes, hypertension, HIV/AIDS, and asthma so that adherence can be enhanced.

Diabetes

Successful management of diabetes requires the patient to adhere to a collection of self-care behaviors, including dietary activity, exercise, medication taking, blood glucose monitoring, and foot care (59), as well as attending regular follow-up visits with diabetes providers and having appropriate medical tests (60). Patients who are adherent in one area of self-care may not be adherent in others (61, 62). In a review of adherence studies among patients with insulin-dependent or non-insulin-dependent diabetes mellitus, Johnson (60) reports that patients tend to be most adherent to medication recommendations (published adherence rates are as high as 90%), and less adherent to dietary (60%–75% adherent), exercise (around 50%

adherent), and blood/urine glucose testing (28%–64% adherent) recommendations.

In recognition of the adherence challenges faced by diabetes patients, both the National Diabetes Education Program (NDEP) (42, 62, 63) and the American Diabetes Association (ADA) (43, 62, 63) highlight the need for providers to deliver patient-centered care that involves patients in decision making and is tailored to their individual needs. In a recent report on their Web site (62, 63), the NDEP (42) recommends that providers focus on four primary strategies when communicating with diabetes patients to improve self-care behavior. First, respect patients' values, preferences and needs by involving patients in shared decision making and developing cultural competence. Second, start each medical visit by asking patients what they would like to discuss and accomplish during the visit. Third, discuss diabetes self-management tasks with patients at each medical visit to identify and address problems that patients may be having with adherence. Fourth, consider using patient-centered communication, motivational interviewing (see chap. 2), and stages of change approaches to patient counseling and education (see chap. 2) about diabetes self-care. Although these communication approaches have a solid theoretical basis, empirical evidence linking specific aspects of provider–patient communication (e.g., specific provider and patient behaviors) to adherence to diabetes treatment regimens is somewhat limited.

Several observational studies have linked patient perceptions of providers' communication skills and behavior to adherence to diabetes self-care behaviors. Heisler et al. (64) found that patient satisfaction with providers' communication efforts, and to a lesser extent patient ratings of providers' participatory decision-making style (PDM style), were associated with higher levels of adherence to self-reported behaviors including diet, exercise, medication, blood glucose monitoring, and foot care. Uhlmann et al. (65) found that patients' perceptions of the extent to which their providers fulfilled their medical and psychosocial requests were related to greater reliability with self-reported timing of insulin injections and fewer severe insulin reactions. However, the same study found that patient perceptions of request fulfillment were not related to adherence to other aspects of diabetes regimens, including insulin administration, glucose monitoring, and dietary guidelines. Viinamaki et al. (66) reported that patients' perceptions of the "self-esteem enhancing" quality of their relationship with their provider were positively related to concurrent glycemic control, whereas general perceptions of the provider–patient relationship, satisfaction with the place of treatment, and perceptions of the safety and trust of the provider–patient relationship were not significantly associated with glycemic control.

Some researchers have uncovered relationships between observed provider communication behaviors and patient glycemic control, and have hypothesized that this association operates through patient adherence to self-care regimens. Schillinger et al. (67) found that observations of providers' assessment of patient recall and comprehension of new concepts introduced in diabetes visits were positively correlated with concurrent glycemic control. Street et al. (68) reported that patients had worse subsequent glycemic control when nurses were more controlling and directive during diabetes visits, even after controlling for a variety of possible confounders.

In addition, other studies have linked patient communication skills and behaviors when interacting with their providers to more favorable adherence behavior and glycemic control. Amir et al. (69) found that patients with more positive cognitive and behavioral coping skills in stressful interactions with providers about diabetes management had better adherence behavior than patients with lower levels of these skills. Street et al. (68) also found that patients who exhibited more negative affect during diabetes visits with nurses had poorer glycosylated hemoglobin levels at follow-up, although this relationship did not remain statistically significant after controlling for possible confounding factors, including nurses' controlling behavior.

In summary, observational studies suggest that the specific provider behaviors that may play an important role in determining patient adherence to diabetes self-care regimens include fulfillment of patient requests, assessment of patient recall and comprehension, and use of a more participatory and less controlling communication style. Patients' ability to cope both cognitively and behaviorally during stressful interactions with medical providers may also play a role.

Hypertension

According to a recent report from the World Health Organization's (WHO) International Society of Hypertension (70), successful management of hypertension involves an individualized treatment plan in which the patient undergoes regular monitoring of blood pressure and other risk factors, follows a diet low in salt and alcohol, exercises regularly, reduces body weight if appropriate, and follows a medication regimen if prescribed. However, the Joint National Committee on Prevention, Detection, Evaluation, and Treatment of High Blood Pressure (71) recognizes adherence to antihypertensive therapy as "a major therapeutic challenge" and emphasizes the importance of providers fully informing patients and encouraging patients to actively participate in their hypertension care.

The provider–patient relationship is often recognized in the hypertension adherence literature as playing an important role in determining adherence to antihypertensive therapy (72–74) and several studies have attempted to describe *how* patients and providers communicate about adherence (75, 76). However, observational studies demonstrating empirical relationships between provider–patient communication and adherence specifically in hypertensive patient populations are relatively limited in number. Some of these studies have also found mixed results when attempting to link particular aspects of provider–patient communication and adherence to antihypertensive therapy. In addition, the literature does not provide much guidance for providers with regard to specific communication strategies that may facilitate patient adherence to antihypertensive therapy.

However, a few studies do provide some evidence for a relationship between specific provider and patient communication behaviors and subsequent patient adherence behavior. In a 2-year longitudinal study of patients with chronic diseases including hypertension, diabetes, and heart disease (13), DiMatteo et al. found that after controlling for an array of provider and patient characteristics, several aspects of the provider–patient relationship were related to subsequent self-reported adherence. They found that providers who reported that they always fully answer patients' questions had patients who were more adherent to exercise recommendations. In addition, providers who ordered more follow-up tests at medical visits had patients who were subsequently more adherent to dietary recommendations. Similarly, providers who scheduled future appointments with patients at medical visits had patients who scored higher on a subsequent measure of general adherence to provider recommendations. In a study of primarily low-income, minority hypertensive patients (77), Orth et al. found that the frequency of patient information giving about medical history and symptoms at office visits was related to a subsequent decrease in systolic blood pressure. They also found that the percentage of provider talk devoted to providing information about illness and treatment at office visits was related to lower subsequent blood pressure, but not a decrease in blood pressure from office visits to follow-up. The authors hypothesized that these provider–patient communication factors had an effect on blood pressure through improvements in adherence, although they did not test this mechanism directly.

In addition to patient and provider behavior, patient perceptions of certain aspects of provider–patient relationships have been explored with regard to adherence. In a cross-sectional study of elderly hypertensive patients (18), McLane, Zyzanski, and Flocke found that the patient's perception of the amount of time spent with their provider was positively related to self-reported adherence to hypertensive medication, after controlling for demographics, disease history, quality of life, and hypertension knowledge. Stanton found in unadjusted analyses that patient perceptions of provider emotional support were positively related to medication adherence (78). However, structural equation modeling failed to show that provider–

patient communication measured in this way was an important factor in determining medication adherence.

In summary, observational studies have identified several provider behaviors that may play an important role in determining patient adherence to hypertension treatment regimens, including answering questions, scheduling future tests and appointments at medical visits, providing more information about the illness and treatment, and spending more time with the patient. The amount of information patients share with providers about their medical history and symptoms may also facilitate adherence to self-care behaviors.

HIV/AIDS

Provider–patient communication factors that effect adherence to antiretroviral therapy (ART) have primarily been studied only since the introduction of highly active antiretroviral therapy (HAART) (79–97). Widespread use of HAART, which occurred around 1996, for the first time prolonged and improved the quality of the lives of people living with HIV (80–86, 98). However, researchers now recognize that patients probably need to maintain exceptionally high levels of ART adherence to prevent treatment failure (79–97). Although, on average, patients with HIV attain higher levels of adherence than patients on other chronic medical therapy, these levels are still suboptimal to maintain treatment success (86). As a result, a great deal of attention has been directed recently toward improving adherence in the treatment of HIV/AIDS. In fact, the Centers for Disease Control and Prevention (CDC) and the U.S. Department of Health and Human Services (U.S. DHHS) National Treatment Guidelines now recommend that medical providers routinely assess, reinforce, and support patient adherence to complex antiretroviral regimens using a patient-centered communication approach (99–101).

Furthermore, these guidelines promote not only regimen-oriented and patient-related strategies, but also, specific "clinician and health team" strategies to improve (99–101). These include: (a) establishing a trusting relationship, (b) assessing the client's readiness to adhere prior to initiating treatment, (c) providing patient education and information regarding ART and the effects of suboptimal antiretroviral adherence, (d) giving patients access to providers to address medication problems that arise between visits, (e) monitoring ongoing adherence with intensification of adherence management when adherence is suboptimal, (f) use of a health care team approach that includes case managers, pharmacists, nurses, physicians, providers, and peer educators, and (g) close consideration of the impact of new diagnoses such as depression, chemical dependency, or liver disease on adherence to ART.

Few data exist to indicate precise communication behaviors that effectively influence ART adherence. Rather, recommendations to use client-centered clinician-based strategies are founded upon evidence of associations that exist between aspects of provider–patient communication and adherence. Qualitative studies have documented that patients themselves perceive that the doctor–patient relationship is an important factor that influences their adherence (102–104). A few cross-sectional and prospective quantitative studies have assessed aspects of the provider–patient communication that are associated with adherence. One study, conducted among women with HIV receiving prenatal care, found that women who perceived that they had a more positive relationship with their provider had a greater intent to adhere to their regimens (105). In other studies, patients who trusted their provider more at baseline were more adherent at follow-up, although this relationship was not consistently maintained after controlling for other factors (106–107). Several studies have demonstrated that patients whose regimen fits with their lifestyle are more likely to adhere to that regimen (98) and that when patients' self-efficacy or confidence to take medications is enhanced, patients can improve their adherence (108, 109). Thus, guidelines instruct providers to focus their communication with patients on assessing patients' daily routines and enhancing patient confidence to take the regimen by helping them develop specific strategies to fit it into other activities (110). One study also showed that patients who had greater knowledge of their regimen were more likely to adhere to that regimen (29). Thus, guidelines recommend that providers spend adequate time educating patients about the specific requirements of their regimen and assessing their understanding.

Studies have also assessed the extent to which current provider ART adherence-related practices fit with current guidelines. Although guidelines recommend that providers estimate patient adherence, several studies have demonstrated that when providers estimate their HIV-infected patients' adherence, these estimate are highly inaccurate compared with more objective measures, with providers most often overestimating patient adherence (29, 86, 87). Some of the reasons for this misunderstanding can be explained by qualitative studies showing that what was perceived as patients' overreporting of their adherence to interviewers was found to actually reflect differences in patient and provider understandings of what was meant by *adherence*. Other studies have shown that although most providers carry out some adherence communication with their patients with HIV/AIDS, the degree and type of communication varies widely and most providers do not provide the comprehensive patient-centered services recommended (111, 112). In one study, not only did providers report not counseling their HIV-positive patients comprehensively about ART adherence, but, in addition, large percentages felt that they did not have adequate skill, space, time, or reimbursement to conduct adherence counseling (111). These findings suggest that providers caring for patients with HIV/AIDS may need more training and time allocated to provide patient-centered antiretroviral adherence communication and counseling services (111, 112).

Asthma

Lack of treatment adherence is common among a large percentage of asthmatic patients (113, 114). For example, Haby et al. (114) found that 60% of children with persistent or frequent asthma were not using regular preventive medicine. Part of the asthma management program presented in the *Global Strategy for Asthma Management and Prevention NHLBI/WHO Workshop Report* (115) emphasizes that in the provider–patient relationship there is a need to (a) educate patients to develop a partnership in asthma management and (b) establish individual medication plans for long-term management. The clinical practice guidelines of the National Asthma Education and Prevention Program of NHLBI (National Heart, Lung, and Blood Institute) reemphasize these points (116). They also emphasize the importance of *jointly* determining the goals of treatment with patients and their families (117). In addition, Clark et al. (11) found that adult asthmatic patients expressed a desire for a relationship with their providers that involved mutual respect and a sense of partnership.

Prior research has in fact shown that adherence to asthma medications is related to provider–patient communication (118–120). Chambers et al. (118) found that adult asthmatic patients were more likely to report regular use of inhaled corticosteroids, if they saw themselves as active participants in their treatment planning. Apter et al. (119) found that poor patient ratings of provider–patient communication about asthma were related to poor adherence to inhaled corticosteroids (taking less than 70% of prescribed doses). Smith et al. (120) found that better adherence (percentage of prescribed doses taken) to asthma medications was related to perceiving the provider as being interested and approachable and one who gave clear and adequate information.

Wissow et al. (121) found that if emergency room providers used more patient-centered styles with children with asthma, parents rated the providers higher on providing "good care." Smith et al. (120) found that asthmatic children who had parents who were more satisfied with the asthma care they received were more adherent to their asthma medications. Parent satisfaction was related to current medication adherence as well as future asthma medication adherence (120). These prior research findings suggest the importance of examining satisfaction with asthma visits and how satisfaction is related to asthma treatment adherence.

Summary

In summary, there is a fair amount of evidence from a wide variety of observational studies that effective provider–patient communication can have a positive impact on treatment adherence. For treating diabetes, communication that focuses on assessing patient's recall and recollection, fostering patient participation in decision making, answering patient questions and concerns, and using a less controlling style of communication can increase adherence to diabetes self-care. As for hypertension, communication that focuses on answering patient questions and concerns, providing additional information about hypertension and its treatment, and spending more time with a patient can increase adherence. As for treating patients with HIV/AIDS, communication that focuses on establishing a trusting relationship with a patient, assessing patient comprehension and recall of information, and providing education and counseling regarding HIV/AIDS and its treatment can help improve adherence. Finally, for treating asthma, communication that focuses on assessing patient recall and recollection, fostering patient participation in decision making, and developing mutual rapport with patients can help improve adherence.

COMMUNICATION SKILLS FOR SPECIAL POPULATIONS

The previous sections have identified how specific aspects of provider–patient communication are thought to affect adherence and reviewed evidence from observational studies conducted with patients with common chronic conditions. Although the aspects of provider–patient communication discussed previously are thought to be important when working with all types of patients, distinct characteristics of certain patient populations can affect the quality of provider–patient communication and present unique barriers and challenges to effective communication. In the following section, we discuss some unique challenges to effective provider–patient communication that are encountered by providers when working with three special patient populations: patients from diverse cultural backgrounds, patients with low health literacy, and elderly patients.

Cultural Competence

The United States is becoming increasingly culturally diverse. In percentage terms, Asians are the most rapidly growing minority group, whereas in absolute numbers, Hispanics are the most rapidly growing group. According to the U.S. Census, by 2020 (120, 122, 123), Asians will comprise 6.5% and Hispanics 16% of the U.S. population. One implication of this increasing cultural diversity is that health care providers will increasingly need to provide care to individuals from different cultural backgrounds.

To successfully provide care to all patients, providers need to attempt to understand each person's cultural frame of reference. The word *culture* means "patterns of human behavior including thoughts, actions, customs, values, and beliefs that can bind a racial, ethnic, religious, or social group within society" (124). Cultural competence is a complex integration of knowledge, attitudes, and skills that enhances cross-cultural communication and appropriate interactions with others. Cultural competence includes at least two perspectives: (a) knowledge of the effects of culture on others' beliefs and behaviors and (b) an awareness of one's own cultural attributes and biases and their impact on others (125).

Patients from different ethnic groups may have different beliefs about their medical conditions and the treatments for them. For example, research has shown that African Americans rate spiritual factors as more important in treating mental-health problems than do Whites (126). Despite the fact that patients may belong to different ethnic groups, all ethnic groups are extremely diverse, which is why it is important to ask questions to better understand each patient's health beliefs and attitudes toward treatment, because a patient's health beliefs and attitudes can impact their treatment adherence.

Because of cultural differences, providers and patients face great challenges when trying to communicate effectively with one another and attain good adherence to medical regimens. There is an abundant literature that discusses specific strategies providers can use to communicate more effectively patients from different cultures (125–140). For example, Anand (125) suggests that providers pay greater attention when obtaining a patients medical history and physical complaints to ensure that the provider does not misinterpret the information. Prieto et al. (137) and Sue and Sue (140) suggest that it is important when talking to patients that providers explain the causes and treatments associated with a patient's illness within the patient's cultural views. In addition, providers should pay close attention to a patient's nonverbal cues as well as situational contexts (125, 141).

Based on the cultural competence literature, researchers recommend many promising communication strategies (see Table 11.4). Although these strategies certainly have the potential to enhance communication with patients from different cultures, it is important to keep in mind that providers should avoid generalizing about a patients' belief system based solely on the patients' race and ethnicity (130, 131, 134).

TABLE 11.4
Commonly Recommended Strategies for Communicating
With Patients From Different Cultures

- Be aware of your own cultural values and biases and the impact that these can have on diverse patients (125, 127, 128, 138–140).
- Avoid medical jargon and abstract language (127, 136, 137).
- Attend to nonverbal cues and situational contexts (125, 137, 141).
- Explanations of etiology, causes, and treatment associated with illness should be explained within patients' cultural views (126, 129, 130, 132–135, 140, 141).
- Elicit patient attitudes, values, and assumptions about the way patient makes decisions (125, 132, 141)

Health Literacy

According to the National Adult Literacy Survey (NALS), almost half of all the U.S. adult population is either functionally illiterate or demonstrates marginal literacy (142). Functional health literacy is a specific domain of literacy and has been defined as "the ability to perform basic reading and numerical tasks required to function in the health care environment." Given the high rates of functional illiteracy, it is not surprising that two recent studies of health literacy, one conducted in a managed care plan serving Medicare patients (142) and one at two urban public hospitals (143), found that approximately one third of English-speaking patients and more than 50% of Spanish-speaking patients demonstrated inadequate or marginal health literacy.

Previous research has suggested that achieving both high levels of adherence to medical regimens and effective provider–patient communication may be more challenging when working with patients with low health literacy. In one study, patients with low literacy reported having committed serious medication errors because of an inability to read medication labels (144). Low literacy has also been identified as an independent predictor of worse adherence to HIV medication regimens (142, 145). Studies of functional health literacy also suggest that providers face greater challenges to enhancing patient understanding, recall, and participation in medical decision making when working with less literate patients compared to more literate patients. Knowledge and understanding can be hampered by patients' lack of appropriate vocabulary and ability to ask questions to clarify points of confusion (146, 147), difficulty in organizing their thoughts about information presented (146, 148), and difficulty in understanding written information presented by providers (148), as well as providers' use of highly technical vocabulary and medical terminology (148). Recall of information presented in medical visits, which is generally low overall for all patients (149), is also likely more difficult to attain in patients with low functional health literacy. Patients with low functional health literacy rely heavily on oral explanations and demonstrations that occur during medical visits (144), and can make use of few written patient education materials or labels to enhance recall after visits with providers. Finally, patient participation in interactions with providers can be hampered by barriers commonly faced by patients with low literacy skills, including a lack of understanding of what providers need and want to know (148), a lack of appropriate vocabulary to give information to and ask questions of providers (148), as well as shame and fear of revealing their lack of literacy and understanding (150).

In addition to experiencing more barriers to understanding, recall, and active participation, a recent study also suggests that patients with lower health literacy have less favorable perceptions of the overall quality of their communication with providers than do patients with higher health literacy (151). Patients reported less favorable perceptions of providers' general clarity, explanation of the patient's condition, and explanations of processes of care, all features of provider communication having great relevance to patient self-care behaviors (151).

There is a great need for more research to identify effective strategies that may help providers communicate more effectively with less literate patients and ultimately affect their adherence to medical regimens (142, 148). Though research in this area has been limited, a few studies have found empirical evidence for specific strategies providers can use to communicate more effectively with less literate patients. For example, Schillinger et al. (67) found that providers' application of the interactive communication loop, whereby the provider routinely asks patients to restate information and instructions, was associated with better glycemic control among diabetic patients with low literacy. Davis et al. (152) also found that using written patient education materials that were specifically tailored to patients with low literacy, by relying on many graphics and very simple language, resulted in better comprehension than using a standard brochure. In addition, providers' use of visual aids, such as pictographs and videos, has been linked to improved recall (153) and adherence (146) among patients with low literacy.

Despite the relative lack of research, health literacy researchers have used what is known about provider–patient communication, health literacy, and adult education to recommend many promising communication strategies (see Table 11.5). Although these strategies certainly have the potential to enhance communication with less literate patients, it is important to keep in mind that the effectiveness of many of these strategies in enhancing patient knowledge, understanding, recall, participation, and ultimately adherence is largely unknown.

TABLE 11.5
Commonly Recommended Strategies for Enhancing
Communication With Patients Demonstrating Low Health Literacy

- Take time to assess patients' literacy skills by paying attention to subtle hints (e.g., avoid reading in front of others, fail to complete forms, regularly bring others to visits who help with reading) (148).
- Limit advice and instruction to key information the patient needs (147, 148, 229).
- Try to avoid medical terminology (148).
- Partition information into small parts (229).
- Use visual aids (e.g., pictographs) (148, 229).
- Repeat instructions in several different ways (147).
- Make instructions interactive by asking patients to demonstrate what they've been told (147, 148, 150).
- Provide examples of concepts that are meaningful to patients' unique situation (147, 229).
- If using written materials, use only those developed by experts and tailored to low-literacy patients (148).
- Include family members in visits whenever possible, with patients' consent (147, 148).
- Exhibit a respectful, encouraging, positive attitude (147, 148).

Elderly Patients

Previous research has suggested that achieving adherence with elderly patients is more difficult for providers, especially those not trained in geriatric medicine (154). Although elderly patients have many of the same problems facing them as do all other populations, the high prevalence of multiple chronic conditions among elderly patients makes adherence in this population especially important (155). Therefore, promoting adherence among elderly patients is an important aspect of geriatric care (156).

Although an abundance of information is available to elderly patients, research has shown that providers spend little to no time with elderly patients discussing medicines and their purposes (18). In addition, even when providers and patients talk about treatments, very few elderly patients are able to recall information about the medicines after leaving their providers (157). Furthermore, elderly patients report that when talking with their providers, many questions and concerns about their illness and its treatment are never mentioned.

In addition to the lack of understanding of medications as well as the number of unvoiced concerns about treatments, the complexity of treatment regimens for elderly patients is another barrier to adherence (157, 158). As with all issues of medicine complexity, the increase number of prescriptions often results in greater chance for unwanted side effects as well as confusion as to which drug to take and how much of it (18, 155, 158).

Unquestionably, providers and elderly patients face great challenges when trying to communicate effectively with one another and attain good adherence to medical regimens (155, 158–165). There is a great need for more research to identify effective strategies that may help providers communicate more effectively with elderly patients and ultimately affect their adherence to medical regimens (142, 148, 155, 156, 160). Though research in this area has been limited, a few studies have found empirical evidence for specific strategies providers can use to communicate more effectively with elderly patients. For example, Coe (160) found that by asking direct questions to elderly patients about their life context (e.g., daily activities, diet, living arrangements, possibly physical and/or mental limitations) providers were able to elicit more unexpressed concerns about a patient's treatment regimen. By discovering these unexpressed concerns, providers were able to tailor the patient's treatment regimen to their specific life context. Thus, providers were able to reduce the number of different medications and treatments as well as reduce the number of times a day that a patient needed to take their medications. By reducing treatment complexity, providers were able to increase overall adherence. In addition to reducing treatment complexity, providers' use of written instructions (155, 156) and incorporation of the elderly patient's caregiver (162) into the medical encounter has been linked to improved adherence among elderly patients.

Despite the relative lack of research, researchers have used what is known about provider–patient communication and elderly patients to recommend many promising communication strategies (see Table 11.6). Although these strategies certainly have the potential to enhance communication with less literate patients, it is important to keep in mind that not all elderly patients will respond in similar ways and that providers should be

TABLE 11.6
Commonly Recommended Strategies for Enhancing
Communication With Elderly Patients

- Elicit and explore patient's life context (155, 160, 164).
- Reduce treatment complexity by reducing the number of different medications or treatments prescribed whenever possible (155, 159).
- Reduce the number of times a day that medicine needs to be taken (158, 160).
- Explain the reason for specific treatments and what the patient needs to do to adhere to treatment (155, 158).
- Elicit patient's concerns and beliefs about their illness and its treatment (155, 158).
- Ask direct questions to elicit unexpressed concerns (161, 165).
- Try to avoid medical terminology (155, 165).
- Reinforce important points (155, 160).
- Include family members in visits whenever possible (155, 162).
- Provide written instruction (155, 160).
- Communicate respect (155, 158).

careful not to overgeneralize what works with certain elderly patients to what works with all elderly patients (166).

INTERVENTION STUDIES

As mentioned earlier, perhaps the most important way to improve treatment adherence is through effective provider–patient communication. Although it is known that better communication increases adherence, only a handful of intervention studies have been conducted. Researchers have utilized four different approaches to investigate the best way to improve provider–patient communication. One approach has attempted to improve the way providers communicate with patients by using physician education programs, whereas a second approach has attempted to train patients on how to communicate more effectively with their providers. A third approach has attempted to improve provider–patient communication by designing health care consultations as ancillary to the medical visit. A fourth approach has utilized motivational interviewing (MI) as a strategy for communicating with patients.

Physician Education Programs

Some preliminary research suggests that teaching physicians how to communicate more effectively can increase patient adherence to medical treatments (see Table 11.7) (167, 168). In one study, a 1–2 hour educational program designed to help physicians improve their skills at identifying nonadherence and discussing ways to control hypertension had higher rates of patient adherence compared to those patients whose physicians did not receive the educational training (167). In the educational program, physicians were taught communication skills designed to elicit patients' attitudes and beliefs about their illness. Compared to physicians who did not participate in the educational training, physicians who received the training reported more conversations with patients about their understanding of their illness and its treatment, as well as discussing ways to adhere to dietary recommendations. In addition, patients whose physicians received communication training reported that their beliefs and attitudes about their illness had changed since talking with their physician, and also reported a better understanding of their illness and its treatment. Finally, patients whose physicians received training were more adherent to their dietary recommendations, medication intake, and appointment keeping.

In another study, an educational program was designed to help pediatricians teach strategies to improve mothers' adherence to their children's medical regimen (168). Specifically, pediatricians attended a 5-hour tuto-

TABLE 11.7

Intervention Studies That Trained Physicians How to Better Communicate With Patients

Study	Physician and Patient Populations	Randomized, Controlled Trial	Type of Intervention	Adherence Outcome	Effect
Inui et al. (167)	62 physicians who saw 219 hypertension patients	Yes	Physicians in the intervention group went to tutorials to improve their effectiveness as managers and educators of patients with essential hypertension.	Proportion of patients taking 75% of pills 2 months after	Observed
				Proportion of patients adherent to their diets 2 months after	Not observed
				Proportion of patients who kept appointments	Not observed
Joos et al. (170)	42 physicians who saw 348 continuity care patients	Yes	Physicians received 4.5 hours of training on eliciting and responding to patient concerns and requests.	Self-report of patients' compliance with medication 3 months later	Not observed
				Follow-up appointments for 12-month period after the intervention	Not observed
Ley et. al. (169)	4 physicians	No	Trained physicians on how to increase the clarity of communication	Proportion of adherent patients	Not observed
Maiman et al. (168)	90 pediatricians and 771 mothers whose children were being treated for otitis media	Yes	Physicians assigned to: Tutorial plus printed materials Printed materials only Control group	Use of medication was measured by counting pills and/or liquid medicine remaining in prescription.	Observed
				Mothers' self-report of no missed doses	Observed
				Physician's self-report of patients who keep follow-up appointments	Observed

rial on chronic pediatric conditions, where they were taught communication skills designed to help improve parents' recall and understanding of information and modify parents' beliefs and attitudes about their children's illness. The results indicated that pediatricians that went through communication training had higher levels of adherence to medicine and keeping follow-up appointments.

Although some studies found that improving physician communication did successfully increase patient adherence, not all interventions were successful at improving adherence (169, 170). An educational program designed to help physicians improve their ability to identify patients' beliefs toward their illness, as well as answer patients' medical questions concerning their illness, did not improve overall patient adherence (170). In a small study, training physicians on how to increase the clarity of their communication did not improve overall patient adherence.

Patient Education Programs

Only a handful of studies have looked at ways to improve patient adherence by training patients on how to communicate with their providers (see Table 11.8) (40, 171, 173). In one study, geriatric patients learned communication skills by using a computer-based educational program developed to teach them about their illness, its treatment, and ways to communicate more effectively with their providers (172). The program was available at 13 centers across Canada for patients who had either hip or knee osteoarthritis. While waiting to see their provider, patients accessed the computer program at the medical center. Results of the intervention showed that patients who completed the computer-based program demonstrated a higher level of medical adherence compared to patients who did not receive the computer-based education.

Although there is some research that suggests that training patients to communicate more effectively in their medical visit can improve their treatment adherence, not all forms of patient communication training have been effective at improving all types of treatment adherence. The results of one study suggest that providing written communication training is not sufficient for improving medication adherence (although adherence to other forms of treatments such as diet, exercise, and appointment keeping was improved) (171). In their study, Cegala et al. (171) provided patients with a training booklet by mail shortly before their medical visit that was designed to teach patients ways to raise important questions and concerns about their medical treatment. The booklet contained various information on what types of questions are important to discuss. Although the booklet contained a great deal of useful information, the results of the study were that the booklets helped patient adhere to follow-up appointments and behav-

TABLE 11.8

Intervention Studies That Trained Patients to Be More Actively Involved During Their Medical Visits

Study	Patient Populations	Random Controlled Trial	Type of Intervention	Adherence Outcome	Effect
Cegala et al. (171)	150 patients	Yes	"Trained" group received a 14-page training booklet in the mail 2 to 3 days before the scheduled visit. "Informed" group received a brief written summary of the major points contained in the training booklet while in the room prior to the scheduled appointment. "Untrained" group received no communication intervention.	Self-report medication compliance	Not observed
				Self-reported behavioral compliance (diet exercise, smoking cessation)	Trained more compliant than untrained but trained not more compliant than informed
				Follow-up appointments and referrals All measured 2 weeks after the visit	Trained more compliant than untrained but trained not more compliant than informed
Edworthy, Devin et al. (172)	252 patients over age 50 years with hip or knee osteoarthritis	Yes	Patients used computer program that provided information about their illness and its treatment as well as information on how to become more involved in treatment.	Appropriate utilization of medication Measured 8 weeks after	Observed

| Greenfield et al. (40) | 59 adult diabetic patients | Yes | 20-minute educational session on patient's disease before a medical visit where research assistant encourages patient to use information gained to negotiate medical decisions with the doctor | Blood sugar control Measured 8–12 weeks later | Observed |
| Tieffenberg et al. (173) | 355 Spanish-speaking children with moderate to severe asthma or epilepsy | Yes | Five weekly meetings of children and parents: children were trained to assume a leading role in health; parents learn to be facilitators | Emergency visits for asthma Asthma crises Emergency visits for epilepsy Epilepsy crises All measured 12 months after the start of the study. | Observed Observed Observed Observed |

ioral modifications, such as diet and exercise, but it did not successfully improve adherence to prescribed medication.

Health Care Consultations

Prior research suggests that pharmaceutical consultations can improve medical adherence (see Table 11.9) (174–176). Patients who receive pharmaceutical consultations report higher levels of medical adherence compared to patients who do not receive the consultations (174–176). Geriatric patients prescribed three or more medications who received pharmacist consultations prior to leaving the hospital were more adherent to treatment regimens compared to patients who did not receive pharmacist consultations (175). Hypertension patients who were given pharmaceutical consultations, written educational and nutritional information, and monthly written reminders were more adherent to their prescribed medications compared to patients who did not receive any additional information (174). Although no control group was used in their study, Burnier et al. (176) found that hypertension patients who received pharmaceutical consultation were more adherent to their prescribed medications compared to the average adherence rate for patients taking hypertension medications.

Although much of the research has shown that pharmaceutical consultations improve adherence, one study did not replicate these findings (177). The results of Weinberger et al.'s pharmaceutical care program found that medication adherence for patients with asthma or chronic obstructive pulmonary disease (COPD) did not improve. The authors point out that part of the lack of success of the intervention was most likely because they recruited pharmacies into the study rather than pharmacists, and not all pharmacists were enthusiastic about helping with the intervention.

Prior research also suggests that when patients are assigned to communicate with nurses, medical adherence can be improved (178–180). Morice and Wrench (178) found improved medication use among asthmatic patients who were assigned to talk with a nurse about how to better manage their condition. Peveler et al. (179) found that counseling by a nurse-improved adherence to tricyclic antidepressants compared to patients who received educational leaflets instead. Steckel and Swain (180) found that if hypertensive patients met with nurses and developed a jointly determined contract about adherence behaviors to work on, blood pressure control and weight loss improved.

Motivational Interviews

MI has been used successfully to change patients' adherence to a variety of recommended health behaviors including medication taking (181–198). MI is a counseling style that was originally developed to facilitate behavior

TABLE 11.9

Intervention Studies That Assigned Patient to Additional Providers

Study	Patient Populations	Random, Controlled Trial	Type of Intervention	Adherence Outcome	Effect
Burnier et al. (175)	41 hypertensive patients	No	Electronic monitoring of medicine intake. At 2-month point, pharmacist discussed the adherence report with the patient.	Blood pressure control at 2 and 4 months after enrollment	Not conclusive
Lipton and Bird (175)	706 geriatric hospitalized patients discharged on three or more medications	Yes	Pharmacist consultation with patients at discharge and 3 months thereafter and with physicians	Medication adherence score. Measured 12–14 weeks into the study	Observed
Morice and Wrench (178)	80 patients with acute asthma	Yes	Nurse consultation during hospital admission	Regular use of b-agonist inhaler. Increased use of inhaled corticosteroids. Peak flow monitoring. All measured 6 months after the intervention	Observed Observed Observed
Peveler et al. (179)	250 patients starting treatment with tricyclics	Yes	Education leaflet. Counseling by a nurse. Education leaflet and counseling. Usual care	Adherence to drug treatment by self-report. Measured at 12 weeks	Counseling improved adherence; informational leaflets did not improve adherence.

(Continued)

TABLE 11.9
(Continued)

Study	Patient Populations	Random, Controlled Trial	Type of Intervention	Adherence Outcome	Effect
Sclar et al. (174)	453 HMO patients with hypertension who are on once-a-day atenolol	Yes	Enrollment kit with educational materials	Medication possession ratio (number of days supply obtained during 180-day study period)	Observed
Steckel and Swain (180)	115 hypertensive outpatients	Yes	Contingency contracting with a nurse in addition to routine care & education from a nurse Education with counseling from a nurse in addition to routine care One group received routine care	Blood pressure control Weight loss	Observed in contracting group compared to other two groups Patients who specifically contracted to lose weight did so compared to all other patients
Weinberger et al. (177)	1113 patients with active COPD or asthma	Yes	Pharmaceutical-care program Peak exploratory rate monitoring control group Usual-care control group	Medication adherence through patient self-report at 6 and 12 months Breathing-related ED or hospital visits for 12 months	Not observed Not observed

change among problem drinkers (183). It is a patient-centered yet directive approach that includes five key principles: (a) expressing empathy, (b) developing discrepancies, (c) avoiding argumentation, (d) rolling with resistance, and (e) supporting self-efficacy (1, 197–199).

In MI, the provider uses patient-centered counseling methods, like reflective listening, drawn from the work of Carl Rogers (200), to help patients become aware of their motivations and health-related behaviors. MI, itself, is not a specific technique or set of techniques, but rather, represents a style of counseling (197). Using this style, a key role of the provider is to help patients to recognize and resolve their feelings of ambivalence about unhealthy behaviors (197–199, 201). MI offers a highly tailored means to assess a patient's inclination to change a health-related behavior and to address changing that behavior based on how ready that individual is to change (181–198, 201). Thus, this approach does not assume that the patient has a current commitment to change behavior (199, 202). By listening openly and reflecting back what is said, the provider creates a nonjudgmental, supportive atmosphere. This atmosphere allows patients to express their feelings regarding both their motivation and their resistance to change their behavior. In the MI session, patients are active participants because the MI style is intended to involve them in setting the agenda for the session. Through reflective listening, the provider helps patients raise their awareness of the discrepancies that exist between their current and desired behavior, between their current behavior and their values (199, 201). During MI, the provider often will provide nonjudgmental, objective feedback about a number of parameters, such as giving data regarding physiologic, neurological, or psychosocial assessments to enhance a patient's motivation to change. Providing objective facts, which is the provider's job, is distinguished from interpreting the personal implications of those facts, which is the role of the patient (198). The patient is also encouraged and facilitated to identify barriers to achieving the desired behavior themselves as well as to develop their own strategies for changing their behavior.

Most of the evidence showing that MI can facilitate medication adherence comes from a series of studies conducted by Kemp and colleagues (184, 201, 202). In two studies, patients with psychosis who received six MI sessions to improve their medication adherence demonstrated significantly greater improvement in their attitudes toward the medications as well as in their medication adherence than did controls receiving only supportive counseling (184, 202). Briefly, MI-style interventions have also been used among patients with HIV to improve adherence to anti-HIV medication (201–203). Patients receiving the MI-styled intervention improved their adherence to anti-HIV medication at a faster rate than did a control group (203). In addition to medication adherence, improvements in other health-related behaviors have been achieved using MI. For example, three of five studies that tested MI interventions addressing HIV risk behaviors of at-risk HIV-negative people significantly improved adherence to condom use and/or unprotected sexual intercourse compared with controls (187, 202, 204–206). In other studies, persons receiving telephone-based MI improved their healthy vegetable intake more than did controls (207). MI has also successfully been used to improve adherence to a behavioral weight control program among older obese women with type 2 diabetes mellittus (208) as well as for smoking cessation (206, 209). For example, in one pragmatic randomized trial in 21 general practices in South Wales, 536 cigarette smokers were randomized to receive motivational consulting or brief advice during one consultation. At 6-month follow-up, significantly more patients in the motivational consulting group reported not smoking in the previous 24 hours compared with controls (206). These data suggest that motivational interviewing is an effective means to promote behavior change related to health, including adherence to medical recommendations; however, more studies are needed to determine the frequency and duration of MI that is needed to achieve specific behavioral goals (198).

Measuring Communication

In all the intervention studies, communication was examined through provider and patient self-reports. Although the aim of the intervention studies was to examine how communication influenced adherence, none of the studies examined the actual communication process that occurred between the patients and their providers. Most of the interventions were set up so that either providers or patients went through training on how to communicate differently; however, when it came time to look at the provider–patient encounters, there were no direct observations of the actual conversations. By not having audiotapes, videotapes, or other forms of direct observations of the provider–patient interaction, it is difficult to assess how well (or poorly) the providers and/or patients were able to actually communicate during the encounter, which is necessary to determine whether or not specific communication skills occurred during the interaction.

Although no intervention studies have analyzed provider–patient communication and adherence by recording the actual conversations, there are a number of useful coding systems a research could use for analyzing these conversations. For coding "patient-centered communication," there is a useful coding system developed by Stewart et al. (7) based on a series of observational studies (Medical Outcomes Study) that looked at the association between patient-centered communication in primary-care visits and subsequent health and medical care utilization (8, 210–212). Their coding system consists of three components of patient-centered care: (a) "exploring the disease and the illness experience," (b) "understanding the whole person," and (c) "finding common ground." For each component, there are a series of subcategories that coders rate (see Stewart et al. for a complete list of subcategories). Then, after coding all the subcategories, coders provide an overall summary score from 0 (not at all patient centered) to 100 (very patient centered) based on their observations.

In addition to the Stewart et al. coding scheme, other communication coding systems exist that could also be easily incorporated into intervention studies that assess provider–patient communication, such as Roter Interaction Analysis System (RIAS) (213), and Empathic Communication Coding System (ECCS) (214). In addition there are a number of useful coding systems that exist that look at the communication the patient uses as well as systems that look at both the provider and the patient's communication (215–218).

LIMITATIONS

Although current research sheds some light on how provider–patient communication can influence patient adherence, a number of limitations exist in this area of research. In fact, in many ways, this area of study is still in its infancy. In particular, our understanding of how to define and measure provider–patient communication is limited and has attenuated our ability to fully elucidate the relationship between such communication and adherence for a number of reasons.

First, a greater conceptual understanding and theoretical cohesion among researchers working in the area of provider–patient communication would facilitate our ability to explore its influence on adherence (219). The research to understand provider–patient communication has been undertaken by workers in many different disciplines who have not always built upon prior work, resulting in a widely dispersed and poorly integrated literature (219, 220). Whereas some behavioral scientists have focused on affective components of communication, others focus on verbal behaviors, and still others, nonverbal communication. Even among those who focus on verbal behaviors, a consensus does not exist regarding the specific verbal behaviors that are most salient (8, 221–224). Greater understanding of how to conceptualize and define provider–patient communication is needed.

Second, the lack of consensus about the theoretical basis for understanding provider–patient communication has contributed to measurement problems in this line of research. A lack of methodological cohesion exists across provider–patient communication studies regarding what constructs to measure and how to measure them. Differing approaches to measuring provider–patient communication have made comparisons across studies difficult and have limited the ability to draw reliable conclusions. Many studies have also inadequately measured the more subtle nuances of provider–patient interactions. For example, with one exception none (48) of currently available instruments captures more subtle aspects of conversations such as the sequences of speech or takes into consideration the segment of the conversation in which specific behaviors occur. Instead, most currently available measures of provider–patient communication that code conversations either directly or from audiotapes or videotapes merely count the number of categories of communication behaviors that occur in a medical visit (such as open-ended questions, interruptions, psychosocial statements, etc.) (8, 221–224). In addition, measurement of patient involvement in decision making, an aspect of provider–patient communication believed to play a key role in patient adherence, has been inadequate. A recent systematic review showed that existing communication instruments do not measure patient involvement accurately (225). Many measures, although they assess the degree of patient-centeredness in an interaction, do not actually measure the level or manner in which the patient is involved in the decision-making process (225). This omission in measurement makes it difficult to assess whether shared decision making does facilitate adherence and, if so, which aspects of it are most influential (225). As our understanding of how to measure more complex aspects of communication grows, in the future, more subtle communication behaviors that reliably influence patients' adherence may be identified.

Third, the majority of the studies that assess the relationship between provider–patient communication and adherence have been cross-sectional. Studies are needed that assess how communication between providers and patients over time is related to adherence. The effect of continuity of care on adherence may be an important factor. In addition, we need better information about the prospective influence of interventions to improve adherence through enhancing specific aspects of provider–patient communication.

Fourth, studies of the relationship between provider–patient communication and adherence have been somewhat narrow, and could be broadened in a number of ways. For example, little is known about the role played by patient companions and/or family members during medical visits (227) and how their involvement in medical visits may impact patient adherence to treatment regimens. Studies that further explore the role of family members and surrogates in facilitating both communication and adherence will likely shed light on additional communication interventions to enhance adherence. Also, research in this area needs to be conducted with more culturally diverse samples of providers and patients to understand better how to implement culturally appropriate interventions to enhance adherence (227, 228). Furthermore, the field has been largely dominated by studies of provider–patient communication and patient adherence; more work needs to examine how other types of provider–patient relationships impact adherence (e.g., pharmacists, nurses). Finally, the majority of previous studies have examined only medication adherence. Future work needs to examine how provider–patient communication impacts adherence to other types of treatment regimens, such as diet or exercise.

REFERENCES

1. Kjellgren KI, Ahlner J, Saljo R. Taking antihypertensive medication: controlling or co-operating with patients? *Int J Cardiol.* 1995;47:257–268.
2. Kaplan SH, Greenfield S, Ware JE Jr. Assessing the effects of physician-patient interactions on the outcomes of chronic disease. *Med Care.* 1989;27:S110–S127.
3. DiMatteo MR. Enhancing patient adherence to medical recommendations. *JAMA.* 1994;271:79–83.
4. DiMatteo MR. Future directions in research on consumer–provider communication and adherence to cancer prevention and treatment. *Patient Educ Counsel.* 2003;50:23–26.
5. DiMatteo MR. Patient adherence to pharmacotherapy: the importance of effective communication. *Formulary.* 1995;30:596–598, 601–602, 605.
6. DiMatteo MR. *The Psychology of Health, Illness, and Medical Care: An Individual Perspective.* Pacific Grove, CA: Brooks/Cole; 1991.
7. Stewart M, Brown JB, Donner A, et al. The impact of patient-centered care on outcomes. *J Fam Pract.* 2000;49:796–804.
8. Stewart MA. Effective physician–patient communication and health outcomes: a review. *CMAJ.* 1995;152:1423–1433.
9. Sbarbaro JA. The patient–physician relationship: compliance revisited. *Ann Allergy.* 1990;64:325–331.
10. Ley P. Satisfaction, compliance and communication. *Br J Clin Psychol.* 1982;21:241–254.
11. Clark NM, Nothwehr F, Gong M, et al. Physician–patient partnership in managing chronic illness. *Acad Med.* 1995;70:957–959.
12. Blackwell B. From compliance to alliance: a quarter century of research. *Neth J Med.* 1996;48:140–149.
13. DiMatteo MR, Sherbourne CD, Hays RD, et al. Physicians' characteristics influence patients' adherence to medical treatment: results from the Medical Outcomes Study. *Health Psychol.* 1993;12:93–102.
14. Waitzkin H. Information giving in medical care. *J Health Soc Behav.* 1985;26:81–101.
15. Svarstad BL. Physician–patient communication and patient conformity with medical advice. In: Mechanic D, ed. *The Growth of Bureaucratic Medicine.* New York: Wiley; 1976:220–238.

16. O'Brien MK, Petrie K, Raeburn J. Adherence to medication regimens: updating a complex medical issue. *Med Care Rev.* 1992;49:435–454.

17. Garrity TF. Medical compliance and the clinician–patient relationship: a review. *Soc Sci Med.* 1981;15:215–222.

18. McLane CG, Zyzanski SJ, Flocke SA. Factors associated with medication non-compliance in rural elderly hypertensive patients. *Am J Hypertens.* 1995;8: 206–209.

19. Hausman A. Taking your medicine: relational steps to improving patient compliance. *Health Market Q.* 2001;19:49–71.

20. Sanson-Fisher RW, Campbell EM, Redman S, Hennrikus DJ. Patient–provider interactions and patient outcomes. *Diabetes Educ.* 1989;15:134–138.

21. Ley P. Doctor–patient communication: some quantitative estimates of the role of cognitive factors in non-compliance. *J Hypertens.* 1985;3:S51–S55.

22. Ley P. *Communicating With Patients: Improving Communication, Satisfaction, and Compliance.* London: Croom Helm; 1988.

23. Hall JA, Roter DL, Katz NR. Meta-analysis of correlations of provider behavior in medical encounters. *Med Care.* 1988;26:657–675.

24. Beisecker A, Beisecker TD. Patient information-seeking behaviors when communicating with doctors. *Med Care.* 1990;28:19–28.

25. Waitzkin H. On studying the discourse of medical encounters. *Med Care.* 1990;28:473–488.

26. Cassileth B. Information and participation preferences among cancer patients. *Ann Intern Med.* 1980;92:832–836.

27. Roter DL, Hall J. *Doctors Talking With Patients/Patients Talking With Doctors.* Westport, CT: Auburn House; 1993.

28. Ende J, Kazis L, Ash A, Moskowitz MA. Measuring patients' desire for autonomy: decision-making and information-seeking preferences among medical patients. *J Gen Intern Med.* 1989;4:24–30.

29. Miller LG, Liu H, Hays RD, et al. Knowledge of regimen dosing and medication adherence: a longitudinal study of antiretroviral medication use. *Clin Infect Dis.* 2003;36:514–518.

30. Cameron C. Patient compliance: recognition of factors involved and suggestions for promoting compliance with therapeutic regimens. *J Adv Nurs.* 1996;24: 244–250.

31. Lewis FM, Morisky DE, Flynn BS. A test of the construct validity of health locus of control: effects on self-reported compliance for hypertensive patients. *Health Educ Monogr.* 1978;6:138–148.

32. Poll IB, De-Nour AK. Locus of control and adjustment to chronic haemodialysis. *Pscyhol Med.* 1980;10:153–157.

33. Schlenk EA, Hart LK. Relationship between health locus of control, health value, and social support and compliance of persons with diabetes mellitus. *Diabetes Care.* 1984;7:566–574.

34. Hussey LC, Gilliland K. Compliance, low literacy, and locus of control. *Nurs Clin North Am.* 1989;24:605–611.

35. Mikhail B. The health belief model: a review and critical evaluation of the model, research, and practice. *Adv Nurs Sci.* 1981;4:65–82.

36. Golin CE, DiMatteo MR, Gelberg L. The role of patient participation in the doctor visit: implications for adherence to diabetes care. *Diabetes Care.* 1996;19:1153–1164.

37. Eisenberg DM, Davis RB, Ettner SL, et al. Trends in alternative medicine use in the United States, 1990–1997: results of a follow-up national survey. *JAMA.* 1998;280:1569–1575.

38. Adams RJ, Smith BJ, Ruffin RE. Impact of the physician's participatory style in asthma outcomes and patient satisfaction. *Ann Allergy Asthma Immunol.* 2001;86:263–271.

39. Bultman DC, Svarstad BL. Effects of physician communication style on client medication beliefs and adherence with antidepressant treatment. *Patient Educ Counsel.* 2000;40:173–185.

40. Greenfield S, Kaplan SH, Ware JE, et al. Patients' participation in medical care: effects of blood sugar control and quality of life in diabetes. *J Gen Intern Med.* 1988;3:448–457.

41. Strassler HE. Post-treatment instructions often go in one ear and out the other. *Dental Assisting.* 1991;11:4.

42. Smith RC, Hoppe RB. The patient's story: integrating the patient- and physician-centered approaches to interviewing. *Ann Intern Med.* 1991;115:470–477.

43. Brody DS. The patient's role in clinical decision-making. *Ann Intern Med.* 1980;93:718–722.

44. Bird JA, Cohen-Cole SA. The three function model of the medical interview: an educational device. In: Hale M, ed. *Models of Teaching Consultation-Liaison Psychiatry.* Basel: Karger; 1991:65–88.

45. Cohen-Cole SA. *The Medical Interview: The Three Function Approach.* St. Louis, MO: Mosby-Year Book; 1991.

46. Benarde MA, Mayerson EW. Patient–physician negotiation. *JAMA.* 1978;239:1413–1415.

47. Greenfield S, Kaplan S, Ware JE Jr. Expanding patient involvement in care: effects on patient outcomes. *Ann Intern Med.* 1985; 102:520–528.

48. Byrne PS, Long BEL. *Doctors Talking to Patients.* London: HMSO; 1976.

49. Chewning B, Sleath B. Medication decision-making and management: a client-centered model. *Soc Sci Med.* 1996;42:389–398.

50. Kinnersley P, Stott N, Peters TJ, et al. The patient-centredness of consultations and outcome in primary care. *Br J Gen Pract.* 1999;49:711–716.

51. Lowes R. Patient-centered care for better patient adherence. *Fam Pract Manage.* 1998;5:46–47, 51–54, 57.

52. Weston W, Brown J, Stewart M. Patient-centered interviewing: understanding patients' experiences. *Can Fam Physician.* 1989;35:147–151.

53. Kaplan SH, Gandek B, Greenfield S, Rogers W, Ware JE. Patient and visit characteristics related to physicians' participatory decision-making style. Results from the Medical Outcomes Study. *Med Care.* 1995;33:1176–1187.

54. Kaplan RM. Health-related quality of life in patient decision making. *J Soc Issues.* 1991;47:69–90.

55. Strull W, Lo B, Charles G. Do patients want to participate in medical decision making? *JAMA.* 1984;252:2990–2994.

56. Ende J, Kazis L, Moskowitz M. Preferences for autonomy when patients are physicians. *J Gen Intern Med.* 1990;5:506–509.

57. Kravitz R, Cope D, Bhrany V, et al. Internal medicine patients' expectations for care during office visits. *J Gen Intern Med.* 1994;9:75–81.

58. Blanchard C. Information and decision-making preferences of hospitalized adult cancer patients. *Soc Sci Med.* 1988;27:1139–1145.

59. Glasgow R. Compliance to diabetes regimens: conceptualization, complexity, and determinants. In: Cramer JA, Spilker B, eds. *Patient Compliance in Medical Practice and Clinical Trials.* New York: Raven Press; 1991:209–221.

60. Johnson SB. Methodological issues in diabetes research: measuring adherence. *Diabetes Care.* 1992;15:1658–1667.

61. Orme CM, Binik YM. Consistency of adherence across regimen demands. *Health Psychol.* 1989;8:27–43.

62. National Diabetes Education Program. Making systems changes for better diabetes care web site. Available at: http://www.betterdiabetescare.org/index.htm#. Accessed October 9, 2003.

63. American Diabetes Association. Standards of medical care for patients with diabetes mellitus. *Diabetes Care.* 2003;26:S33–S50.

64. Heisler M, Bouknight RR, Hayward RA, Smith DM, Kerr EA. The relative importance of physician communication, participatory decision making, and patient understanding in diabetes self-management. *J Gen Intern Med.* 2002;17:243–252.

65. Uhlmann RF, Inui TS, Pecoraro RE, Carter WB. Relationship of patient request fulfillment to compliance, glycemic control, and other health care outcomes in insulin-dependent diabetes. *J Gen Intern Med.* 1988;3:458–463.

66. Viinamaki H, Niskanen L, Korhonen T, Tahka V. The patient–doctor relationship and metabolic control in patients with type 1 (insulin-dependent) diabetes mellitus. *Int J Psychiatr Med.* 1993;23:265–274.

67. Schillinger D, Piette J, Grumbach K, et al. Closing the loop: physician communication with diabetic patients who have low health literacy. *Arch Intern Med.* 2003;163:83–90.

68. Street RL, Jr., Piziak VK, Carpentier WS, et al. Provider–patient communication and metabolic control. *Diabetes Care.* 1993;16:714–721.

69. Amir S, Rabin C, Galatzer A. Cognitive and behavioral determinants of compliance in diabetics. *Health Soc Work.* 1990;15:144–151.

70. World Health Organization. 1999 World Health Organization: International society of Hypertension guidelines for the management of hypertension. *Blood Press Suppl.* 199;1:9–43.

71. Anonymous. The sixth report of the Joint National Committee on prevention, detection, evaluation, and treatment of high blood pressure. *Arch Intern Med.* 1997;157:2413–2446.

72. Betancourt JR, Carrillo JE, Green AR. Hypertension in multicultural and minority populations: linking communication to compliance. *Curr Hypertens Rep.* 1999; 1:482–488.

73. Sanson-Fisher RW, Clover K. Compliance in the treatment of hypertension: a need for action. *Am J Hypertens.* 1995;8:S82–S88.

74. Coleman VR. Physician behavior and compliance. *J Hypertens.* 1985;3:S69–S71.

75. Kjellgren KI, Svensson S, Ahlner J, et al. Antihypertensive medication in clinical encounters. *Int J Cardiol.* 1998;64:161–169.

76. Steele DJ, Jackson TC, Gutmann MC. Have you been taking your pills? The adherence-monitoring sequence in the medical interview. *J Fam Pract.* 1990;30: 294–299.

77. Orth JE, Stiles WB, Scherwitz L, Hennrikus D, Valibona C. Patient exposition and provider explanation in routine interviews and hypertensive patients' blood pressure control. *Health Psychol.* 1987;6:29–42.

78. Stanton AL. Determinants of adherence to medical regimens by hypertensive patients. *J Behav Med.* 1987;10:377–394.

79. Montessori V, Heath B, Yip R, et al. Predictors of adherence with triple combination antiretroviral therapy. Paper presented at: 7th Conference on Retroviruses & Opportunistic Infections, February 2000.

80. Markowitz M, Saag M, Powderly WG, et al. A preliminary study of ritonavir, an inhibitor of HIV-1 protease, to treat HIV-1 infection. *N Eng J Med.* 1995;333: 1534–1539.

81. Danner SA, Carr A, Leonard JM, et al. A short-term study of the safety, pharmacokinetics, and efficacy of ritonavir, an inhibitor of HIV-1 protease: European-Australian collaborative ritonavir study group. *N Eng J Med.* 1995;333:1528–1533.

82. Collier AC, Coombs RW, Schoenfeld DA, et al. Treatment of human immunodeficiency virus infection with saquinavir, zidovudine, and zalcitabine: AIDS Clinical Trials Group. *N Engl J Med.* 1996;334:1011–1017.

83. Gulick RM, Mellors JW, Havlir D, et al. Simultaneous vs sequential initiation of therapy with indinavir, zidovudine, and lamivudine for HIV-1 infection: 100-week follow-up. *JAMA.* 1998;280:35–41.

84. Gulick RM, Mellors JW, Havlir D, et al. Treatment with indinavir, zidovudine, and lamivudine in adults with human immunodeficiency virus infection and prior antiretroviral therapy. *N Eng J Med.* 1997;337:734–739.

85. Mathez D, Truchis P, Gorin I, et al. Ritonavir, AZT, DDC, as a triple combination in AIDS patients. Paper presented at: 3rd Conference Retrovirus & Opportunistic Infections, 1996; Washington, DC.

86. Paterson DL, Swindells S, Mohr J, et al. Adherence to protease inhibitor therapy and outcomes in patients with HIV infection. *Ann Intern Med.* 2000;133:21–30.

87. Bangsberg DR, Perry S, Charlebois ED, Clark R, Robertson M, Moss AR. Adherence to HAART predicts progression to AIDS. Paper presented at: 8th Conference on Retroviruses and Opportunistic Infections, 2001.

88. Carpenter CC, Fischl MA, Hammer SM, et al. Antiretroviral therapy for HIV infection in 1998: updated recommendations of the International AIDS Society-USA Panel. *JAMA.* 1998;280:78–86.

89. Chow R, Chin T, Fong IW, Bendayan R. Medication use patterns in HIV-positive patients. *Can J Hosp Pharm.* 1993;46:171–175.

90. Reichman LB. Compliance with zidovudine therapy. *Ann Intern Med.* 1990;113:332–333.

91. el-Farrash MA, Kuroda MJ, Kitazaki T, et al. Generation and characterization of a human immunodeficiency virus type 1 (HIV-1) mutant resistant to an HIV-1 protease inhibitor. *J Virol.* 1994;68:233–239.

92. Ho DD, Toyoshima T, Mo H, et al. Characterization of human immunodeficiency virus type 1 variants with increased resistance to a C2-symmetric protease inhibitor. *J Virol.* 1994;68:2016–2020.

93. Jacobsen H, Yasargil K, Winslow DL, et al. Characterization of human immunodeficiency virus type 1 mutants with decreased sensitivity to proteinase inhibitor Ro 31-8959. *Virology.* 1995;206:527–534.

94. Kaplan AH, Michael SF, Wehbie RS, et al. Selection of multiple human immunodeficiency virus type 1 variants that encode viral proteases with decreased sensitivity to an inhibitor of the viral protease. *Proc Natl Acad Sci USA.* 1994;91:5597–5601.

95. Knobel H, Carmona A, Grau S, Pedro-Botet J, Diez A. Adherence and effectiveness of highly active antiretroviral therapy. *Arch Intern Med.* 1998;158:1953.

96. Liu H, Golin CE, Miller LG, et al. A comparison study of multiple measures of adherence to HIV protease inhibitors. *Ann Intern Med.* 2001;134:968–977.

97. Lin Y, Lin X, Hong L, et al. Effect of point mutations on the kinetics and the inhibition of human immunodeficiency virus type 1 protease: relationship to drug resistance. *Biochemistry.* 1995;34:1143–1152.

98. Gifford AL, Bormann JE, Shively M, et al. Predictors of self-reported adherence and plasma HIV concentration in patients on multidrug antiretroviral regimens. *J Acquir Immune Defic Syndr.* 2000;23:386–395.

99. Panel on Clinical Practices for the Treatment of HIV. Guidelines for using antiretroviral agents among HIV-infected adults and adolescents. Recommendations of the Panel on Clinical Practices for Treatment of HIV. *Morbidity & Mortality Weekly Report Recommendations & Reports.* 2002;51:1–55.

100. Weinstein MC, Goldie SJ, Losina E, et al. Use of genotypic resistance testing to guide HIV therapy: clinical impact and cost-effectiveness. *Ann Intern Med.* 2001;134:440–450.

101. Henry K. The case for more cautious, patient-focused antiretroviral therapy. *Ann Intern Med.* 2000;132:306–311.

102. Meystre-Agustoni G, Dubois-Arber F, Cochland P, Telenti A. Antiretroviral therapies from the patient's perspective. *AIDS Care.* 2000;12:717–721.

103. Roberts KJ. Barriers to and facilitators of HIV-positive patients' adherence to antiretroviral treatment regimens. *AIDS Patient Care STDS.* 2000;14:155–168.

104. Golin C, Isasi F, Bontempi JB, et al. Secret pills: HIV-positive patients' experiences taking antiretroviral therapy in North Carolina. *AIDS Educ Prev.* 2002;14:318–329.

105. Sowell RL, Phillips KD, Murdaugh C, Tavokali A. Health care providers' influence on HIV-infected women's beliefs and intentions related to AZT therapy. *Clin Nurs Res.* 1999;8:336–354.

106. Golin CE, Liu H, Hays RD, et al. A prospective study of predictors of adherence to combination antiretroviral medication. *J Gen Intern Med.* 2002;17:756–765.

107. Chesney MA. Factors affecting adherence to antiretroviral therapy. *Clin Infect Dis.* 2000;30:S171–S176.

108. Smith SR, Rublein JC, Marcus CM, Brock T, Chesney M. A medication self-management program to improve adherence to HIV therapy regimens. *Patient Educ Couns.* 2003;50:187–199.

109. Gifford AL, Bormann JE, Shively M, et al. Effects of group HIV patient education on adherence to antiretrovirals: a randomized controlled trial. Paper presented at: 8th Conference on Retroviruses and Opportunistic Infections, 2001; Chicago.

110. http://www.aidsinfo.nih.gov/guidelines/adult\AA_071403.pdf.

111. Golin CE, Smith S, Reif S, et al. Usual care adherence counseling practices of generalists and specialists caring for patients with HIV in North Carolina. *J Gen Intern Med.* In press.

112. Roberts KJ. Physician belief about antiretroviral adherence communication. *AIDS Patient Care & Standards.* 2000;14:477–484.

113. Warman KL, Silver EJ, McCourt MP, Stein RE. How does home management of asthma exacerbations by parents of inner-city children differ from NHLBI guideline recommendations? National Heart, Lung, and Blood Institute. *Pediatrics.* 1999;103:422–427.

114. Haby MM, Powell CV, Oberklaid F, Waters EB, Robertson CF. Asthma in children: gaps between current management and best practice. *J Paediatr Child Health.* 2002;38:284–289.

115. National Heart Lung and Blood Institute/World Health Organization Report. *Global Strategy for Asthma Management and Prevention.* NIH, National Heart Lung and Blood Institute; January 1995:Publication Number 95-3659.

116. National Asthma Education and Prevention Program. *Expert Panel Report: Guidelines for the Diagnosis and Management of Asthma: Update on Specific Topics (02-5075).* Washington, DC; 2002.

117. National Heart Lung and Blood Institute. *Guidelines for the Diagnosis and Management of Asthma: Expert Panel Report 2.* NIH, National Heart Lung and Blood Institute; April 1997.

118. Chambers CV, Markson L, Diamond JJ, Lasch L, Berger M. Health beliefs and compliance with inhaled corticosteroids by asthmatic patients in primary care practices. *Respir Med.* 1999;93:88–94.

119. Apter AJ, Reisine ST, Affleck G, Barrows E, Zuwallack RL. Adherence with twice-daily dosing of inhaled steroids: socioeconomic and health-belief differences. *Am J Respir Crit Care Med.* 1998;157:1810–1817.

120. Smith NA, Seale JP, Ley P, Shaw J, Bracs PU. Effects of intervention on medication compliance in children with asthma. *Med J Aust.* 1986:144:119–122.

121. Wilson BM. Promoting compliance: the patient–provider partnership. *Adv Ren Replace Ther.* 1995;2:199–206.

122. Guzman B. The Hispanic population. Census 2000 Brief. Available at: http://www.census.gov/prod/2001pubs/c2kbr01-3.pdf. Accessed May 10, 2002.

123. Humes K, McKinnon J. *The Asian and Pacific Islander Population in the United States: March 1999*. Washington, DC: U.S. Census Bureau; 2000.

124. Carrillo JE, Green AR, Betancourt JR. Cross-cultural primary care: a patient-based approach. *Ann Intern Med*. 1999; 130:829–834.

125. Anand R. *Cultural Competence in Health Care: A Guide for Trainers*. 2nd ed. Washington, DC: NMCI Publications; 1999.

126. Millet PE, Sullivan BF, Schwebel AI, et al. Black Americans' and White Americans' views of the etiology and treatment of mental health problems. *Community Men Health J*. 1996;32:235–242.

127. Pedersen P. Ten frequent assumptions of cultural bias in counseling. *Journal of Multicultural Counseling & Development*. 1987;15:16–24.

128. Carter RT. Cultural values: a review of empirical research and implications for counseling. *Journal of Consulting & Development*. 1991;70:164–173.

129. Mull JD. Cross-cultural communication in the physician's office. *West J Med*. 1993;159:609–613.

130. Ivey A, Ivey M, Simek-Morgan L. *Counseling and Psychotherapy: A Multicultural Perspective*. 3rd ed. Boston: Allyn & Bacon; 1993.

131. Ridley CR, Mendoza DW, Kanitz BE, Angermeier L, Zenk R. Cultural sensitivity in multicultural counseling: A perceptual schema model. *J Counsel Psychol*. 1994;41:125–136.

132. Pachter LM. Culture and clinical care: folk illness beliefs and behaviors and their implications for health care delivery. *JAMA*. 1994;271:690–694.

133. Rose LE, Kim MT, Dennison CR, et al. The contexts of adherence for African Americans with high blood pressure. *J Adv Nurs*. 2000;32:587–594.

134. Kleinman A, Eisenberg L, Good B. Culture, illness, and care: clinical lessons from anthropologic and cross-cultural research. *Ann Intern Med*. 1978;88: 251–258.

135. Sugarman J, Butters RR. Understanding the patient: medical words the doctor may not know. *N C Med J*. 1985;46:415–417.

136. Tring FC, Hayes-Allen MC. Understanding and misunderstanding of some medical terms. *British Journal of Medical Education*. 1973;7:53–59.

137. Prieto LR, Miller DS, Gayowski T, et al. Multicultural issues in organ transplantation: the influence of patients' cultural perspectives on compliance with treatment. *Clin Transpl*. 1997;11:529–535.

138. Lingard L, Tallett S, Rosenfield J. Culture and physician–patient communication: a qualitative exploration of residents' experiences and attitudes. *Ann R Coll Physicians Surg Can*. 2002;35:331–335.

139. Sodowsky GR, Lai EW, Plake BS. Moderating effects of sociocultural variables on acculturation attitudes of Hispanics and Asian Americans. *J Counsel Development*. 1991;70:194–204.

140. Sue DW, Sue D. *Counseling the Culturally Different: Theory and Practice*. 3rd ed. New York: Wiley & Sons; 1999.

141. Win D, Brawer R, Plumb J. Cultural factors in preventive care: African-Americans. *Prim Care Clin Office Pract*. 2002;29:487–493.

142. Ad Hoc Committee on Health Literacy for the Council on Scientific Affairs, American Medical Association. Health literacy: report for the AMA Council on Scientific Affairs. *JAMA.* 1999;281:552–557.

143. Williams MV, Parker RM, Baker DW, et al. Inadequate functional health literacy among patients at two public hospitals. *JAMA.* 1995;274:1677–1682.

144. Baker DW, Parker RM, Williams MV, et al. The health care experience of patients with low literacy. *Arch Fam Med.* 1996;5:329–334.

145. Kalichman SC, Ramachandran B, Catz S. Adherence to combination antiretroviral therapies in HIV patients of low health literacy. *J Gen Intern Med.* 1999;14: 267–272.

146. Hussey LC. Minimizing effects of low literacy on medication knowledge and compliance among the elderly. *Clinical Nursing Research.* 1994;3:132–145.

147. Mayeaux EJ, Murphy PW, Arnold C, Davis TC, Jackson RH, Sentell T. Improving patient education for patients with low literacy skills. *Am Fam Physician.* 1996;53:205–211.

148. Williams MV, Davis T, Parker RM, Weiss BD. The role of health literacy in patient-physician communication. *Fam Med.* 2002;34:383–389.

149. Ong L, Haes JD, Hoos A, et al. Doctor–patient communication: a review of the literature. *Soc Sci Med.* 1995;40:903–918.

150. Doak C, Doak L, Root J. *Teaching Patients With Low Literacy Skills.* Philadelphia: J.B. Lippincott; 1985.

151. Schillinger D, Bindman A, Wang F, Stewart A, Piette J. Functional health literacy and the quality of physician-patient communication among diabetes patients. *Patient Educ Couns.* 2004;52(3):315–323.

152. Davis TC, Jackson RH, Bocchini JA, Arnold C, Mayeaux EJ, Murphy P. Comprehension is greater using a short vaccine information pamphlet with graphics and simple language. *J Gen Intern Med.* 1994;9:103.

153. Houts PS, Witmer JT, Egeth HE, Tringali CA, Bucher JA, Localio RA. Using pictographs to enhance recall of spoken medical instructions II. *Patient Educ Couns.* 2001;43:231–242.

154. Haug M. Doctor-patient relationships and their impact on elderly self-care. In: Dean K, Hickley T, Holstein B, eds. *Self-Care and Health in Old Age.* London: Croom Helm; 1986:230–250.

155. Stewart M, Meredith L, Brown JB, Galajda J. The influence of older patient-physician communication on health and health-related outcomes. *Clin Geriatr Med.* 2000;16:25–36.

156. Brown JB, Stewart M, Ryan BL. Outcomes of patient-provider interaction. In: Thompson TL, Dorsey AM, Miller KI, et al., eds. *Handbook of Health Communication.* Mahwah, NJ: Lawrence Erlbaum Associates; 2003:141–161.

157. Cochrane RA, Mandal AR, Ledger-Scott M, Walker R. Changes in drug treatment after discharge from hospital in geriatric patients. *BMJ.* 1992;305: 694–696.

158. Salzman C. Medication compliance in the elderly. *J Clin Psychiatry.* 1995;56: 18–23.

159. Baile WF, Gross RJ. Hypertension: psychosomatic and behavioral aspects. *Prim Care.* 1979;6:267–282.

160. Coe RM, Prendergast CG, Psathas G. Strategies for obtaining compliance with medications regimens. *J Am Geriatr Soc.* 1984;32:589–594.

161. Greene MG, Adelman RD, Friedmann E, Charon R. Older patient satisfaction with communication during an initial medical encounter. *Soc Sci Med.* 1994;38: 1279–1288.

162. Greene MG, Majerovitz SD, Adelman RD, Rizzo C. The effects of the presence of a third person on the physician-older patient medical interview. *J Am Geriatr Soc.* 1994;42:413–419.

163. Greene MG, Adelman RD, Charon R, Friedmann E. Concordance between physicians and their older and younger patients in the primary care medical encounter. *Gerontologist.* 1989;29:808–813.

164. Tennstedt SL. Empowering older patients to communicate more effectively in the medical encounter. *Clin Geriatr Med.* 2000;16:61–70, ix.

165. Vieder JN, Krafchick MA, Kovach AC, et al. Physician–patient interaction: what do elders want? *J Am Osteopath Assoc.* 2002;102:73–78.

166. Greene MG, Adelman R, Charon R, Hoffman S. Ageism in the medical encounter: an exploratory study of the doctor–elderly patient relationship. *Lang Commun.* 1986;6:113–124.

167. Inui TS, Yourtee EL, Williamson JW. Improved outcomes in hypertension after physician tutorials: a controlled trial. *Ann Intern Med.* 1976;84:646–651.

168. Maiman LA, Becker MH, Liptak GS, Nazarian LF, Rounds KA. Improving pediatricians' compliance-enhancing practice: a randomized trial. *Am J Dis Child.* 1988;142:773–779.

169. Ley P, Whitworth MA, Skilbeck CE, et al. Improving doctor-patient communication in general practice. *J R Coll Gen Pract.* 1976;26:720–724.

170. Joos SK, Hickam DH, Gordon GH, Baker LH. Effects of a physician communication intervention on patient care outcomes. *J Gen Intern Med.* 1996;11: 147–155.

171. Cegala DJ, Marinelli T, Post D. The effects of patient communication skills training on compliance. *Arch Fam Med.* 2000;9:57–64.

172. Edworthy SM, Devins GM. Improving medication adherence through patient education distinguishing between approximate and inappropriate utilization. *J Rheumatol.* 1999;26:1793–1801.

173. Tieffenberg JA, Wood EI, Alonso A, Tossutti MS, Vicente MF. A randomized field trial of ACINDES: a child-centered training model for children with chronic illnesses (asthma and epilepsy). *J Urban Health.* 2000;77:280–297.

174. Sclar DA, Chin A, Skaer TL, Okamoto MP, Nakahiro RK, Gill MA. Effect of health education in promoting prescription refill compliance among patients with hypertension. *Clin Ther.* 1991;13:1–7.

175. Lipton HL, Bird JA. The impact of clinical pharmacists' consultations on geriatric patients' compliance and medical care use: a randomized controlled trial. *Gerontologist.* 1994;34:307–315.

176. Burnier M, Schneider MP, Chiolero A, et al. Electronic compliance monitoring in resistant hypertension: the basis for rational therapeutic decisions. *J Hypertens.* 2001;19:335–341.

177. Weinberger M, Murray MD, Marrero DG, et al. Effectiveness of pharmacist care for patients with reactive airways disease: a randomized controlled trial. *JAMA.* 2002;288:1594–1602.

178. Morice AH, Wrench C. The role of the asthma nurse in treatment compliance and self-management following hospital admission. *Respir Med.* 2001;95: 851–856.

179. Peveler R, George C, Kinmonth AL, et al. Effect of antidepressant drug counselling and information leaflets on adherence to drug treatment in primary care: randomised controlled trial. *BMJ.* 1999;319:612–615.

180. Steckel SB, Swain MA. Contracting with patients to improve compliance. *Am J Nurs.* 1977;51:81–83.

181. Rollnick S, Heather N, Bell A. Negotiating behaviour change in medical settings: the development of brief motivational interviewing. *J Mental Health.* 1992;1:25–37.

182. Shinitzky HE, Kub J. The art of motivating behavior change: the use of motivational interviewing to promote health. *Public Health Nurs.* 2001;18:178–185.

183. Miller WR. Motivational interviewing with problem drinkers. *Behav Psychother.* 1983;11:147–172.

184. Kemp R, Hayward P, Applewhaite G, Everitt B, David A. Compliance therapy in psychotic patients: randomised controlled trial. *BMJ.* 1996;312:345–349.

185. Kalichman SC, Nachimson D. Self-efficacy and disclosure of HIV-positive serostatus to sex partners. *Health Psychol.* 1999;18:281–287.

186. Simoni J, Mason H, Marks G, Ruiz MS, Reed D, Richardson JL. Women's self-disclosure of HIV infection: rates, reasons and reactions. *J Consult Clin Psychol.* 1995;63:474–478.

187. NIMH Multisite HIV Prevention Trial Group. The NIMH multisite HIV prevention trial: reducing HIV sexual risk behavior. *Science.* 1998:1889–1894.

188. Marks G, Bingman C, Duval S. Negative affect and unsafe sex in HIV-positive men. *AIDS Behav.* 1998;2:89–100.

189. Davidson S, Dew MA, Penkower L, Becker KT, Kingsley L. Substance use and sexual behavior among homosexual men at risk for HIV infection: psychosocial mediators. *Psychol Health.* 1995;7:259–272.

190. Kennedy CA, Skurnick J, Wan J, et al. Psychological distress, drug and alcohol use as correlates of condom use in HIV-serodiscordant heterosexual couples. *AIDS.* 1993;7:1493–1499.

191. Flom PL, Friedman SR, Kottiri BJ, et al. Stigmatized drug use, sexual partner concurrency, and other sex risk network and behavior characteristics of 18- to 24-year-old youth in a high-risk neighborhood. *Sex Transm Dis.* 2001;28: 598–607.

192. Baker A, Healther N, Wodak A, Dixon J, Holt P. Evaluation of a cognitive-behavioral intervention for HIV prevention among injection drug users. *AIDS.* 1993;7:247–256.

193. Belcher L, Kalichman S, Topping M, et al. A randomized trial of a brief HIV risk reduction counseling intervention for women. *J Consult Clin Psychol.* 1998; 66:531–541.

194. Harding R, Dockrell MJD, Dockrell J, et al. Motivational interviewing for HIV risk reduction among gay men in commercial and public sex settings. *AIDS Care.* 2001;13:493–501.

195. Resnicow K, Dilorio C, Soet J, Ernst D, Borrelli B, Hecht J. Motivational interviewing in health promotion: it sounds like something is changing. *Health Psychol.* 2002;21:444–451.

196. Yahne CE, Miller WR, Irvin-Vitela L, et al. Magdalena Project: motivational outreach to substance abusing women street sex workers. *J Subst Abuse Treat.* 2002;23:49–53.

197. Miller W. Motivational interviewing: research, practice, and puzzles. *Addict Behav.* 1996;21:835–842.

198. Emmons KM, Rollnick S. Motivational interviewing in health care settings: opportunities and limitations. *Am J Prev Med.* 2001;20:68–74.

199. Miller W, Rollnick S. *Motivational Interviewing: Preparing People to Change Addictive Behavior.* New York: Guilford Press; 1991.

200. Rogers CR. The underlying theory: drawn from experience with individuals and groups. *Counseling and Values.* 1987;32:38–46.

201. Dilorio C, Resnicow K, McDonnell M, Soet J, McCarty F, Yeager K. Using motivational interviewing to promote adherence to antiretroviral medications: a pilot study. *J Assoc Nurses AIDS Care.* 2003;14:52–62.

202. Picciano JF, Roffman RA, Kalichman SC, Rutledge SE, Berghuis JP. A telephone based brief intervention using motivational enhancement to facilitate HIV risk reduction among MSM: a pilot study. *AIDS Behav.* 2001;5:251–262.

203. Adamian MS, Golin CE, Shain LS, DeVellis B. Motivational interviewing to improve adherence to antiretroviral therapy: development and pilot evaluation of an intervention. *AIDS Patient Care STDs.* 2004;18(4):229–238.

204. Kelly JA, Kalichman SC. Behavioral research in HIV/AIDS primary and secondary prevention: recent advances and future directions. *J Consult Clin Psychol.* 2002;70:626–639.

205. Kamb ML, Fishbein M, Douglas JM, et al. Efficacy of risk-education counseling to prevent human immunodeficiency virus and sexually transmitted diseases: a randomized controlled trial. *JAMA.* 1998;280:1161–1167.

206. Rollnick S, Butler CC, Stott N. Helping smokers make decisions: the enhancement of brief intervention for general medical practice. *Patient Educ Couns.* 1997;31:191–203.

207. Resnikow K, Jackson A, Wang T, et al. A motivational interviewing intervention to increase fruit and vegetable intake through Black churches: results of the Eat for Life trial. *Am J Public Health.* 2001;91:1686–1693.

208. Smith DE, Heckemeyer CM, Kratt PP, Mason D. Motivational interviewing to improve adherence to a behavioral weight-control program for older obese women with NIDDM: a pilot study. *Diabetes Care.* 1997;20:52.

209. Butler C, Rollnick S, Cohen D, et al. Motivational counseling versus brief advice for smokers in general practice: a randomized trial. *Br J Gen Pract.* 1999;49: 611–616.

210. Henbest RJ, Stewart M. Patient-centeredness in the consultation: does it really make a difference? *Fam Pract.* 1990;7:28–33.

211. Brown JB, Weston WW, Stewart MA: Patient-centered interviewing: 2. Finding common ground. *Can Fam Physician.* 1989;35:153–157.

212. Brown JB, Stewart M, Tessier S. *Assessing Communication Between Patients and Doctors: A Manual for Scoring Patient-Centered Communication.* London, Ontario: University of Western Ontario, Centre for Studies in Family Medicine; 1995.

213. Roter D, Larson S. The Roter interaction analysis system (RIAS): utility and flexibility for analysis of medical interactions. *Patient Educ Couns.* 2002;46: 243–251.

214. Bylund CL, Makoul G. Empathetic communication and gender in the physician–patient encounter. *Patient Educ Couns.* 2002;48:207–216.

215. Bales RF. *Interaction Process Analysis.* Cambridge, MA: Addison-Wesley; 1950.

216. Cegala DJ. A study of doctors' and patients' communication during a primary care consultation: implications for communication training. *J Health Commun.* 1997;2:169–194.

217. Street RL, Millay B. Analyzing patient participation in medical encounters. *Health Commun.* 2001;13:61–73.

218. Stiles WB. *Describing Talk: A Taxonomy of Verbal Response Modes.* Newbury Park, CA: Sage; 1992.

219. Kreps GL, Arora NK, Nelson DE. Consumer/provider communication research: directions for development. *Patient Educ Counsel.* 2003;50:3–4.

220. Kreps GL. Consumer/provider communication research: a personal plea to address issues of ecological validity, relational development, message diversity, and situational constraints. *J Health Psychol.* 2001;6:597–601.

221. Roter DL. *The Roter Method of Interaction Process Analysis.* Baltimore: Johns Hopkins University, Department of Health Policy and Management; 1991.

222. Street RJ. Communicative styles and adaptations in physician-patient consultations. *Soc Sci Med.* 1992;34:1155–1163.

223. Calahan EJ, Bertakis KD. Development and validation of the Davis Observation Code. *Fam Med.* 1991;5:19–24.

224. Stiles WB, McDaniel SH, McGaughey K. Verbal response mode correlates of experiencing. *J Consult Clin Psychol.* 1979;47:795–797.

225. Elwyn G, Edwards A, Mowle S, et al. Measuring the involvement of patients in shared decision-making: a systematic review of instruments. *Patient Educ Couns.* 2001;43:5–22.

226. Bensing J, van Dulmen S, Takes K. Communication in context: new directions in communication research. *Patient Educ Counsel.* 2003;50:27–32.

227. Roter DL. Observations on methodological and measurement challenges in the assessment of communication during medical exchanges. *Patient Educ Couns.* 2003;50:17–21.

228. Ramirez AG. Consumer-provider communication research with special populations. *Patient Educ Couns.* 2003;50:51–54.

229. Doak CC, Doak LG, Friedell GH, Meade CD. Improving comprehension for cancer patients with low literacy skills: strategies for clinicians. *CA Cancer J Clin.* 1998;48:153–162.

Chapter 12

Physician Adherence to Clinical-Practice Guidelines

Morris Weinberger
Talya Salz

Regardless of the disease or condition, one universal truism appears to be that physicians vary in the way they practice medicine. This is not a new observation. In *The Doctor's Dilemma*, written in 1906, George Bernard Shaw wrote:

> During the first great epidemic of influenza towards the end of the 19th century, a London evening paper sent round a journalist-patient to all great consultants of the day, and published their advice and prescriptions, a proceeding passionately denounced by the medical papers as a breech of confidence of these eminent physicians. The case was the same, but the prescriptions were different, and so was the advice. Now a doctor cannot think his own treatment right and at the same time think his colleague right in prescribing a different treatment when the patient is the same.

Since the 1970s, Wennberg and his colleagues demonstrated that physicians did not practice consistently either within small areas (i.e., variation based on individual physician practices) or across large areas (i.e., community standards); identifying practice variation may represent opportunities to reduce inappropriate care (1, 2). Since these seminal studies, practice variation has been observed across many medical and surgical treatments in countries throughout the world. During the 1980s, concerns about rising health care costs, an aging population, ubiquitous practice variation, and reports of inappropriate use of health care services gave rise to the effective-

373

ness movement; that is, two alternative clinical strategies were unlikely to be equal in terms of *both* their effectiveness and costs (3). With the effectiveness movement came the consideration of strategies to reduce observed practice variation and inappropriate care.

The introduction of clinical-practice guidelines represents one strategy designed to reduce practice variation. The Institute of Medicine defined clinical-practice guidelines as "systematically developed statements to assist practitioner and patient decisions about appropriate health care for specific clinical circumstances" (4). Clinical-practice guidelines are intended to: improve knowledge by making clinicians aware of recommendations, change attitudes about the standard of care, shift practice patterns, and, ulimately, enhance patient outcomes (3, 5). To the extent that guidelines are evidence based, one would expect practitioners to adhere to these guidelines to maximize the quality of care provided to their patients. However, a recent national study found that Americans received 55% of recommended care, with little difference among preventive, acute, or chronic care recommendations (6). An important question for researchers and policymakers is why physicians fail to adhere to clinical-practice guidelines if those guidelines represent high-quality care.

With this background, this chapter reviews: (a) the development of clinical-practice guidelines, (b) issues related to defining and measuring adherence to guidelines, (c) strategies that have been successful or unsuccessful in increasing adherence to guidelines, and (d) challenges for researchers and policymakers interested in evaluating and/or implementing innovative strategies to enhance adherence to guidelines. Because clinical-practice guidelines are generally intended for physicians, we limit this chapter to this group of practitioners.

DEVELOPMENT OF CLINICAL-PRACTICE GUIDELINES

Concerns about rising health care costs, observed practice variation, and reports about inappropriate care contributed to the rise of the effectiveness initiative in the United States (3, 5). Clinical-practice guidelines were viewed as a strategy to enhance the effectiveness of health care delivery by: (a) improving physicians' knowledge and awareness of current recommendations, (b) changing attitudes about the standard of care, (c) shifting practice patterns to be more consistent with evidence, and (d) improving patient outcomes (7). Desirable attributes of clinical-practice guidelines include their validity, reliability and reproducibility, clinical acceptability, clinical flexibility, clarity, documentation, development by a multidisciplinary process, and plans for review (8). More recently, the Conference on Guideline Standardization has published a checklist that provides a framework to support more comprehensive documentation of clinical-practice guidelines (9).

Clinical-practice guidelines can benefit *patients* through: (a) improving health outcomes by promoting effective, and discouraging ineffective, interventions, (b) increasing consistency of care (i.e., reduce variation), (c) informing patients and the public about the quality of care, and (d) influencing public policy. For *health care professionals,* clinical-practice guidelines may: (a) improve quality of care when the individual physician is uncertain, (b) support quality improvement efforts by helping decide how patients should be treated, and (c) identify gaps in the literature that need further study. Finally, for *health care systems,* clinical-practice guidelines may: (a) improve efficiency and optimize value received for resources (money and personnel), (b) prevent costly events (e.g., hospitalization and/or readmission), and (c) improve public image (5).

Various strategies have been used to develop clinical-practice guidelines, including:

- *Informal consensus development:* This approach uses the judgment of expert panel members to make recommendations. Though scientific evidence often forms the basis for discussion, little methodological information is provided to assure readers that the science was reviewed without bias. And, there are no criteria that describe the process by which consensus was achieved. Although this strategy is simplest, it produces guidelines that often have poor quality and are least trusted by clinicians (10).

- *Formal consensus development:* In this model, an expert panel is provided with relevant articles that review existing evidence for a practice or procedure. Before the first meeting, panel members rate appropriateness of a procedure for a specific action (clearly inappropriate to clearly appropriate). The panel reviews distribution of ratings, compares ratings with their own scores, and discusses reasons for differences. The process is repeated as necessary, and the result is a list of procedures and indications coupled with recommendations. The methodological rigor of the study is formally considered. Although this offers some advantages over informal consensus, formal consensus development is cumbersome and difficult to apply in practice (10).

- *Evidence-based guideline development:* Sponsored by organizations such as the U. S. Preventive Services Task Force and the Canadian Task Force on the Periodic Health Exam, guidelines are accompanied by background articles that describe in detail the evidence for each recommendation and the quality of the methods on which the recommendations are based. These reports are typically published in major journals and more regularly accepted by physicians because the process for guideline development is clear. However, because the evidence for the strongest recommendations has such high methodological standards, recommendations are often neutral. Furthermore, most practices cannot be assessed due to lack of high-grade evidence (10).

- *Explicit guideline development:* This strategy uses scientific evidence and formal analytical models that is supplemented with expert opinion. After selecting a topic, expert panel members are provided the purpose of the guidelines (e.g., types of patients, setting). Then, they are asked to assess the scientific evidence, consider expert opinion, and draft guidelines based on a summary of benefits and harms. This process is complex and time-consuming, and the methods behind the guidelines may not be intuitive to practicing physicians (10).

With the promulgation of clinical-practice guidelines came many issues that affected their acceptance by the medical community (5, 11). Specifically, there are many questions about the validity of clinical-practice guidelines. Several factors may contribute to practitioners' questioning their validity.

First, there is often *inconsistency across guidelines.* That is, there are often several, sometimes contradictory, guidelines being recommended for the same clinical scenario (e.g., frequency of eye examinations for patients with diabetes). In part, this may be caused by differences in the strategies used to develop the guidelines and/or the interpretation of published studies. In addition, sponsoring agencies (e.g., federal government, medical societies, insurers, private sector) and/or experts may have differences of opinion regarding the interpretation of evidence. Whatever the reason, inconsistencies across guidelines create confusion about recommended clinical practice (3, 5).

Second, physicians may believe that the evidence for a guideline is *not applicable to their patients.* When selecting the best available research on which to base guidelines, the strongest evidence comes from randomized controlled trials. This is because trials are the gold standard for establishing causality. However, trials emphasize efficacy over effectiveness. Thus, patients enrolled in these trials are often not representative of those seen in typical practices. For example, many studies of medications are conducted with highly selected patients that physicians rarely see in their practice (e.g., no comorbid conditions) (12).

Third, guidelines may be based on *outdated or poor-quality studies.* If guidelines are not based on the most current evidence, they can cause harm to patients. Situations that might require clinical guidelines to be updated include: (a) changes in evidence on the existing benefits and harms of interventions, (b) changes in outcomes considered important, (c) changes in available interventions, (d) changes in evidence that current practice is optimal, (e) changes in values placed on outcomes, and (f) changes in resources available for health care (13). A recent review suggested that more than 75% of guidelines developed by the Agency for Healthcare Research and Quality need updating; the authors recommend that guidelines should be reassessed for validity every 3 years (14).

DEFINING AND MEASURING ADHERENCE TO CLINICAL-PRACTICE GUIDELINES

As with any scientific endeavor, a valid operational definition of adherence is central to conducting research on adherence to clinical-practice guidelines. However, assessing adherence to clinical-practice guidelines differs from studies of patient adherence to their regimens. For example, what is an appropriate level of adherence for a particular recommendation? In the case of patient adherence to medications, one assumes that the goal is for patients to take their medication exactly as prescribed, that is, 100% adherence. This is generally not the case for physician adherence to clinical-practice guidelines. Even for guidelines for which there is general consensus, some patients will not be eligible for the recommended care. For example, there may be a contraindication to a recommended medication (a patient with a history of gastrointestinal bleeding may not be able to tolerate aspirin) or diagnostic test (e.g., screening mammography is not appropriate for women with a double mastectomy). This can create a measurement nightmare for investigators. Even with sophisticated medical record systems, researchers are unlikely to be able to determine the denominator (i.e., which patients are eligible for a specific guideline) because relevant information (e.g., history, contraindications for a medication) is not readily available. Carrying this one step further, the goal of perfect adherence to a clinical-practice guideline may actually credit physicians for adhering to a guideline that is inappropriate for a specific patient (although one generally assumes that adherence to guidelines reflects better quality care).

STRATEGIES TO ENHANCE ADHERENCE TO CLINICAL-PRACTICE GUIDELINES

Strategies that seek to increase physician adherence to clinical-practice guidelines employ models in which enhancing knowledge (e.g., medical education) will lead to improved attitudes toward the guidelines (e.g., acceptability), which, in turn results in behavioral changes (i.e., adoption of guidelines) and, ultimately, improved patient outcomes (7, 12). In an excellent literature review on barriers to physician adherence to clinical-practice guidelines, Cabana et al. develop a model in which behavioral changes (in this case, physicians' adherence to guidelines) would be most sustainable if physicians possessed the requisite knowledge and attitudes to support adherence (12). In their model, barriers to *knowledge* include *lack of awareness* and/or *lack of familiarity* with a guideline. Specific barriers include the sheer volume of information, the time needed to stay informed, and the accessibility of guidelines. Developing *attitudes* that support physicians' adherence to guidelines must overcome: (a) *lack of agreement with a specific guideline*, which may be a function of physicians' interpretation of the evidence, the guideline's applicability to their own patients, or the sponsor of the guideline; (b) *lack of agreement with guidelines in general*, for example, viewing guidelines as "cookbook medicine," too rigid, or not feasible to be useful in clinical practice; (c) *lack of outcome expectancy*—that is, they do not believe that adhering to guidelines will lead to the desired outcome; (d) *lack of self-efficacy* or physicians not believing that they can perform what is required by the guideline; and (e) *lack of motivation due to inertia of previous practice*. Finally, there exist external barriers that also affect attitudes (and ultimately behaviors). These *external barriers* may involve patient factors (e.g., patient preferences), guideline factors (e.g., contradictory guidelines), and environmental factors, including lack of time, inadequate resources, or lack of reimbursement (12).

In the sections that follow, we review a series of strategies that attempted to increase physicians' adherence to clinical-practice guidelines.

Continuing Medical Education

In order to deliver high-quality care (including following clinical-practice guidelines), physicians must know what to do. Therefore, it is not surprising that traditional continuing medical education has been a mainstay among strategies to disseminate current knowledge. Strategies may include grand rounds, peer-reviewed journals, mailings, and didactic classes. Formal literature syntheses have consistently demonstrated that traditional continuing medical education is ineffective in improving the processes or outcomes of care (15–17). These findings should not be interpreted to mean that adequate knowledge is unnecessary to produce behavioral changes such as adherence. Rather, the lack of effectiveness of traditional continuing medical education likely occurs because knowledge is necessary, but not sufficient, to influence physicians' attitudes and behavior. Strategies that provide the requisite knowledge, in combination with other strategies (such as the ones reviewed later), are likely to be far more effective in promoting adherence to clinical-practice guidelines (12, 15–17).

Academic Detailing

For years, the pharmaceutical industry has used "detailing," in which pharmaceutical sales representatives make visits to physicians' offices to promote their company's products. In the 1980s, it was estimated that the pharmaceutical industry spent $5,000 per physician annually on this very effective strategy (18). The question is whether one could adapt these principles by using academic detailing to encourage physicians to engage in activities that are consistent with high-quality care. With academic detailing, pharmacists, physicians, or other health care professionals become educators who work individually with physicians to change their behavior. The authors outlined a series of detailing strategies that could be adapted to promote change in physician behavior in the realm of improving quality of care: (a) defining specific problems and objectives; (b) performing "market research" to better understand physicians' motives; (c) establishing credibility, for example, by associating with reputable medical groups; (d) identifying, targeting, and involving "high potential" physicians, that is, those with particular utilization problems for whom intervention is likely to make a large difference; (e) identifying and involving local medical opinion leaders who may influence the practice of others; (f) using two-sided communication in which both sides of an issue are presented and counterarguments are made; (g) encouraging physicians' active learning (e.g., asking focused questions); (h) repeating and reinforcing important concepts; (i) distributing brief print materials, including graphics; (j) offering practical alternatives to usual practice; and (k) selecting and training detailers who can be effective in communication and persuasion (18).

Using these recommended strategies for academic detailing, Avorn and Soumerai successfully reduced excessive prescribing of three drugs by 14% in comparison with controls (19). More recently, Solomon and colleagues (20) conducted a randomized, controlled trial to evaluate whether academic detailing could reduce inappropriate use of antibiotics. Academic detailers in the study, who were clinician-educators, infectious-disease physicians, and a pharmacist, were trained to approach physicians who were targeted for suboptimal prescription of antibiotics. The authors found that physicians in the intervention group were significantly less likely to prescribe unnecessary antibiotics or use antibiotics for an inappropriately long duration. Although effective, this strategy is very labor intensive (20).

Opinion Leaders

"Opinion leaders are not necessarily innovators or authority figures, but are trusted by their colleagues to evaluate new information and assess the value of new medical practices in the context of local group norms; are approached frequently for clinical advice; have good listening skills; and are perceived as clinically competent and caring" (21). Given these attributes, these individuals should be in an excellent position to influence their colleagues to adhere to clinical-practice guidelines that are consistent with high-quality care. Literature syntheses suggest that opinion leaders are generally effective in increasing adherence to clinical-practice guidelines (15, 17). The strongest evidence to date comes from a randomized controlled trial in which opinion leaders were involved in disseminating information on adherence to a guideline on the pharmaceutical treatment of acute myocardial infarction (21). After surveying physicians in hospitals to identify those physicians who were trusted by their peers as leaders, cardiologists met once with opinion leaders in the intervention group. The cardiologists distributed slides, brochures, and educational support that the opinion leaders helped to create. The leaders then returned to their practices and organized educational sessions in small groups. Intervention hospitals showed a significant improvement in delivering appropriate care in cases of acute myocardial infarction (21).

Clinical Decision Support Systems

Clinical decision support systems are "any software designed to directly aid in clinical decision-making in which characteristics of individual patients are matched to a computerized knowledge base for the purpose of generating patient-specific assessments or recommendations that are then presented to clinicians for consideration" (22). Clinical support systems that have the capability to integrate the medical literature and evidence-based medicine with physicians' practice and patient information have become increasingly common in promoting adherence to guidelines. A pioneering clinical decision support system is provided through the Regenstrief Medical Record System. Developed by McDonald and his colleagues in the 1970s, this is one of the oldest, largest, and most comprehensive electronic medical record systems in the country (23, 24). It has been the site of more controlled trials and epidemiologic investigations than any other such system (25, 26), particularly to improve the quality of care delivered (27–35). The Regenstrief Medical Record System stores nearly 30 years of longitudinal data, including health services utilization, medication histories, clinical outcomes, results of all tests and procedures, and diagnoses made in the outpatient, emergency room, and inpatient settings. An important reason for the success of the Regenstrief Medical Record System is its ability to generate computerized reminders. That is, it has the potential to define standards of care (i.e., clinical-practice guidelines), determine whether these standards are being met for individual patients, and generate reminders to physicians at the time the patient has a clinic visit with the physician. In one randomized trial that was initiated in the late 1970s, computerized reminders improved adherence to treatment recommendations (27). Notably, when the reminders were removed, physician adherence returned to baseline rates (27). Thus, reminders are a prompt to action, rather than a tool that increases physicians' knowledge.

Computer reminders for preventive care have often been studied in outpatient settings. However, hospitalization represents a potential opportunity to deliver preventive care. So, the question is whether computer reminders to implement preventive care guidelines can be effective during hospital stays. Using the Regenstrief Medical Record System, Overhage and his colleagues were unable to increase the provision of preventive care while patients are hospitalized (28). A subsequent study in this same setting found that the majority of hospital patients were eligible for preventive-care strategies, and that reminders to initiate preventive care were effective (29). The authors attribute the success of the latter study to having the computer display full prewritten orders, repeating the order up to four times during the admission, and making it easier for physicians to order the preventive-care strategy.

There have been rigorous studies of clinical decision support systems to assist physicians with drug dosing, diagnosis, prevention (including screening), and other aspects of medical care (e.g., managing specific diseases). A systematic review of these systems (22) found that: (a) dosing systems that help physicians determine the appropriate dosage of potentially toxic drugs had inconsistent effects in changing physician behavior; (b) diagnostic aids were rarely studied and demonstrated mixed effects; (c) prevention systems, particularly reminder systems, were the most consistently effective in changing physician behavior (74% of studies showed a positive effect); and (d) computerized assistance with other aspects of medical care demonstrated an overall positive effect on the process of care that was similar in magnitude to reminder systems (73% improved significantly). The authors found: (a) great variability across studies, (b) that systems that work in one setting, may not work in others, and (c) that the effect of clinical decision support systems on patient outcomes has not been adequately studied (22). Steinberg suggested that the increased use of computerized reminders could be particularly effective in improving quality of care because, as the number of medical interventions and guidelines increase over time, reminder systems could assist physicians in remembering to implement appropriate preventive care sequentially (36).

Finally, computer reminders typically use objective data contained in many electronic medical record systems. However, an important question is whether providing physicians with data on their patients' symptoms would affect physician behavior. Because clinical-practice guidelines for heart failure recommend adjustments based on patients' symptoms (e.g., shortness of breath), heart failure is an ideal model to test such a strategy. Using a randomized trial, physicians were randomized to receive care suggestions generated with electronic medical record data and symptom data obtained from recent questionnaires or to receive suggestions generated by electronic medical record data alone. The results found no difference between groups, suggesting that the addition of symptom information to computer-generated heart failure care suggestions did not improve physicians' treatment decisions or patients' outcomes (37).

Feedback

Feedback systems represent another strategy to improve adherence to guidelines. Feedback can be provided in many forms, but all involve providing physicians with data about the care they provide compared to others. The Regenstrief Medical Record System, described previously, has been used in multiple creative ways to provide feedback to physicians. Tierney and his colleagues compared the effects of supplying physicians with *monthly feedback reports* of their adherence to preventive-care guidelines with providing them *specific reminders* at the patients' visits (30). Both strategies had a positive effect on adherence to preventive-care protocols, but the effect of providing specific reminders was greater (30). Subsequently, this group evaluated whether displaying past test results would influence physician behavior (31). When intervention physicians ordered laboratory tests, a window opened that provided them with previous test results and the time interval between first and last test. Physicians were then asked whether they still wished to order a test. Presenting physicians with previous results reduced test ordering by 13% (32). In a later study, the investigators used predictive models derived from their own databases to determine whether displaying the probability that the next test would be positive changed physician behavior. After seeing the predicted probability of an abnormal test result, physicians were again asked whether they still wanted to order the test. The intervention group had a significant reduction in charges (9%) compared to the control group (32). In a subsequent investigation, these investigators also found that displaying charges for diagnostic tests significantly reduced the number and costs of tests ordered in the outpatient setting, especially during scheduled appointments (33). As with studies of computer reminders, when the intervention was discontinued, test ordering returned to baseline levels (33).

Feedback that provides comparison with national standards may not provide a useful goal or motivation for change. Kiefe and colleagues conducted a randomized controlled trial to evaluate "achievable benchmarks," that is, providing physicians with local rather than national averages to address potential differences in patients or practice settings (38). This innovative strategy used benchmarks that were attained by physicians within their practice; that is, they were achievable by their own colleagues. Physicians in the intervention group were given feedback on their performance in addition to information on their performance in relation to achievable benchmarks established by their peers. Physicians in the control group received feedback without information about the achievable benchmark. The achievable benchmark intervention resulted in a significant increase (33% to 57%) in appropriate care for diabetic patients as compared to controls (38).

Beyond these specific studies, Jamtvedt and colleagues performed a systematic review of feedback use for the Cochrane Collaboration, an international group that focuses on synthesizing up-to-date studies of health care interventions (39). Studies that used feedback in relation to guidelines or peers, or both, generally had a small, but positive, effect. The greatest effects were observed in situations where the baseline level of physician adherence was low (39). Davis et al. (17) described the effectiveness of feedback as greater than traditional continuing medical education, but less than academic detailing and opinion leaders. Of 24 studies, 10 had positive outcomes; the positive outcomes were associated with feedback delivered in the form of chart review (17). Greco and Eisenberg reviewed studies of feedback and found that whereas some feedback interventions did change physician behavior, others did not; few studies addressed patient outcomes (40). The authors attributed the relative failure of some feedback interventions to the physicians' belief that the process being assessed, such as drug prescribing, did not need to be changed. Additionally, the authors hypothesized that in cases where physicians felt unable to implement the appropriate change (a lack of self-efficacy barrier) in a timely manner, feedback was not effective in changing behavior (40).

Continuous Quality Improvement

Studies have consistently suggested that adherence to clinical-practice guidelines requires an organizational structure that promotes adherence (12, 15–17). Continuous quality improvement (CQI) is an approach that is rooted in industrial/management models. This approach suggests that achieving quality requires a continuous effort by all members of an organization to meet the needs and expectations of the customers. Once a specific quality problem is identified as important, appropriate organizational members plan and implement carefully conceived strategies and use empirical data to determine the effect of the strategy. Through these rapid "plan-do-study-act" cycles, there is a continuous effort to improve quality based on input from many members of the organization. Required elements of CQI include active managerial leadership for change, a focus on processes as the object of improvement, elimination of unnecessary variation, and revised strategies for personnel management. CQI principles have been used to increase physicians' adherence to clinical-practice guidelines (41).

There are two general approaches to evaluating any intervention, including CQI. One option is to use *nonexperimental* methods. That is, an organization (e.g., a hospital or health care system) introduces a CQI program and evaluates changes by making pre–post comparisons. As with any nonexperimental design, inferring causality is difficult. Some threats to making causal inferences include: (a) the possibility of a Hawthorne effect, that is, knowledge that the organization is being observed may change behavior; (b) history (influences other than the intervention may be causing observed changes), which threatens internal validity; (c) that generalizability may be limited, as such investigations often occur in atypical, highly motivated organizations.

Alternatively, one could conduct a *randomized trial* to evaluate the effectiveness of CQI programs. Philbin and his colleagues conducted a randomized trial to evaluate whether organizing and implementing a voluntary, regional, collaborative multihospital CQI program would result in more favorable changes in process and outcomes than usual care (42). They reported that their CQI intervention had a negligible effect on the care or outcomes (42). In another randomized trial, Solberg and his colleagues examined whether systems created by CQI intervention led to significantly higher rates of offering and performing preventive services; this CQI intervention also did not result in clinically important increases in preventive service delivery rates (43). Given that randomized trials are the gold standard by which to evaluate the effectiveness of interventions, are we to conclude that CQI is ineffective?

Before doing so, it is important to discuss the inherent problems associated with conducting randomized trials of CQI interventions (44). First, trials typically demand that the investigator provide a precise *specification of the intervention,* that is, defining exactly what was done, to whom, and with what frequency. CQI interventions cannot be specified with that precision. Instead, CQI is a management process and philosophy that offers principles to guide specific interventions. Second, there are issues related to the *target population.* In order to be enrolled in a trial of CQI, organizations will typically need to make commitments (e.g., identifying a local opinion leader who is provided the time and financial resources to implement the intervention). If randomized to the control group, one cannot assume that the organization will remain stagnant. Indeed, one can assume that the organization will take steps to implement quality improvement activities. To the extent this occurs, differences between the intervention and control groups will be small. Finally, the *duration* of a trial to evaluate a CQI program is likely to be quite long, and the costs may be prohibitive.

Thus, evaluating CQI programs involve trade-offs between trials and single-site studies. Difficulties in identifying comparable control groups make interpretation difficult. It is recommended that, when possible, multiple strategies are used to evaluate CQI initiatives. If results across complementary methods in different settings provide consistent results, conclusions about the effectiveness of CQI activities would be enhanced. An excellent example of such an approach attributed the high quality of care in the VA (Department of Veterans Affairs) to the quality improvement strategies the VA implemented (45).

Summary

Increasing physician adherence to clinical-practice guidelines is important to improve the quality and outcomes of care. Specific strategies, such as those described earlier, have been the subject of multiple literature syntheses. The consistent theme of these reviews is that increasing physician adherence is a complex issue with multiple barriers. Thus, efforts to overcome these barriers with single-component interventions are likely to be less effective than interventions that combine multiple strategies (7, 12, 15–17). For example, using local opinion leaders, CQI, and computer reminders may represent a cohesive and complementary package of strategies that would be very effective in increasing physician adherence to clinical-practice guidelines. From a research and policy perspective, evaluating multi-component interventions involves a trade-off. Though combining multiple interventions may be the most potent strategy, one will not be able to identify the single effective component. This is particularly important if certain components are expensive (e.g., a sophisticated electronic medical system) and health care systems wish to make resource allocation decisions based on the benefits relative to the marginal costs of a strategy.

CLINICAL, RESEARCH, AND POLICY IMPLICATIONS: CHALLENGES TO RESEARCHERS AND DECISION MAKERS

Physician adherence to clinical-practice guidelines is essential to improving the quality of care delivered and, ultimately, patient outcomes (46, 47). Clinical-practice guidelines are ubiquitous and are now considered part of the landscape in American medicine. Indeed, physician refusal accounts for a relatively small proportion of nonadherence to clinical-practice guidelines (48). However, to realize their benefits, investigators and decision makers interested in promoting physician adherence to these guidelines face some important issues.

One set of barriers that mitigate physician adherence is related to the guidelines themselves. To be accepted by physicians, guidelines must be clinically sensible, based on current empirical evidence, capture appropriate clinical nuances, and allow for flexibility and clinical judgment (47, 49). There must be strategies developed to ensure that current clinical-practice guidelines are maintained (13, 14). Health care systems should be allowed to take into account the local practice environment and patients when implementing national guidelines locally. To the extent that physicians view guidelines as impinging, rather than supporting, the care they deliver, they develop the attitudes that decrease the likelihood of adherence.

The more important barriers may be related to designing systems that foster adherence to clinical-practice guidelines. A key issue is how to disseminate effective strategies that improve adherence to guidelines into real-world practices (50). Some of the barriers that must be considered are outlined next.

Data Issues. The data required to assess adherence to clinical-practice guidelines are often lacking or difficult to access (e.g., clinical status), and the accuracy and validity of the data are unknown. Electronic medical records help, but are not the panacea. Furthermore, electronic medical record systems represent a sizable investment. Adding to the data-related concerns is the Health Insurance Portability and Accountability Act (HIPAA): HIPAA was enacted to provide national standards to protect the privacy of personal health information. These standards provide patients with access to their medical records and more control over how personal health information is used and disclosed. HIPAA provides guidance on how medical data can be shared, both on paper and electronically. The Institute of Medicine and other influential organizations advocate the centrality of electronic medical records to enhance quality of care, including adherence to clinical-practice guidelines. Although the technology may exist to allow physicians access to more complete clinical data upon which to make decisions (and adhere to clinical-practice guidelines), strategies must recognize any constraints imposed by HIPAA.

Incentives. There is a simultaneous increase in the demand on physicians to see more patients and do more in a visit. Implementing guidelines requires time, and current incentives do not support this. Thus, an important challenge is aligning incentives to support physicians' adherence to clinical-practice guidelines.

The Role of Patients. There are many who espouse increasing patients' involvement in care and empowering then to demand care that is consistent with clinical-practice guidelines. If this is correct, there is much work to be done. First, we must educate patients so that they understand what clinical-practice guidelines are. To the extent that report cards are based, in part, on adherence to clinical-practice guidelines, we must develop report cards that present data in a way that is understood by patients; unless patients are fully informed, it will be difficult for them to use report cards to find a physician and/or health care system that deliver high-quality care. Next, assuming they have identified a physician who delivers high-quality care (i.e., high adherence to clinical-practice guidelines), patients must understand that not all guidelines apply to all patients, and their clinical and demographic characteristics may influence whether their physicians adhere to a specific guideline to them. Assuming physicians adhere to guidelines, the system must identify strategies to overcome barriers (financial and otherwise) to ensure that patients can follow recommendations.

Legal Issues. The question of how clinical-practice guidelines can be used within the legal system is complex. On the one hand, clinical-practice guidelines are, by definition, intended to provide suggestions to physicians regarding the care they provide. There is some concern that they may be used in litigation when, perhaps, care was delivered that is not consistent with guidelines. However, this may be more of a theoretical concern than an actual one. If the data exist to drive the guideline, the guidelines can be used to show that a physician did the right things.

These are some of the many issues that clinicians, researchers, and decision makers will need to address as we search for effective ways to increase physician adherence to clinical-practice guidelines.

REFERENCES

1. Wennberg J. Dealing with medical practice variations: a proposal for action. *Health Aff Millwood.* 1984;3:271–297.

2. Wennberg JE, Gittelsohn A. Variations in medical care among small areas. *Sci Am.* 1982;246:120–134.

3. Woolf SH. Practice guidelines: a new reality in medicine: I: recent developments. *Arch Intern Med.* 1990;150:1811–1818.

4. Field MJ, Lohr KN, eds. *Clinical Practice Guidelines: Directions for a New Program.* Washington, DC: National Academy Press, 1990.

5. Woolf SH, Grol R, Hutchinson A, Eccles M, Grimshaw J. Potential benefits, limitations and harms of clinical guidelines. *BMJ.* 1999;18:527–530.

6. McGlynn EA, Asch SM, Adams J, et al. The quality of health care delivered to adults in the United States. *New Engl J Med.* 2003;348:2635–2645.

7. Woolf SH. Practice guidelines: a new reality in medicine: III: impact on patient care. *Arch Intern Med.* 1993;153:2646–2655.

8. Field MJ, Lohr KN. *Guidelines for Clinical Practice: From Development to Use.* Washington, DC: National Academy Press, 1992.

9. Shiffman RN, Shekelle P, Overhage JM, Slutsky J, Grimshaw J, Deshpande AM. Standardized reporting of clinical practice guidelines: a proposal from the conference on guideline standardization. *Ann Intern Med.* 2003;139:493–498.

10. Woolf SH. Practice guidelines: a new reality in medicine: II: methods of developing guidelines. *Arch Intern Med.* 1992;152:946–952.

11. Lohr KN, Eleazer K, Mauskopf J. Health policy issues and applications for evidence-based medicine and clinical practice guidelines. *Health Policy.* 1998;46: 1–19.

12. Cabana MD, Rand CS, Powe NR, et al. Why don't physicians follow clinical practice guidelines? A framework for improvement. *JAMA.* 1999;282:1458–1465.

13. Shekelle PG, Eccles MP, Grimshaw JM, Woolf SH. When should clinical guidelines be updated? *BMJ.* 2001;323:155–157.

14. Shekelle PG, Ortiz E, Rhodes S, et al. Validity of the Agency for Healthcare Research and Quality clinical guidelines: how quickly do guidelines become outdated? *JAMA.* 2001;286:1461–1467.

15. Davis DA, Taylor-Vaisey A. Translating guidelines into practice: a systematic review of theoretic concepts, practical experience and research evidence in the adoption of clinical practice guidelines. *Can Med Assoc J.* 1997;157:408–416.

16. Davis DA, Thomson MA, Oxman AD, Haynes RB. Evidence for the effectiveness of CME: a review of 50 randomized controlled trials. *JAMA.* 1992;268:1111–1117.

17. Davis DA, Thomson MA, Oxman AD, Haynes RB. Changing physician performance: a systematic review of the effect of continuing medical education strategies. *JAMA.* 1995;274:700–705.

18. Soumerai SB, Avorn J. Principles of educational outreach (academic detailing) to improve clinical decision making. *JAMA.* 1990;263:549–556.

19. Avorn J, Soumerai SB. Improving drug-therapy decisions through educational outreach. A randomized controlled trial of academically based "detailing." *N Engl J Med.* 1983;308:1457–1463.

20. Solomon DH, Van Houten L, Glynn RJ, et al. Academic detailing to improve use of broad-spectrum antibiotics at an academic medical center. *Arch Intern Med.* 2001;161:1897–1902.

21. Soumerai SB, McLaughlin TJ, Gurwitz JH, Guadagnoli E, Hauptman PJ, Borbas C. Effect of local medical opinion leaders on quality of care for acute myocardial infarction. *JAMA.* 1998;279:1358–1363.

22. Hunt DL, Haynes RB, Hanna SE, Smith K. Effects of computer-based clinical decision support systems on physician performance and patient outcomes: a systematic review. *JAMA.* 1998;280:1339–1346.

23. McDonald CJ, Blevins L, Tierney WM, Martin DK. The Regenstrief Medical Records. *MD Computing.* 1988;5:34–47.

24. McDonald CJ, Tierney WM, Martin DK, Overhage JM. The Regenstrief Medical Record System: 20 years' experience in hospital outpatient clinics and neighborhood health centers. *MD Computing.* 1992;9:206–217.

25. Haynes RB, Walker CJ. Computer-aided quality assurance: a critical appraisal. *Arch Intern Med.* 1987;147:1297–1301.

26. Johnson ME, Langton KB, Haynes RB, Mathieu A. Effects of computer-based clinical decision support systems on clinician performance and patient outcome: a critical appraisal. *Ann Intern Med.* 1994;120:135–142.

27. McDonald CJ, Hui SL, Smith DL, et al. Reminders from an introspective medical record: a two-year randomized trial. *Ann Intern Med.* 1984;100:130–138.

28. Overhage JM, Tierney WM, McDonald CJ. Computer reminders to implement preventive care guidelines for hospitalized patients. *Arch Intern Med.* 1996;156: 1551–1556.

29. Dexter PR, Perkins S, Overhage JM, Maharry K, Kohler RB, McDonald CJ. A computerized reminder system to increase the use of preventive care for hospitalized patients. *New Engl J Med.* 2001;345:965–970.

30. Tierney WM, Hui SL, McDonald CJ. Delayed feedback of physician performance versus immediate reminders to perform preventive care: effects on physician compliance. *Med Care.* 1986;24:659–666.

31. Tierney WM, McDonald CJ, Martin DK, Hui SL, Rogers MP. Computerized display of past test results: effects on outpatient testing. *Ann Intern Med.* 1987;107: 569–574.

32. Tierney WM, McDonald CJ, Hui SL, Martin DK. Computer predictions of abnormal test results: effects on outpatient testing. *JAMA.* 1988;259:1194–1196.

33. Tierney WM, Miller ME, McDonald CJ. The effect on test ordering of informing physicians of the charges for outpatient diagnostic tests. *New Engl J Med.* 1990;233:1499–1504.

34. Tierney WM, Overhage JM, Takesue BY, et al. Computerizing guidelines to improve care and patient outcomes: the example of heart failure. *J Am Med Inform Assoc.* 1995;2:316–322.

35. Tierney WM, Overhage JM, McDonald CJ. Toward electronic medical records that improve care. *Ann Intern Med.* 1995;122:725–726.

36. Steinberg EP. Improving the quality of care—can we practice what we preach? *N Engl J Med.* 2003;348:2681–2683.

37. Subramanian U, Fihn SD, Weinberger M, et al. A controlled trial of including symptom data in computer-based care suggestions for managing chronic heart failure. *Am J Med.* 2004;116(6):375–384.

38. Kiefe CI, Allison JJ, Williams OD, Peson SD, Weaver MT, Weissman NW. Improving quality improvements using achievable benchmarks for physician feedback: a randomized controlled trial. *JAMA.* 2001;285:2871–2879.

39. Jamtvedt G, Young JM, Kristoffersen DT, Thomson O'Brien MA, Oxman AD. Audit and feedback: effects on professional practice and health care outcomes. *Cochrane Database Syst Rev.* 2003;3:CD000259.

40. Greco PJ, Eisenberg JM. Changing physicians' practices. *New Engl J Med.* 1993; 329:1271–1274.

41. Kritchevsky SB, Simmons BP. Continuous quality improvement: concepts and applications for physician care. *JAMA.* 1991;266:1817–1823.

42. Philbin EF, Rocco TA, Lindenmuth NW, Ulrich K, McCall M, Jenkins PL. The results of a randomized trial of quality improvement in the care of patients with heart failure. *Am J Med.* 2001;109:443–449.

43. Solberg LI, Kottke TE, Brekke ML, et al. Failure of a continuous quality improvement intervention to increase the delivery of preventive services: a randomized trial. *Effective Clin Pract.* 2000;3:105–115.

44. Samsa G, Matchar D. Can continuous quality improvement be assessed using randomized trials? *Health Serv Res.* 2000;35:687–700.

45. Jha AK, Perlin JB, Kizer KW, Dudley RA. Effect of the transformation of the Veterans Affairs health care system on the quality of care. *New Engl J Med.* 2003;348: 2218–2227.

46. Grimshaw J. Effect of clinical guidelines on medical practice: a systematic review of rigorous evaluations. *Lancet.* 1993;342:1317–1322.

47. Grimshaw J, Russell I. Achieving health gain through clinical guidelines. I: developing scientifically valid guidelines. *Qual Health Care.* 1993;2:243–248.

48. Ellrodt AG, Conner L, Riedinger M, Weingarten S. Measuring and improving physician compliance with clinical practice guidelines. *Ann Intern Med.* 1995; 122:277–282.

49. Katz DA. Barriers between guidelines and improved patient care: an analysis of AHCPR's unstable angina clinical practice guidelines. *Health Serv Res.* 1999;34: 377–390.

50. Grimshaw J, Russell I. Achieving health gain through clinical guidelines. II: ensuring guidelines change medical practice. *Qual Health Care.* 1994;3:45–52.

Part IV

METHODOLOGICAL ISSUES AND TREATMENT ADHERENCE

Treatment Adherence at the Community Level: Moving Toward Mutuality and Participatory Action

Alice Ammerman
Mansoureh Tajik

There have been dramatic advances in our knowledge regarding the treatment and prevention of many chronic diseases such as obesity, diabetes, heart disease, and various forms of cancer. However, the rates of many of these illnesses continue to rise, particularly among minority and vulnerable populations(1–4). There is a considerable gap between the findings from efficacy studies of interventions targeting many of those chronic diseases and the findings from effectiveness studies (5, 6). Treatment and prevention programs with high efficacy in a tightly controlled clinical trial with strict inclusion/exclusion criteria and significant resources for implementation are often ineffective when tested under real-world circumstances. Some researchers attribute this ineffectiveness to reluctance or inability of individuals to properly and thoroughly follow the recommendations of the medical and public health professionals, a phenomenon generally known as noncompliance or nonadherence (7). Others consider the inability of the health care system and our broader sociopolitical culture to adequately reach and affect over time the behaviors, organizations, and policies that facilitate compliance or adherence as the cause of the failure (8, 9).

We begin with reviewing some of the current semantics in the field of intervention adherence before we introduce a more comprehensive community-based model. *Compliance* is generally defined as the extent to which the patient's or the targeted population's behavior corresponds to medical or health advice (10). *Adherence* has come to reflect a greater degree of mutual responsibility between the provider and patient (11). Still, both terms assume primarily an individual-level interaction and fail to consider the broader ecologic influences on both patient and provider behaviors (7, 12). Here, we argue for an additional semantic progression in the field of treatment adherence. We recommend borrowing the term *mutuality* from the literature regarding patient–provider interactions to describe a truly equal relationship and distribution of power between recipient(s) and provider(s) of health care and intervention programs. In this context, the recipient of an intervention may be an individual patient, a group of people sharing similar characteristics, or a community. We would also argue that the definition of provider be extended to a much wider field of players including public health professionals and organizations as well as community advocates. In addition, we suggest the notion of mutuality be extended throughout all facets of interaction, from identification and prioritization of health concerns, to decision making regarding treatment plans, to implementation, to outcome evaluation and treatment plan revision. In this capacity, we make the assumption that the recipients of health care and intervention programs have expert knowledge about their existing capabilities (e.g., economic capability—to be able to afford a given treatment) and context (e.g., community characteristics and the built environment—access to healthy food and opportunities for physical activity) and the providers have the expert knowledge about available, effective, and appropriate treatment options that correspond to the recipients' particular circumstances and needs.

In light of the vital role of the community in creating healthier environments, we recommend the term *participatory action* to describe a more ecological approach to treatment adherence. We believe this approach will help the field of adherence evolve from focusing mainly on the individual patient as the source of nonadherence toward a collective responsibility for change.

This chapter primarily addresses initiating and maintaining community-level lifestyle modification in the areas of nutrition and physical activity, crossing various age groups. Our focus on lifestyle intervention is due to the fact that obesity has now reached epidemic proportions. Although there are a number of unique aspects to lifestyle interventions, many of the issues related to nutrition and physical activity should be applicable to adherence in a number of other health domains. The current chapter differs from chapters 3 (exercise) and 4 (diet) in that three theoretical frameworks are presented that consider adherence at multiple levels of a continuum rather than exclusively at the individual level. They are the socioecologic framework, the RE-AIM model, and Community-Based Participatory Research (CBPR). As such, the frameworks have implications not only for the design and conduct of treatment and intervention programs but also for how we study the relevant processes.

First, the socioecologic framework provides a multilevel model that describes impact on individual and group behaviors at various levels of influence: individual (intra- and interpersonal) level, organizational level, community and environmental level, and finally policy level. Moving "upstream" from individual- to policy-level influences, the model increasingly addresses the role of factors outside traditional "patient compliance" that have a significant impact on whether an individual, a group, or a community is able to follow an intervention plan.

Second, the RE-AIM model, developed by Glasgow and colleagues (6, 13), addresses translation of "proven" interventions to everyday settings. This model integrates the elements of *reach* (proportion of the intended population participating in the intervention program), *efficacy or effectiveness* (success rate of the program if implemented), *adoption* (proportion of delivery organizations adopting the intervention), *implementation* (extent to which the intervention is delivered as intended), and *maintenance* (sustainability of the intervention over time). RE-AIM provides a framework to identify the gaps between efficacy and effectiveness and raises questions about the most appropriate intervention design strategies to advance the field of adherence.

Third, Community-Based Participatory Research (CBPR) is an approach to study conceptualization, design, implementation, and impact that engages communities and researchers in a collaborative process designed to reach a broader population more effectively and have a meaningful and sustainable impact on adherence at multiple levels over time (14). Implemented properly, CBPR culminates in participatory action to directly implement research findings at all levels of the socioecologic framework and shift the balance toward a shared responsibility for change.

THE SOCIOECOLOGIC MODEL—INTERSECTING INFLUENCES

Bosworth (7) describes the need for an ecological approach to adherence, arguing that "treatment adherence research has typically neglected to consider the multiple layers of the patients' social context and its influence on their treatment adherence." The socioecologic model (SEM) developed by McLeroy and others (15) considers influences on health-related behaviors ranging from individual-level attitudes, beliefs, and behaviors to policy influences. However, in the adherence literature, this still assumes primarily a unidirectional approach, evaluated by the degree to which the behavior of patients or study participants corresponds to medical advice or treatment.

The socioecologic framework considers the multiple layers of intersecting influence between patients, providers, communities, and the health

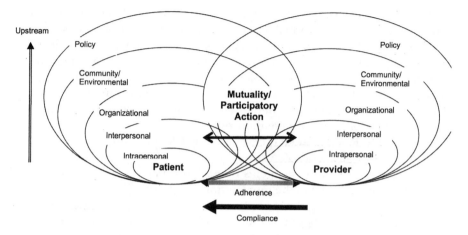

FIG. 13.1. Intersecting socioecologic frameworks.

care system. Figure 13.1 illustrates such a framework, beginning at the intrapersonal level where individual-level factors such as patient knowledge, attitudes, and behaviors interface with provider characteristics, such as counseling skill, cultural competence, or personal biases about health behaviors or patient characteristics (e.g., a provider's lack of tolerance for obese patients).

Intrapersonal Factors and Adherence

The intra- and interpersonal levels of the socioecological model are inextricably related and have generally been addressed more fully in the adherence literature. However, some of these factors are rooted in broader societal influences and norms and thus can be influenced at a more "upstream" level of the model. For example, health literacy has been shown to influence adherence to a variety of medical therapies (16, 17). Low literacy skills can be viewed either as a "characteristic" of an individual patient or as a broader social factor that must be considered by the health care system. Numerous studies demonstrate a wide gap between the literacy level required to comprehend health education materials and the reading level of most patients seeking health care (18). Other studies show that the majority of health education materials are written at a level above the average reading level of the U.S. population (19). In this case, a systematic approach to producing educational tools that accommodate limited literacy skills, and thus meet the needs of the majority of the population, would seem the best course of action to take in order to improve adherence.

Similarly, gender and racial concordance between patient and provider has been associated with improved health outcomes and adherence, presumably due to increased cultural sensitivity and improved communication (20). Matching patients with providers of similar gender and ethnicity is not a practical solution, but including diversity training for individuals and health care organizations has the potential for broader and more long-term societal benefits. In a study by Ammerman and colleagues (21), physicians and nurses serving predominantly lower income patient populations reported very limited confidence in the likelihood that their patients would respond to counseling by improving dietary and physical-activity practices related to cardiovascular disease prevention (21, 22). Provided with culturally relevant and literacy-appropriate tools, however, many providers reported an increase in their counseling self-efficacy as well as greater confidence in the willingness of their patients to adhere to lifestyle recommendations. The adherence factors in this case could be described at the intrapersonal level as factors associated with patient "compliance" but also associated with provider counseling confidence and skill. On the other hand, this could be considered an issue at the organizational or policy level if one considers that health care training and delivery systems must support practitioners in meeting the needs of patients from diverse backgrounds.

Interpersonal Factors and Adherence

The interpersonal level of the socioecological model is defined by interactions among individual patients, providers, and other members of the patients' social network. Moving to the interpersonal level, there is a growing literature in patient–provider communication that links characteristics of this therapeutic relationship with health outcomes (see ref. 23 and chap. 11, this volume).

Roter and Hall describe four archetypal forms of doctor–patient relationships: paternalism, consumerism, mutuality, and default, reflecting combinations of high and low patient and physician control (24). Paternalism represents high physician control and low patient control. Whereas this can be beneficial in times of severe illness, it is less likely to empower individuals to take responsibility for their own health. The opposite of paternalism is consumerism, where patients challenge unilateral decision making by the provider and take a much more active, if not directive, role in health care decisions. Mutuality is a more moderate alternative than the two extremes of paternalism and consumerism, where the power relationship is more equal and decisions are made jointly. As stated earlier, the term mutuality may serve to best describe the next logical linguistic step in the evolution of the term compliance to adherence. Figure 13.1 illustrates through the direction and width of the arrows how this progression moves to a more balanced position of communication and authority between patient and provider. Mutuality reflects a greater interface between the socioecologic influences on both the patient and provider, ultimately leading to the potential for participatory action to address health concerns as described more in later sections.

Other interpersonal relationships can have an important influence on medical regimen adherence or more general health promotion advice as well. In the church environment, for example, it is well known that "pleasing the pastor" with one's cooking is a desired outcome. In the PRAISE! project, a National Cancer Institute–funded study, 60 African American churches were included in the design to reduce cancer risk through dietary change (25). The participants indicated that (a) being known as a good cook was more important than all other domestic skills, (b) pastors were among those individuals that participants most desired to please with their cooking, and (c) whereas pastors frequently complimented good cooks among the parishioners, few made a point of commending them for preparing healthier foods. Health Promotion Workshops for Pastors were part of the study intervention, where pastors role-played offering compliments for healthier dishes without offending those bringing the traditional foods. At the end of the study, participants reported an increase in pastor support for bringing healthy foods to church functions (25). Though it is impossible to sort out the effect of this interpersonal dynamic relative to other components of the intervention, one could imagine a positive impact on adherence to dietary change advice.

Organizational Factors and Adherence

Organizational factors associated with the patient's school, work, or faith-based organizations also have the potential to influence treatment adherence. We have already mentioned a number of organizational influences on adherence in the context of what may first appear as inter- or intrapersonal factors, such as the example in an earlier section regarding increased counseling self-efficacy/confidence of physicians and nurses serving predominantly lower income patient populations when supplied by their organization with appropriate counseling tools. Organizational factors may either support or diminish an individual's ability to adopt and maintain medical or lifestyle change regimens that improve health outcomes.

In *schools*, controversy exists about the selling of soft drinks, unhealthy snacks, and other foods that contribute to the national epidemic of obesity. A recent survey of pediatricians revealed that 76% of the responding doctors identify the school food environment and 74% cite the school physical-exercise environment as significant barriers to obesity management (26). Not surprisingly, facing these obstacles, 85% of responding pediatricians reported they felt significantly less able to manage obesity than asthma, and 80% reported less ability to manage obesity than attention-deficit hyperactivity disorder. Clearly, the organizational environment and policies of the school can have an impact on the patient's ability to comply with the provider's recommendations and indirectly interferes with the provider's ability to successfully deliver the counseling guidance recommended by their professional organizations. Focusing only on the pediatrician or child fails to recognize broader socioecologic influences on treatment adherence. Figure 13.2 illustrates the complex set of factors influencing a child's dietary behaviors and attitudes, where parental and environmental influences may directly and indirectly outweigh the influence of the pediatric office or primary-care provider in the more traditional adherence relationship.

At the *work site*, a number of intervention studies have been developed and tested that use organizational-level change to promote healthier lifestyles in hopes of preventing chronic disease that can result in significant health insurance costs to the company. A common theme derived from these workplace projects includes the need for a multilevel strategy (27). Baranowski and colleagues emphasize that obesity prevention and control efforts will be most successful when they are theoretically driven and address multiple levels of the socioecologic framework (28). Work sites can be thought of as small "communities" where interventions are possible at various levels, including: intrapersonal (individual employee health), interpersonal (employee–supervisor, employee–coworker relations), organizational (social and

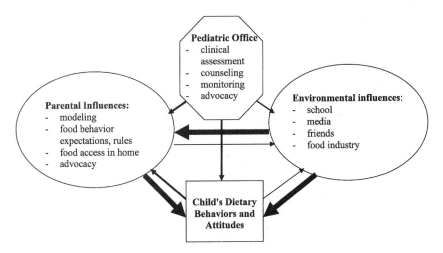

FIG. 13.2. Influences on adherence to pediatrician advice: overweight children. From ref. 50. Copyright 2005 by Mosby. Adapted by permission.

physical environment, work practices/policies), community (organizational–community linkages), and policy (policies internal or external to the workplace that influence worker health).

Work site interventions may address the social environment (norms, culture, and networks), physical environment (facilities, structures or systems such as cafeterias, fitness facilities, etc.), or policy (internal to organization or external/societal). They may encourage healthy diet and activity behaviors by promoting access to safe physical-activity opportunities and/or access to healthy foods. Biener and colleagues found that work site environments with greater numbers of healthy foods, better labeling of food content, and improved employee awareness of these healthy changes were associated with self-reported changes in better eating habits (e.g., eating lower fat and high-fiber foods) (29).

As an example of the influence of the work environment on adherence to recommendations for increased physical activity, in some work sites, stairwells have been made more appealing by adding artwork, carpeting, and piped-in music. This, along with promotional campaigns to use the steps, resulted in a significant increase in stairwell over elevator use (30). One could imagine that an employee at this work site would have more opportunities for success in adhering to her physician's recommendations to get more exercise.

Regarding primary health care organizations, there is a growing body of literature on system-level change in primary-care practices that can support a wide variety of clinical and preventive interventions (31). A practice as simple as routinely documenting and plotting body mass index (BMI) in a pediatric patient's chart can alert the provider to weight trends that may raise concerns about obesity risk. Similarly, office support staff reinforcing simple messages about healthy eating and exercise can supplement the 7–10 minutes most providers have for an entire patient visit. Again, a failure to recognize these organizational factors in the "adherence equation" is likely to lead to ineffective efforts to improve health outcomes.

Community/Environmental Factors and Adherence

Although they are less often examined in the context of treatment adherence, community and environmental factors greatly influence the potential for treatment adherence. Community influences on adherence to healthy diet and physical activity are two areas that have received recent attention. Some research has addressed the impact of residential proximity to exercise facilities on levels of physical activity (32). The presence of neighborhood trails and general access to places for exercise has been positively associated with physical-activity levels (33). In addition, there is evidence of a strong association between distribution of food stores and income, with greater access to healthy foods (particularly fresh fruits and vegetables) in higher socioeconomic status communities (34, 35).

Many factors in the community environment can impact the degree to which community members of all age groups adhere to dietary and physical activity recommendations that lead to a healthier lifestyle. For example, though many communities provide services through a parks and recreation department, programming generally emphasizes competitive sports, ranging from basketball in the winter to baseball in the spring. Often absent are affordable and diverse programs that appeal to youth of both genders, or to those who may not be confident of their athletic abilities, and thus are probably at greatest risk for inactivity and consequently obesity. Because these services are created to meet the needs of local taxpayers, lobbying local community members, organizations, and public health professionals for alternative programming can support the efforts of local pediatricians and family physicians who are urging their patients to be more physically active. It is difficult for the overweight child to adhere to such a recommendation when few opportunities in the community meet their needs.

Similarly, public schools represent a shared community resource, and could be used much more effectively to promote physical activity outside of the traditional school day and population. In many cities, schools are opening their tracks and gyms to the broader community during nonschool times, providing exercise opportunities for those who can not afford a health club membership. Again, health care providers might have more impact on adherence to exercise recommendations by advocating for the opening of these facilities.

Policy Factors and Adherence

The emerging field of policy and environmental change has been spawned, in part, by the frustration of public health and health care professionals with their inability to influence meaningful lifestyle change required to stem the tide of many of the chronic diseases that are the leading causes of death in the United States. The ultimate goal of environmental and policy change is to make the environment more conducive to adopting healthier lifestyles—to make it easier for an individual to make healthier choices. For example, to facilitate adherence to exercise recommendations among those living in high-traffic or high-crime neighborhoods, it may be most effective to pass a local ordinance for traffic-calming mechanisms and security at local parks. Similarly, rather than rely on intensive nutrition education programs in schools, it may be more useful to support the school lunch program at a level that allows school cafeterias to "take risks" in terms of introducing healthier food choices.

Too often, individuals and communities perceive policy-level change as unattainable and influenced only by those in legislative positions. However, micro or macro policy change can be implemented all along the socio-ecologic continuum and is within the grasp of individuals and community organizations. At the most downstream level, family policy may take the form of household "rules" requiring equal time spent in active play as on the computer or watching television. Moving to organizational-level policy examples, some churches involved in the PRAISE! project (25) implemented an informal church policy to serve water at all church functions and, though not eliminating fried chicken, agreed to serve smaller pieces of chicken at the *end* of the buffet line. In this way, plates were full of healthier foods, leaving limited room for the fried chicken.

Similarly, work site health and wellness committees are more common and have begun working with the organization's leadership to implement policies regarding flex time for exercise as well as healthier food options available at staff meetings and in vending machines. Policies for incentive and benefits packages can reinforce healthier lifestyles by rewarding those who quit smoking or maintain a healthy weight.

Policies at a more macro level can affect the "built environment" (structural factors that can affect a person's behavior that are physically external to that person) to mandate zoning and development approaches that facilitate more physical activity through traffic-calming mechanisms, sidewalks, and neighborhood designs laid out in grid patterns rather than cul de sacs, which tend to discourage walking for transportation. In a study by Eyler and Vest (36), six focus groups were conducted with women age 20–50 years who were not currently regular exercisers. Women reported that the environmental and policy barriers such as lack of access to places to exercise and safety concerns had a strong impact on their physical activity level. In a cross-sectional study conducted from 1999 to 2000 among U.S. adults, neighborhood characteristics such as the presence of sidewalks, enjoyable scenery, and slower traffic speeds were positively associated with physical activity (37).

To address nutrition, some municipal areas are now deciding to subsidize grocery stores in lower income neighborhoods based on the epidemiologic evidence that individuals in these communities have significantly less access to good-quality fruits and vegetables, low-fat milk, and other food products deemed important to a healthy diet. Community gardens are another venue where nutrition and physical activity are enhanced. In California Healthy Cities and Communities, for example, cities have enacted policies for interim land and complimentary water use and ultimately improved access to fresh produce through community garden initiatives (38).

There is much opportunity at the state and national level to implement and enforce standards regarding foods served in schools, but the economic and political "will" must be behind these policies. In 1994, regulatory changes proposed by the U.S. Department of Agriculture promised to bring progressive changes to school meals. However, lobbying by interest groups resulted in substantial changes to the final rule. A retrospective analysis of the federal school meals policymaking process during 1992 to 1996 demonstrated a strong influence by the interest groups in affecting the shape, pace, and direction of the policy (39). Although this may seem far removed from adherence by an individual overweight child to the dietary recommendations of their doctor, the influence can be significant.

A common thread through all the policy options just described is that each of these policies ultimately increases the likelihood that an individual can "adhere" to recommendations from a health care provider to improve their diet and exercise habits. The effects of any one policy on any individual are likely to be too small to measure, but collectively they can make a difference.

THE RE-AIM MODEL: TRANSLATING THEORY INTO PRACTICE

In an effort to diminish the translation gap between research and public health practice, Glasgow and colleagues have developed a model challenging the assumption that effective real-world interventions logically and seamlessly flow from efficacy studies (13, 40, 41). They define efficacy studies as intensive, specialized interventions designed to maximize effect size in highly standardized and controlled studies. In contrast, effectiveness studies involve brief, feasible interventions not requiring great expertise to deliver and adaptable to a variety of settings. The RE-AIM model (Table 13.1) places responsibility on the larger public health system to assure that interventions are designed appropriately for the intended audience, delivered through systems and channels with the greatest potential for reaching this audience (**R**each), are evidence and theory based to maximize likelihood of success (**E**fficacy/**E**ffectiveness), can be adopted by a variety of organizations and implemented as designed (**A**doption, **I**mplementation), and are designed for long-term maintenance of positive impact (**M**aintenance). The RE-AIM model shifts the burden of responsibility for adherence from the individual alone to the interface of that individual with the design and delivery system of the intervention. Table 13.1 describes in detail the five RE-AIM components and how they compare across efficacy and effectiveness studies. Table 13.2 offers a fictitious example of the dissemination of a "magic diet pill" to illustrate how even an intervention as desirable as this may become an "adherence failure" due to the combined effects of limited reach, adoption, implementation, and maintenance, even though it

TABLE 13.1
RE-AIM Model and Characteristics of Components
in Efficacy and Effectiveness Studies

RE-AIM Component	Description	Efficacy Studies	Effectiveness Studies
Reach	Proportion of the target population that participated in the intervention	Homogeneous, highly motivated sample; exclude those with complications, other comorbid problems	Broad, heterogeneous, representative sample: often from a defined population re ethnicity, gender, and so on
Efficacy or effectiveness	Success rate if implemented as in guidelines; defined as positive outcomes minus negative outcomes	Intensive, specialized interventions that attempt to maximize effect size; highly standardized, randomized designs	Brief, feasible interventions not requiring great expertise; adaptable to setting; randomized, time series, or quasi-experimental designs
Adoption	Proportion of settings, practices, and plans that will adopt this intervention	Often one setting to reduce variability; settings with many resources and expert staff	Appeal to and work in multiple settings; able to be adapted to fit setting
Implementation	Extent to which the intervention is implemented as intended in the real world	Implemented by research staff closely following a specific protocol	Implemented by variety of different staff with competing demands, using adapted protocol
Maintenance	Extent to which a program is sustained over time	Few or no issues; focus on individual level	Major issues; setting-level maintenance is as important as individual-level maintenance

Note. From ref. 48. Copyright 2003. Adapted with permission from Elsevier.

is effective in 50% of the population who use it (high by most diet therapy standards). Table 13.2 presents a systemwide failure versus a failure of the individual pill taker alone.

Reach

The reach component of RE-AIM refers to the proportion of the target population that participates in the intervention. As illustrated in the diet pill model, Reach starts with the ability to engage the health care system and providers in the process of intervention delivery. In this case, the pa-

TABLE 13.2
Stages of Translating an Efficacious Program
Into Real-World Settings: Example

The Magic Diet Pill		
Dissemination Step	*RE-AIM Concept*	*Cumulative "Adherence"*
50% of Clinics use	Adoption	50%
50% of Clinicians prescribe	Adoption	25%
50% of patients accept medication	Reach	12.6%
50% follow regimen correctly	Implementation	6.2%
50% of those taking correctly benefit	Effectiveness	3.2%
50% continue to benefit after 6 months	Maintenance	1.6%

Note. From ref. 49. Copyright 2004. Adapted with permission from Elsevier.

tient has no potential to adhere, and cannot be "reached" unless the clinics and clinicians have first adopted the intervention. Many efficacy studies, by nature of exclusion criteria and recruitment approaches, include a primarily homogeneous and highly motivated sample with few medical problems other than the specific health concern being studied. In reality, however, most patients receiving clinical care or desiring to take the "magic diet pill" are likely to be very heterogeneous, significantly less motivated, and face multiple interrelated health problems. It is easy to see how adherence rates plummet when moving from the efficacy to effectiveness level.

Adoption/Implementation

Before either the provider or the patient can implement a treatment approach or intervention, the organization or setting that brings them together must make a commitment to implement it. Increasingly, practitioners have available evidence reviews from the U.S. Preventive Services Task Force Guide to Clinical Services and the parallel Guide to Community Services from CDC. The evidence-based recommendations of health professional organizations are often generated from these reviews and disseminated to the relevant health care providers. Unfortunately, however, adoption of such guidelines is far from universal (26) and often requires substantial commitment from health care agencies to provide the necessary resources or allow time for the providers to implement them.

As an example of the difficulties of adopting guidelines, in a recent study, Perrin and colleagues (26) tested the degree to which primary-care pediatricians' use of body mass index (BMI) screening charts would result in a greater likelihood of identifying obesity or risk for obesity among patients. Few pediatricians reported using BMI screening charts, but those who did were more likely to correctly identify a weight concern. Currently the American Academy of Pediatrics (AAP) recommends BMI assessment on an annual basis (42). Although the survey by Perrin was conducted just prior to this recommendation, subsequent qualitative data collection reveals many office-based barriers to assessing BMI despite the AAP recommendations. Often the BMI charts are not available, there is no simple tool provided to calculate or plot BMI, and it is difficult to interpret the results to patients and families. Perhaps the most significant barriers reported, however, are that providers feel they have virtually nothing to offer families of patients who are identified as obese, and if they did, there would be no reimbursement for such services.

Where does the responsibility lie for a child's obesity? With the family that faces many environmental forces encouraging unhealthy eating and a sedentary lifestyle? With the pediatrician who does not have the time or resources to offer screening and treatment? With the clinic that does not consistently provide these resources? With the public health and research communities that have been unable to identify and translate key intervention strategies? With the health care insurance system that fails to recognize obesity as a significant health problem for which intervention services should be reimbursed? Of course, all of these parties bear some responsibility, but it is clear that adherence by the child and family to provider recommendations is a small piece of the puzzle, especially when one factors in socioecologic influences beyond the health care system.

Efficacy or Effectiveness

The efficacy or effectiveness component of RE-AIM measures the success rate of interventions if implemented as intended by practice guidelines, and represents positive minus negative outcomes. Efficacy studies are often designed in a way to greatly facilitate adherence at both the organization and individual level. Unfortunately, however, these approaches are rarely translatable in the real-world environment of effectiveness studies, so we often see a dramatic drop in effect sizes of the outcome measures. In other words, though a certain approach to lifestyle modification may appear highly effective when reported in the scientific literature or popular press, the average member of the community is likely to receive substantially less benefit.

The fact that efficacy studies are far more successful in impacting health outcomes than effectiveness or community-based studies raises the question of whether participants in efficacy studies are more "compliant" with the treatment than those in effectiveness studies. Are more "compliant" individuals more willing to be recruited and participate in efficacy studies? Are interventions tested in efficacy studies better designed to overcome the usual barriers to compliance? Perhaps both are true. Often, however, adherence research fails to recognize that the study design may contribute to the answer as much as the interaction between patient and provider.

There have been many successful interventions to improve treatment adherence for specific diseases. For example, high-tech pocket devices have increased the degree to which complex pharmacologic regimens are followed by HIV-positive patients by prompting them to take medications at the proper time. In an investigational study of an HIV adherence device, it was demonstrated that the device can keep patients on track with their antiretroviral therapy more effectively than a monthly educational session. The pocket-size device, called the Disease Management Assistance System, electronically tells patients when to take their medications and what side effects to monitor (43). Similarly, in the Diabetes Prevention Program (DPP) (44), study participants had extensive one-on-one counseling by trained therapist, participated in frequently held group sessions, and were assigned the equivalent of a personal trainer to monitor their progress and troubleshoot as needed (44). As a result, the lifestyle intervention reduced the development of diabetes by 58% (44). Though some of these innovations can be translated into everyday patient care, few individuals can afford an expensive electronic device to remind them to take their pills and even fewer can afford a personal trainer at the level of time required for the DPP study. However, there are promising recent developments among federal funding agencies recognizing the gap between research and practice. There are now a few entire study sections at the National Institutes of Health devoted to translational research. A paper by Garfield et al. (45), for example, quotes Allen Spiegel, director of the National Institute of Diabetes and Digestive and Kidney Diseases (NIDDK), as saying, "NIDDK's mission is to conduct and support research on diseases such as diabetes in order to increase knowledge to improve the public's health. NIDDK's goals will not be completely achieved until the knowledge gained from the research it supports is translated and fully applied."

Maintenance

Even with the best of efforts and support by a health care agency to adopt and implement an approach to lifestyle intervention, rarely are these interventions able to help individuals maintain positive lifestyle changes over time even if initially successful. Part of the problem is that maintenance interventions are almost always focused at the downstream or individual level. Few children can maintain weight loss resulting from an intensive clinical program in the face of constant availability of high-calorie, low-nutrient-dense foods and ever more limited opportunities to build physical activity into everyday living. Most intervention programs last for a fixed number of visits or weeks and participants commonly relapse after that point. The Ushaped weight curve almost seems inevitable. Once again, the likelihood of maintaining positive lifestyle change, or longer term adherence, is highly dependent on a multitude of other factors along the socioecologic chain as well as the degree to which interventions are designed to account for these factors, as described in the RE-AIM model.

COMMUNITY-BASED PARTICIPATORY RESEARCH: AN APPROACH TO ENHANCING MUTUALITY AND PARTICIPATORY ACTION

Improving adherence requires not only development and implementation of treatment approaches to increase the likelihood of individuals and populations performing the health behaviors intended, but also improved research strategies to correctly identify the factors that affect these behaviors. There is growing interest in various methods of participatory research, now generally described by the term *community-based participatory research* or CBPR. By involving research participants in the design and conduct of the study, there are a number of potential benefits to the quality of the research as well as increased likelihood that the research will result in adherence-promoting strategies that are well designed for the population being served (14).

The authors of a recent systematic evidence review describe CBPR as: (a) colearning and reciprocal transfer of expertise by all research partners, (b) shared decision-making power, and (c) mutual ownership of the process and products of the research enterprise (46). The end result of CBPR is application of the knowledge gained to social or political action designed to positively influence health outcomes. If conducted as intended, CBPR benefits participants and researchers, enhancing the conduct and validity of the research as well as its impact on health outcomes. Table 13.3 describes the critical elements of CBPR, ranging from assembling the research team to manuscript writing and translating research findings into health action. Application of each element has the potential to bring benefits to the community as well as the researcher. Potential research challenges presented by this relatively innovative approach are also described.

Assembling a Research Partnership, Collaborative Decision Making, and Defining the Question.   The most effective approach to CBPR is through long-standing research partnerships between communities and universities that exist independent of a specific funded effort. Throwing together a "partnership" in response to a funding announcement is unlikely to create the meaningful levels of trust and reciprocity required for true CBPR.

TABLE 13.3

Critical Elements in Community-Based Participatory Research (CBPR)

CBPR Implementation and Potential Impact

Research Element	CBPR Application	Community Benefits	Research Benefits	Research Challenges
Assembling a research team of collaborators with the potential for forming a research partnership	Identifying collaborators who are decision makers that can move the research project forward	Resources can be used more efficiently	Increases the probability of completing the research project as intended	Time to identify the right collaborators and convincing them that they play an important role in the research project
A structure for collaboration to guide decision making	Consensus on ethics and operating principles for the research partnership to follow, including protection of study participants	The beginning of building trust and the likelihood that procedures governing protection of study participants will be understood and acceptable	An opportunity to understand each collaborator's agenda, which may enhance recruitment and retention of study participants	An ongoing process throughout the life of research partnerships that requires skills in group facilitation, building consensus, and conflict accommodation
Defining the research question	Full participation of community in identifying issues of greatest importance; focus on community strengths as well as problems	Problems addressed are highly relevant to the study participants and other community members	Increased investment and commitment to the research process by participants	Time consuming; community may identify issues that differ from those identified by standard assessment procedures or for which funding is available

(Continued)

TABLE 13.3
(Continued)

CBPR Implementation and Potential Impact

Research Element	CBPR Application	Community Benefits	Research Benefits	Research Challenges
Grant proposal and funding	Community leaders/members involved as a part of the proposal-writing process	Proposal is more likely to address issues of concern in a manner acceptable to community residents	Funding likelihood increases if community participation results in tangible indicators of support for recruitment and retention efforts, such as writing letters of support, serving on steering committee or as fiscal agents or co-investigators	Seeking input from the community may slow the process and complicate the proposal development effort when time constraints are often present
Research design	Researchers communicate the need for specific study design approaches and work with community to design more acceptable approaches, such as a delayed intervention for the control group	Participants feel as if they are contributing to the advancement of knowledge, as if they are passive research "subjects," and that a genuine benefit will be gained by their community	Community is less resentful of research process and more likely to participate	Design may be more expensive and/or take longer to implement
Possible threats to scientific rigor
Participant recruitment and retention	Community representatives guide researchers to the most effective way to reach the intended study participants and keep them involved in the study	Those who may benefit most from the research are identified and recruited in dignified manner rather than made to feel like research subjects	Facilitated participant recruitment and retention, which are among the major challenges in health research	Recruitment and retention approaches may be more complex, expensive, or time consuming

Formative data collection	Community members provide input to intervention design, barriers to recruitment and retention, and so on, via focus groups, structured interviews, narratives, or other qualitative method	Interventions and research approach are likely to be more acceptable to participants and thus of greater benefit to them and the broader population	Service-based and community-based interventions are likely to be more effective than if they are designed without prior formative data collection	Findings may indicate needed changes to proposed study design, intervention, and timeline, which may delay progress
Measures, instrument design, and data collection	Community representatives are involved in extensive cognitive response and pilot testing of measurement instruments before beginning formal research	Measurement instruments are less likely to be offensive or confusing to participants	Quality of data is likely to be superior in terms of reliability and validity	Time consuming; possible threats to scientific rigor
Intervention design and implementation	Community representatives are involved with selecting the most appropriate intervention approach, given cultural and social factors and strengths of the community	Participants feel the intervention is designed for their needs and offers benefits while avoiding insult; provides resources for communities involved	Intervention design is more likely to be appropriate for the study population, thus increasing the likelihood of a positive study	Time consuming; hiring local staff; may be less efficient than using study staff hired for the project

(Continued)

TABLE 13.3
(Continued)

CBPR Implementation and Potential Impact

Research Element	CBPR Application	Community Benefits	Research Benefits	Research Challenges
Data analysis and interpretation	Community members are involved regarding their interpretation of the findings within the local social and cultural context	Community members who hear the results of the study are more likely to feel that the conclusions are accurate and sensitive	Researchers are less likely to be criticized for limited insight or cultural insensitivity	Interpretations of data by nonscientists may differ from those of scientists, calling for thoughtful negotiation
Manuscript preparation and research translation	Community members are included as coauthors of the manuscripts, presentations, newspaper articles, and so on, following previously agreed-upon guidelines	Pride in accomplishment, experience with scientific writing, and potential for career advancement; findings are more likely to reach the larger community and increase potential for implementing or sustaining recommendations	The manuscript is more likely to reflect an accurate picture of the community environment of the study	Time consuming; requires extra mutual learning and negotiation

Note. From ref. 46. Copyright 2004. Adapted with permission from Elsevier.

CBPR in its purest form allows the community to define the research question. Residents living near a waste dump, for example, might bring their concerns to an epidemiologist if they become aware of an unusually large number of cancer deaths in their community. Clearly, the likelihood of this happening is enhanced by an existing partnership where trust has been developed. The benefits of community-generated research questions are that the problems addressed are highly relevant to the community. This in turn benefits the researcher in terms of greater investment and commitment to the research process, which is likely to increase adherence to study protocols and interventions. The challenge of this approach to researchers is that categorical, disease-specific funding sources rarely allow the investigator the flexibility of responding directly to community-identified concerns.

Research Design and Measurement, Intervention Implementation. Interventions designed in consultation with members of the intended participant group are more likely to be responsive to the cultural factors, economic challenges, and logistical barriers relevant to the study population. Although this may result in improved levels of participant adherence, it may have less to do with the "adherence levels" of individual study participants than with the appropriateness of the intervention design. Similarly, recruitment and retention strategies designed in conjunction with individuals similar to those whose participation is desired may facilitate greater community "buy-in" and thus improved participation. Measures of adherence may elicit more honest and less socially desirable responses if they have been reviewed by community members to assess cultural sensitivity. Finally, intervention approaches to promote adherence that are more responsive to the real-world challenges faced by participants are more likely to have a positive effect. Researchers must be prepared to accept the fact that the point of intervention may need to be much further "upstream" on the socioecologic framework (i.e., organizational and policy change) in order to ultimately make it more possible for the individual to "comply."

Data Interpretation and Dissemination of Research Findings. Few researchers would consider involving research participants in data analysis and dissemination of research findings. However, interpreting psycho-social data without considering the community and cultural context can be seriously flawed. The CBPR approach suggests that community participants be involved in "making sense" of the study findings, taking care to protect confidentiality at the individual level.

Implemented fully, CBPR involves application of research findings to address the originally identified health concern. This often requires dissemination of study results well beyond the traditional academic venues. Of increasing concern to the health care community is the ability to "translate" the findings of clinical studies to real-world application. As discussed earlier, there is a growing emphasis on "translational research," which represents the transition from efficacy to effectiveness trials (47).

The challenge of translational research then is to design ways that an intervention like the DPP, discussed earlier, can be implemented in a cost-effective and sustainable manner. CBPR could facilitate such a design by identifying innovative community-based approaches to intervention delivery, blending the strengths of the health care system with the often untapped resources of the community. For example, community diabetes advisers (community members having personal experience with the disease) could be called on to reinforce messages of health care professionals and help patients navigate the support systems that are available but often underused.

SUMMARY AND CONCLUSIONS

There are many factors contributing to nonadherence associated with lifestyle recommendations and interventions. The vast majority of the literature on adherence and nonadherence to date has been focused at the individual or perhaps individual and provider level. Using the perspective of the socioecologic model, it becomes clear that both patients and providers are influenced by a complex web of factors that significantly complicate the ability of providers to offer the most useful interventions and for patients to alter their behaviors in positive ways.

The RE-AIM model forces one to consider issues well beyond whether an intervention or treatment program is effective in a highly controlled and structured clinical trial. It offers a framework to guide those who are pursuing models for longer term sustainable change rather than short-term adherence to a specific intervention. Similarly, CBPR has the potential to hold researchers accountable, both for more valid research findings and interpretation as well as for whether their research ultimately results in positively impacting the initial health problem identified.

The mutuality model that combines the three models and approaches discussed in this chapter can serve as an overarching guideline for health care providers and researchers in devising effective intervention programs. In the mutuality model (Fig. 13.3), both the recipient of care (i.e., individual patient or a community) and the health care provider (i.e., physician, public health worker, or researcher) are experts: One is an expert on the immediate environment and the capabilities required to meet the demands of an intervention program; the other is an expert on the most up-to-date

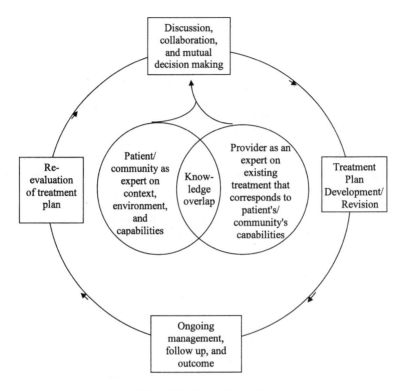

FIG. 13.3.   Mutuality model.

scientific findings that correspond to the given environment and capabilities. This is a small but important overlap of knowledge between the two. Naturally, any intervention program would require mutuality throughout the process from identifying the health concern to devising and implementing an effective intervention program. We assert that it is the mutuality and equal partnership throughout the process that encourages individual patients and communities to have ownership and be invested in seeing that intervention and treatment programs succeed. Mutuality and participatory action represent shared responsibility for adherence at multiple levels of influence within the community.

REFERENCES

1. Ritchie LD, Ivey SL, Woodward-Lopez G, Crawford PB. Alarming trends in pediatric overweight in the United States. *Soz Praventivmed.* 2003;48:168–177.

2. Nzerue CM, Demissochew H, Tucker JK. Race and kidney disease: role of social and environmental factors. *J Natl Med Assoc.* 2002;94:28S–38S.

3. Pradhan AD, Skerrett PJ, Manson JE. Obesity, diabetes, and coronary risk in women. *J Cardiovasc Risk.* 2002;9:323–330.

4. Singh GK, Hoyert DL. Social epidemiology of chronic liver disease and cirrhosis mortality in the United States, 1935–1997: trends and differentials by ethnicity, socioeconomic status, and alcohol consumption. *Hum Biol.* 2000;72:801–820.

5. Clarke GN. Improving the transition from basic efficacy research to effectiveness studies: methodological issues and procedures. *J Consult Clin Psychol.* 1995;63:718–725.

6. Glasgow RE, Vogt TM, Boles SM. Evaluating the public health impact of health promotion interventions: the RE-AIM framework. *Am J Public Health.* 1999;89:1322–1327.

7. Bosworth HB. Treatment adherence. In: Miller JR, Lerner RM, Schiamberg LB, Anderson PM, eds. *The Encyclopedia of Human Ecology.* Santa Barbara, CA: ABC-Clio; 2003:686–690.

8. Goldman DP, Smith JP. Can patient self-management help explain the SES health gradient? *Proc Natl Acad Sci USA.* 2002;99:10929–10934.

9. van Ryn M, Burke J. The effect of patient race and socio-economic status on physicians' perceptions of patients. *Soc Sci Med.* 2000;50:813–828.

10. Haynes BR, Taylor WD, Sackett DL. *Compliance in Health Care.* Baltimore: Johns Hopkins University Press, 1979.

11. Rudd P, Marshall G. Medication taking in hypertension. In: Brenner B, Laragh JH, eds. *Hypertension: Pathophysiology, Diagnosis, and Management.* New York: Raven Press; 1990:2309–2327.

12. Wallack L, Winkleby M. Primary prevention: a new look at basic concepts. *Soc Sci Med.* 1987;25:923–930.

13. Glasgow RE, Bull SS, Gillette C, Klesges LM, Dzewaltowski DA. Behavior change intervention research in healthcare settings: a review of recent reports with emphasis on external validity. *Am J Prev Med.* 2002;23:62–69.

14. Israel BA, Schultz AJ, Parker EA, Becker AB. Critical issues in developing and following community based participatory research principles. In: Minkler M, Wallerstein N, eds. *Community-Based Participatory Research for Health.* San Francisco: Jossey-Bass; 2003:56–76.

15. McLeroy KR, Bibeau D, Steckler A, Glanz K. An ecological perspective on health promotion programs. *Health Educ Q.* 1988;15:351–377.

16. Schillinger D, Piette J, Grumbach K, et al. Closing the loop: physician communication with diabetic patients who have low health literacy. *Arch Intern Med.* 2003;163:83–90.

17. Kalichman SC, Ramachandran B, Catz S. Adherence to combination antiretroviral therapies in HIV patients of low health literacy. *J Gen Intern Med.* 1999;14:267–273.

18. Doak CC, Doak LG, Root JH. *Teaching Patients With Low Literacy Skills.* 2nd ed. Philadelphia: J. B. Lippincott Company; 1996.

19. U.S. Department of Education. *National Adult Literacy Survey.* Washington, DC: National Center for Education Statistics; 1993.

20. Cooper-Patrick L, Gallo JJ, Gonzales JJ, et al. Race, gender, and partnership in the patient–physician relationship. *JAMA.* 1999;282:583–589.

21. Ammerman AS, DeVellis RF, Carey TS, et al. Physician-based diet counseling for cholesterol reduction: current practices, determinants, and strategies for improvement. *Prev Med.* 1993;22:96–109.

22. Jilcott SB, Macon ML, Rosamond WD, et al. Implementing the WISEWOMAN program in local health departments: staff attitudes, beliefs, and perceived barriers. *J Women's Health.* 2004;13(5):598–606.

23. Kaplan SH, Greenfield S, Ware JE Jr. Assessing the effects of physician–patient interactions on the outcomes of chronic disease. *Med Care.* 1989;27:S110–S127.

24. Roter DL, Hall JA. Patient–provider communication. In: Glanz K, Lewis FM, Rimer BK, eds. *Health Behavior and Health Education: Theory, Research, and Practice.* 2nd ed. San Francisco: Jossey-Bass Publishers; 1997:206–226.

25. Ammerman A, Washington C, Jackson B, et al. The PRAISE! project: a church-based nutrition intervention designed for cultural appropriateness, sustainability, and diffusion. *Health Promot Pract.* 2002;3:286–301.

26. Perrin EM, Flower KB, Ammerman AS. Body mass index charts: useful yet underused. *J Pediatr.* 2004;144:455–460.

27. Linnan LA, Harden EA, Bucknam L, Carleton RA. Marketing cardiovascular disease risk reduction programs at the workplace. The Pawtucket Heart Health Program experience. *AAOHN J.* 1990;38:409–418.

28. Baranowski T, Cullen KW, Nicklas T, Thompson D, Baranowski J. Are current health behavioral change models helpful in guiding prevention of weight gain efforts? *Obes Res.* 2003;11:23S–43S.

29. Biener L, Glanz K, McLerran D, et al. Impact of the Working Well Trial on the worksite smoking and nutrition environment. *Health Educ Behav.* 1999;26: 478–494.

30. Blamey A, Mutrie N, Aitchison T. Health promotion by encouraged use of stairs. *BMJ.* 1995;311:289–290.

31. Ockene IS, Hebert JR, Ockene JK, et al. Effect of physician-delivered nutrition counseling training and an office-support program on saturated fat intake, weight, and serum lipid measurements in a hyperlipidemic population: Worcester Area Trial for Counseling in Hyperlipidemia (WATCH). *Arch Intern Med.* 1999;159:725–731.

32. Sallis JF, Hovell MF, Hofstetter CR, et al. Distance between homes and exercise facilities related to frequency of exercise among San Diego residents. *Public Health Rep.* 1990;105:179–185.

33. Huston SL, Evenson KR, Bors P, Gizlice Z. Neighborhood environment, access to places for activity, and leisure-time physical activity in a diverse North Carolina population. *Am J Health Promot.* 2003;18:58–69.

34. Reidpath DD, Burns C, Garrard J, Mahoney M, Townsend M. An ecological study of the relationship between social and environmental determinants of obesity. *Health Place.* 2002;8:141–145.

35. Morland K, Wing S, Diez Roux A, Poole C. Neighborhood characteristics associated with the location of food stores and food service places. *Am J Prev Med.* 2002;22:23–29.

36. Eyler AA, Vest JR. Environmental and policy factors related to physical activity in rural white women. *Women Health.* 2002;36:111–121.

37. Brownson RC, Baker EA, Housemann RA, Brennan LK, Bacak SJ. Environmental and policy determinants of physical activity in the United States. *Am J Public Health.* 2001;91:1995–2003.

38. Twiss J, Dickinson J, Duma S, Kleinman T, Paulsen H, Rilveria L. Community gardens: lessons learned from California Healthy Cities and Communities. *Am J Public Health.* 2003;93:1435–1438.

39. Hobbs SH, Ricketts TC, Dodds JM, Milio N. Analysis of interest group influence on federal school meals regulations 1992 to 1996. *J Nutr Educ Behav.* 2004;36: 90–98.

40. Dzewaltowski DA, Estabrooks PA, Klesges LM, Bull S, Glasgow RE. Behavior change intervention research in community settings: how generalizable are the results? *Health Promot Int.* 2004;19:235–245.

41. Bull SS, Gillette C, Glasgow RE, Estabrooks P. Work site health promotion research: to what extent can we generalize the results and what is needed to translate research to practice? *Health Educ Behav.* 2003;30:537–549.

42. Krebs NF, Jacobson MS. Prevention of pediatric overweight and obesity. *Pediatrics.* 2003;112:424–430.

43. Andrade A. HIV adherence strategies take a high-tech route. *Aids Alert.* 2001;16: 97–98.

44. Diabetes Prevention Program Research Group. The Diabetes Prevention Program (DPP): description of lifestyle intervention. *Diabetes Care.* 2002;25:2165–2171.

45. Garfield SA, Malozowski S, Chin MH, et al. Considerations for diabetes translational research in real-world settings. *Diabetes Care.* 2003;26:2670–2674.

46. Viswanathan M, Ammerman A, Eng E, et al. *Community-Based Participatory Research: Assessing the Evidence.* Evidence Report/Technology Assessment No. 99. AHRQ Pub. No. 04-E022-2. Rockville, MD: July 2004.

47. National Institutes of Health, Centers for Disease Control and Prevention. *From Clinical Trials to Community: The Science of Translating Diabetes and Obesity Research.* Bethesda, MD: Natcher Conference Center, National Institutes of Health; 2004.

48. Glasgow RE, Lichtenstein E, Marcus AC. Why don't we see more translation of health promotion research to practice? Rethinking the efficacy-to-effectiveness transition. *Am J Public Health.* 2003;93:1261–1267.

49. Dzewaltowski DA, Estabrooks PA, Glasgow RE. The future of physical activity behavior change research: what is needed to improve translation of research into health promotion practice? *Exerc Sport Sci Rev.* 2004;32:57–63.
50. Ammerman A, Perrin E, Flower K. Promoting healthy nutrition (p. 194). In: Osborn L, DeWitt T, First L, Zenel J, eds. *Pediatrics.* Philadelphia: Mosby; 2005.

Chapter 14

Implications of Nonadherence for Economic Evaluation and Health Policy

Courtney Harold Van Houtven
Morris Weinberger
Tim Carey

Clinical and health services researchers interested in studying nonadherence must be cognizant of costs for several reasons. First, on the patient level, adherence to prescribed regimens is a critical mediating variable when seeking to improve many patient outcomes. Thus, nonadherence to prescribed regimens reduces the efficacy of medical care and may limit patients from receiving the full benefit of their treatment. To the extent that patients pay for these treatments, their investment in health may be compromised. Second, beyond the effect on individual patients, nonadherence can be costly to health care providers, insurers, and society. For example, to the extent that following appropriate treatment regimens results in preventable emergency department visits and hospitalizations, nonadherence can result in substantial costs that might otherwise be averted. One dated study estimated that the cost of nonadherence in the United States, including hospital and nursing home admissions, lost productivity, premature deaths, and excessive treatments surpassed $100 billion per year (1). Another estimated that patient nonadherence accounted for between 2% and 6.5% of all hospital admissions (2). Finally, policymakers must also recognize the impact of costs on nonadherence. That is, patients who lack the resources to obtain prescribed treatments are at increased risk of nonadherence. Unfortunately, those who lack these (often financial) resources (e.g., socioeconomically disadvantaged, older adults) are at greater risk of poor health outcomes and use of costly health care services.

Clinical and health services researchers often seek to develop interventions to improve patients' outcomes, including clinical markers and health-related quality of life. These interventions can be heterogeneous, including medications, new technologies, and the structure of care. However, common to these varied interventions is that improving patients' outcomes often requires patients' adherence to a specific treatment. This is particularly true as investigators move from efficacy studies (i.e., estimating the effect of the intervention on patients' outcomes under ideal circumstances, including adherent patients) to effectiveness studies (the impact of the intervention under real-world conditions). For example, knowing that a medication, if taken as prescribed, lowers blood pressure when patients are observed in a clinical research unit is important information. However, it is unlikely that a similar benefit will be conferred to patients when primary-care physicians prescribe this same medication; nonadherence is one factor that mitigates the benefit of efficacious interventions.

Health services researchers and behavioral scientists face similar issues in the design of their interventions ranging from disease management to self-efficacy programs. According to a recent *Cochrane Review*, even the most effective strategies designed to help patients follow medication regimens led to modest improvements in adherence for chronic disease; most strategies were ineffective (3). Thus, to improve patients' outcomes, investigators must design and evaluate pragmatic strategies that patients are willing to adopt (i.e., adherence). Otherwise, patients and payers will be unlikely to pay for these strategies and outcomes will suffer.

Researchers must consider the cost of nonadherence explicitly when drawing conclusions about feasibility, bias, and the potential impact of an intervention. For example, concluding that there is "inadequacy of treatment" in the intervention group (4) may actually be explained by nonadherence; that is, nonadherence makes the intervention group and control groups look similar. This phenomenon can be observed in health services research studies as well as clinical studies. For example, an intervention designed to integrate mental-health nurse specialists in the care of primary-care patients with depression had no effect on patients' outcomes; on closer inspection, the nurses' nonadherence to the study protocol (one that they were involved in designing) led to the observation of no difference between groups (5). When determining that the lack of between-group differences is due to nonadherence, researchers must decide whether to: (a) abandon further study of the intervention or (b) develop strategies that may enhance implementation and improve adherence. The decision may well depend on the cost of the intervention itself and/or the strategies that would be required to enhance adherence. This decision requires careful consideration of costs. And, regardless of the intervention (e.g., medication, technology, structure of health care), clinical and health services researchers would be well advised to consider the costs and effects of nonadherence in their research design and analysis. Currently many clinical trials do not assess treatment adherence, much less consider the costs of nonadherence behavior.

Policy analysts and policymakers must also consider nonadherence. Failing to do so may lead to endorsing a program in which the projected benefits are over stated or neglect a policy option whose benefits are understated. Furthermore, when considering two different policy options, policymakers should recognize that if the adherence rates are different enough to change health outcomes, the cost-effectiveness ratios might also change. Ignoring nonadherence costs can ultimately distort policymaking and lead to net welfare losses to society.

In this chapter we use patient adherence to medications as a model to illustrate how researchers might consider the cost of nonadherence in their work. Though we have chosen to focus on medications, the same issues apply to other strategies that target patients (e.g., diet, exercise, smoking cessation) or providers (e.g., strategies to enhance adherence to clinical practice guidelines). In addition, we focus on chronic disease, because the costs of nonadherence are more profound in chronic disease and because much of the research on adherence behavior has focused on chronic disease. The same costing considerations are applicable to the study of medications used for acute problems (e.g., short-term antibiotics for infections).

In this chapter we:

- Review the economics literature on studies of nonadherence.
- Review economic evaluation methods and health utility preference measures.
- Describe the mechanics of adapting the cost-effectiveness calculation to incorporate nonadherence.
- Present a template of costs and effects that researchers should consider, including how these considerations influence the study design and interpretation.
- Discuss methodological issues surrounding economic evaluations (especially how they apply to studies of nonadherence).
- Describe some of the special considerations related to studies of medication nonadherence.
- Discuss the implications of considering nonadherence costs in health policy.

NONADHERENCE IN THE ECONOMICS LITERATURE

What have health economists found thus far about the net costs and effects of nonadherence? The main message in the scant economics literature on adherence is that there is not enough being done to understand the costs of nonadherence. For example, researchers at the University of Bologna, Italy, write "Conventional economic studies in well controlled clinical trial settings have not adequately assessed factors such as nonadherence, switching and discontinuation of treatment which have an important impact on the costs of antihypertensive therapy in actual clinical practice" (6).

We presume that the cost of nonadherence is high and that there are negative effects of nonadherence on health outcomes. But the cost being high has not been established due in large part to the lack of empirical studies. For example, in a review by Hughes et al. (7), the cost of nonadherence was ambiguous even though the health effects were not. The evidence from 22 studies showed that the rate of adherence falling consistently leads to falling benefits of the intervention. There is no consistency, however, in the effect on costs. In some cases decreased adherence leads to decreased costs but in others it leads to increased costs. The uncertainty surrounding the net effect of nonadherence behavior on costs is summed up well by Cleemput and Kesteloot (4). According to them, costs associated with nonadherence include additional diagnostic and treatment costs for the initial disease and new diseases. By contrast, nonadherence might lead to savings if the cost of unprovided treatment offsets the cost of increased morbidity. The net effect might be positive, no effect, or negative (4). In some instances nonadherence with very expensive and relatively ineffective treatments may be cost saving (7), but most studies to improve adherence show that there are clinical benefits from even modest gains in nonadherence. More effort should be devoted to assessing the cost-effectiveness of such efforts.

Investigators can draw from existing bodies of health economics and health services to learn about the cost of nonadherence in some cases because lack of access to care and medication clearly affects treatment adherence. Much work in health economics and health services research has focused on access to care and how lack of access to care affects subsequent health outcomes. One of the most famous studies, the RAND Health Insurance Experiment, carefully documented how the cost of health care affects demand and outcomes (see ref. 8 for an example on prescription drugs). Other studies have focused on low-income or uninsured populations because of their well-known barriers to care. In a recent article in the *American Economic Review,* for example, Case and colleagues (9) carefully laid out the negative relationship between a child's family income and child health status. Independent of income, there is also a large literature on access to care problems for racial and ethnic minorities (ref. 10, for example), which can affect treatment adherence as well. Drawing from studies of access to care and access to drugs could be important sources when considering how best to examine the economic barriers to adherence even though these studies do not address adherence directly. Finally, we know from health services research that differences in the health care payment system can affect adherence. *A Cochrane Review* article showed that compliance with a recommended number of visits to a provider was higher under fee-for-service systems compared with capitated payment systems (11). This finding reiterates the importance of investigators considering individual patient issues as well as system issues when approaching nonadherence.

There is an older body of literature that examines how adherence affects hospitalization rates for given diseases (see ref. 2 for a recent example; ref. 12 for depression; ref. 13 for diabetes). Although these studies focus on other reasons for hospitalization, the general consensus is that poor adherence leads to unnecessary hospitalization. More recent examples of how drug nonadherence affects costs and medical outcomes for a particular disease (where medical outcomes are measured as subsequent utilization and the drug is dilantin for epilepsy) can be found in Singer (14) or by visiting the International Society for Pharmaceutical Outcomes Research Web site (www.ispor.org).

The studies highlighted focus on a tallying of costs and effects for a given disease or intervention and do not include multivariate modeling. More general multivariate studies of how adherence affects subsequent utilization for less narrow patient populations would help fill a gap in the health services research and health economics literature. Most approaches to examine the costs of nonadherence are limited to one aspect of health economics work, cost-effectiveness analysis, which is also commonly used by clinical researchers and trialists. We discuss cost-effectiveness analysis and other economic evaluation methods in the next section.

ECONOMIC EVALUATION METHODS AND HEALTH UTILITY PREFERENCES MEASURES

Economic Evaluation Methods

To quantify the costs and consequences of treatment nonadherence, researchers may use four main economic evaluation methods: cost-minimization analysis, cost-effectiveness analysis, cost–utility analysis, and cost–benefit analysis (15, 16). For a discussion of partial economic evaluation methods, see Drummond et al. (15). For more extensive discussion of economic theory behind economic evaluation, see Johannesson (17) or Sloan (18).

When considering an economic evaluation, "effects" can be used broadly to encompass any health outcome that the investigator hypothesizes as being attributed to the intervention under study. Effects are also referred to in the literature as health outcomes, health consequences, or health benefits; effects may include quality-adjusted life years, clinical measures, and/

or patient-centered measures. Because the majority of economic evaluations in health are called "cost-effectiveness studies" (despite the fact that they may be technically cost–utility or cost-minimization studies), we refer to economic evaluation studies as cost-effectiveness analyses generically throughout the chapter. Common to all of these economic evaluation methods is that researchers compare one strategy or program against another or others; for example, the intervention group compared to the control group. Comparing the additional costs of one treatment over another is known as the *incremental* or *marginal* costs of that treatment. In the discussion that follows, we use the following notation: total cost of program for intervention group (TC_I); total cost of program for control group (TC_C); total effects for the intervention group (TE_I); total effects for the control group (TE_C).

Cost-Minimization Analysis. In cost-minimization analysis, one directly compares two programs or strategies and selects the one with the least cost. Cost-minimization analysis is appropriate when two interventions or two technologies are expected to be equally effective. Cost-minimization is also appropriate when each of two interventions has met the predetermined objective, but researchers are interested in identifying the least costly strategy (15). For example, if there were strong evidence that two smoking cessation programs were equally effective (i.e., they had similar adherence rates), then a health planner would want to implement the program that is least costly. In cost-minimization analysis, the relevant comparison is $TC_I - TC_C$.

Cost-Effectiveness Analysis (CEA). In CEA, researchers compare costs of two strategies to some common effect or outcome. CEA is quite flexible, as it can be applied to a wide range of effects, for example, life years gained, reductions in viral load, blood pressure, or proportion of patients cured (7). The relevant comparison is $(TC_I - TC_C)/(TE_I - TE_C)$. Notably, CEA allows researchers to compare either alternative therapies for a given disease, or to compare gains from therapies for totally different diseases (as long as the effects use the same metric). For example, one can compare cost per life year gained from a diet intervention for obese patients to cost per life year gained of a drug therapy intervention for stroke patients. This type of analysis can be used to allocate finite budget resources within a hospital or health care system.

Cost–Benefit Analysis (CBA). In CBA, all costs and benefits associated with a strategy are expressed in monetary terms; an incremental cost–benefit ratio is calculated. The advantages of CBA are that all effects are translated to monetary terms, creating a numerator and denominator that are both in dollars. This is useful when effects cannot be measured by a single metric, such as life years saved (19). Additionally, CBA allows researchers to choose the program with the largest net benefit. Yet, CBA is not commonly used in health care because it is the most difficult both to understand conceptually and to estimate empirically (19). Conceptually, CBA frames benefits in terms of cost saving (e.g., treatment costs averted), which is conceptually difficult to grasp (20). Empirically, how does one place a dollar value on the loss of a person's life? One could use a human capital approach, in which the loss of life is valued as the individual's estimated future earnings; this approach places a lower dollar value on the life of older persons and those who have low-paying jobs (16). Alternatively, the value of a statistical life (VSL) can be calculated based on people's willingness to pay to reduce their risk of premature death (19); the willingness-to-pay (WTP) approach is discussed in a subsequent section of this chapter. Briefly, the VSL could be calculated as the willingness to pay to increase life expectancy by a preset unit of time, or willingness to pay to avoid morbidity.

Cost–Utility Analysis (CUA). In economics, utility means happiness. In the health field, utility refers to a specific health state, so is often called health utility. Goldstein (21) refers to utility as *desirability* or *preference*, that is, the preferences individuals or society may have for any particular set of health outcomes. CUA allows researchers to compare the costs and utility of an intervention. It is based on the notion that the utility is different from the outcome, effect, or level of health status itself (15). In CUA, utility is usually measured in terms of quality-adjusted life years (QALYs), a measure that takes into account simultaneously both the quality and quantity of an individual's health. In the case of medication adherence, QALY can account for both reductions in health utility from side effects or unpleasantness of taking the drug, as well as improvements in health utility from the drug treatment. Thus, one advantage of CUA over CEA is that researchers can compare the value attached to a change in health status, rather than a change in health status itself. The disadvantage, not surprisingly, is that techniques used to elicit utilities are difficult and controversial.

To calculate the QALY value, one first estimates the total life years gained from a treatment and then weights each year with a health-related quality of life (HRQOL) score for that year. CUA assumes that the utility of *any* health state can be expressed on a scale from 0 (dead) to 1 (perfect health) (19). Table 14.1 shows an example of a QALY calculation using QALYs over one's lifetime. Further adjustments to the QALY value can be made to incorporate the probability of being alive in a given time period and the discount rate.

The HRQOL score (q_i in Table 14.1), also called a utility index, is intended to reflect the HRQOL in a given time period. To calculate an HRQOL score, researchers can turn to general or disease-specific indices,

TABLE 14.1
Example of a QALY Calculation

Let the **quality-of-life score** for health state i = q_i
Let N_i = number of years in health state i

So one's Lifetime Health Profile = $(N_1, N_2, N_3, \ldots N_n)$
which is simply the number of years in each health state

QALY = $(q_1 \times N_1) + (q_2 \times N_2) + (q_3 \times N_3) + \ldots + (q_n \times N_n)$
which is simply the number of *quality adjusted* years in each health state

---

Note. From ref. 19. Copyright 2003. Adapted by permission.

or construct a score through interviews with respondents. Each approach has relative advantages and disadvantages. General or generic HRQOL indices allow comparability across studies and patient populations. The most widely used generic HRQOL measure, which is actually a health status measure, is the SF-36, which provides scores along eight dimensions that are considered to be important to all patients, regardless of their disease (22). The EuroQol, Quality of Well-Being Scale (23), Health Utilities Index, and CDC HRQOL-14 are a few of the off-the-shelf general indices that can be used. In a comparison of five scales (EuroQol, Health Utility Index, 15D, Rosser Scale, Quality of Well-Being Scale), Brazier and colleagues (24) rated the EuroQol and the Health Utility Index as superior indices because they used choice-based techniques to elicit preferences. Choice-based techniques rely on the willingness of respondents to trade risk of death or life years in order to improve their state of health, so are more consistent with consumer theory (24).

Disease-specific measures are intended for a specific disease or population. Thus, they are likely to be more responsive and sensitive to changes and side effects. Examples of disease-specific indices include the Q-utility index (25) for cancer clinical trials or the Beck Depression Inventory for depression patients. Other tailored indices target specific populations, such as women or children (26). Incidentally, the Panel on Cost Effectiveness recommends that researchers wishing to use disease-specific indices also consider including a general HRQOL index to allow cross-study comparisons (16).

Recall that utility is different from the health outcome itself. Hence, in order to compare different treatments and different diseases, it is important for HRQOL indices to work across different health states and to assess preferences (21). That is, not only do HRQOL indicators need to reflect a person's health status, such as the SF-36, they need to assess how the individual values a particular health state. For more on measuring health and

HRQOL, see McDowell and Newell (27). Next we discuss methods for assessing HRQOL using interviews with respondents.

Health Utility Preference Measures

Sometimes existing HRQOL indices, even disease-specific ones, will not accurately assess health utility. Because side effects and adverse outcomes from treatment can be specific to a given regimen and condition, this may be particularly true when examining nonadherence behavior and costs. Several methods exist to elicit utility directly from respondents. Among the most common are the visual analog scale, magnitude estimation, standard gamble, time trade-off, and WTP methods (Table 14.2). For a hypothetical patient with hypertension, we describe how utility preferences would be elicited when considering two alternative treatment options to avoid stroke: surgery or multiple drugs with side effects. The respondent would most likely not have hypertension him or herself. Hence, in framing this scenario the patient would be told about side effects of the drugs, as well as what it would be like to experience hypertension, take multiple drugs, and receive surgery before he or she is asked to consider the options. Some of the possible side effects associated with a regime of hypertension drugs are frequent urination, erectile dysfunction, cough, fatigue, and constipation, among others. Depending on the method, the person would also be told about different risks associated with the two alternatives (Table 14.2). By the complexity of the scenarios, it becomes clear that communicating the health states involved in different treatment options quickly becomes complex, especially as one moves from conceptually intuitive visual analog scales to those that involve making trade-offs.

The *visual analog scale* is a common and simple method for respondents to understand. People simply rank different health states on a scale: from 0 to 10 or from 0 to 100. In some cases faces can be used to indicate different health states, ranging from a deep frown on the left-hand side of the scale to a large smile on the right-hand side. *Magnitude estimation* is similar to the *visual analog scale,* but respondents have to relate two conditions to each other using ratios so it requires more math skills. In our example, surgery is viewed to be 4 times worse than drug therapy.

The *standard gamble* is the method most grounded in economic theory; it seems particularly useful when considering drug adherence. For example, with many drug regimens with adverse side effects, the consequence of not adhering is uncertain. It can increase the risk of death in the future or may have no effect on health. Because there is uncertainty surrounding whether a person will have a stroke, the bad side effects of a drug may dominate a person's choices. For other diseases, such as human immunodeficiency virus (HIV) disease, the story may be starkly different. For HIV, there is much

TABLE 14.2
Common Methods Used in Health State Valuation

Scenario:	Imagine you are a patient with severe hypertension with two choices: 1. Surgery to relieve blockage and help avoid stroke 2. A regimen of four drugs per day to help avoid stroke (with side effects)

Visual Analog Scale	Respondent asked to place health states on a scale, ranked from 0, the worst imaginable health state, to 100, the best imaginable. *Surgery given a score of 20 and drug option a score of 80.*
Magnitude Estimation	Respondent asked to assign ratios to the undesirability of the health states. *Surgery ranked as 4 times more undesirable than the drug option.*
Standard Gamble	Respondent given two alternatives. One has an x percent chance of normal health and living for an additional x years and a y percent chance of dying immediately (in our case from surgery). Two leads to the certain outcome of life in a given health state (controlled hypertension with drugs) for z years. Probabilities associated with the two outcomes in alternative one would be varied in order to find the point at which the patient is indifferent between the two alternatives. *After changing the probabilities associated with the outcomes in alternative one, the point of indifference between drugs and surgery occurred when surgery had a 1% risk of death and a 99% chance of full recovery.*
Time Trade-Off	Respondent given two alternatives. One is living with a particular health condition followed by death at time t. Two is living in perfect health for a set period of time less than time t, the time of death. *In this example, after altering the time lived in perfect health, the point of indifference is living with chronic hypertension and drugs for 20 more years versus living in perfect health for 15.*
Person Trade-Off	Respondent informed of two groups of people in two different adverse health states and has to decide which group to help. The number of people in one of the groups would be altered iteratively until the respondent is indifferent between helping either group. *For the hypertension example, respondent would be told about the uncertainty surrounding surgery and the differences in costs of the two alternatives (given that limited resources are why you can only help one group). After altering the number of persons able to receive surgery, the point of indifference arises when there are 50 people in the surgery group and 120 people in the drug group.*
Willingness to Pay	Respondent would be given information on a health condition. Then using different probabilities and monetary values, the respondent would arrive at the value he or she would be willing to pay to avoid the condition. Trade-offs could be made between treatments as well. *This could be approached a couple of ways in our example. (1) Given that a person has hypertension (and they have been told of risk of stroke from it), they would be willing to pay $10,000 a year to get rid of it. (2) A patient without hypertension would be willing to pay $8,000 a year to avoid getting hypertension (ex ante). It is unclear which willingness to pay values would be higher in the ex post versus ex ante approaches.*

Note. Information on methods draws heavily from ref. 24. Hypothetical examples constructed by the authors.

less uncertainty surrounding the bad health outcome—not adhering to medication regimens almost certainly leads to death. Still, using standard gamble can help reveal how patients weigh potentially bad side effects from a treatment against a potentially bad health outcome.

The *person trade-off* method is the newest method, and may be appropriate in allocating scarce public health resources among different programs or initiatives (see Table 14.2). Including possible adherence behavior in the scenarios would more accurately guide respondents in choosing the group they wish to help. Adherence differences, because they will affect the effectiveness of the program, could be as influential to a respondent as the number of people in each group. For more information on these methods, including a discussion of their validity, see chapter 4 of Brazier et al. (24).

WTP scenarios can be useful when considering costs of nonadherence and predicting adherence behavior. For example, people often make trade-offs between the cost of a drug, the potential side effects, the administration of the drug (oral vs. injection), the quantity and frequency of dose, and the prescription duration in determining how they will adhere. WTP methodologies could be used to not only assess how much patients are willing to pay to avoid harsh side effects of drugs, but to determine how willing patients are to adhere given that there are harsh side effects. Learning about trade-offs through WTP can help researcher efforts to minimize nonadherence. They can also be used to predict adherence behavior and hence adherence costs. There are many technical issues surrounding WTP methodologies that cannot be discussed here, including whether or not ability to pay interferes with eliciting unbiased WTP values (28). For more information on health care applications of WTP methodologies, including approaches to control for starting point bias, information on test–retest reliability and examples of different bidding games, see O'Brien et al. (29) or Hirth et al. (30). For information on how patients' value alternative interventions using WTP methods, see Donaldson (31).

In all of the methods discussed for assessing utility, there are complex and unresolved issues surrounding whose preferences to elicit (e.g., persons with or without the disease) and what kinds of scenarios to use to best communicate the health state trade-offs. For one thing, it is difficult to convey the health state information to the respondent so that you give them enough information to understand the health state without biasing their responses (32). For more information on some of the controversies surrounding utility measurement and some useful comparisons, see Lenert and Kaplan (33).

To summarize, there are four basic economic evaluation methods used in health care. CEA and CUA are most common, but all of these economic evaluation methods could be used to examine costs of nonadherence. If the CUA requires QALYs, researchers have several options to measure utility, from existing general and disease-specific HRQOL indices to utility elicitation methods like those in Table 14.2. The method a researcher chooses depends on the objectives and the perspective of the study. Next we discuss the calculation of cost-effectiveness ratios and the implications of imperfect adherence on these calculations.

MECHANICS OF COST-EFFECTIVENESS CALCULATIONS

The nuts and bolts of calculating cost-effectiveness ratios are simple accounting; issues surrounding the difficult question of which costs and effects to measure are discussed later in this section. The average cost-effectiveness ratio is the cost of the intervention divided by the effects of the intervention (TC_I/TE_I). Considering the average does not help decide between two programs, which is why economists prefer examining the incremental or marginal costs and effects. The incremental cost-effectiveness ratio provides information on the additional costs of one treatment over another and the additional effects associated with one treatment over the other ($TC_I - TC_C)/(TE_I - TE_C$). Researchers can examine the incremental cost-effectiveness ratio to decide between different treatment choices or to set priorities for funding decisions (34).

To be a sound analysis, the cost-effectiveness calculations must carefully account for adherence changes in the control group as well as the intervention group. Table 14.3 shows explicitly how to calculate an incremental cost-effectiveness ratio given imperfect adherence. The justification for breaking out the nonadherence specific costs and effects is to allow one to examine what the incremental effect of nonadherence is to the study. For example, if utilization changes a great deal based on an intervention, it would be useful to ascertain how much of the utilization change can be attributed to the intervention and how much can be attributed to nonadherence behavior. For example, take a care manager intervention program for patients with depression (35). Initially patients in the treatment group may have more visits if the case manager notices a problem with the medication prescribed or the dose and the patient gets the medication changed during a follow-up doctor's visit. Three months later, however, doctor's visits may go down due in part to the appropriate adjustment of medications and in part to improved adherence behavior because of the weekly calls with the care manager. Attributing some of the utilization changes to the intervention effects and some to better adherence may be useful when analyzing the intervention.

TABLE 14.3
Calculating an Incremental Cost-Effectiveness
Ratio Given Imperfect Adherence

Costs	Effects
Let TC_I = total cost of the intervention Let CI = cost of the intervention Let CI_{AD} = cost of nonadherence for intervention group	Let EI = health effect of the intervention Let EI_{AD} = health effect of nonadherence for intervention group Let TEI = total health effect of the intervention
Let TCC = total cost of the comparison group Let CC = cost of the comparison group Let CC_{AD} = cost of nonadherence	Let TEC = total health outcome of the comparison group Let EC = health outcome of the comparison group Let EC_{AD} = health outcome from nonadherence
Then $TCI = CI + CI_{AD}$ $\quad\ TCC = CC + CC_{AD}$ The incremental costs are, $IC_I = CI - CC$ $\quad\quad\quad\quad\ IC_{AD} = CI_{AD} - CC_{AD}$	Then $TEI = EI + EI_{AD}$ $\quad\ TEC = EC + ECAD$ And $\ IE_I = EI - EC$ $\quad\ IE_{AD} = EI_{AD} - EC_{AD}$

Incremental Cost-Effectiveness Ratio Accounting for Nonadherence

$$\frac{CI + CI_{AD} - CC - CC_{AD}}{EI + EI_{AD} - EC - EC_{AD}} = \frac{(TCI - TCC)}{(TEI - TEC)} = \frac{IC_I + IC_{AD}}{IE_I + IE_{AD}} = \frac{IC}{IE} = \frac{C}{E}$$

Note. Adapted from Table 3.1 of ref. 16 to include costs and effects adherence. Copyright 1996 by Oxford University Publishing.

Standard Considerations in CEA

As described earlier, much of the actual calculation of CEA ratios involves relatively simple accounting methods. However, there exist some issues that researchers must consider explicitly and in advance in order to make these calculations. We describe some of these here and some more controversial issues next.

Constant Dollars. All costs and effects should be reported in constant dollars. For example, if the cost of a drug therapy occurs in 2003 but the utilization costs occur in 2004, the researcher will need to convert costs in 2004 to 2003 dollars or vice versa.

Discounting. All costs and effects should be discounted; that is, one must explicitly recognize that the value of a dollar today is not the same as the value of a dollar in 10 years. The Panel on Cost-Effectiveness prefers the use of a 3% discount rate (16). However, because researchers commonly use 5%, the Panel recommends discounting health effects and costs at both 3% and 5% in order to ensure comparability. Whatever discounting rate is selected, researchers can use a technique known as sensitivity analysis to determine how much the assumptions about discounting affect their conclusions; sensitivity analyses are discussed later in this chapter.

Time Horizon. Sometimes the costs of nonadherence are realized during the study, but the effects are not seen until long after the study is completed. For example, short-term effects of nonadherence to diuretics for hypertension may lead to an increase in blood pressure or to an increase in QALY due to an alleviation of side effects like frequent urination. It may not be until 5 years later, when a stroke occurs, that the true loss in a person's QALY score may occur. The same logic can be applied to costs. If a person stops taking diuretics, it saves the health plan money in prescriptions initially; however, the costs to a health plan may be realized later, when it pays for hospital services and rehabilitation from stroke. Hence, it is very important to define the time horizon of a study. Having a 5-year followup period on costs and effects may be prohibitive, but it is important to define up front what the short-term and long-term considerations are and whether the time horizon allowed by the study will capture these or not.

Other Considerations in CEA

Time costs and unrelated future costs of health care are more thorny issues in CEA. We briefly discuss them here, but for more information, see Gold et al. (16).

Time Costs. There is some controversy surrounding how researchers account for time costs because of the potential to double count them as costs and effects. It is generally agreed that travel time to and from appointments should be counted as a cost. Considering time spent sick due to side effects of a drug, however, should instead be incorporated into the QALY calculation. Consider HIV antiretroviral drugs and the fact that perfect adherence can improve life expectancy. These drugs can also cause substantial side effects ranging from nausea, shortness of breath, or rashes, to longer term effects such as kidney stones or hypercholesterolemia (36). So in the short term, perfect adherence may lead to bad side effects, so bad that a person misses work for a week. A researcher may tally this cost in the numerator (lost productivity, an indirect cost, or lost wages, a direct cost). It could be argued that tallying the work lost is incorrect because the side effect will reduce the QALY by reducing quality of life. Hence, including it in the numerator would be double counting (argument drawn from ref. 16). Because work time lost also affects other people, mainly the employer, one would want to include the external costs to the employer from the lost work due to side effects, especially if they had to hire more labor. And the new laborers may introduce friction costs, that is, costs associated with training them and the start-up costs of them learning the job.

How should researchers account for time working at low productivity due to side effects of a drug? Lost productivity due to morbidity should not be counted in costs because it will be incorporated into the QALY calculation (Luce et al. in ref. 16). However, if an employer has to hire replacement workers or make direct expenditures, these would be considered as costs. Likewise, if an employee misses wages from treatment, the lost wages should be included in the cost calculation.

Unrelated Future Costs of Health Care.   Similar to the time horizon issue discussed earlier, by increasing life expectancy (or decreasing time spent ill) interventions can produce future costs (and effects) that have nothing to do with the intervention. For example, say an intervention for hypertension is found to be effective in reducing blood pressure to healthy levels if patients adhere to treatment. A proportion of adherent study participants will avoid stroke because of the study, and yet a proportion of the stroke avoiders will experience new conditions because they live longer. There may be additional cases of cancer for a number of them or additional cases of Alzheimer's to treat, to name a couple. Generally it is recommended that researchers *include* future health-related costs that arise from the benefits of the intervention in the numerator. That is, for the adherent study participants who avoid stroke, there may be higher health care costs associated with their living longer. Researchers should also include future QALY gains that stem from the intervention. If other future costs are truly unrelated to the intervention, then they may be omitted (16). Many studies do not consider costs and effects that accrue far into the future, but doing so meets the Panel's recommendation that CEA consider the full economic perspective (16). The full economic perspective, simply put, is the costs and effects that all members of society incur.

TEMPLATE OF COSTS AND EFFECTS WHEN CONSIDERING TREATMENT NONADHERENCE

Carefully cataloging all of the costs and benefits of treatment nonadherence can help researchers perform full economic evaluations of their studies. In this section we present a full range of direct and indirect costs and effects that may be associated with a drug therapy intervention and then discuss how the costs and effects for each stakeholder may change by considering nonadherence. First we define some more terminology.

Direct Versus Indirect Costs.   Costs in CEA are often classified as direct and indirect costs. Direct costs are expenditures on health care; these are often separated into two categories—direct medical costs and direct non-medical costs. Examples of direct medical costs are cost of a lab test, staff costs of examining the patient, or other medical equipment costs. Direct nonmedical costs can include transportation costs incurred by the patient to get to an appointment or lost wages due to treatment time. Indirect costs are nonpecuniary costs or, in economic terms, opportunity costs (i.e., the cost of using the resource compared to its next best use). It may be easier to think of these as nonmonetary costs or nonmonetary losses. For example, if a patient has to spend an hour to travel to an appointment, one might value her time as the amount of money she would have earned for her time if she had remained at work (15).

Table 14.4 classifies costs according to the different stakeholders involved: patients, providers, insurers, employers, family members, and society. Many of the stakeholders incur direct and indirect costs. For example, costs of drugs are direct costs borne by both the individual and the insurer, whereas lost productivity at work is an indirect cost borne by both the patient and the employer. There is a whole host of costs specific to delivering the intervention as well. For example, research personnel needed to deliver the intervention, space and equipment needed, drugs, and so forth. We do not include the intervention costs explicitly in the table but researchers will need to decide how to account for such costs in advance of performing an economic evaluation of the intervention. Ignoring intervention costs would bias the findings. As investigators embark on CEAs, several other important considerations must be made in advance and explicitly.

Perspective of the Analysis.   The perspective adopted by the investigator will influence how cost is measured and, ultimately, the cost-effectiveness analyses and conclusions. The Panel on Cost Effectiveness in Health and Medicine (16) recommends using the societal perspective at least to develop a reference case. In the societal perspective, "the analyst considers everyone affected by the intervention and counts all significant health outcomes and costs that flow from it, regardless of who experiences the outcomes or costs" (16). One approach to adopting a societal perspective is to consider all stakeholders in Table 14.4 and the exhaustive list of costs and effects to each stakeholder. Cleemput and Kesteloot (4) point out that the effectiveness of interventions should be assessed in the light of both individual patient-related and public health nonadherence, because these may have far-reaching societal consequences.

There are other perspectives as well. For example, a health care system will make decisions on investing dollars based on its return to the system. For example, if the Department of Veterans Affairs (VA) health care system

TABLE 14.4
Incorporating Adherence Behavior Into Economic Evaluations

Intervention Costs and Effects	Nonadherence Costs and Effects
Net Change in Costs (IC$_I$)	Net Change in Costs (IC$_{AD}$)
Patient	
Out-of-pocket drug costs	Onset of new conditions
Out-of-pocket utilization costs	Increased visits from added morbidity
Health care costs of living longer	Changes in length of life from interven-
Expenditure on transportation to visit	tion
Lost wages for treatment	
Opportunity cost for time in treatment	
Provider	
Provider share of cost of the visit	Increased utilization due to side effects
Staff time spent with patient, materials	Increased staff time due to complications
Insurer	
Insurer's share of utilization costs	Increased utilization
Insurer's share of cost of the drug	Decreases in intervention drug
Opportunity cost of patient resources	Increases in other drugs or future drugs
Employer	
Expenditures due to absenteeism, hiring	Changes in absenteeism
temporary workers	Changes in productivity, other friction
Productivity changes in patient from absence	costs
or morbidity	
Changes in premiums	
Family members & caregivers	
Share of cost of the visit and/or drugs	Share of increased visits
Expenditures associated with transport	More expenditures and help w/ transport
Time spent helping patient get to treatment	
Society	
Opportunity cost of patient resources	Changes resources available to others
Research	
Materials	
Personnel	
Net Change in Health From Intervention (IE$_I$)	Net Change in Health Adherence (IE$_{AD}$)
Patient	
Health status or health utility	Increase in short-term health status
Productivity from change in health status	Decrease in longer term health status/
Intrinsic value of health	death
Family members & caregivers	
Health status	Change in health status
Society	
Public health effects	Effects on herd immunity, antibiotic re-
Welfare changes to others	sistance, disease communicability

Note. Adapted from conceptual frameworks in refs. 15, 16, 19, and 47, as well as from unpublished slides.

is considering the adoption of a new medical technology, the relevant costs are those that the health care system would incur directly. The management would not consider costs occurring outside of their health care system. Because the VA is likely to be responsible for the care of its patients for the remainder of their lives, they may use different inputs than health care systems with high turnover. For example, if a health care system estimates that they will not provide care to 50% of its patients 5 years from now, they will need a faster return on investment in drawing conclusions about the cost-effectiveness of a particular strategy or intervention.

If one were considering a vaccination campaign, the perspective would be more broadly focused on the public health costs and effects of the intervention. In addition to the cost of the vaccine and clinic costs, and the positive (from avoided future disease) and negative side effects and adherence rate (because most childhood vaccines take more than one dose there will be some parents who do not adhere to the subsequent doses), the investigator would consider factors such as herd immunity in the measure of the effects. Herd immunity is the resistance of a group to a pathogen due to immunity of a large proportion of the group to that pathogen (37). This means that a nonimmunized child, or a child whose parents do not adhere to the full number of vaccination doses will benefit from having many children around him or her vaccinated. In terms of the economic evaluation of the vaccination campaign then, there are benefits that reach beyond the patients who are actually vaccinated in the study. Increasing herd immunity, the group, say a neighborhood, school, or other definition of community, reduces the community's chance of contracting the disease. The same could be true of a program that aims to increase patient adherence to antibiotic drug regimens. Disease strains resistant to antibiotics can affect society broadly as well.

These two examples center on how a patient's behavior affects public health. But the effects on the public from treatment nonadherence do not always come from patients being nonadherent. For example, physicians who prescribe ineffective antibiotic therapies (4) or who prescribe antibiotics indiscriminately even when not indicated can affect the public as well. These behaviors would not be captured unless the investigator adopts a full societal perspective of costs and effects of an intervention.

In addition, we can imagine a study that is undertaken strictly from the patient's perspective. Patients make trade-offs all the time about whether and how much they are willing to pay for a medication given all of the other things they want to spend their money on. For a government considering offering discounted HIV drugs, for example, it would be important to first know the amount patients are willing to pay out of pocket for the drug. Using this information could allow an efficient subsidy to be implemented: The net cost to patients would not impinge upon treatment adherence but would be high enough to ensure that the subsidy could be offered to the highest number of patients (38).

Defining Adherence. Finally, to measure the costs of treatment adherence well it is important for the researchers to establish a clinically or economically relevant definition of adherence for a given study *a priori.* Medication adherence can be measured many ways (see chap. 6 for more details). Researchers can assess discontinuation rates or drug regimen nonadherence (7), or more sophisticated measures such as the "medication possession ratio" (MPR) (39). The MPR is defined as the days supply of medication divided by the days between refills. Alternatively, adherence to drugs can be measured using the number of unused drugs returned to the pharmacy (40). All methods of measurement have drawbacks that need to be considered. For example, the MPR method misses nonadherence from people not fulfilling prescriptions in the first place, and does not measure whether people actually take the drugs that are filled, so the method may overstate adherence. Considering these drawbacks in sensitivity analyses can help bind the estimates.

In addition, one should consider at what phases to measure treatment nonadherence behavior. It may be that the effect for the study is a "QALY at month 12 of the intervention." Yet to consider the effect of nonadherence behavior, it may make sense to consider nonadherence effects at different time phases: acceptance of drug treatment and regimen during initial consultation, adherence with dosing regimen, and persistence with therapy (7). Or in the case of exercise, it may make sense to assess adherence at the time of acceptance of an exercise regimen, adherence to the regimen in the short term, and the maintenance of activities after completion of the intervention.

METHODOLOGICAL ISSUES SURROUNDING ECONOMIC EVALUATIONS

How Nonadherence Affects the Calculation of Costs and Effects. The left-hand column of Table 14.4 provides an exhaustive list of incremental costs and effects. These are the net costs and effects that arise after subtracting the control group costs and effects from the intervention group costs and effects. In order to do this in a study methodically it may be necessary to obtain estimates of relevant categories in Table 14.4 separately for the control and intervention groups; these would serve as inputs into the incremental cost-effectiveness calculation. Later, we discuss net changes between the intervention and control group. This table is intended to offer a menu of costs and effects for researchers to choose from. Considering all of the items would provide a societal perspective.

Looking down the left-hand column, there are costs to all of the stakeholders, medical and nonmedical direct costs and indirect costs. Based on the study perspective the researcher would compile a list of items to include in the calculation. Costs to family members and caregivers, though not trivial in some cases, or costs to employers, such as the hiring of temporary workers due to absenteeism, may or may not be considered for a particular study.

Further down the left-hand column are the incremental effects of the intervention. The patient's health effects could be measured by changes in QALYs, or some other measure of health status such as life years saved or an improvement in a clinical test. Reverting to the example on hypertension, reducing 50% of the treatment group's blood pressure to 130 may translate to an increase of 0.1 in the overall QALY score (or the effectiveness measure could simply be "under 130 or above 130," a dichotomous measure). In addition, there may be health effects of family members and/or society to consider depending on the perspective of the study.

Considering treatment nonadherence, in the right-hand column of Table 14.4, it is clear that there are diverse consequences of nonadherence behavior. In addition to concrete costs such as net changes in health care costs from not taking one's medicine (could save out-of-pocket drug expenditures while increasing utilization due to nonadherence), a patient could require more staff time at the doctor's office due to complications, could lose productivity at work or have more absences, or could require more intensive caregiving from family members.

In terms of nonadherence effects on health, at the bottom of the right-hand column, not only could a patient's QALY score change from both short-term and long-term changes in health status, but also a researcher may want to consider the societal changes from the nonadherence behavior. Most common considerations are when nonadherence behavior affects others indirectly by changing the herd immunity of a community, by contributing to antibiotic resistance, or by spreading disease to others directly. Also, for particular diseases the societal effects are very different. Consider a schizophrenic patient who does not adhere and has a psychotic break. His or her subsequent behavior can affect society on many levels, including harming others, becoming homeless and using more social services (say a homeless shelter), or no longer supporting his or her family so that they have to use more social services. This is very different from HIV nonadherence in which the effects could be on increased infection directly through sex, and indirectly through the development of drug-resisting HIV strains.

In calculating the net costs and effects, it may not be possible to establish the causal pathway between treatment nonadherence and the observed changes. Does a person's QALY score change because they stopped taking their medication, or did they stop taking their medication because their QALY score had changed, say from side effects? For the economic evaluation the goal is to record all of the costs and effects as accurately as possible and causality can be addressed using other research tools. Next we discuss some further considerations to make in an economic evaluation in order to achieve this goal.

Aggregation. In addition to aggregating all relevant costs and effects in the first column of Table 14.4, ultimately all of the costs and consequences of nonadherence will be aggregated once for the intervention group and once for the control group in order to get the incremental cost-effectiveness ratio of nonadherence (called IC_{AD} and IE_{AD} in Table 14.2). Aggregation may differ based on the intervention because nonadherence behavior can be manifested in several ways. For example, all patients could be nonadherent for part of the time. Alternatively, only a portion of the patients could be nonadherent.

Even if two individuals are equally nonadherent, outcomes may be affected in different ways, which creates interesting issues for aggregation. For example, if two patients both neglect to take their HIV drug cocktail for 1 week, it may have a linear relationship with the outcome, say risk of viral resistance. For the other patient, however, the effect on the outcome may be a multifold increase in the risk of viral resistance.

Not aggregating over the full time period may lead to differences in costs of adherers and nonadherers. In the short term, a patient who is totally nonadherent may not incur any costs. They are not going into the doctor for follow-up care; they are not filling the prescription; they are not missing time off work to go to appointments. Aggregating across all patients over the full time horizon of the study will allow for the full picture to emerge.

Sensitivity Analyses. Difficulties in aggregating costs and effects of nonadherence are one of many reasons to perform sensitivity analysis on the cost-effectiveness results. Sensitivity analysis allows researchers to ascertain how sensitive outcomes are to changes in the assumptions and adds robustness to the results (for an example with HIV drugs, see Freedberg et al., ref. 41). Changing key assumptions (such as changes in risk of viral resistance or changes in the discount rate) will establish a confidence interval around one's cost-effectiveness results. In addition to changing the discount rate and the future costs of the intervention, altering adherence rates and the adherence definition could provide useful information. Sensitivity analysis can also be performed using simulation techniques such as Monte Carlo Estimation. For example, the results of the analysis may change depending on whether the investigator calculates nonadherence behavior as: (a) 50% of patients are completely adherent and 50% are not at all adherent or (b) 100% of the patients are adherent 50% of the time. The simulated health outcomes and the costs may both be different.

Sensitivity analysis on the adherence rates in a randomized controlled trial can also help predict what might happen if the intervention is adopted into the practice setting, because adherence usually falls outside of a randomized controlled trial.

SPECIAL CONSIDERATIONS WHEN STUDYING MEDICATION NONADHERENCE

The costs and consequences of nonadherence are not uniform. Adherence problems occur more with some types of medications or treatment regiments than others, and the consequences will vary with characteristics of the disease and patient. For the purposes of this discussion, we assume that we are dealing only with chronic diseases. Adherence is a substantial problem with medication for acute illnesses such as acute bacterial infections (e.g., urinary tract infections), but the consequences are similarly relatively acute and easily understood. Chronic diseases such as hypertension, asthma, diabetes, HIV, and tuberculosis are the greatest challenges at present. The second assumption is that the medications used are effective in ameliorating symptoms, delaying morbidity, improving function, and so on. Ineffective or marginally effective medications will of course lead to cost savings if they are not taken. In this section, we discuss four areas that may influence adherence: the characteristics of the medication prescribed, the characteristics of the disease being treated, the characteristics of the patient, and the characteristics of the study design.

Characteristics of the Medications. The characteristics of the prescribed medications influence the rate of nonadherence. It is difficult to isolate the role of the medication in nonadherence, because such characteristics often interact with the other special considerations discussed in this section, especially the disease. For example, the pharmaceutical industry would never consider testing a medication that had substantial side effects and could only be delivered by injection when the disease being treated was allergic rhinitis. Diseases with modest health consequences are generally treated with medications with modest side effect profiles. However, within a given disease, some medications will be more likely to lead to nonadherence than other medications. Empiric data on this topic are relatively scant. Medications with more side effects are going to be more likely to result in nonadherence than medication with few side effects. This issue is magnified in chronic diseases in which the patient may have few, if any symptoms. For example, patients with hypertension or hyperlipidemia (elevated LDL cholesterol) generally have no symptoms at all. Any adverse reaction may be viewed with concern by the patient, because the outcome to be prevented (stroke or myocardial infarction) may not occur until years in the future, if at all. Factors such as taste, pill size, cost, and whether or not the medication needs to be taken with meals or other medications may all influence treatment adherence. The need for multiple doses each day may be a significant factor leading to reduced adherence. Though adherence for twice daily dosing may be only marginally reduced, if a medication is required four times a day adherence may be substantially reduced. The increased availability of extended-release preparations can ameliorate this problem.

Characteristics of the Disease.   Diseases such as hyperlipidemia and hypertension are the most pertinent examples of diseases that may have more serious consequences for nonadherence costs compared to other diseases because they are essentially asymptomatic for a period of years (for more on chronic asymptomatic diseases and adherence, see Miller, ref. 42). The out-of-pocket costs of the medication, and the disutility of administration in time and concurrent side effects must then be weighed against future benefit. Type 2 diabetes may be either symptomatic or asymptomatic. With increased emphasis on early detection and recently emphasis on more aggressive glycemic control, diabetes is now a chronic disease that is often asymptomatic. Early-stage HIV may similarly manifest few symptoms. As the CD-4 count drops and HIV progresses, the disease will of course become much more symptomatic.

The consequences of nonadherence with a medication regimen may of course vary substantially as well. For some diseases, morbidity may ensue within weeks or months of cessation or reduction in medication. Tuberculosis is the most typical example of rapid occurrence of morbidity from nonadherence, and HIV has demonstrated that it has similar characteristics (this is exacerbated for persons with HIV who have contracted tuberculosis, which is a serious problem throughout the world). Conversely, the consequences of cessation of HMG-CoA lipid-lowering agents ("statins") may not be observable for months, years, or ever. Clinical epidemiologists employ a standard metric for such circumstances, the "number needed to treat" (NNT). The NNT is simply 1/Absolute Risk Reduction. In words, the NNT is the number of patients with disease X who must be treated in order to prevent one morbid (or mortal) event. If the absolute risk reduction from an intervention is 0.2, then the NNT = 5, meaning that five patients must be treated in order to benefit one. The same agent may have different NNT depending on the disease being treated. For example, statins are used both for treatment of primary hyperlipidemia (primary prevention) and for secondary prevention after a myocardial infarction (MI) or episode or unstable angina. The NNT for primary prevention is about 140 over 5 years (43) and for secondary prevention is 30 over 5 years (44). The consequences of nonadherence are therefore quite different because the baseline rate of the same event (MI or cardiac death) is so different in the two circumstances. The costs of nonadherence will therefore be much greater when the rate of events is greater, and when the time to the event is sooner rather than later. Where the consequences of nonadherence are mild, such as the recurrence of symptomatic allergic rhinitis, adherence behavior will be expected to be somewhat worse.

Characteristics of the Patient. Nonadherence costs will also differ depending on patient characteristics. Patients who have multiple comorbidities are an interesting case in point. The risk of adverse cardiac events (cardiac death or MI) in the setting of hyperlipidemia is much greater if comorbidities of preexisting angina and/or diabetes and/or hypertension are present. Though the proportional reduction in risk from a given medication is often similar between high-comorbidity and low-comorbidity patients, the absolute reduction in risk may be much greater. For example, if taking an HMG-CoA reductase inhibitor reduces cardiac event risk by 25%, the absolute risk reduction to the patient with a 1% cardiac event risk/year in the subsequent 4 years will be one event prevented for every 100 patients treated. If a patient has multiple comorbidities or advanced age and has an 8% annual risk, then that patient's cardiac event risk over the next 4 years will be approximately 32%. A 25% reduction in that risk will prevent eight events for every 100 patients treated. The cost and health consequences of nonadherence are therefore much greater for the higher risk patients with multiple comorbidities. Over a relatively brief time horizon, the cost-effectiveness of many treatments for patients with multiple concurrent conditions is more than for patients with single conditions.

Patients with multiple comorbidities and some demographic characteristics such as advanced age may inhibit adherence. Patients with diabetes and common comorbidities now commonly take eight different medications (three medications for glucose control, three antihypertensive agents, aspirin for cardiac protection, plus a cholesterol-lowering agent). Even absent payment problems, the difficulties of remembering to take the medications, keep up with refills, and so on, are substantial. Even when patients are insured, many plans will only allow a 1-month supply of medication. Refilling multiple medications on time is complex and can lead to reduced adherence. In addition, as we mentioned earlier, the more frequent the dose, the less likely it will be taken.

Clearly, economic barriers to drugs exist for some low-income persons (e.g., those not on Medicaid or elderly who are only on Medicare). Many health insurance plans, including Medicare (as of 2003), do not provide any assistance in purchasing medications. Cost issues may be pertinent for a single medication, and these issues are multiplied when a patient requires multiple medications for multiple conditions. Prescriptions may not be filled, or they may be "stretched" by taking medications only every other day instead of every day. Such issues are not present in standard randomized clinical trials, because the medication is almost always supplied at no cost to the patient. Medication costs should not be dichotomized into "insurance–no insurance" but exist on a continuum. Patients with insurance may have a variety of deductibles and copayment options, which may be substantial in situations such as "reference-based pricing," where one medication in a class may have a different copayment structure than another. Collection of information on the amount of copayment in addition to the presence or absence of any insurance or insurance for medications is important when assessing the determinants of drug adherence.

Patient preferences may also play some role in adherence. Such preferences will vary markedly from patient to patient, with patients sometimes having to make choices between purchasing medications for chronic conditions and other essential purchases such as food or housing. Without insurance, in the case of a diabetic with comorbid conditions, out-of-pocket costs will easily amount to several hundred dollars per month.

Institutional factors such as poor continuums of care or lack of communication between primary-care and specialty doctors can lead to little oversight on number of drugs someone is taking and hence nonadherence behavior (bad outcomes, more side effects, etc.). Clearly there are many more provider and institutional issues that investigators should consider in a given study if provider and organizational issues could affect nonadherence and costs from nonadherence.

Study Design. Beyond the characteristics of the medications, disease, and patients, the research design influences aspects of conducting CEAs. For example, patients receiving usual care within a trial may be quite different than the patients who would receive the intervention (if effective). Patients who are excluded from the trial due to, for example, age, comorbidity, or refusal would potentially receive efficacious interventions. The impact of restricted eligibility criteria can be seen in trials of medications, where trials are often conducted with pristine patients not commonly seen in most primary-care practices. Yet, these medications may be included in clinical practice guidelines for all patients with a specific disease. Patients in randomized control trials are generally healthier and more adherent than patients in usual practice (45).

Randomized trials are often conducted with a "run-in period." The run-in is a period during which patients take the study medication prior to randomization to study medication or placebo. During the run-in, adherence is assessed, as is tolerability of the study medication. Individuals with high rates of nonadherence will be identified through the surveillance and excluded from the trial. This decision makes sense from the perspective of establishing efficacy, and such exclusions do not decrease the internal validity of the trial. But, if nonadherence will ultimately be prevalent for an efficacious medication, the potential effect would be overestimated (and resulting cost-effectiveness ratio understated). Finally, the high degree of intensive surveillance and the offer of incentives to participate in a treatment trial may artificially increase adherence to the regimens. This may, again, impact the magnitude of the effect that would be observed when the intervention is applied outside of the trial.

NONADHERENCE IN HEALTH POLICY

We can offer many examples of how nonadherence can affect cost-effectiveness estimates for a health policy. Prescription drug coverage for patients on Medicare may be the single most discussed policy in health care for the past decade. Because the high prevalence of chronic disease increases with age, Medicare recipients are prescribed far more medications than non-Medicare recipients. However, unless Medicare beneficiaries have supplemental insurance, they must pay for their outpatient medications using their own financial resources (at the writing of this chapter The Medicare Prescription Drug, Improvement, and Modernization Act of 2003 had just passed, hence prescription-drug coverage will begin in 2006).

The cost of the prescription-drug program is likely to be substantial. Estimates in 2003 in the popular press are upwards of $400 billion; however, estimating the costs and impact of this policy is substantially affected by patient adherence. Certainly, health economists can make estimates about the average number of drugs that will be prescribed to each Medicare recipient, as well as the cost. However, it is more difficult to estimate the cost implications of this program because questions related to costs and adherence become important:

- Will physicians prescribe drugs to Medicare recipients? On the patient side, doing so will require that he or she visit the physician. And, once there, physicians must prescribe the medications.
- Assuming this barrier is overcome, how many Medicare patients will actually obtain these medications? The answer to this will depend on other barriers to filling prescriptions (e.g., out-of-pocket costs from copayments and deductible, transportation barriers). It is interesting to note that, should the program increase access for only the most af-

fluent patients, it may have less impact upon individuals with the greatest need (and potential benefit) for this program.

- Assuming patients fill their medication prescriptions, will they actually adhere to prescribed medications? As the degree of nonadherence increases, society is faced with a cost that may have no benefit.
- How will a prescription-drug program influence the cost of medications? This will be a function of factors such as increased demand, ability of the participating private plans to negotiate price, and manufacturers' ability to lower the profit margin per drug when the number of medications sold increases.
- Finally, assuming the aforementioned issues are resolved, what will be the net benefit of increasing prescription-drug coverage on our society? Will there be a cost offset in that subsequent health services utilization is reduced?

Clearly, one policy change can have complicated effects on adherence behavior and subsequent costs. This can be applied to any health policy change being considered and can be useful when debating two different policy options. For example, Medicare prescription-drug legislation with less privatization may have had differential effects on access to prescription drugs and adherence than legislation with a great deal of privatization because access to care for sick elders or copays may be different. There is a risk for cherry picking healthier patients into privatized plans, which in turn can create barriers to access for more-sick elderly patients. Taking a societal perspective, having lower adherence to needed drugs in a highly privatized plan may have changed the relative cost-effectiveness of the two proposals.

Besides considering new health policies, investigators may need to examine how existing policies contribute to nonadherence costs. For example, say a national HIV drug trial shows a highly efficacious treatment for HIV patients, yet in the South there is a steep step-down in efficacy in the practice setting. This regional step-down in efficacy may be explained by health policy and adherence behavior. Why? Historically public money for AIDS care has gone primarily to New York, Los Angeles, and other metropolitan areas because in the early years of the epidemic AIDS hit those cities hard. But currently the disease is hitting rural areas and Black communities in the South, where money for care is lacking (46). In fact, due to lack of funding North Carolina recently started putting HIV patients on waiting lists to get help with HIV drugs so adherence is expected to fall. Such considerations, though outside the normal scope of factors explaining nonadherence, can be useful for the clinical investigator in order to disentangle why adherence rates are poor for a given treatment regimen.

SUMMARY

This chapter has provided an overview of how researchers can account for nonadherence costs and effects in their clinical and health services research. We used patient adherence to medications and chronic diseases as our guiding example in addressing the costs of nonadherence. We reviewed the scant economic literature on the cost of nonadherence, discussed the most common economic evaluation methods that are available to approach nonadherence costs, and described health utility preference measures as they relate to nonadherence. We discussed the mechanics of cost-effectiveness given imperfect adherence behavior and provided a template of costs and effects that researchers should consider in their work. We also laid out standard methodological considerations needed for performing sound economic evaluation studies of nonadherence costs. In addition we presented special cases when adherence would be expected to differ, and discussed the implications of considering nonadherence costs in health policy.

A resounding theme emerged in this chapter—despite knowing that nonadherence can lead to poor patient outcomes, we lack information on the *costs* of nonadherence behavior. The few studies that exist focused on treatment nonadherence leading to increased hospitalization. Few economic evaluations of interventions explicitly consider the costs and effects of nonadherence behavior, and few studies in the health economics or health services literature have used multivariate modeling techniques to estimate the costs of nonadherence for a broad population of patients. Despite this, nonadherence continues to be a significant clinical problem in medicine and shows no sign of abating (3). Hence, we hope that researchers can use the economic evaluation methods described in this chapter as a first step toward incorporating nonadherence costs into their work.

REFERENCES

1. Berg JS, Dischler J, Wagner DJ, Raia JJ, Palmer-Shevlin N. Medication compliance: a healthcare problem. *Ann Pharmacother.* 1993;27(Suppl):1–24.
2. Iskedjian M, Addis A, Einarson TR. Estimating the economic burden of hospitalization due to patient nonadherence in Canada. In: *1998 International Society for Pharmaceutical and Outcomes Research Conference.* 1998.
3. Haynes R, McDonald H, Garg AX, Montague P. Interventions for helping patients to follow prescriptions of medications. (Cochrane Review). In: *The Cochrane Library.* 2003.
4. Cleemput I, Kesteloot K. Economic implications of non-compliance in health care. *Lancet.* 2002;359(9324):2129–2130.

5. Swindle RW, Rao JK, Helmy A, et al. Integrating clinical nurse specialists into the treatment of primary care patients with depression. *Int J Psychiatry Med.* 2003;33:17–37.

6. Ambrosioni E. Pharmacoeconomic challenges in disease management of hypertension. *J Hypertens.* 2001;19(Suppl 3):33–40.

7. Hughes DA, Bagust A, Haycox A, Walley T. The impact of non-compliance on the cost-effectiveness of pharmaceuticals: a review of the literature. *Health Econ.* 2001;10:601–615.

8. Leibowitz A, Manning WG Jr., Newhouse JP. The demand for prescription drugs as a function of cost sharing. *Soc Sci Med.* 1985;21:1063–1070.

9. Case A, Lubotsky D, Paxon C. Economic status and health in childhood: the origins of the gradient. *American Economic Review.* 2001;92(5):1308–1334.

10. Ashton C, Haidet P, Pateniti DA, et al. Racial and ethnic disparities in the use of health services: bias, preferences, or poor communication? *J Gen Intern Med.* 2003;18(2):146–152.

11. Gosden T, Forland F, Kristiansen IS, et al. Impact of payment method on behaviour of primary care physicians: a systematic review. *Journal of Health Services Research Policy.* 2001;6(1):44–55.

12. Green JH. Frequent rehospitalization and noncompliance with treatment. *Hospital Community Psychiatry.* 1988;39(9):963–966.

13. Fishbein HA. Precipitants of hospitalization in insulin-dependent diabetes mellitus (IDDM): a statewide perspective. *Diabetes Care.* 1985;8(Suppl 1):61–64.

14. Singer ME. Medical and economic outcomes of noncompliance with dilantin in adult Medicaid epileptics. *Value Health.* 1998;1(1):47.

15. Drummond MF, O'Brien B, Stoddart GL, Torrance GW. *Methods for the Economic Evaluation of Health Care Programmes.* 2nd ed. New York: Oxford Medical Publications; 1997.

16. Gold MR, Siegel JE, Rossell LB, et al. *Cost-Effectiveness in Health and Medicine.* Weinstein M, ed. New York: Oxford University Press; 1996.

17. Johannesson M. *Theory and Methods of Economic Evaluation of Health Care.* Dordrecht, the Netherlands: Kluwer Academic Publishers; 1996.

18. Sloan FA, ed. *Valuing Health Care: Care, Costs and Benefits of Pharmaceuticals and Other Medical Technologies.* New York: Cambridge University Press; 1995.

19. Van Houtven G. *Lecture Notes on Economic Evaluation Methods.* In: Marisa Domino's health economics course. University of North Carolina; 2003.

20. McIntosh E, Donaldson C, Ryan M. Recent advances in the methods of cost–benefit analysis in healthcare. *Pharmacoeconomics.* 1999;15(4):357–367.

21. Goldstein MK. Introduction to patient preferences and utility assessment. In: *Health Economics Research Group Health Economics Research Course.* Menlo Park, CA: VA Palo Alto Health Care System; 2003.

22. Ware JE, Sherbourne CD. The MOS 36-item short-form health survey (SF-36): I. conceptual framework and item selection. *Med Care.* 1992;30:473–483.

23. Kaplan RM, Anderson JP. A general health policy model: update and applications. *Health Serv Res.* 1988;June 23:203–235.

24. Brazier J, Deverill M, Green C. A review of the use of health status measures in economic evaluation. *Health Technol Assess.* 1999;3(9):i–ix;1–164.

25. Weeks J, O'Leary J, Fairclough D, et al. The Q-tility Index: a new tool for assessing healthrelated quality of life and utilities in clinical trials and clinical practice. *Proceedings of the American Society of Clinical Oncology.* 1994;13:436.

26. American Thoracic Society. *Quality of Life Indicators.* http://www.thoracic.org.

27. McDowell I, Newell C. *Measuring Health: A Guide to Rating Scales and Questionnaires.* 2nd ed. New York: Oxford University Press; 1996.

28. Donaldson C. Valuing the benefits of publicly provided health care: does "ability to pay" preclude the use of "willingness to pay"? *Soc Sci Med.* 1999;49(4):551–563.

29. O'Brien B, Viramontes J. Willingness to pay: a valid and reliable measure of health state preference? *Med Decis Mak.* 1994;14(3):290–297.

30. Hirth RA, Chernew ME, Miller EA, Fendrick AM, Weissert WG. Willingness to pay for a quality-adjusted life year: in search of a standard. *Med Decis Mak.* 2000;20(3):332–342.

31. Donaldson C. Eliciting patients' values by the use of "willingness to pay": letting the theory drive the method. *Health Expect.* 2001;4(3):180–188.

32. Goldstein MK, Michelson DG, Clarke AE, et al. A multimedia preference-assessment tool for functional outcomes. In: *17th Annual Symposium on Computer Applications in Medical Care.* New York: McGraw-Hill; 1993.

33. Lenert L, Kaplan RM. Validity and interpretation of preference-based measures of health-related quality of life. *Med Care.* 2000;38(Suppl 9):138–150.

34. Keilhorn A, Graf von der Schulenburg JM. *The Health Economics Handbook.* 2nd ed. Chester: Adis International; 2000.

35. *Macarthur initiative on depression and primary care at Dartmouth and Duke Web sites.* Respect-depression randomized controlled trial.

36. Toronto General Hospital. http://uhn.ca/tgh/.

37. *Hyperdictionary.* http://www.hyperdictionary.com.

38. Whittington D, Matsui O, Freiberger J, Van Houtven G, Pattanayak S. Private demand for a HIV/AIDS vaccine: evidence from Guadalajara, Mexico. *Vaccine.* 2002;20(19/20):2585–2591.

39. Blandford L, Dans PE, Ober JD, Wheelock C. Analyzing variations in medication compliance related to individual drug, drug class, prescribing physician. *J Manag Care Pharm.* 1999;5(1):47–51.

40. Bronder E, Klimpel A. Unused drugs returned to the pharmacy—new data. *Int J Clin Pharmacol.* 2001;39(11):480–483.

41. Freedberg KA, Losina E, Weinstein MC, et al. The cost effectiveness of combination anti-retroviral therapy for HIV disease. *N Engl J Med.* 2001;344(11):824–831.

42. Miller N. Compliance with treatment regimens in chronic asymptomatic diseases. *Am J Med.* 1997;201(2A):43–49.

43. Simes J, Furburg CD, Braunwald E, et al. Effect of pravastatin on mortality in patients with and without coronary heart disease across a broad range of cholesterol levels. The Prospective Pravastatin Pooling Project. *Eur Heart J.* 2001;23:207–215.

44. Pedersen TR, Olsson AG, Faergeman O, et al. Lipoprotein changes and reduction in the incidence of major coronary heart disease events in the Scandinavian Simvastatin Survival Study. *Circulation.* 1998;97:1453–1460.
45. Rosser WW. Application of evidence from randomized controlled trials to general practice. *Lancet.* 1999;353:661–664.
46. Avery S. NC aid for HIV will run short: state to put people on a waiting list. In: *News and Observer.* 2003.
47. Luce BR, Manning WG, Siegel JE, et al. Estimating costs in cost-effectiveness analysis. In: Gold MR, Siegel JE, Russell LB, Weinstein MC, eds. *Cost-Effectiveness in Health and Medicine.* New York: Oxford University Press; 1996.

Chapter 15

Estimating Causal Effects in Randomized Studies With Imperfect Adherence: Conceptual and Statistical Foundations

Kevin J. Anstrom
Kevin P. Weinfurt
Andrew S. Allen
Duke University

Other chapters in this volume describe nonadherence's impact on health treatment and describe methods for its prevention. In this chapter, we describe the impact of nonadherence on the interpretations of clinical study findings. This newer statistical literature is characterized by a wide diversity of methods not easily implemented using standard software packages. Accordingly, our intent in this chapter is to convey key statistical concepts using simple examples without focusing on computational and implementation issues. Readers interested in a more technical discussion will find references to more advanced treatments toward the end of this chapter. The reader will also find a glossary of key terms at the end of this chapter.

To better understand the statistical issues underlying interpretation of studies with imperfect adherence, we review the findings from a randomized study comparing the effect of a vitamin supplement versus a control on 1-year mortality. A prior series of observational studies of Javanese children had suggested a link between excess mortality and vitamin A deficiency (1, 2). As with all observation studies, these findings were subject to potential selection biases such as access to medical treatment, family motivation, and dietary differences. Therefore, a randomized study was designed to test the hypothesis that vitamin A supplementation would decrease mortality in these children (3).

A total of 450 villages were randomized to either a vitamin A supplementation arm or a control arm. For reasons related to the method of vitamin A administration, randomization was conducted at the village level rather than the child level. Children in the 229 villages in the vitamin A arm were scheduled to receive two doses of vitamin A; the first dose was scheduled to be administered between 1 and 3 months following randomization and the second dose was planned for approximately 6–8 months thereafter (3). For local regulatory reasons, children in the 221 villages randomized to the control arm received usual care rather than placebo. All children were scheduled to be followed for at least 12 months. The primary response variable was survival at 1-year postrandomization.

A summary of the data comparing mortality by treatment arm is shown in Table 15.1. To be included in the data presented in Table 15.1, children had to have been alive at 4 months postrandomization, which would have allowed them enough time to have received their initial vitamin A supplementation. A comparison of mortality rates suggests that children in the vitamin A arm had lower mortality (0.38% vs. 0.64%). The estimated risk ratio for mortality comparing vitamin A children to control children was 0.59 = (.0038/.0064). Alternatively, the risk difference estimated by the difference between was .26% favoring those children randomized to vitamin A supplementation.

Do the data in Table 15.1 suggest the mortality benefit of receiving vitamin A supplementation? The answer is yes and no. The data do provide strong statistical evidence ($p < .05$) that survival was better among children *randomized* to vitamin A. So yes, there is a suggestion that receiving vitamin A is associated with lower mortality. However, before addressing the question of what impact vitamin A has on reducing infant mortality, we should mention that not every child in the vitamin A arm actually received the supplements. Consider data shown in Table 15.2, where children in the vitamin A arm are described as adherent if they received at least one dose of vitamin A and not adherent otherwise. For children randomized to the control arm we know that they did not receive vitamin A but we do not know if they would have received vitamin A if it was offered. This lack of information is displayed in Table 15.2 using dashes and in Fig. 15.1 using dotted lines. We observe that 20% of children (or 2,419 of the 12,094) randomized to vitamin A never received the supplement. From Table 15.2, we also

TABLE 15.1
Data From the Vitamin A Study

	Randomized to Control Arm		Randomized to Vitamin A Arm	
	# of Children	% of Children	# of Children	% of Children
Alive	11,514	99.36%	12,048	99.62%
Dead	74	0.64%	46	0.38%
Total	11,588	100.00%	12,094	100.00%

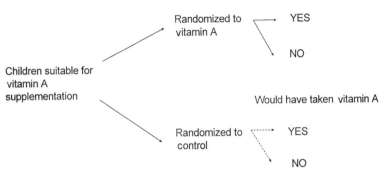

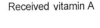

FIG. 15.1. Illustration of observed and counterefactual adherence data.

TABLE 15.2
The Vitamin A Study Mortality Data Stratified by Adherence Status

Study Group	Adherence Status	# of Children	# Alive	# Dead	Mortality Rate
Control	No	—	—	—	—
	Yes	—	—	—	—
	Total	11,588	11,514	74	0.64%
Vitamin A	No	2,419	2,385	34	1.41%
	Yes	9,675	9,663	12	0.12%
	Total	12,094	12,048	46	0.38%

see a suggestion that the 20% of nonadherent children in the vitamin A arm are somehow different than the children in the control arm. In fact, the mortality rate among the nonadherent children in the vitamin A arm is more than twice as high as the overall mortality rate in the control arm (1.41% vs. 0.64%). What, then, is the proper way to conceptualize the effect of vitamin A on mortality?

Prior to going deeper into the analysis and interpretation of the vitamin A study, we describe a statistical framework that will allow us to describe the assumptions required to estimate the effects of treatment. In the statistical literature, the term *compliance* is commonly used to describe a patient's adherence to treatment. Throughout this chapter, we use the term *adherence* except when describing a proper term from the statistical literature.

After reading this chapter, we hope that readers are able to understand and answer the following questions:

1. Why do regulatory agencies encourage intention-to-treat (ITT) analyses? Is this reasonable?

2. Can't we just take the children that received vitamin A and compare them with controls? Why not?

3. What would have been the effect of the vitamin A supplementation if every child had received the supplement as planned?

4. Would changing the method of vitamin A administration alter the observed benefit? Why?

5. How are we to interpret the effects of studies in which people do not have perfect adherence?

APPROACHES TO RANDOMIZED STUDIES

Although there are many ways to design a clinical study to address questions of causal efficacy, the randomized clinical trial method is regarded as most scientifically valid (4). Considered one of the 20th century's great scientific advances, the process of randomization guarantees that all baseline variables, both measure and unmeasured, are balanced on average between groups assigned to different interventions (5). Thus, in a properly controlled study, any observed difference in outcomes between two or more randomized groups can be attributed to the actions (e.g., taking medications, exercising regularly) that followed randomization.

One type of randomized trial is the clinical trial, which is designed to address certain types of questions. In an oft-cited paper by Schwartz and Lellouch, a distinction was made between so-called "explanatory" and "pragmatic" approaches to conducting clinical research (6). An explanatory approach can be described as an attempt to understand and test hypotheses concerning the biological action of the treatment (7). In a drug trial, for example, the explanatory question would address the pharmacologic effect of the drug. On the other hand, a pragmatic approach can be described as an attempt to understand the effects of a treatment regime when it is taken in the context of usual practice. This approach focuses on public health questions with the hope that the clinical studies will provide information necessary to improve and change health policy. For many studies, the question of interest is how effective a treatment would be in normal practice.

A more recent version of the distinction just described, and the one that we adopt for the remainder of this chapter, is from the work of Sheiner and Rubin (8). These authors consider two ways to evaluate the effectiveness of treatment. *Use-effectiveness* measures the impact of therapy assignment on response, also known as the programmatic effectiveness or effectiveness (9). *Method-effectiveness* measures the impact of the actual therapy administered on response, also known as the biological efficacy or efficacy. Sheiner and Rubin stress that both use- and method-effectiveness are important to demonstrate. The authors suggest that once a therapy has been shown to work under ideal circumstances (method-effectiveness), then it is reasonable to test the use-effectiveness.

The most widely accepted approach to analyzing clinical trials, the ITT strategy, is also assumed to be an estimate of the use-effectiveness. In an ITT analysis, comparisons among patients are made based on their *nominal* treatment group—that is, the group to which they were randomized. As shown in Fig. 15.1, the children in the vitamin A study receive their nominal treatment strategies once they are randomized. So, in the context of the vitamin A study, the ITT paradigm tests the statistical hypothesis that *randomization to treatment* is statistically independent of (i.e., has nothing to do with) the children's survival 1 year later.

Many statisticians and researchers have discussed the properties of the ITT approach(5, 8, 10–18) Briefly, the strengths of ITT include:

- Maintains the benefits of randomization; namely, that treatment comparisons are balanced based on prerandomization factors.
- Provides an unbiased estimate of use-effectiveness within the conditions of care observed in the specific trial. To the degree that the trial is representative of usual care outside of the trial, ITT provides an estimate of use-effectiveness for contexts outside of the trial.
- Is a simple analysis that uses all patients' data and makes few assumptions (compared to modeling). ITT does not require modeling, which creates uncertainty and the need for sensitivity analyses.

Some weaknesses of the ITT approach are that:

- If the conditions of the trial deviate significantly from routine care, ITT will not provide a good use-effectiveness estimate. A variety of factors may cause differences between clinical trials and standard practice. These include the individual's rate of adherence level, access to medical staff, level of motivation, and awareness that they may be receiving a placebo.
- The results may be misinterpreted as unbiased estimates of method-effectiveness, when in fact they are not necessarily good estimates.
- The analyses create confusion when the null hypothesis is not rejected. Was the lack of a statistically significant result due to an ineffective drug or was it due to high rates of nonadherence and crossover?
- For many investigators, it seems illogical to treat individuals who have not received the intervention as if they have or to count individuals known to have received the intervention as controls.

Depending on the precise question being asked, ITT may or may not be the best approach. In particular, the type of analysis should match the study question. With respect to nonadherence, ITT is not especially helpful if (a) adherence in the trial does not reflect adherence under conditions of routine care, and/or (b) we are primarily interested in estimating the method-effectiveness of the intervention.

POTENTIAL OUTCOMES AND RUBIN'S CAUSAL MODEL

Clinical investigators may seek to make causal statements about randomization to an intervention or actual receipt of the intended intervention. The causal effect of randomization is a quantity more relevant for use-effectiveness whereas the causal effect of actual receipt of intervention is more relevant for method-effectiveness. In the causal effect of intervention receipt, we seek to know whether a particular patient will respond differently if they receive or do not receive the intervention.[1] These hypothetical data are referred to as potential outcomes. With data from a clinical trial, we are not able to observe what would happen to each person if they tried one, then another treatment. Instead, we observe what happens to each patient when they receive the condition to which they were assigned. To directly answer our causal question, then, we need access to data that do not exist. We can, however, indirectly answer our question by making some assumptions about the study design, treatments, and people's behavior. The Rubin causal model (RCM) helps us to identify those assumptions required for us to estimate causal effects. Specifically, the RCM allows us to estimate the *average* causal effect for some population of patients—that is, if we had to pick one number to use to guess each person's causal effect, the average causal effect would be our best guess. In randomized studies with nonadherence, we restrict average causal effect estimates to the subset of individuals that would have altered their behavior, depending on the treatment assignment.

To define average causal effect, we first define the ideal case (i.e., pretend that we observe potential outcomes). This allows us to formally state the causal effect we'd like to estimate. Then, we specify equation(s) for estimating the effect of interest, given the trial's observed data. In the following sections, we define variables that assist in describing the ideal case and in characterizing different approaches to analyzing trial data within the RCM. In a later section, we present an example using the vitamin A study that in-

---

[1] As a general rule, if you can not imagine a patient receiving either treatment then use of the potential outcomes framework is not valid (19). For example, applying causal-inference techniques to estimate benefits of surgery compared with medical therapy with a patient population that includes some individuals with contraindications for surgery would not be appropriate.

cludes an equation to estimate an average causal effect of interest based on the RCM.

As the previous section illustrated, nonadherence can complicate the interpretation of clinical trial results. An additional complexity is the fact that patients may be nonadherent for different reasons, and those different reasons may lead us to treat them differently. In the end, we want to estimate the causal effect of the intervention for the average person. To do this, we need to identify possible types of nonadherence within a principled statistical framework. The RCM (sometimes referred to as the potential outcomes or counterfactual framework) is applicable to various disciplines (e.g., economics, social sciences) and methodologies (e.g., randomized vs. nonrandomized studies) (20). Furthermore, the model assists us in conducting sensitivity analyses to judge how changing assumptions might change our results.

To describe the model, we define variables corresponding to: (a) the treatment assignment, (b) the treatment or dose actually received, and (c) the response that would have occurred under conditions that could be manipulated by the experimenter. In the simplest case, we consider two possible treatments, two possible levels of adherence, and a binary response variable. In a study with perfect compliance, the treatment received would always be the same as the nominal treatment. In other words, if a child was randomized to the vitamin A then they would receive the supplements; if they were randomized to control then they would not receive the supplements. In the vitamin A example, we can think of two levels of potential outcomes: (a) the potential receipt of vitamin A depending on treatment assigned and (b) the potential survival at 1 year depending on the treatment assigned and receipt of the supplement. In actuality, each child is randomized to only one of the treatments. If a child is randomized to vitamin A, we are able to observe whether they received vitamin A and whether they survived beyond 1 year. The other potential outcomes, the treatment receipt and response if assigned to control, are not observed and we refer to those quantities as counterfactual (or contrary to fact). For no child in the study do we get to see both sets of potential outcomes.

In the RCM, causal effects are defined as differences between potential outcomes. For example, the causal effect of randomization on receipt of vitamin A is given by the difference between the potential outcomes (e.g., receipt of vitamin A if randomized to vitamin A and receipt of vitamin A if randomized to control). In Table 15.3, the possible adherence combinations are displayed. A child would be labeled an *always-taker* (or *never-taker*) if they would always (never) receive vitamin A regardless of the randomization. A child would be labeled a *complier* if their actual receipt of vitamin A would correspond to their treatment assignment. A child would be labeled *defier* if their receipt of vitamin A was always discordant with their treatment assignment. We note that the groups are not observable quantities and are

TABLE 15.3.
Definitions for Compliers, Never-Takers, Defiers, and Always-Takers.

		Randomized to Control	
		Didn't Receive Vitamin A	Did Receive Vitamin A
Randomized to Vitamin A	Didn't receive Vitamin A	Never-taker	Defier
	Did receive Vitamin A	Complier	Always-taker

regarded as latent (or unobservable) variables. The adherence categories are considered latent baseline factors.

Similarly, the causal effect of randomization on 1-year mortality is given the difference between "alive if randomized to vitamin A" and "alive if randomized to control." In the RCM, estimation of average causal effects focuses on subgroups of individuals that would be induced to change their treatment status. The average causal effect defined over the subset of participants labeled *complier* is referred to as the complier average causal effect or CACE (21). Among the subset of participants labeled *defier*, the average causal effect is referred to as the defier average causal effect or DACE. For the two other adherence types, the always-takers and the never-takers, the average causal effects are not defined because the participant's behavior would not be changed regardless of the treatment assignment. In the vitamin A study, the focus would be on the subset of children that would take the supplement if offered but wouldn't take it if they were assigned to the control group. For general purposes, we would consider never-takers, defiers, and always-takers to be non-adherent. In the vitamin A study, we make the additional assumption that children in the control villages would never have had the opportunity to have taken vitamin A. This assumption rules out the possibility of defiers and always-takers.

Several assumptions are required to identify RCM average causal effects estimators for method effectiveness.

1. *Stable unit treatment value assumption* (SUTVA) (22): This assumption states that potential outcomes for each person are unrelated to other individuals. Potential outcomes for one child don't interfere with those from another child. An example of where the SUTVA might be violated is in a vaccination trial where a person's risk of infection might depend on whether other people were vaccinated.

2. *Randomization*[2]: This assumption states that children in both groups are comparable based on the baseline risk factors.

---

[2]This assumption can be weakened to allow various forms of conditional independence.

3. *Exclusion restriction*: This assumption states that the effect of randomization on response is through the effect of randomization on exposure (see Fig. 15.2). In the vitamin A study, this assumption implies that children who never take vitamin A supplement have the same response regardless of the randomization assignment. The exclusion restriction could be violated if medical personnel in villages randomized to receive vitamin A supplements detected and treated other diseases unrelated to vitamin A deficiency during their study-related visits. The exclusion restriction implies that always-takers and never-takers have an average causal effect of zero.

4. *Randomization has a nonzero effect on exposure*: This assumption implies that, on average, children in villages assigned to the vitamin A arm are more likely to receive vitamin A.

5. *Monotonicity*: This assumption implies that every child is at least as likely to receive vitamin A if they are randomized to the vitamin A arm compared to the control arm. Monotonicity implies that there are no defiers.

Having presented the assumptions of the RCM, we can now turn to consider the mostly commonly applied estimators of method-effectiveness in the medical literature: the as-treated (AT) and per-protocol (PP) analyses (17, 23, 24). Using the RCM, we can now quantify the potential bias of these approaches. As opposed to an ITT analysis, the AT and PP analyses do not make comparisons based on groups that are defined at the time of

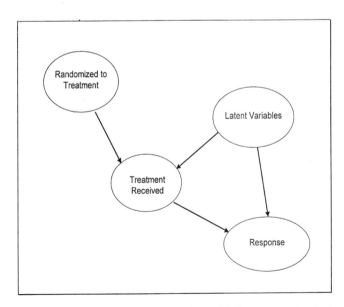

FIG. 15.2. Causal diagram illustrating relationship between randomization, treatment received, and response.

randomization (25). A PP analysis excludes the individuals who were not adherent with the treatment protocol. In the vitamin A example, a PP analysis would remove those children in the vitamin A arm that didn't receive the supplements but would not exclude any of the children in the control arm. An AT analysis assigns each individual the treatment that they received rather than the one to which they were randomized. In the vitamin A study, an AT analysis would not exclude any children; rather, the children in the vitamin A arm who didn't receive supplements would be relabeled as controls. By not excluding any children, an AT analysis attempts to capture some of the statistical power lost from removing patients in the PP analysis (17).

To simplify the calculations, we make the assumption that children in the control arm have no access to vitamin A. This implies that there are no defiers and no always-takers. This leaves the never-takers as the only remaining type of nonadherence. Furthermore, we assume that never-takers would have had the same response regardless of the randomization. This is an example of the restriction exclusion assumption. Remembering that randomization guarantees all baseline factors are balanced between treatment groups and that the adherence categories are unobservable baseline variables, we know that the proportion of compliers (and never-takers) is identical in both treatment groups. We denote the proportion of compliers using the symbol π. We define the average response among compliers randomized to vitamin A to be μ_A and the average response among compliers randomized to the control group to be μ_C. Among the never-takers, we define the average response to equal $\mu_C + \delta_C$. Because the never-takers would not change their behavior regardless of the randomization, we focus on estimating the average causal effect among the compliers or the CACE, which equals $\mu_E - \mu_C$.

Under these assumptions, the ITT estimate is a weighted average of responses among the compliers and the never-takers. Both the vitamin A and the control arms are a mix of $100\pi\%$ "compliers" and $100(1 - \pi)\%$ never-takers. In the vitamin A arm, the treatment average is given by $\pi \mu_A + (1 - \pi)(\pi_C + \delta_C)$. In the control arm, the treatment average is given by $\pi \mu_C + (1 - \pi)(\mu_C + \delta_C)$. Therefore, the ITT estimand is given by the difference of the treatment arm-specific averages, which simplifies to $\pi(\mu_A - \mu_C)$. In the previous calculation, the terms involving the average response among the never-takers cancel each other out, illustrating the exclusion restriction assumption. As shown earlier, ITT does not accurately estimate method-effectiveness unless there is perfect adherence (e.g., $\pi = 1$) or no treatment effect (e.g., $\mu_A - \mu_C = 0$).

 In general, the use-effectiveness estimand is the method-effectiveness estimand multiplied by π. With less than perfect adherence, estimates of the use-effectiveness will be closer to the null value of zero treatment effect than estimates of the method-effectiveness. Within the context of any particular randomized trial, an ITT analysis provides an unbiased estimate of use-effectiveness. As noted, however, in the earlier discussion of ITT's weaknesses, an ITT analysis does not necessarily provide a valid estimate of use-effectiveness when applied to routine practice (26).

With the AT approach, children in the vitamin A villages that didn't receive the supplements were treated as controls. According to the AT approach, the vitamin A treatment average is simply the μ_A from the compliers. The control treatment average is a weighted average of the compliers randomized to control (e.g., 100 π % of children randomized to control) and all of the never-takers (e.g., $100[1 - \pi]$% of children in both treatment arms). The AT treatment average for the control group is given by $[\pi \mu_C + 2 (1 - \pi) (\mu_C + \delta_C)] / [\pi + 2(1 - \pi)]$. After some algebra, the AT estimand simplifies to $(\mu_A - \mu_C) + 2 (1 - \pi) \delta_C / (2 - \pi)$, which will be biased for method-effectiveness unless there is perfect adherence (e.g., $\pi = 1$) or never-takers have the same response as compliers randomized to control (e.g., $\delta_C = 0$).

In a PP analysis, the $100(1 - \pi)$% of children assigned to vitamin A arm are eliminated from the analysis. The PP treatment average for the vitamin A arm is simply μ_A, which is identical to the AT vitamin A arm treatment average. For the control group, the PP treatment average equals $\pi \mu_C + (1 - \pi)$ $(\mu_C + \delta_C)$, which is identical to the ITT control arm treatment average. By taking the difference between the treatment averages, the PP estimand equals $(\mu_E - \mu_C) - (1 - \pi) \delta_C$, which will be biased for method-effectiveness in the same situations as the AT estimand.

In this section, we formally described the problem of estimating causal effects in the context of nonadherence; we described ITT, AT, and PP in terms of the RCM and examined their potential weaknesses. The next sec-

TABLE 15.4
The Assumed Vitamin A Study Mortality Data
Under the Rubin Causal Model

Study Group	Adherence Status	Percentage of Children	# Alive	# Dead	Mortality Rate
Control	Never-takers	20.0%[a]	2,285.2	32.6	1.41%[b]
	Compliers	80.0%	9,228.8	41.4	0.45%[c]
	Total	100%	11,514	74	0.64%
Vitamin A	Never-takers	20.0%[a]	2,385	34	1.41%[b]
	Compliers	80.0%	9,663	12	0.12%[d]
	Total	100%	12,048	46	0.38%

[a]The proportion of never-takers is balanced by randomization. [b]The mortality rate for never-takers is identical for both treatments (e.g., the exclusion restriction assumption). [c]The mortality rate for compliers randomized to control. [d]The mortality rate for compliers randomized to vitamin A supplementation.

tion uses the RCM—which describes unobservable events (e.g., potential outcomes, compliers, and defiers)—to develop statistical approaches that use observable data to estimate the method-effectiveness.

STATISTICAL METHODS FOR ADDRESSING NONADHERENCE

By applying RCM assumptions, we are able to fill in the unobserved data describing the adherence status and mortality rates for children in the control group. In Table 15.4, the rows of data shown in italics are calculated by assuming that randomization balances all factors at baseline and that the children's (potential outcome) response did not depend on the randomization after accounting for treatment received. Based on the assumption of randomization, we have estimated that 20% of children would have been never-takers and 80% would have been compliers. The estimated mortality rate for the never-takers of 1.41% was based on the observed data from the vitamin A arm children that did not receive the supplements. Our estimate of method-effectiveness, the average causal treatment effect among compliers, is estimated to be –0.32% (=0.12% – 0.45%) indicating a lower mortality rate favoring vitamin A supplementation.

As noted in a previous section, the method-effectiveness estimate typically is $1/\pi$ times the use-effectiveness estimate. The instrumental variable (IV) method allows the exploitation of this relationship to obtain a valid estimate of method effectiveness.[3] Sommer and Zeger used an instrumental variables analysis to estimate the effect of vitamin A supplementation on mortality (27). In the simplest settings, the instrumental variable estimate is obtained by calculating the ITT estimate of randomization on mortality and dividing that quantity by the ITT estimate of randomization on treatment received. The ITT estimate of randomization on mortality is given by 0.38% – 0.64% = –0.26%. Because we have made the assumption that no children in the control arm could have received vitamin A, the ITT estimate of randomization on treatment receipt is 80.0%. This implies that the instrumental variable estimate equals –0.0026/0.80 = –0.32%, which is identical to the previous estimate of method-effectiveness.

For comparison's sake, we calculate the AT and PP estimates that we already know typically are not valid estimators of method-effectiveness. In Table 15.5, we arranged the data to indicate that children randomized to the

---

[3]In economics, instrumental variables are an important tool for estimating the causal effects of treatments (19, 21). In statistics, randomization is typically the mechanism used to make causal inference. A seminal paper by Angrist, Imbens, and Rubin (19) compared the economic and statistical approaches used to make causal inference and made explicit the assumptions required for inference.

TABLE 15.5
Vitamin A Study Mortality Data Under the As-Treated Approach.

As-Treated Group	# of Children	# Alive	# Dead	Mortality Rate
Randomized to control	11,588	11,514	74	0.64%
Randomized to vitamin A—				
never received supplements	2,419	2,385	34	1.41%
Control group total	14,007	13,899	108	0.77%[a]
Randomized to vitamin A—				
received supplements	9,675	9,663	12	0.12%[b]

[a]AT average mortality rate for the control group. [b]AT average mortality rate for the vitamin A group.

TABLE 15.6
Vitamin A Study Mortality Data Under the Per-Protocol Approach

Per-Protocol Group	# of Children	# Alive	# Dead	Mortality Rate
Randomized to control	11,588	11,514	74	0.64%[a]
Randomized to vitamin				
A—received supplements	9,675	9,663	12	0.12%[b]

[a]PP average mortality rate for the control group. [b]PP average mortality rate for the vitamin A group.

vitamin A group but not receiving supplements were shifted to the control group. The AT estimate of –0.65% (=0.12% – 0.77%) implies that the magnitude of benefit received from vitamin A is twice as large as the instrumental variable estimate. In Table 15.6, we show the data required to calculate the PP estimate (i.e., where children randomized to vitamin A and not receiving the supplements are excluded). The PP estimate of –0.52% favoring vitamin A supplementation is between the instrumental variable and AT estimates.

All methods attempting to estimate method-effectiveness with less-than-perfect compliance must rely upon assumptions that cannot be tested using observed data. Thus, any analysis that estimates the method-effectiveness of a treatment should be accompanied by sensitivity analyses. This process might involve both qualitative and quantitative assessments. The key assumption of the method-effectiveness estimator is that never-takers are assumed to have equivalent survival experience regardless of the treatment to which they are assigned (e.g., the exclusion restriction assumption). In the vitamin A study, it is possible that this assumption was violated because the children in the control group knew that they were not receiving the supplements. The psychological impact of this might be very different than in a double-blind placebo-controlled trial where the patients and study personnel do not know who is on the active compound.

For a more quantitative assessment, Balke and Pearl developed a method based on nonlinear programming that uses the observed data from a randomized study to calculate theoretical limits (e.g., sharp bounds) for the parameter estimate (28). These authors applied their approach to the vitamin A study and determined bounds on the method-effectiveness parameter of (−19.46%, 0.54%). This result indicates that the supplement could increase mortality by as much as 19.46% and does not reduce mortality by more than 0.54%. Clearly, the ITT and IV method-effectiveness estimates of 0.26% and 0.32% are very close to the upper limit of the bound. At first glance, this is a surprising and possibly disappointing result. However, the lower-bound estimate is based on the extreme assumptions that (a) every child who took vitamin A would have lived even if they had not and (b) the 20% of children assigned to the vitamin A arm that didn't take the supplement would have died had they taken the supplement. With this sensitivity analysis as with any other, an assessment must be made as to the likelihood of the various scenarios. Interestingly, the AT approach to estimate method-effectiveness provides an estimate that is outside of the theoretical bounds. Clearly, the AT estimate is not valid in this example.

EXTENSIONS

Even in a fairly simple trial such as the vitamin A study, adherence is a multidimensional quantity. According to the study design, children in the vitamin A arm were supposed to receive two vitamin A doses, the first dose scheduled at 1–3 months and the second dose 6–8 months later (3). Some children did in fact receive both doses, others received only the initial dose, others received only the second dose, and some missed both doses. In fact, a small number of children (~1%) from the control villages received vitamin A supplementation (27). Furthermore, verification that children received the supplements was not straightforward. Three methods were used to assess whether the children had received the supplements: note cards to households, interrogation of the children's guardians or relatives, and report forms from the vitamin administrators. Of those methods, interrogation of guardians was deemed to be the most accurate source of information and was used in the data analysis.

When children randomized to the control arm receive vitamin A, it is a type of nonadherence referred to as crossover or contamination. As one might imagine, estimating biological effects of vitamin A are more complicated when children in the control villages have access to vitamin A. Cuzick et al. have proposed an IV-type approach to estimate method-effectiveness in studies with contamination and binary measures of treatment received and response (29).

The estimates presented in the previous section have assumed (a) that measurements of adherence are known without error and (b) that there is no clustering of responses within villages. Dunn proposed a measurement error model to obtain valid estimates and account for the possibility that measures of adherence are not perfectly accurate (e.g., measurement error) (30). This approach requires that more than one method is used to assess the individual's adherence. In many statistical problems, the failure to account for this source of error will result in biased parameter estimates. Albert (31) and Loeys et al. (32) suggested methods to adjust for a possible correlation within villages. Results from Albert's analysis of the vitamin A study found that the correlations within the villages were very small and the confidence intervals for the efficacy estimates were only slightly wider than the simple analysis not accounting for correlations. However, in other simulation studies Albert found that correlations as small as 0.02 resulted in nonstatistically significant 95% confidence intervals for the efficacy parameter. The findings of Albert and Dunn suggest that even small deviations in the model assumptions (e.g., measurement error and correlation) can result in biased parameter estimates and confidence intervals.

In the analysis of the vitamin A study presented in this chapter, we have treated adherence as a binary event. However, this is not always the case. In studies of drugs taken over an extended period of time, compliance is often summarized using the percentage of doses taken (26, 33, 34). Using a different approach, Efron and Feldman (26) developed an estimator that incorporated continuous adherence information and examined measured changes in a continuous response variable. Although adherence to treatment varied widely between drugs, Efron and Feldman were able to estimate the biological efficacy of the drug by assuming that adherence had a structural ranking (i.e., if patients A and B were assigned to the same treatment and patient A was observed to have better adherence, then patient A would have had at least as good of compliance as patient B if they had been randomized to the other treatment). Another approach using a continuous measure of adherence was taken by Goetghebeur and Lapp (34), who measured adherence in the active-treatment group but not in the placebo-controlled group.

For time-to-event outcomes, Mark and Robins (35) and Robins and Tsiatis (36) have proposed rank-preserving structural-failure time models to estimate method-effectiveness in randomized studies with nonadherence. These estimators have several favorable properties: (a) under the null hypothesis of no treatment effect, they are identical to a log-rank test from an ITT analysis and (b) under the alternative hypothesis, they estimate the hazard ratio corresponding to the difference that would have been observed under full adherence.

We conclude this section on extensions by highlighting two methodologies that have relevance for treatment adherence researchers and are easily implemented using standard statistical software. Robins and colleagues developed the inverse probability of censoring weighted (IPCW) estimators method (37–39). In these models, censoring weights are calculated by modeling the probability that an individual will be censored given their observed data up to that point in time. For our purposes, the time of censoring might be considered the time when the individual stopped the protocol-dictated treatment or crossed over to the other treatment. Within each treatment arm, these analyses are considered observational but the overall comparison protects randomization. These estimators are also particularly useful for estimating average causal effects in observational studies (39). For the inverse probability of censoring weighted estimators, several sensitivity analyses methods have been suggested (28, 37, 38, 40, 41).

The second methodology involves modeling approaches based on the compliance score (42–44). For binary treatments, the compliance score is the randomization effect on the proportion of compliers with a given covariate level. In this situation, the compliance score has an interpretation similar to the propensity score (43). Standard propensity score techniques such as matching, stratifying, and regression models can be used to compare individuals with similar compliance scores but different observed adherence.

The "run-in" study is a design technique frequently used in drug trials to identify and remove individual's unlikely to adhere to the proposed treatment regimes (45–51). Typically, a run-in study involves giving all potential study participants a placebo treatment for the short period of time. Individuals that are observed to have poor adherence on placebo are then excluded from the study. The remaining group is then randomized to their treatments. Depending on the setting, run-ins are thought to decrease the costs and increase the statistical power to detect treatment differences. In a clever study design, Davis and colleagues used a run-in placebo period but did not exclude the less adherent individuals from the study (52). Rather, they conducted the analysis using the entire study population and then acted as if the less adherent individuals in the run-in phase had been excluded. The results of both analyses (with and without less adherent individuals) were virtually identical and it was concluded that exclusions based on the run-in period would have decreased the statistical power and increased the study duration and costs. The benefits of a run-in study need to be assessed on a case-by-case basis. A rule of thumb is that if the adherence during the run-in phase is highly predictive of the future adherence then the run-in is likely to be more beneficial.

CONCLUSION

When nonadherence occurs, care must be taken in interpreting the clinical trial results. This chapter has presented several frameworks for understanding the complexities associated with this situation. We have demonstrated that in some instances it is more important to understand the biological effect of the treatment rather than the effect of treatment randomization. However, ITT and the associated use-effectiveness estimates are still necessary. Regulatory agencies, such as the U.S. Food and Drug Administration, typically expect the primary analysis to be conducted using an ITT strategy. And, a strong and reasonable argument for the necessity of ITT was made by Begg (18):

> To understand the more compelling motivation for the ITT approach we must look to arguments that are based more on the philosophy of science, and cn the realities of the pressures facing the sponsors of new medical interventions, including both career academic researchers and commercial sponsors in the private sector. (p. 242)

It's important to remember that the ITT approach has its limitations. For adherence researchers, if you consider making adherence improvement methods part of the intervention being tested, you should know that will influence the generalizability of the trial's results. ITT estimates provide valid estimates of use-effectiveness within the randomized study; however, the generalizability of the results will depend on the similiarity between trial conditions and routine care.

Some new methods of analyzing trial data with nonadherence rely on the presence of variables collected at baseline to help understand who will and will not comply. Adherence researchers can make a unique contribution to trial methodology by helping to identify factors that are related to nonaherence. For example, the inverse probability of censoring weighted estimators of Robins and colleagues relies directly on adherence predictions internal to the trial to obtain valid estimates of method-effectiveness (38, 39); whereas, the instrumental variable method-effectiveness estimates rely on compliance rates that could be estimated from an external source.

In addition to providing better estimates of method-effectiveness, the collection of detailed adherence data using multiple methods increases the likelihood of identifying subsets of individuals likely to have difficultly adhering to treatment due to side effects. Goetghebeur and Shapiro argued that collection and interpretation of adherence data is crucial to the understanding of clinical findings. Furthermore, they argued that it is our "ethical imperative" to make the best use of data collected from individuals who have given their time and resources to participate in the research (53).

If we fail to collect adherence data, we are left with few options other than the default ITT analysis with its associated limitations. Regarding the potential pitfalls of ignoring adherence data, Sheiner and Rubin write "blind adherence to the ITT paradigm becomes a self-fulfilling prophecy: The data that would help estimate method-effectiveness are not gathered, and one has little recourse but to settle for estimates of use-effectiveness, which might be of little value for projecting use-effectiveness in the future" (p. 8). With the goal of identifying and estimating method-effectiveness, statisticians and other researchers are encouraged to develop studies that are more likely to carefully monitor patients. The tools necessary to obtain valid estimates of method-effectiveness are currently available. With these new tools, we recommend that the standard AT and PP analyses should never be used as a basis for estimating method-effectiveness.

GLOSSARY

As-treated: an analysis strategy comparing groups based on the treatment that was actually received.

Average causal effect: the population average difference of potential outcomes between two possible treatment strategies.

Counterfactual outcome: an outcome that would have been observed if the experimenter had randomized the individual to a treatment different that the observed randomization.

Explanatory approach to clinical trials: a view common to laboratory sciences, highly structured treatment strategies, ideal conditions, focused on isolating the "biologic" effect of a therapy.

Instrumental variables: variables that are related to the outcome of interest exclusively through their relationship to the treatment of interest. Instrumental variable estimation techniques are popular in the econometric literature.

Intent-to-treat: an approach to the design and analysis of clinical trials that preserves the benefits gained through randomization. Comparisons between groups are based on the treatment assigned at the time of randomization. This strategy is sometimes referred to as an *as-randomized* analysis

Method-effectiveness: an approach for estimating the biological effects of a treatment strategy that attempts to remove the study-specific contextual factors. Considered synonymous with the explanatory approach to clinical trials.

Model-based approach to noncompliance: the use of statistical models to estimate the average causal effect of a treatment on response.

Nominal treatment: the label representing the treatment strategy that the experimenter has assigned to the study participant.

Per-protocol analysis: an analysis strategy that excludes all individuals that did not adhere to the intended treatment strategy. Typically, estimators deriving under this philosophy are biased for both use-effectiveness and method-effectiveness.

Potential outcomes: a key ingredient to Rubin's Causal Model. These variables correspond to the vector of outcome variables that would be observable under different randomization settings.

Pragmatic approach to clinical trials: a public health view of clinical trials focused on estimating treatment effects that would be observed under normal conditions.

Rubin's Causal Model: a framework based on potential outcomes that allows for the definition of causal effects. This approach extends to observational studies. Frequently, parameters of interest are estimated using Bayesian statistical methods.

Subgroup analysis: an analytic approach that focuses on a subset of the study population. These analyses are subject of potential biases because they either ignore randomization or rely on assumptions that are not testable.

Use-effectiveness: an approach for estimating the entire effects of a treatment strategy, which includes biologic, contextual, and psychological effects. Considered synonymous with the pragmatic approach.

REFERENCES

1. Sommer A, Tarwotjo I, Hussaini G, Susanto D. Increased mortality in children with mild vitamin A deficiency. *Lancet.* 1983;2(8350):585–588.
2. Sommer A. Mortality associated with mild, untreated xerophthalmia. *Trans Am Ophthalmol Soc.* 1983;81:825–853.
3. Sommer A, Tarwotjo I, Djunaedi E, et al. Impact of vitamin A supplementation on childhood mortality. A randomised controlled community trial. *Lancet.* 1986;1(8491):1169–1173.
4. Davis CE. Generalizing from clinical trials. *Control Clin Trials.* 1994;15:11–14.
5. Lachin JM. Statistical considerations in the intention-to-treat principle. *Control Clin Trials.* 2000;21:167–189.
6. Schwartz D, Lellouch J. Explanatory and pragmatic attitudes in therapeutical trials. *J Chron Dis.* 1967;20:637–648.
7. Armitage P. Attitudes in clinical trials. *Stat Med.* 1998;17:2675–2683.
8. Sheiner LB, Rubin DB. Intention-to-treat analysis and the goals of clinical trials. *Clin Pharmacol Ther.* 1995;57:6–15.
9. Zeger SL. Adjustment for noncompliance. In: Armitage P, Colton T, eds. *Encyclopedia of Biostatistics.* Chichester, England: John Wiley & Sons Ltd.; 1998: 3006–3009.
10. Wright CC, Sim J. Intention-to-treat approach to data from randomized controlled trials: a sensitivity analysis. *J Clin Epidemiol.* 2003;56:833–842.

11. Sheiner LB. Is intent-to-treat analysis always (ever) enough? *Br J Clin Pharmacol.* 2002;54:203–211.

12. Salsburg D. Intent to treat: The reductio ad absurdum that became gospel. *Pharmacoepidemiol and Drug Saf.* 1994;3:329–335.

13. Montori VM, Guyatt GH. Intention-to-treat principle. *CMAJ.* 2001;165:1339–1341.

14. Hollis S, Campbell NR. What is meant by intention to treat analyses? Survey of published randomised controlled trials. *BMJ.* 1999;319:670–674.

15. Heitjan DF. Causal inference in a clinical trial: A comparive example. *Control Clin Trials.* 1999;20:309–318.

16. Goetghebeur E, Loeys T. Beyond intention to treat. *Epidemiol Rev.* 2002;24:85–90.

17. Ellenberg JH. Intention-to-treat analysis versus as-treated analysis. *Drug Information Journal.* 1996;30:535–544.

18. Begg CB. Ruminations on the intention-to-treat principle. *Control Clin Trials.* 2000;21:241–243.

19. Angrist JD, Imbens GW, Rubin DB. Identification of causal effects using instrumental variables (with discussion). *J Am Stat Assoc.* 1996;91:444–472.

20. Holland P. Statistics and causal inference. *J Am Stat Assoc.* 1986;81:945–970.

21. Imbens GW, Rubin DB. Bayesian inference for causal effects in randomized experiments with noncompliance. *Annals of Statistics.* 1997;25:305–327.

22. Rubin DB. More powerful randomization-based p-values in double-blind trials with noncompliance. *Stat Med.* 1998;17:371–385.

23. Peduzzi P, Wittes J, Detre K., Holford T. Analysis as-randomized and the problem of non-adherence: an example from the Veterans Affairs Randomized Trial of Coronary Artery Bypass Surgery. *Stat Med.* 1993;12:1185–1195.

24. Lee JL, Ellenberg JH, Hirtz DG, Nelson KB. Analysis of clinical trials by treatment actually received: Is it really an option? *Stat Med.* 1991;10:1605.

25. Rochon J. Supplementing the intention-to-treat analysis: Accounting for covariates observed postrandomization in clinical trials. *J Am Stat Assoc.* 1995;90:292–300.

26. Efron B, Feldman D. Compliance as an explanatory variable in clinical trials. *Journal of the American Statistical Association.* 1991;86:9–17.

27. Sommer A, Zeger SL. On estimating efficacy from clinical trials. *Stat Med.* 1991;10:45–52.

28. Balke A, Pearl J. Bounds on treatment effects from studies with imperfect compliance. *J Am Stat Assoc.* 1997;92:1171–1176.

29. Cuzick J, Edwards R, Segnan N. Adjusting for non-compliance and contaminations in randomized clinical trials. *Stat Med.* 1997;16:1017–1029.

30. Dunn G. The problem of measurement error in modelling the effect of compliance in a randomized trial. *Stat Med.* 1999;18:2863–2877.

31. Albert JM. Estimating efficacy in clinical trials with clustered binary responses. *Stat Med.* 2002;21:649–661.

32. Loeys T, Vansteelandt S, Goetghebeur E. Accounting for correlation and compliance in cluster randomized trials. *Stat Med.* 2001;20:3753–3767.

33. Goetghebeur E, Molenberghs G. Causal inference in a placebo-controlled clinical trial with binary outcome and ordered compliance. *J Am Stat Assoc.* 1996;91: 928–934.

34. Goetghebeur E, Lapp K. The effect of treatment compliance in a placebo-controlled trial: Regression with unpaired data. *App Stat.* 1997;46:351–364.

35. Mark SD, Robins JM. A method for the analysis of randomized trials with compliance information: an application to the Multiple Risk Factor Intervention Trial. *Control Clin Trials.* 1993;14:97.

36. Robins JM, Tsiatis AA. Correcting for non-compliance in randomized trials using rank preserving structural failure time models. *Communications in Statistics.* 1991;20:2609–2631.

37. Scharfstein D, Rotnitzky A, Robins JM. Adjusting for nonignorable drop-out using semiparametric nonresponse models. *J Am Stat Assoc.* 1999;94:1096–1120.

38. Rotnitzky A, Scharfstein D, Su T-L, Robins JM. Methods for conducting sensitivity analysis of trials with potentially nonignorable competing causes of censoring. *Biometrics.* 2001;57:103–113.

39. Robins JM. Correction for non-compliance in equivalence trials. *Stat Med.* 1998; 17:269–302.

40. Jo B. Model misspecification sensitivity analysis in estimating causal effects of interventions with non-compliance. *Stat Med.* 2002;21:3161–3181.

41. Matsuyama Y. Sensitivity analysis for the estimation of rates of change with nonignorable drop-out: an application to a randomized clinical trial of the vitamin D3. *Stat Med.* 2003;22:811–827.

42. Joffe MM, Ten Have TR, Brensinger C. The compliance score as a regressor in randomized trials. *Biostatistics.* 2003;4:327–340.

43. Rosenbaum PR, Rubin D. The central role of the propensity score in observational studies for causal effects. *Biometrika.* 1983;70:41–55.

44. Follmann DA. On the effect of treatment among would-be treatment compliers: an analysis of the Multiple Risk Factor Intervention Trial. *Journal of the American Statistical Association.* 2000;95:1101–1109.

45. Shumaker SA, Dugan E, Braun TJ. Enhancing adherence in randomized controlled clinical trials. *Control Clin Trials.* 2000;21:226S–232S.

46. Brittain E, Wittes J. The run-in period in clinical trials. The effect of misclassification on efficiency. *Control Clin Trials.* 1990;11:327–338.

47. Lang JM. The use of a run-in to enhance compliance. *Stat Med.* 1990;9:87–95.

48. Lang JM, Buring JE, Rosner B, Cook N, Hennekens CH. Estimating the effect of the run-in on the power of the Physicians' Health Study. *Stat Med.* 1991;10: 1585–1593.

49. Schechtman KB, Gordon ME. A comprehensive algorithm for determining whether a run-in strategy will be a cost-effective design modification in a randomized clinical trial. *Stat Med.* 1993;12:111–128.

50. Buring JE, Hennekens CH. Cost and efficiency in clinical trials: the U.S. Physicians' Health Study. *Stat Med.* 1989;9:29–33.

51. Jo B. Statistical power in randomized intervention studies with noncompliance. *Psychol Methods.* 2002;7:178–193.

52. Davis CE, Applegate WB, Gordon DJ, Curtis RC, McCormick M. An empirical evaluation of the placebo run-in. *Control Clin Trials.* 1995;16:41–50.

53. Goetghebeur E, Shapiro SH. Analysing non-compliance in clinical trials: ethical imperative or mission impossible? *Stat Med.* 1996;15:2813–2826.

Chapter 16

Improving Adherence With Clinical Guidelines

David B. Matchar
Meenal B. Patwardhan
Gregory P. Samsa

BACKGROUND

Over the past several decades, there has been a dramatic rise in the number of clinical guidelines (1), especially those "evidence-based guidelines" that make the link to the best scientific evidence both consistent and explicit (2, 3). Yet, establishing standards is but the first step in improving medical practice. Research indicates that simply making providers aware of a clinical guideline is a disappointingly weak strategy for inducing adherence with clinical guidelines. This holds true for continuing medical education (CME), printed educational materials, and academic detailing using opinion leaders (4–9). (See chap. 13 for more details on opinion leaders.) Such strategies can be successful in encouraging providers to *want* to change, but unless the system of care is modified in a way that helps them to *act* on these new beliefs, permanent change is unlikely.

LESSONS FROM THE LITERATURE

Various system-level intervention strategies have been tried to promote adherence with clinical guidelines (Table 16.1). Excellent reviews are available elsewhere (4–15), the main conclusions being that:

- No single approach works in all circumstances.

- Strategies with multiple elements are more likely to be effective than more narrowly based approaches, particularly when the interventions in question address the multiple levels of the provider, the patient, and the system.

- Tailoring interventions to the individual and local context has considerable potential, although the best way to accomplish this tailoring has yet to be determined.

- Perhaps most important, like any complex system, the system of medical care is more difficult to change than might naively be assumed.

A potential deficiency with the approaches outlined in Table 16.1 is that the tools tend to be *prespecified* rather than tailored to local resources and con-

TABLE 16.1
Taxonomy of Implementation Tools

Implementation Tool	*Definition*
I) Chart reminder	Placing a colorful sticker or comprehensive checklist of relevant services, including lab monitoring, in patients' charts.
II) Computerized record reminder	Using software programmed to determine the date tests/treatments are due, and then print computer-generated reminder messages for patients with appointments.
III) Standing orders	Implementing a written order stipulating that all persons meeting certain criteria should be tested/treated, thus eliminating the need for individual physician's orders for each patient.
IV) Performance feedback	Motivating providers by reporting their performance rate in delivering clinical-practice guidelines' (CPG) recommended tests/treatments; thereby inspiring personal challenges or friendly competition.
V) Patient education	Providing patients with an information sheet to review and prompting them to tell the doctor or office staff if they feel they are indicated for any of the tests/treatments in the CPG.
VI) Personal health records	Issuing personal health records (PHR) to patients that contain a care schedule, including recommended times to receive tests/treatments.
VII) Mailed/Telephoned patient reminders	Calling with, or mailing a reminder to a patient that a test/treatment is due.
VIII) Expanding access in clinical settings	Making CPG-related activities more convenient by reducing the distance patients must travel, offering more convenient hours or locations, and/or reducing administrative hassle.

Note. Adapted from the American College of Physicians' taxonomy of tools (15).

straints. One strategy for tailoring involves the use of process reengineering techniques such as total quality management or one of its variants. Briefly, total quality management involves the development of a team with some degree of training in data collection and analysis using prescribed techniques. Illustrated in Fig. 16.1, total quality management begins with a detailed understanding of the current local process of care. The result of this exploration is a clarification of the goals of the process (what may be called the "functional specifications"), and points at which the current process is failing. This leads to development and implementation of an intervention plan, and follow-up evaluation with modifications based on insights from this follow-up. A core concept of total quality management is that a detailed understanding of the current local process of care and local process failures is the key to tailoring the intervention. This set of activities must occur locally, as designated by the box surrounding the total quality management steps.

The practical results of total quality management–based initiatives in health care settings have been mixed, however, with studies of wide-scale implementation of total quality management as a management philosophy tending to be negative (16), and the results of individual interventions inspired by the principles of total quality management faring significantly

TQM

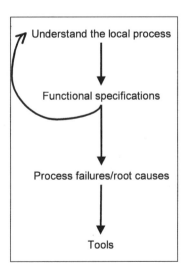

FIG. 16.1. Schematic of a total quality management approach to local practice improvement. The box indicates that the entire process occurs at the local level.

better (17). One reason for this discrepancy pertains to the substantial requirements: Large-scale, unsupervised implementation of total quality management is essentially (to paraphrase a leading practice improvement researcher, Dr. Harold Goldberg) "an under-funded and otherwise undersupported form of health services research practiced by amateurs." Additional structure is needed; in particular, a structure of *facilitated* process improvement that can effectively transmit what is known about process improvement to local personnel whose intentions are excellent but whose experience level and other resources may be limited.

Taking all of the aforementioned into account, our experience has been that, rather than utilizing either prespecified intervention tools in the absence of a process reengineering plan, or an undirected total quality management–based approach that requires an unrealistic level of commitment from local personnel, what is most likely to succeed in promoting adherence with clinical guidelines is an approach that combines the principles of total quality management and a range of potential tools in a way that supports and simplifies local tailoring. In the next section we describe such an approach, termed *facilitated process improvement*. Following this, we illustrate this approach using our recent work with the Renal Physicians Association to develop a tool kit to promote conformance with guidelines for care of patients with advanced chronic kidney disease.

SYNTHESIS: FACILITATED PROCESS IMPROVEMENT

Our goal is an approach to developing a set of tools (perhaps on behalf of a professional organization) that a practice could easily tailor in order to implement guidelines for care of a specific type of patient. Toward that aim we propose a general-purpose solution (Fig. 16.2) based on the key concept in total quality management that all activities are processes that can be improved. However, unlike total quality management, instead of requiring that all the program development be done by local providers, we note that much of the preliminary work to setting up a practice improvement intervention is similar from site to site and thus propose that an external group perform this formative work. The result of this formative work is a procedure that should allow clinicians to accomplish process improvement without being subjected to the demands imposed by conventional total quality management.

Our starting point is an explicit *functional specification* of what the care process is intended to accomplish. This functional specification does not make reference to the means by which they will be accomplished (i.e., as long as the functional specifications are satisfied, the care process would be deemed acceptable). Next, we investigate the processes of care in a variety

Facilitated
Process Improvement

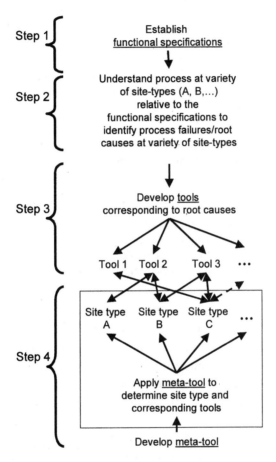

Step 1 — Establish functional specifications

Step 2 — Understand process at variety of site-types (A, B,...) relative to the functional specifications to identify process failures/root causes at variety of site-types

Step 3 — Develop tools corresponding to root causes

Tool 1   Tool 2   Tool 3   ...

Site type A   Site type B   Site type C   ...

Step 4 — Apply meta-tool to determine site type and corresponding tools

Develop meta-tool

FIG. 16.2. Schematic of the facilitated process improvement approach. The box indicates activities that occur at the local level.

of sites in order to understand the ways and reasons why process may fall short of satisfying the functional specifications. Third, we develop a variety of *tools* to attack the root causes of specific process failures (noting that in many cases several types of sites may have a similar root cause for failure and thus may benefit from a similar or identical tool). Finally, we develop a tool to guide the local selection of tools (what we term the *meta-tool*). The application of the meta-tool (as well as the actual implementation of the tools) is a local activity, as indicated in Fig. 16.2 by the box surrounding a subset of the facilitated process improvement steps.

In the following subsections, we describe in more detail the three elements that serve as the nuts and bolts of the facilitated process improvement approach: (a) the functional specifications, (b) the tools, and (c) the meta-tool. By developing these elements as an extension of the guidelines, say by the sponsoring professional society, practitioners will be able to engage in more sophisticated and effective forms of process improvement than would have been possible if they had been left to their own devices. Before proceeding to a more detailed example of facilitated process improvement, we clarify definitions, using a simple example of blood pressure management.

The Functional Specifications.   Well-formed clinical guidelines consist of actionable statements in the form of "when X is true Y should be done." Such a statement provides the foundation of the functional specifications of a guideline. A complete functional specification includes, in generalizable terms, the process by which X is determined to be true and Y is accomplished. For example, the statement "all hypertensive patients should maintain a record of their own blood pressure readings between clinic visits" leads to the following functional specification, here listed as actions (what needs to be done), and prerequisites (things needed to do the action):

1. The patient is identified as being hypertensive.
   - A definition of "hypertensive patient" is established.
   - The provider is aware that the patient is hypertensive.
2. The need to measure interval blood pressures is communicated.
   - The patient is educated about the need to measure blood pressure.
   - The patient understands the means by which blood pressure will be measured.
3. The patient measures and records their blood pressure.
   - The patient has the means to measure blood pressure.
   - The patient has a place to record blood pressure measurements.
   - The patient has a reminder mechanism.

Note that the functional specifications are necessary and sufficient: Failure to follow any element of the specification would lead to nonadherence and following all elements of the specification will assure adherence.[1] Furthermore, note that the specifications do not provide specific details about *how* they should be fulfilled; this is the role of the tools.

---

[1]Of course, this is within the limits of the provider's sphere of influence. Nothing that the provider can (ethically) do will guarantee patient adherence.

The Tools. Tools in this context denote the means for accomplishing the functional specifications. Without belaboring the point, the wide variety of tool types noted in the initial section of this chapter (Table 16.1) can be considered tool templates and they can be endlessly modified to suit a specific circumstance. Apropos to the blood pressure example, tools to consider in a general tool set include information sheets summarizing the essential elements of the guideline for physicians, providers, and patients, chart stickers, computerized reminders, reminder postcards, a preprinted patient diary, a list of pharmacies with free blood pressure measurement equipment, and so on.

Unlike the functional specifications, the tool set contains a variety of tool types. Some will be highly appropriate for a specific circumstance, others less so or not at all. Though it is well accepted by experts in guideline adherence that interventions must be tailored to local circumstances, there is little empirical data to support a specific strategy for accomplishing the tailoring. At the outer reaches of practice improvement research, we advocate the development of what we term a meta-tool—a tool that allows local users to select the most appropriate tools from the set.

The Meta-Tool. The term meta-tool is used here to indicate a rational procedure an end user can apply to select tools.[2] The meta-tool could be the element that completes a kit that would be distributed by a professional society, allowing the broadest possible range of providers to implement a guideline effectively. It facilitates implementation thereby improving adherence.

Because a meta-tool is intended to be "general purpose," it should take into account the wide range of practice contexts. This requires an understanding of the processes that are followed in those contexts, so that one can provide useful advice about which tools should be used to satisfy the guideline functional specifications. In the simple example of interval blood pressure monitoring, such a meta-tool could be as basic as a brief paragraph describing the types of tools to use in common situations. In a more complex situation in which "optimal" tool selection depends on several patient, provider, and system characteristics, the meta-tool may need to take a more structured form, such as a written algorithm.

Illustration: The Advanced Chronic Kidney Disease Practice Improvement Tool Kit

To better describe the process of meta-tool development in the context of more involved guidelines, we consider the entire process of kit making (the

---

[2]To our knowledge, this is a newly coined term; we selected this as more stylish than alternatives considered such as "tool tool."

functional specifications, the tools, and the meta-tool) using an ongoing effort by the Renal Physicians Association (RPA) to improve the care of patients with advanced chronic kidney disease for illustration.

Advanced chronic kidney disease is a progressive medical condition in which the ability of the kidney to eliminate waste is diminished, short of requiring replacement therapy via dialysis or transplantation. It has become increasingly evident that a substantial number of individuals have relatively advanced chronic kidney disease that is either unrecognized, or recognized and inadequately managed (18–26). Furthermore, epidemiological studies are pointing to a beneficial effect of early and aggressive care of patients with advanced chronic kidney disease (26–28). The RPA, a leading professional society, has been actively pursuing a systematic effort to improve care of individuals with advanced chronic kidney disease, based on evidence-based recommendations. In conjunction with the Duke Center for Clinical Health Policy Research, the RPA has disseminated a comprehensive literature review on the care of people with advanced chronic kidney disease, not yet on dialysis. This evidence report, *Appropriate Patient Preparation for Renal Replacement Therapy* (29), was used to construct a clinical-practice guideline and performance measures (3). The next step, described here, is to create a set of tools to be distributed to clinicians that would improve clinical practice in a measurable way.

The RPA tool development effort was grounded in three basic steps of process improvement, supplemented by a fourth step aimed at tailoring. These steps are (a) understand the process, (b) identify process failures and root causes, (c) develop tools to attack root causes, and (d) establish a tailoring strategy.

Note that Steps 1 through 3 lead to a tree of elements (the process has subprocesses, each subprocess can be associated with a failure and a root cause, and multiple tools can be created to attack each root cause.) For clarity of exposition, we limit the illustration to representative paths on this tree (Fig. 16.3).

Step 1. Understand the Process. All activities can be characterized by a process by which they are accomplished. Because the objective of the entire exercise is to understand how the process can be improved, viz., recommended practice, this step involves establishing the functional specifications of a process that successfully leads to the outcome recommended by the guideline.

This first step was accomplished by convening focus groups of referring physicians and nephrologists from diverse geographic and work environments. We initiated this process by asking practicing physicians to reflect on details about current practice patterns, likely opportunities for practice improvement, points of maximum leverage for improving practice, and so

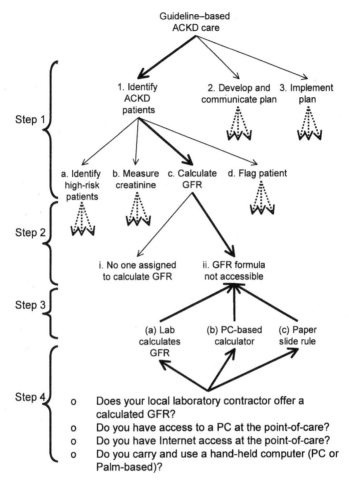

FIG. 16.3. Illustration of the application of the facilitated process improvement steps to the task of promoting guideline-based care of patients with advanced chronic kidney disease. ACKD—advanced chronic kidney disease; creatinine—an indirect serum measure that is elevated with diminished kidney function, as well as other factors such as muscle mass; GFR—glomerular filtration rate, a direct measure of kidney function that can be estimated from creatinine and other factors other than kidney function that raise or lower creatinine; PC—personal computer.

forth. Special emphasis was made to capture all the social, ethical, regulatory, and financial barriers that physicians perceive in the implementation of the guidelines.

We also performed face-to-face interviews with patients with chronic kidney disease, and summarized patients' views regarding the tools that they believe would be most effective in order to involve them in the process of their care. We included patients who were already on dialysis, as well as those who were not yet on any form of renal replacement therapy. This afforded us a complete spectrum of patients' views and perceptions about the care they were receiving, had received, or would have liked to receive during the course of their disease.

These data provided substantial insight into the process of advanced chronic kidney disease care in typical practice environments. It was evident that the process involved a large number of tasks and to make tool development more tractable, we chose to subdivide each step by separately considering each of the following three major task categories: (a) Identify the patient with advanced disease; (b) develop and communicate a management plan specific to the patient; and (c) implement the plan.

Specifically for Step 1, understand the process, we first considered major task category (a) identify the patient with advanced disease. This is a problem because advanced chronic kidney disease is frequently without symptoms until function is substantially reduced (and dialysis is imminent). From the patients and physicians, we developed a detailed list of subtasks; here patients at high risk for advanced chronic kidney disease based on risk factors (e.g., diabetes and hypertension) are identified; high-risk patients have creatinine measured (creatinine being a standard, easily obtained laboratory test that is affected by kidney function as well as other factors such as muscle mass); glomerular filtration rate is calculated (where glomerular filtration rate is a direct reflection of kidney function but is difficult to measure; glomerular filtration rate can be estimated from creatinine and other factors using a standard formula); and patients with advanced disease are flagged for special management. The same Step 1 exercise was repeated for major task category (b) develop and communicate a management plan specific to the patient—and for major task category (c) implement the plan.

Step 2. Identify Process Failures and Root Causes. To illustrate Step 2, we focus on the subtask "glomerular filtration rate calculated" within major task category (a). Why might this not happen? In this case, possible root causes include (a) no one is assigned the task of performing the calculation and (b) the standard formula is not readily accessible.[3]

Step 3. Develop Tools to Attack Root Causes. The goal here is to identify for each root cause a practical tool to address the problem. It may be, as in the case of the root problem "glomerular filtration rate formula is not

---

[3]Tasks, subtasks, and root causes are typically interrelated in a weblike fashion. Strategies for uncovering these relationships are well described in the process improvement literature. Interested readers are directed to the textbook *Theory of Constraints* (30).

readily available," that several tools exist. Because the standard formula for calculation is based only on creatinine and race, the laboratory contractor can report estimated glomerular filtration rate by race. Other available options include a pocket slide rule, and several calculators available on the Web, directly (31) or for downloading to a personal digital assistant (32). In some cases, a new tool may need to be developed. For example, for the root problem "no mechanism is in place for assuring that a person identified as high risk has specific labs ordered," one can develop a reminder card for the provider or triage nurse to be posted at their workstation, a computer-based reminder, or an addition to existing flowcharts for patients with diabetes mellitus and hypertension.

Step 4. Establish a Tailoring Strategy. The objective here is to develop the meta-tool— ideally in the form of brief, easy-to-use instructions for practitioners or (more or less formal) quality improvement teams. To accomplish this, one must first characterize the variety of target practices in terms that clarify which tools make the most sense for a given practice environment. The specific characteristics relate to the resources and constraints that influence whether a specific tool is suitable for satisfying a specific task in the functional specifications.

In the case of the RPA initiative, we relied heavily on the input of experts and focus group participants to develop a general taxonomy that could guide tool selection. In this regard, we took two approaches. First, to assure a reasonable level of completeness, we constructed an algorithm corresponding to each major task. The algorithm consists of a series of questions that serve as a guide to the type of tool that would take advantage of the available resource and/or overcome the constraints in that practice. Once the tool type is identified, the user is guided to tools of that type.

We recognize that many providers will not have the inclination to use a series of algorithms to guide tool selection. Therefore, we also took a second approach: We identified several vignettes, and identified a set of tools that would be suitable for that situation. This is akin to the "quick start" instructions provided with software, to be used by those practices that recognize themselves to be typical of one of the vignettes.

In this case, we identified four major vignettes that captured most of the practice situations described by our experts and focus group participants:

1. Busy primary provider; no interest or particular knowledge about advanced chronic kidney disease.
2. Small primary provider in a rural community who must provide comprehensive services.
3. Nephrologist; good communication with referring providers; overloaded with patients.

4. Nephrologist; loose relationship with community physicians; not too many referrals for advanced chronic kidney disease; referrals are late.

For Vignette 1, the busy primary-care provider with few resources to support ongoing care of patients with advanced chronic kidney disease, tools focus on patient identification and referral. For Vignette 2, the isolated primary-care provider, an additional set of tools will be needed to negotiate comanagement with a distant nephrologist consultant, and to provide appropriate care within that arrangement. For Vignette 3, the nephrologist who is currently above capacity who is concerned about a host of new referrals of advanced chronic kidney disease patients, tools are needed to more efficiently manage the ongoing care of such patients, perhaps with the development of a specialized clinic with an advanced practice nurse or physician assistant. Finally, for Vignette 4, the nephrologist who has not developed a strategy for coordinating with referring physicians, relevant tools would promote education of and communication with non-nephrologists (e.g., education programs for grand rounds, a "Dear Colleague" letter, a fax-back consult form requesting basic referral data, or a template consultation form to assure that plans and expectations are clarified).

DISCUSSION

Despite initial hope that developing and disseminating evidence-based guidelines would be followed painlessly by practice improvement, this has not been the case. Medical care is embedded in a complex system that exists in a dynamic equilibrium—significant changes from that equilibrium require more than a bit of well-intentioned jiggering.

Substantial efforts have been made to find tools that will improve adherence with guidelines, and many are creative solutions to specific barriers to practice improvement.

Individual, one-size-fits-all tools are still not sufficient and we must move beyond treating individual tools as the "fix." We need to facilitate the development of coherent efforts that have a reasonable probability of success in a range of typical practice settings. Total quality management is conceptually an appropriate approach, but it is expensive and has not proved easily generalizable in the medical context.

In this chapter, we have described one approach to practice improvement that builds on the general principles of total quality management for process improvement, with the added component of facilitated implementation (facilitated process improvement) based on a preestablished set of functional specifications (goals of care), tools (means for accomplishing those goals in different settings), and a meta-tool (procedure for tailoring tools to specific practice settings.) The approach we recommend is detailed in Fig. 16.1 for a specific application, practice improvement in the care of advanced chronic kidney disease.

Our experience here has made it abundantly clear that developing a tool kit based on the notion of facilitated implementation is by no means simple and, of course, the point was to address the complex issues up front so as to free clinicians to do what they do best. This complex exercise has involved many months of intensive participation by community clinicians, patients, nephrology experts, and representatives of professional organizations. Others considering this approach should first consider the importance of the effort, the degree of commitment from supporting organizations, and the adequacy of funding.

We are planning to test this approach in typical practice settings. The subsequent broad rollout will be linked to a broad educational effort initiated through professional organizations, including presentations at clinical meetings and workshops to "train the trainers." The success of this approach is not a forgone conclusion; the history of guideline adherence initiatives teaches us to never underestimate the challenge.

REFERENCES

1. National Guideline Clearinghouse. Agency for Healthcare Research and Quality. Available at: http://www.guideline.gov. Accessed January 5, 2004.
2. Woolf SH. Evidence-based medicine and practice guidelines: an overview. *Cancer Control.* 2000;7(4):362–367.
3. Renal Physicians Association—Clinical Practice Guideline #3: Appropriate Patient Preparation for Renal Replacement Therapy. Available at: https://www.renalmd.org/publications/index.cfm. Accessed January 5, 2004.
4. Grimshaw JM, Russell IT. Effect of clinical guidelines on medical practice: a systematic review of rigorous evaluations. *Lancet.* 1993;342(8883):1317–1322.
5. Davis DA, Taylor-Vaisey A. Translating guidelines into practice. A systematic review of theoretic concepts, practical experience and research evidence in the adoption of clinical practice guidelines. *CMAJ.* 1997;157(4):408–416.
6. Oxman AD, Thomson MA, Davis DA, Haynes RB. No magic bullets: a systematic review of 102 trials of interventions to improve professional practice. *CMAJ.* 1995;153:1423–1431.
7. *Effective Health Care: Getting Evidence Into Practice.* Feb 1999;5(1):1–16.
8. Grol R. Implementing guidelines in general practice care. *Qual Health Care.* 1992;1:184–191.
9. Trowbridge R, Weingarten S. Educational techniques used in changing provider behavior. In: *Making Health Care Safer: A Critical Analysis of Patient Safety Practices.* Available at: http://www.ahcpr.gov/clinic/ptsafety/chap54. Accessed January 5, 2004.

10. Eagle KA, Lee TH, Brennan TA, Krumholz HM, Weingarten S. 28th Bethesda Conference. Task Force 2: Guideline implementation. *J Am Coll Cardiol.* 1997; 29(6):1141–1148.

11. Bero LA, Grilli R, Grimshaw JM, Harvey E, Oxman AD, Thomson MA. Closing the gap between research and practice: an overview of systematic reviews of interventions to promote the implementation of research findings. The Cochrane Effective Practice and Organization of Care Review Group. *BMJ.* 1998;317 (7156):465–468.

12. Cabana MD, Rushton JL, Rush AJ. Implementing practice guidelines for depression: applying a new framework to an old problem. *Gen Hosp Psychiatry.* 2002; 24(1):35–42.

13. Szilagyi PG, Bordley C, Vann JC, et al. Effect of patient reminder/recall interventions on immunization rates: a review. *JAMA.* 2000;284(14):1820–1827.

14. Weingarten S. Translating practice guidelines into patient care: guidelines at the bedside. *Chest.* 2000;118(2 Suppl):4S–7S.

15. CDC resources. Strategies for increasing adult vaccination rates. Available at: http://www.cdc.gov/nip/publications/adultstrat.htm. Accessed January 5, 2004.

16. Shortell SM. Bennett CL. Byck GR. Assessing the impact of continuous quality improvement on clinical practice: what it will take to accelerate progress. *Milbank Q.* 1998;76(4):593–624.

17. Samsa G. Matchar D. Can continuous quality improvement be assessed using randomized trials? *Health Serv Res.* 2000 Aug;35(3):687–700.

18. Greene T, Bourgoignie JJ, Habwe V, et al. Baseline characteristics in the Modification of Diet in the Renal Disease Study. *J Am Soc Nephrol.* 1993;4:1221–1236.

19. Woodrow G, Oldroyd B, Turney JH, Tompkins L, Brownjohn AM, Smith MA. Whole body and regional body composition in patients with chronic renal failure. *Nephrol Dial Transplant.* 1996;11:1613–1618.

20. Mailloux Lu, Levey AS. Hypertension in patients with chronic renal disease. *Am J Kidney Dis.* 1998; 32(5 Suppl 3):S120–S141.

21. Bushinsky DA. The contribution of acidosis to renal osteodystrophy. *Kidney Int.* 1995;47:1816–1832.

22. Lin Y, Sheih S, Diang L. Influence of rapid correction of metabolic acidosis on serum osteocalcin level in chronic renal failure. *ASAIO J.* 1994;40:M440–M444.

23. Kopple JD, Greene T, Chumlea WC, et al. Relationship between nutritional status and the glomerular filtration rate; results from the MDRD study. *Kidney Int.* 2000;57:1688–1703.

24. Stack AG, Bloembergen WE. A cross-sectional study of the prevalence and clinical correlates of congestive heart failure among incident dialysis patients. *Am J Kidney Dis.* 2001;38(5):992–1000.

25. Levin A, Singer J, Thompson CR, Ross H, Lewis M. Prevalent left ventricular hypertrophy in the predialysis population: identifying opportunities for intervention. *Am J Kidney Dis.* 1996;27(3):347–354.

26. Nissenson AR, Collins AJ, Hurley J, Petersen H, Pereira BJ, Steinberg EP. Opportunities for improving the care of patients with chronic renal insufficiency: current practice patterns. *J Am Soc Nephrol.* 2001;12(8):1713–1720.

27. Hunsicker LG, Adler S, Caggiula A, et al. Predictors of the progression of renal disease in the Modification of Diet in Renal Disease Study. *Kidney Int.* 1997;51: 1908–1919

28. Pereira BJ. Optimization of pre-ESRD care: the key to improved dialysis outcomes. *Kidney Int.* 2000. 57(1):351–365.

29. McCrory DC, Klassen P, Rutschmann OT, et al. *Evidence Report: Appropriate Patient Preparation for Renal Replacement Therapy.* Rockville, MD: Renal Physicians Association; 2002.

30. Dettmer HW. *Goldratt's Theory of Constraints: A Systems Approach to Continuous Improvement.* Milwaukee, WI: ASQ Quality Press. 1997:2–27

31. National Kidney Disease Education Program: MDRD GFR calculators. Available at: http://www.nkdep.nih.gov/GFR-cal.htm. Accessed January 5, 2004.

32. Renal Physicians Association—PDA downloads. Available at: http://www.renalmd.org/palmdownloads/index.html. Accessed January 5, 2004.

Chapter 17

New Technologies and Their Influence on Existing Interventions

Celette Sugg Skinner
Sarah C. Kobrin
Marci K. Campbell
Lisa Sutherland

How to facilitate adherence to medical regimens is not a new question, but recent answers to the question have incorporated strategies using new technologies. The best of these seek to emulate the old wisdom evidenced among savvy, caring providers who knew that no one approach would be effective for all patients in all situations and, thus, crafted individualized interventions for patients under their care. Perhaps the goal was to convince Mrs. Smith to continue taking her pills once she began to feel better or to help Mr. Jones, who was already convinced of the pill's importance, to remember what time he was supposed to take them. Although "adherence-promoting interventions" may not have been in the lexicon, many a practitioner developed and communicated many a plan for helping patients follow treatment or prevention recommendations.

Today's health care genre presents a challenge for such individualized approaches. Organizations are publishing recommendations for primary and secondary prevention (diet, exercise, smoking cessation, and screening), managed care organizations are dealing with financial incentives for adherence to the guidelines, and average length of time providers can spend in patient visits is shrinking. The need for *individualized* interventions remains, but the feasibility of developing and delivering them is diminished. Still, the question remains, how do we identify and address adherence issues important to individuals without time to craft a separate intervention promoting these behaviors for each one?

One answer to this question has come from the ability of computers to match highly specialized information to a particular patient's needs. Known as "tailoring," this approach approximates the customization of traditional face-to-face interventions and combines it with the time and cost savings of mass production. The underlying concept for tailored interventions is quite simple. Just as a tailor creates clothing by taking numerous measurements and sewing together pieces of fabric to create a custom fit, a computer-tailoring program collects numerous "measurements" by querying patients to determine which issues affect their adherence to the recommendation in question. The "fabric" of the tailored intervention can be composed of many, distinct text, audio, and graphic elements. Both the querying and the resulting tailored intervention can employ nearly any communication medium (print, phone, CD-ROM, DVD, etc.). In their excellent 2000 edition, *Tailoring Health Messages*, Kreuter, Farrell, Olevitch, and Buckholtz define tailored interventions as "Any combination of information or change strategies *intended to reach one specific person*, based on characteristics that are unique to that person, related to the outcome of interest, and have been *derived from an individual assessment*" (1). This definition highlights several features that distinguish tailored interventions from other commonly used approaches: (a) Tailored interventions are unique *collections* of messages or intervention components; (b) each tailored intervention is intended for a particular person rather than a group of persons; and (c) tailored interventions are assembled based on individual-level factors related to the recipient's adherence behavior of interest.

Tailored interventions are composed of multiple elements, combined based on several data points. Elements of the intervention are created to anticipate and address every possible response to the queries. Each of these potential intervention messages is stored in a computer file "library." A system of computer algorithms, generally "if/then" statements, is used to match the appropriate intervention messages to each participant, based on the query responses. Tailoring programs read patients' responses, run responses through the algorithms, and generate a special combination of messages for each intervention recipient.

To continue the clothing analogy, tailored interventions are distinguished from targeted interventions just as custom clothing is distinguished from those sold "off the rack." Tailored interventions—and custom clothing—are intended to fit one particular individual. Targeted interventions—and off-the-rack clothing—are intended to fit any member of a group of people who share some number of common characteristics. As with clothing, a targeted intervention is less likely to suit a particular person's needs than an intervention tailored specifically to that individual.

In the 1990s, tailoring research quickly jumped from controlled comparisons of tailored versus nontailored interventions to assessing many different types of tailored interventions delivered through various media. And, as is the case with a number of research areas, technological capacity to produce tailored interventions has grown at a more rapid pace than understanding of what types of tailored interventions are most effective for influencing what behaviors in what groups. In short, tailoring research has demonstrated more of what is technically feasible than what is most effective.

Chapter Format

Several reviews of tailored intervention trials have been published, and it is not our intention to duplicate them. Rather this chapter surveys how tailoring technology has been used in adherence-promoting interventions, features examples that illustrate various types of tailored interventions studied via randomized controlled trials, and summarizes what we can and cannot conclude about the effectiveness of tailored adherence interventions. We begin with a survey of the earliest tailoring studies that used only the print medium and then move to a discussion of more interactive and technologically advanced media. The chapter is set up to address four questions:

1. Has tailoring been shown to be effective?
2. What do we know about how tailored interventions should be designed (e.g,. variables, media, length, style, etc.)?
3. How do we apply advanced interactive technology to tailoring?
4. What new questions about tailored interventions have been introduced by recent technological advances?

QUESTION 1—HAS TAILORING BEEN SHOWN TO BE EFFECTIVE?

Because print was the first feasible medium for production of computer-tailored interventions, the first controlled trials of tailored versus non-tailored adherence interventions were conducted in the print medium. These tailored interventions produced customized variations of text with simple graphical content (see description in Kreuter et al., 2000) (2). A pair of studies published in 1994 compared, among primary-care patients, adherence to mammography screening and smoking cessation recommendations by receipt of tailored versus nontailored print interventions (3, 4). Samples of patients were contacted by phone "on behalf of" their physicians. Those who agreed to participate were interviewed by phone, then randomly assigned to receive nontailored or tailored print recommendation letters. Consistent with technological development at the time, the method of tailoring was a simple merge program with numerous if/then statements that read individuals' questionnaire data and assembled tailored combinations of print and graphics. The mailings included a cover letter with the recipient's physician's digitized signature, a mammography recommendation newsletter (for female participants over the age of 40), and/or a smoking cessation recommendation newsletter (for all current smokers).

Newsletters for patients assigned to the tailored group had text based on the recipient's interview data regarding some basic constructs from the transtheoretical and health belief models (see chap. 2, this volume). These included: stage of considering behavior change (having a mammogram or stopping smoking); perceived benefits and barriers (related to the behavior); perceived cancer risk and actual risk factors (i.e., number of cigarettes smoked daily; family history of breast cancer); age; race; and, for smokers, reasons attributed to past failed quit attempts. Out of a library of potential messages, appropriate message texts were selected and put together by the tailoring algorithms.

Figure 17.1 shows two examples of these first tailored mammography recommendation newsletters. The digitized photo in the left corner varied by race. Captions varied by the recipient's age and whether she had ever had a mammogram or was considering having one.

Because the goal was to test whether tailored intervention content was more effective than nontailored content for facilitating adherence, these studies were carefully controlled to vary only the content—not the appearance of the printed materials or the experience of tailored and nontailored recipients. Therefore, the nontailored newsletter (shown in Fig. 17.2) was developed to look much like the tailored versions and tailored recipients were given no hint that their newsletters were any different from those of other recipients.

Outcomes compared between tailored and nontailored recipients included changes in adherence and communication "process variables" including whether participants remembered receiving the letters and, of those who remembered, how much they read. Even though the letters' appearance was quite similar and recipients didn't know about the tailoring, there were significant between-groups differences in recall and readership for both mammography and smoking cessation recommendations, such that tailored letter recipients were more likely to have read "most of all." Given that one has to notice and attend to a message for communication to take place, the finding that more women read the tailored recommendations is not trivial.

The ultimate test of an intervention, however, is adherence. Of women nonadherent for mammography at baseline, more tailored than nontailored recipients (44% vs. 31%, respectively) had been screened by 3-month follow-up (3). There were significant interaction effects for intervention group (tai-

Mammography

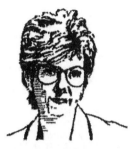

"I've never even thought about having a mammogram to check for breast cancer. I've never even thought about the fact that I need one."

What Are The Facts?

Most women surveyed know that *breast cancer has a good chance of being cured if it is found early*, when it's just getting started, and that mammograms are the best way of finding breast cancer early. In fact, *mammograms can detect breast cancers much smaller than the hand can feel.* They know that regular mammograms are so important they could save your life.

Unfortunately, we found that a lot of patients in our survey have never had a mammogram and are not even thinking about having one any time soon. Are you one of these women?

Any Roadblocks?

You may have heard that mammograms are very expensive. While it's true that certain facilities charge high rates, there are places in the area where mammograms are not expensive. Also, more and more health insurance plans are covering the cost of mammograms. *Don't let the cost hold you back.*

Some women may not think mammography is important because they get physical breast exams by their doctors. Since a breast exam *and* a mammogram is much more likely to find breast cancer than an exam alone, a breast exam should not be considered a substitute for mammography.

Having regular screening mammograms is very important and *could save your life.* That's why the National Cancer Institute and the American Cancer Society recommend getting regular mammograms.

Can it happen to you?

Almost every woman thinks, "I'm not going to get breast cancer". But studies show that one in every ten women in the U.S. (10%) will get breast cancer sometime during her life. The chances of getting breast cancer are even higher for women age 50 and over. If you are over 50, mammograms are especially important for you.

So, the thing to do is to get regular mammograms -- just like regular pap smears -- either to find out you don't have breast cancer or to find it early while there's a good chance for a cure. If you haven't thought about it, please think about it now. You can call our office to arrange for an appointment or to get more information (542-2731).

Chatham Family Physicians   Route 5, Box 7   Pittsboro, North Carolina   27312

FIG. 17.1.   *(Continued).*

Mammography

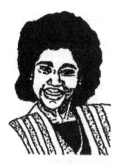

"I've had a mammogram, but it was over two years ago. Since I'm in my 40's, I know I should be checked every 2 years. I've thought about having another mammogram, but I just haven't done it yet."

What Are The Facts?

Most women surveyed know that breast cancer has a good chance of being cured if it is found early, when it's just getting started, and that mammograms are the best way of finding breast cancer early. In fact, mammograms can detect breast cancers much smaller than the hand can feel. They know that regular mammograms are so important they could save your life.

Many patients in our survey had their last mammogram more than two years ago. It's now time for them to have another mammogram. They may be thinking about having another one but they haven't done it yet. Has it been more than two years since *your* last mammogram? Since breast cancer can develop at any time, you should be checked again soon.

Any Roadblocks?

You may have heard that mammograms are very expensive. While it's true that certain facilities charge high rates, there are places in the area where mammograms are not expensive. Also, more and more health insurance plans are covering the cost of mammograms. *Don't let the cost hold you back.*

Some women may not think mammography is important because they get physical breast exams by their doctors. Since a breast exam *and* a mammogram is much more likely to find breast cancer than an exam alone, a breast exam should not be considered a substitute for mammography.

Having regular screening mammograms is very important and *could save your life.* That's why the National Cancer Institute and the American Cancer Society recommend getting regular mammograms.

Can it happen to you?

Almost every woman thinks, "I'm not going to get breast cancer". But studies show that one in every ten women in the U.S. (10%) will get breast cancer sometime during her life.

So, the thing to do is to get regular mammograms -- just like regular pap smears -- either to find out you don't have breast cancer or to find it early while there's a good chance for a cure. If you've had a mammogram, that's a great start. But it may be time for you to have another one. If you've thought about having another mammogram, please go ahead and call our office to arrange for an appointment or to get more information (542-2731).

Chatham Family Physicians　　　Route 5, Box 7　　　Pittsboro, North Carolina　　　27312

FIG. 17.1.　Two samples of tailored newsletters.

Mammography

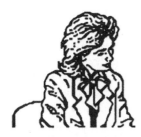

Early detection is the best defense against breast cancer. Mammography is the best method for detecting breast tumors at their earliest stages--before they can be felt and before they have had a chance to spread.

But too few women have been taking advantage of mammograms. They may have heard that mammography is very painful, or that it is expensive, or that it will result in hazardous radiation exposure. For whatever reasons, our best data show that most women are not taking any steps at all to thwart breast cancer.

A woman may feel some momentary discomfort during a mammogram because the breasts must be compressed briefly. Some women will experience more discomfort if they get the examination a few days before their menstrual period.

Costs for mammograms vary, but some insurance policies cover breast examinations, and the American Cancer Society and the American College of Radiology have joined in a program that will reduce mammogram costs.

The amount of radiation a woman's breast is exposed to is, of course, a concern. But the benefits of mammography far outweigh the risk of not being examined. Further, the amount of radiation exposure needed for a mammogram today has been greatly reduced through the use of better film and equipment. In fact, the average amount of exposure has been cut by about 50 percent over the past 15 years.

Women over age 50 have a greater chance of developing breast cancer than women under 50. And the chances of getting breast cancer are even higher for women with a family history of breast cancer. That is, a woman with a relative on her mother's side who has had breast cancer may be twice as likely to develop breast cancer sometime during her life.

Both the National Cancer Institute and the American Cancer Society recommend regular mammograms for all women over age 40. Women between age forty and fifty should have a mammogram every two years while women age 50 and over should have one every year.

There is a considerable amount of encouraging news about breast cancer. For one thing, the five-year survival rate is now slightly above 90 percent. Secondly, not every lump is malignant--indeed, 9 out of 10 aren't. Finally, very small tumors--those that mammography detects--are virtually 100 percent curable without disfiguring surgery. So, if you're a logical candidate, scheduling a mammogram makes sense.

Guilford College
Family Practice
ASSOCIATES

FIG. 17.2.   Nontailored newsletter.

lored vs. nontailored) and two demographic characteristics—minority and low-income status—such that, for women in these subgroups, tailored recipients were significantly more likely to be adherent at follow-up. This finding is important, given that minorities and low–socioeconomic status patients typically present the highest risk of disease and may benefit most from strategies that can effectively increase adherence. For example, Black Americans are 33% more likely than White Americans to die from cancer (5).

Similarly, the smoking cessation newsletters did not produce an overall main effect for quit rates between tailored and nontailored recipients, but letter type interacted significantly with smoking status. Among those who smoked no more than 20 cigarettes per day, recipients of tailored newsletters were more likely to have stopped smoking, at follow up (4). These results, modest in some ways, were remarkable considering the interventions were minimal-contact, one-shot, one-page recommendation letters that neither pointed out to recipients nor capitalized on the fact they were tailored.

As discussed in a 1998 review of "first generation" tailoring research (6), only a few studies sought to replicate this comparison of tailored versus nontailored print (3, 7–10); no others did so with "hidden tailoring." Only five studies measured communication process variables, each finding that tailored print interventions were "better remembered, read, and/or perceived as relevant than nontailored communications" (6). Four studies that compared tailored versus nontailored diet and exercise interventions(7, 9–11) found main effects—tailored intervention recipients were more likely to be adherent than nontailored recipients.

Given that tailored interventions have come to be widely used, one might expect that these are examples from a large literature including carefully controlled trials comparing adherence outcomes of tailored versus nontailored interventions addressing a variety of behaviors, using a variety of tailoring variables, and delivered via a number of media. However, only a few studies have looked at head-to-head comparisons of tailored and nontailored interventions. Results were deemed promising enough to move the field past this basic tailored/nontailored comparison and on to more complex tailored intervention designs and combinations, described later in the chapter. Technology advanced, tailored print showed promise, and researchers were eager to explore the seemingly limitless ways interventions could be tailored.

QUESTION 2—WHAT DO WE KNOW ABOUT HOW TAILORED INTERVENTIONS SHOULD BE DESIGNED?

Tailored interventions can be lengthy or brief; they can be tailored on many types of variables including demographics, cultural characteristics, and behavior theory models outlined in chapter 2, and they can be delivered via a variety of media. What do we know about what works best? Although answers are still not definitive, we have the most data regarding intervention media.

Media

Intervention media can be interactive or noninteractive. The first tailored media comparison studies assessed the noninteractive medium of print versus the interactive medium of telephone counseling. Telephone counseling—without the use of computer-tailoring technology—had shown promise in adherence-promoting intervention trials. It quickly became apparent that the counseling could be streamlined via computer-generated tailored counseling guides. With tailored counseling guides, the phone time could more efficiently be spent addressing—rather than *assessing and addressing*—important issues for each patient being counseled. Whereas tailored telephone counseling was expected to have the advantage of a personal touch (albeit only over a phone line), print had the advantage of including visual elements; print could also be retained by the patient for later review. Because of the personnel time involved, costs for delivering tailored telephone interventions were expected to be higher, but the increased costs might be justified if tailored phone counseling was significantly more effective for facilitating adherence.

Building on results of the 1994 print-tailored mammography intervention study (3), two studies compared phone- and print-tailored media for mammography intervention. Although the studies were similar, there were some important differences that may have affected the slightly different findings they yielded—differences that lead to remaining questions about print- versus phone-tailored interventions.

In the first study, titled *Personally Relevant Information About Mammography* (PRISM), Rimer and colleagues assigned women to receive "usual-care" annual reminder cards, tailored brochure (year 1) and newsletter (year 2), or the brochure and newsletter plus tailored counseling calls both years. The PRISM newsletter's cover page appears in Fig. 17.3. Two rounds of follow-up analyses (12, 13) showed tailored print plus phone significantly outperformed both tailored print alone and the usual-care practice of sending a nontailored card, but the tailored print brochure and newsletter did not outperform the nontailored reminder card. The other study, conducted by Champion and Skinner, also tested tailored print and phone interventions, but differed from PRISM in three ways. First, the intervention content was limited to what would fit on a one-page newsletter. Second, there was a fourth group that received only tailored phone counseling. Finally, the sample was quite demographically diverse (54% African American and 52% income < \$15,000 annually). At 2 months after the first round of interven-

Personally Relevant Information about Screening Mammography

PRISM   A Newsletter Created Just for Taki Sumioshi

More Information Just for YOU

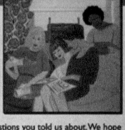

Women need to consider the benefits and limitations of mammograms to make informed choices.

That's where PRISM comes in. PRISM is a program of Duke University Medical Center and Blue Cross and Blue Shield of North Carolina. We are here to help women like you make informed decisions about getting mammograms. The project is for both those women who are getting mammograms and those who are not. It is also for current and past members of Blue Cross and Blue Shield.

Last year, we interviewed you and then created a booklet just for you. This newsletter tells you where you stand on the issues now and what other women in PRISM are doing. It also updates you on your risk and answers any questions you told us about. We hope this newsletter will help you think about getting regular mammograms. Read on to learn the latest! ❂

Taking Steps for Good Health

Could you take more steps to ensure your good health? Yes! A few weeks ago, you told us that you have not had a mammogram in the last one to two years, and that you are not thinking about getting one anytime soon. We'd like you to think again about getting a mammogram as a way to take care of your health.

Most women in their 40s are getting regular mammograms. In fact, almost all women in their 40s who are taking part in PRISM (92%) are thinking about or planning to get a mammogram in the next one to two years. We hope you will join the other women your age who are protecting their health by getting regular mammograms. **So think about it!** ❂

You are here NOW

| Not getting regular mammograms and not thinking about getting them | Not getting regular mammograms but thinking about getting them | Not getting regular mammograms but planning on getting them | Getting mammograms but not definitely planning to continue on a regular basis | Getting mammograms and definitely planning to continue on a regular basis | Most women in PRISM are HERE |

You were here LAST YEAR

FIG. 17.3. PRISM newsletter cover.

500

tion, mammography adherence in all three intervention groups was significantly higher than usual care, but did not differ significantly among intervention groups (14). At the next follow-up, after the second round of intervention, adherence in each of the intervention groups was still significantly higher than usual care. However, the combination of print plus phone emerged as the most effective of the tailored interventions (15). Therefore, findings generally support the combination of tailored phone and print as more effective than tailored print alone—for both very brief and more thorough intervention content—but leave several questions about why some tailored print has been found effective and others have not.

Variables

Another obvious way in which tailored interventions can differ from each other is in the variables on which they are tailored. In general, adherence outcomes for interventions tailored on variables from behavioral theories (see chap. 2) are more positive than interventions tailored only on basic demographic and medical variables, such as those available in electronic medical records or claims data (16). However, as Kreuter and colleagues have noted, most interventions have been tailored only on a collection of variables from "a hand full of behavioral theories."

Despite much discussion among intervention researchers regarding whether there are certain variables particularly important for facilitating certain types of adherence (17, 18) and whether there are potentially important tailoring variables that have not yet been used in interventions (19), only a few studies have sought to systematically examine these issues.

For adherence to smoking cessation recommendations, a team of Dutch researchers (20) compared the long-term effectiveness of computer-generated six-page print feedback tailored on: (a) positive outcomes of stopping smoking, (b) recipients' perceived self-efficacy for being able to successfully quit, and (c) both outcomes and self-efficacy. Findings indicated those who received the combination of tailoring on outcomes and efficacy were significantly more likely than members of the control group to maintain 12-month continuous abstinence (5% vs. 1.6%, respectively; $p < .05$). Neither the interventions tailored on outcomes only or efficacy only was significantly more effective than the control condition for facilitating long-term adherence.

Other researchers have experimented with tailoring on cultural characteristics of intervention recipients. For example, Krueter and colleagues have tested cancer-screening and dietary-change-promoting interventions that are tailored on (a) behavioral constructs (see chap. 2), (b) cultural constructs important among African Americans (21), or (c) both cultural and behavioral variables. Preliminary findings indicate interventions tailored to both cultural and behavioral constructs may be especially effective for facilitating cancer-screening and dietary-change adherence (22).

Length and Type of Content

As discussed previously, the amount of content in tailored adherence interventions tested to date has varied widely. Although at least one study has used preferred amount of information on specific topics as a tailoring variable (23), we know of no published studies that have specifically compared adherence outcomes between patients who received interventions with more versus less tailored content. There are many types of elements that can be included in tailored print interventions—narratives, photos, illustrations, puzzles, cartoons, graphs, and charts. Some of the tailored intervention studies discussed in this chapter have differed widely in the amount of content they included but, because length was only one among a number of differences, any conclusions about the effect produced by amount of content or, for example, the relative amount of text versus graphics, would be speculative.

Intervention Dose

Conventional wisdom suggests that one-shot interventions may produce one-shot adherence and that, to facilitate maintained behavior change, more doses of an intervention may need to be delivered. There is a need for tests of tailored intervention doses in randomized controlled trials. In Champion and colleagues' study of mammography-promoting interventions (described earlier), women in each of three experimental groups all received a first intervention dose but then were randomly assigned to receive or not receive a second "booster" dose the following year. Preliminary findings indicate that women who were screened after the first intervention were more likely to have been rescreened, on schedule, if they received the booster dose ($OR = 1.68$; $p = .03$) but, if women were given a 15-month window for rescreening, the booster dose effect was no longer significant. Eventually—by 15 months postbooster—adherence in the booster/no-booster groups was similar. Furthermore, among those who had not become adherent after the first intervention dose, booster recipients were no more likely to be screened, during the 2nd year, than those who did not receive the booster. These findings suggest that additional doses of interventions that "worked the first time" may have some benefit for facilitating timely adherence whereas giving a booster intervention dose to those for whom the first dose wasn't effective doesn't seem to be a promising strategy (24).

Summary

Answers to the question of what we know about how tailored interventions should be designed—how much content they should include, through which medium or media they should be delivered, on what variables they should be tailored, and how many doses should be delivered—are not very satisfying. There is some evidence that combining tailoring from print and telephone media is more effective than print alone. However, whether print alone or phone alone is effective for facilitating adherence has not produced a well-studied or consistent answer. Nor has which medium or combination is most cost-effective yet been established. These issues continue to be studied; we hope reliable answers will emerge in the next few years.

QUESTION 3—HOW DO WE APPLY ADVANCED INTERACTIVE TECHNOLOGY TO TAILORING?

In all their variations, printed tailored interventions provide one-way communication. Participants give information and the tailoring system responds. Tailored telephone counseling provides two-way communication—interactivity—but requires substantially more time to set up, and then conduct, a live conversation. Technology changed rapidly in the mid–1990s and the emergence of the Internet and the explosion of data storage space available on hard disks and CD-ROMs allowed the development of interactive tailoring that requires as little expert time as printed interventions. (Although there are many other technologies, for the purposes of this chapter we focus on CD-ROM, Web-based, and interactive voice response programs.)

This increased storage capacity means the "library" of potential messages can grow dramatically, allowing for more fine-tuned responses to participants. Interactive tailoring systems can change directions on the spot, modifying both what questions are asked and what feedback is given. For both queries and feedback, the range of formats has expanded substantially. Very creative *printed* feedback might include tailored stories, word puzzles, or expert Q&A; interactive feedback can take forms as varied as live-action soap operas with characters discussing issues a participant just indicated as important, cooking demonstrations featuring the dietary choices suggested for and preferred by an individual participant, and talk shows with experts addressing, for example, factors a user indicates as barriers to adherence (e.g., Campbell et al., ref. 25).

Interactive programs can be made available to participants in many ways. They may be presented in freestanding kiosks or on a laptop computer located in a private clinic or health department. A provider or researcher can recommend a person spend time working on the program just as patients often watch a health education video while at the doctor's office. Or, these programs can be found on a Web site; again, the participant would be recommended to spend time with the program and perhaps to return to it a number of times. Interactive programs, in their many formats, have joined the tools available to help providers and researchers facilitate adherence to medical regimens and preventive behaviors.

FoodSmart: An Interactive Example

An example of a tailored interactive program is FoodSmart, a CD-ROM-based program to improve adherence to nutritional recommendations (25). FoodSmart has been implemented in kiosks in social service and public health settings. Users first log into the system with a unique user name and password; this process (a) creates a record of the participant's use of the program, just as would be done by a data-entry assistant—after the fact—if data were collected on paper; (b) ensures confidentiality; (c) allows the program to recognize the participant again when he or she returns for another session, and (d) is of great value for tracking behavioral changes and progress in adherence.

In some programs, users can choose whether to opt for audio support, whether to use a mouse, keyboard or touch screen, and even in what language the program will appear (26, 27). After introductory screens that explain how the program works, users typically answer a set of questions, which can include demographics, psychosocial variables, current behaviors, and any other data needed to tailor program feedback. Some programs go directly to providing tailored feedback à la an expert system (e.g., "you told us you exercise once a week . . .") whereas others may embed or intersperse the feedback in a game, quiz, story, infomercial, or one of the "edutainment" techniques (i.e., soap opera, cooking show) mentioned before. For example, the FoodSmart program intersperses video soap opera story segments with interactive infomercials that provide the tailored feedback and education. In the first version of FoodSmart, participants were required to proceed linearly through the program's components; a later version allowed participants to choose, from a menu of options, which information or activities they wished to select during that session.

Anticipated Advantages (and Disadvantages)
of Interactive Technology

As described previously, changes in tailored interventions to improve adherence were largely driven by advances in technological capacity rather than conclusions drawn from research. Similarly, the arrival of interactive technology has stimulated a substantial shift in tailoring technology. Interactive tailored technology's anticipated advantages and disadvantages outlined in the following paragraphs have yet to be systematically addressed.

Programs using the new interactive media are anticipated to present significant advantages for participants and researchers. For participants, the assumption is that interactive media will be more engaging and create more sense of control and choice than print interventions because interactivity allows users to navigate the Web site or system, selecting the feedback and topics that are of greatest interest. Such involvement should increase retention of information (28). Finally, interactive media have the potential for widespread dissemination to users anywhere rather than dependence on institutions or private companies to collect data and produce feedback from a central location.

The assumed disadvantages of interactive programs include a dependency on user interest, inclination to seek information, and skill in using programs. (This skill may vary according to age, literacy, and computer experience; see ref. 26). Because they can select or skip various parts of the program, users may not select the information most important or relevant for facilitating adherence. Of course, readers may skip part of a printed text as well, just as viewers may not attend as closely to part of a video. But these varying levels of attention seem different from the option to avoid completely a component of an interactive program. Disadvantages for the researcher include the time and cost of designing, developing, and programming these interventions.

Much of early interactive tailoring has been designed for users with relatively advanced skills—those who were comfortable completing computer-based surveys and using a mouse to navigate fairly text-heavy screens. Tailored programs to reach lower income, minority, and/or low-literacy populations, which require extensive usability testing to ensure that less skilled users are able to log on and navigate the system to get tailored feedback, are currently being evaluated. To reach everyone, interactive systems must be usable by people who are elderly, have low literacy, or lack computer skills. An ironic finding is that individuals with novice skills are less likely to click on help links compared to more skilled users (26)—perhaps because they are less familiar with the existence of "online help." A technique to address this problem is pop-up help information that appears automatically when the user moves the mouse over a word (so-called "mouseover" links). Touch screens are also beneficial for people with low literacy and low computer skills (29), however factors such as the size and placement of buttons and icons may greatly affect usability among certain groups such as the elderly. Finally, even easy-to-use programs may be intimidating to people who are afraid to try "anything on a computer" (29).

QUESTION 4: WHAT NEW QUESTIONS ABOUT TAILORED INTERVENTIONS HAVE BEEN INTRODUCED BY RECENT TECHNOLOGICAL ADVANCES?

Despite the recent proliferation of interactive health communications on CD-ROM and the World Wide Web, few studies have rigorously evaluated effectiveness of interactive media to promote and maintain health behavior changes (30). Among these, several have shown effects on *determinants* of behavior, such as knowledge about and self-efficacy related to healthier eating (25), intentions to change dietary behavior (31), and recall of program content (32), but no effect on behavior (25, 31, 32). A possible explanation of these findings is that participants were less likely to use the interactive program than to read nontailored printed information mailed to their homes (31).

Automated Telephone Systems

The recent ability to link user-originated telephone calls with computer-automated responses has resulted in promising approaches to promoting adherence to medical regimens and preventive behaviors, including those using automated telephone systems. For example, Hyman and others examined the efficacy of an automated telephone system for maintaining adherence to a diet and cholesterol reduction program (33) and concluded that the automated calls were capable of maintaining contact, providing patient feedback, and may have helped in maintaining lower cholesterol levels for some patients. Piette and others have done extensive work on the use of automated telephone systems for diabetes self-management among low-income patients and have shown intervention effects on self-efficacy to perform self-care (34).

The TLC (Telephone-Linked Communications), a computer-based telecommunications system developed by Friedman and colleagues, carries out totally automated telephone conversations with a user (35). Functioning as an at-home monitor, educator, and counselor for reinforcing or changing health-related behaviors, the TLC combines an interactive voice response (IVR) subsystem for generating speech over the telephone, a speech recognition subsystem for recognizing what the participant is saying, a database management system for storing and managing system and user data, and a conversation control subsystem that controls the content and flow of individual TLC conversations with users.

During TLC conversations, the system speaks to participants with computer-controlled prerecorded human speech. Participants communicate with TLC by speaking into any telephone (even a cell phone) or using the touch-tone keypad. During TLC participant conversations—which can take place as often as daily or as infrequently as monthly—TLC assesses behavior, attitudes, and motivations and provides tailored feedback and behavioral counseling. TLC has been developed, tested, and shown to be effective for medication-taking (36), diet (37), exercise (38–40), smoking cessation (41), and screening behaviors (e.g., mammograms) (35). The intervention delivered by TLC is based on social cognitive and goal-setting theories (see chap. 2, this volume, for discussion of theories that can be used to develop interactive interventions) and on heuristics developed by experienced counselors, including telephone counselors; call structure and feedback incorporate principles of motivational interviewing and the transtheoretical model.

Issues for Future Research

The rapid transition to interventions designed around interactive media has left many questions unanswered. Chief among these questions are: (a) What are the effects of interactive technology on the patient–provider relationship? And (b) what dose of an interactive intervention is cost-effective?

Effects of Interactive Technology on the Patient–Provider Relationship. In the United States the average doctor visit lasts between 7 and 21 minutes (42). The Internet has emerged as one way for physicians to provide health information to patients in a time when the pressure is great to reduce costs and increase patient support and provides a venue for patients to participate in decision-making and care processes. A study of patient adherence to congestive heart failure management found that patients using the Internet to communicate with their physicians had significant positive changes in side effect management from medications, quality-of-life scores, and provider communication satisfaction (43). Abel and Painter reported patient–physician relationship, including confidence, trust, and access, to be one of the greatest factors influencing adherence to antiretroviral therapy in women with human immunodeficiency virus (HIV) disease (44). As technology is adopted to deliver health information and behavior change adherence interventions—patients clearly still look to their physicians for expertise, comfort, and healing. Moyer and others concluded that 70% of outpatient clinic patients reported willingness to use e-mail to communicate with their providers; however they also expressed concerns about efficiency, effectiveness, and whether e-mail use would improve their relationship with providers (45). The increase in consumer technology use and decrease in time spent with providers is often referred to as a "hi-tech, low-touch" situation. The Internet should not replace office visits, expert advice, or emotional support. The goal of new technologies should be to enhance the patient–provider relationship and not to diminish patient confidence, interaction, or dependence on providers (46, 47).

Using the Internet to Provide Interactive Adherence Programs

In 2002, more than 100 million Americans searched for health information online—an increase of 13 million from the previous year (48). In the landmark Pew Internet & American Life Project, 41% of those surveyed in 2000 reported the Internet affected their health care decisions (49). Although lower-income and minority populations are increasing rapidly in terms of computer and Internet access, significant gaps still remain; these gaps, sometimes referred to as the "digital divide," are most pronounced in rural areas with limited Internet access and low bandwidth (49).

In a recent nationwide survey of online adults, 90% were interested in communicating with their health care providers via e-mail (50); in contrast, 13% of providers said they used e-mail to communicate with patients in 2001 (51). Barriers to adoption include privacy, security, cost, reimbursement, office staff time, and medical malpractice (51, 52). The American Medical Association has addressed some of these concerns in their issuance of 18 guidelines for physicians communicating with patients by e-mail and separate guidelines for medico-legal and administrative communication. Patt and colleagues (53) reported that of physicians using e-mail to reach patients, e-mail communication fell into four broad categories: (a) e-mail access and content, (b) effects of e-mail on the doctor–patient relationship, (c) managing clinical issues by e-mail, and (d) integrating e-mail into office processes. The most consistent theme was that e-mail communication enhanced chronic-disease management. Many physicians also reported improved continuity of care and increased flexibility in responding to non-urgent issues. Another study concluded that requests for information on medications or treatments, specific symptoms, and requests for actions regarding medications or treatments accounted for 75% of all requests sent via e-mail to their providers. Physicians responded to 80.2% of all these requests (54). Despite barriers, physicians are increasingly using e-mail to communicate with patients. This practice has the potential to enhance patient–physician communication, which, in turn, has been reported to improve patient adherence, provider satisfaction, and health status (55).

Few studies have assessed the Internet's effectiveness for improving patients' medical self-management, health behavior adherence, or clinical outcomes (17). However, several advantages of using the Internet to deliver health care have begun to emerge. In addition to the ability to tailor information, patients report benefits such as increased perceived anonymity, the ability to receive social support 24 hours a day, enhanced patient–provider interaction, and greater access to health information (46, 56). Internet studies that have targeted socioeconomically disadvantaged populations have shown positive effects on behaviors such as medical protocol adherence, decreasing alcohol consumption during pregnancy, and decreasing risky sexual behavior. The impact of increased perceived anonymity has been especially effective in the medical management of patients with sensitive health conditions, such as HIV and mental health (57–59). Studies have also reported that patients accessing health information and drug adherence regimens on the Internet were more likely to disclose their health status, risks, and fears, which leads to increased treatment adherence (60, 61).

Web-based systems may have advantages in terms of offering additional functions that may work together to encourage treatment adherence. For example, the Web provides opportunities for patients to interact with other patients and experts via discussion forums, e-mail, online chat, and links to other recommended sites or programs. These functions may be helpful in promoting adherence by enabling users, for example, to create virtual communities and support groups around specific behaviors or health conditions.

Although many potential benefits have been reported, it is still unclear whether the benefits of using the Internet to deliver adherence interventions outweigh potential harms, including delays in seeking health care, patient self-diagnosis and inappropriate treatment, lack of privacy and confidentiality, and deterioration of the patient–provider relationship (46, 62, 63). Furthermore, it is very hard to track where people go on the Internet and what information they receive once they leave the "home" Web site; each site will likely include links to additional sites. Participants may associate this entire cascade of sites with the adherence-promoting program, assuming— probably erroneously—they all have the same quality and credibility.

Issues for Future Research on Internet-Based Adherence Programs

In response to concerns about potential benefits and harms of Internet-based health information, the U.S. Department of Health and Human Service's Office of Disease Prevention and Health Promotion (ODPHP) convened a science panel, which issued a report in 1999 (46). Panel members unanimously agreed that of all the issues concerning the Internet as a health communication medium, the need for systematic and scientifically based evaluation of Web-based applications is one of the most critical issues that needs to be addressed, and that promoting evaluation should be a central strategy to improving application quality and effectiveness. But, despite this 1999 published report, little research has been conducted on the potential harms of using the Internet to promote health behavior (64).

Effectiveness of Self-Tailoring Versus Program Tailoring

Although recent studies have examined Web tailoring versus print and tailored web sites versus existing Web-based content, we do not have a good understanding of why tailoring on the Web may work. One question yet to be examined is whether patients prefer to seek and read only what is of interest (self-tailoring) or prefer access to a Web site that assesses their needs and delivers tailored content identified by an "expert system" as meeting those needs. One could imagine that an Internet user who has experienced frustration when trying to find a specific piece of health information would embrace a system that requires answering a few questions about information needs and then instantaneously produces tailored output. The flip side of this scenario is that the same large volumes of Web-based health content can be ideal for those who prefer to sort through information themselves and select the most relevant and salient pieces. How issues such as computer skill level, available information, search skills, and the context in which a user seeks information influence these preferences is not clear.

One study by Sutherland and colleagues has compared the impact of tailored Web-based nutrition education content to similar nontailored content available on existing high-quality Web sites (65). Participants were randomized to either a tailored program or a similar home page with selected links to credible nutrition Web sites. Health behavior change adherence was not measured in this study, but mediators known to predict behavior change and adherence—knowledge, self-efficacy, and intent to change— were influenced more significantly by the tailored Web site.

Assessing Web Site Credibility

One issue at the center of debate by patients, providers, and intervention researchers is the quality of consumer health information on the Internet. Health content has been reported to vary widely in terms of accuracy, completeness, and consistency (66–68). More than 80 studies have reported on the quality of content and Web site design characteristics for a myriad of health and medical issues (66); each has employed a different measurement for evaluating Web sites, making it virtually impossible to compare findings or draw any sound conclusions. Gagliardi and Jadad have identified 98 instruments to evaluate Web sites (69, 70). Several organizations, including the American Medical Association, National Cancer Institute, and many universities, have created patient and consumer Web site rating instruments, or guidelines (71–73). Health Web sites have also attempted to establish their credibility as providers of quality content by the adoption of "seals of approval" and "codes of conduct" created by a variety of organizations including the Council of Better Business Bureau, TRUSTe organization, Internet Healthcare Coalition, and Health on the Net Foundation (74).

So, the question remains: How do consumers determine the credibility and trustworthiness of online health information? The majority of studies examining this issue report the source of the Web site as the most important variable to determine credibility. Not surprisingly, personal physicians have emerged as the most trusted source of online health information, followed by large medical universities, and then government sources (75). Web site aesthetics and perceived "professionalism" have also been reported to increase consumer preference and influence site creditability (71)—an interesting finding given that repeated studies have found university and government sites to rate high in content accuracy, but low in usability and aesthetics (76–78). Characteristics such as education, income, health beliefs, and perceived importance of seeking health information have been found to influence which variables people use to determine online health information credibility and trust (75, 79). These differences among different Internet user groups may have far-reaching implications for delivering adherence interventions via the Internet.

CONCLUSION

For the foreseeable future, it is probably safe to assume that technology will continue to develop at the same breakneck speed of recent decades. This pace makes trying to envision the future impractical. Instead, we should focus on seeking answers to questions about current technology—assuming those answers will be applicable to future technology as well—and to making the best use of the many options available to us today.

This chapter has discussed several of these unanswered questions; let us highlight a few crucial ones here. First are the many questions raised by the "black box" of interactive technology, particularly tailoring (17). We know that tailoring often works, but many of the specifics of how, why, and under what circumstances it works best—or at all—are unknown. Without these answers, we cannot move forward to answer other questions, such as what "dose" of an intervention is most cost-effective in a given circumstance or how to apply current knowledge to move from short- to long-term adherence.

Studies to improve treatment adherence and to find the answers to these questions need to be designed to make the best use of technological options available. To do that, investigators should recognize that the latest technology is not always the easiest or most appropriate to a particular situation. New technology always has kinks that need to be worked out; in fact, currently video segments play most smoothly on CD-ROM interventions, despite the apparent promise of greater storage space on the Internet. More important, investigators should pay particular attention to the match between the proposed intervention and the type of technology. Be open to a wide range of options from no-tech (a talk with a provider) to low-tech (paper tailoring) to high-tech (CD-ROM or automated telephone system). Ultimately, the most successful adherence intervention will be the one using the technology best matched to the circumstances, rather than the one using the newest, flashiest technology.

REFERENCES

1. Kreuter M, Farrell D, Olevitch L, Brennan L. *Tailoring Health Messages, Customizing Communication With Computer Technology.* Mahwah, NJ: Lawrence Erlbaum Associates; 2000.
2. Kreuter M, Skinner C. Tailoring: what's in a name? *Health Educ Res.* 2000;15(1): 1–4.
3. Skinner CS, Strecher VJ, Hospers H. Physicians' recommendations for mammography: do tailored messages make a difference? *Am J Public Health.* 1994;84(1):43–49.
4. Strecher VJ, Kreuter M, Den Boer DJ, Kobrin S, Hospers HJ, Skinner CS. The effects of computer-tailored smoking cessation messages in family practice settings [see comment]. *J Fam Prac.* 1994;39(3):262–270.
5. National Cancer Institute. *SEER Incidence 1973–1996.* Surveillance, Epidemiology, and End Results Program, Division of Cancer Control and Population Sciences, 1999.
6. Skinner CS, Sykes RK, Monsees BS, Andriole DA, Arfken CL, Fisher EB. Learn, share, and live: breast cancer education for older, urban minority women. *Health Edu Behav.* 1998;25(1):60–78.
7. Campbell MK, DeVellis BM, Strecher VJ, Ammerman AS, DeVellis RF, Sandler RS. Improving dietary behavior: the effectiveness of tailored messages in primary care settings. *Am J Public Health.* 1994;84(5):783–787.
8. Brinberg D, Axelson M. Increasing the consumption of dietary fiber: a decision theory analysis. *Health Educ Res.* 1990;5(4):409–420.
9. Brug J, Steenhuis I, van Assema P, de Vries H. The impact of a computer-tailored nutrition intervention. *Prev Med.* 1996;25(3):236–242.
10. Brug J, Glanz K, Van Assema P, Kok G, van Breukelen GJ. The impact of computer-tailored feedback and iterative feedback on fat, fruit, and vegetable intake. *Health Educ Behav.* 1998;25(4):517–531.
11. Marcus BH, Emmons KM, Simkin-Silverman LR, et al. Evaluation of motivationally tailored vs. standard self-help physical activity interventions at the workplace. *Am J Health Promotion.* 1998;12(4):246–253.

12. Rimer BK, Halabi S, Sugg Skinner C, et al. The short-term impact of tailored mammography decision-making interventions. *Patient Educ Counsel.* 2001; 43(3):269–285.

13. Rimer BK, Halabi S, Skinner CS, et al. Effects of a mammography decision-making intervention at 12 and 24 months. *Am J Prev Med.* 2002;22(4):247–257.

14. Champion V, Skinner C, Menon U, Seshadri R, Anzalone D, Rawl S. Comparisons of tailored mammography interventions at two months postintervention. *Ann. Behav. Med.* 2002;24(3):211–218.

15. Champion VL, Maraj M, Hui S, Perkins AJ, Tierney W, Menon U, Skinner CS. Comparison of tailored interventions to increase mammography screening in non-adherent older women. *Prev. Med.* 2003;36(2):150–158.

16. Meldrum P, Turnbull D, Dobson HM, Colquhoun C, Gilmour WH, McIlwaine GM. Tailored written invitations for second round breast cancer screening: a randomised controlled trial. *J Med Screen.* 1994;1(4):245–248.

17. Miller S, Bowen DJ, Campbell MK, et al. Current research promises and challenges in behavioral oncology: Report from the American Society of Preventive Oncology annual meeting. *Cancer Epidemiol, Biomarkers Prev.* In press.

18. Ryan EL, Skinner CS. Risk beliefs and interest in counseling: focus-group interviews among first-degree relatives of breast cancer patients. *J Cancer Educ.* 1999; 14(2):99–103.

19. Kreuter MW, Skinner CS, Steger-May K, Holt CL, Bucholtz DC, Cark EM, Haire-Joshu D. Responses to behaviorally vs. culturally tailored cancer communications among African American women. *American Journal of Health Behavior.* 2004;28(3):195–207.

20. Dijkstra A, De Vries H, Roijackers J. Long-term effectiveness of computer-generated tailored feedback in smoking cessation. *Health Educ Res.* 1998;13(2): 207–214.

21. Lukwago SN, Kreuter MW, Bucholtz DC, Holt CL, Clark EM. Development and validation of brief scales to measure collectivism, religiosity, racial pride, and time orientation in urban African American women. *Fam Community Health.* 2001; 24(3):63–71.

22. Kreuter M. *Computer-Tailored Interventions for Health Behavior Change.* St. Louis, MO: Midwest Nursing Research Soicety; 2004.

23. Skinner CS, Schildkraut JM, Berry DA, et al. Pre-counseling education materials for BRCA testing: does tailoring make a difference? *Genet Test.* 2002;6(2):93–105.

24. Skinner CS. *Computer-Tailored Interventions for Health Behavior Change.* St. Louis, MO: Midwest Nursing Research Society; 2004.

25. Campbell MK, Carbone E, Honess-Morreale L, Heisler-Mackinnon J, Farrell D, Demissie S. Development and evaluation of a multimedia tailored nutrition education program for women. *Journal of Nutrition Education and Behavior.* 2004; 36(2):58–66.

26. Sutherland LA, Campbell M, Ornstein K, Wildemuth B, Lobach D. Development of an adaptive multimedia program to collect patient health data. *Am J Prev Med.* 2001;21(4):320–324.

27. Lobach D, Hasselblad V, Wildermuth B. Evaluation of a tool to categorize patients by reading literacy and computer skill to facilitate the computer-assisted patient interview. In: Musen M, ed. *AMIA 2003 Proceedings*. Philadelphia: Hanley & Belfus, Inc; 2003:391–395.

28. Petty R, Cacioppo J. Issue involvement can increase or decrease persuasion by enhancing message-relevant cognitive responses. *J Pers Soc Psychol.* 1979;31(10): 1945–1926.

29. Buchanan A, Skinner C, Rawl S, et al. Patient's interest in discussing cancer risk and risk management with primary care physicians. *Patient Educ Counsel.* In press.

30. Robinson TN, Patrick K, Eng TR, Gustafson D. An evidence-based approach to interactive health communication: a challenge to medicine in the information age. Science Panel on Interactive Communication and Health. *JAMA.* 1998;280(14):1264–1269.

31. Oenema A, Brug J, Lechner L. Web-based tailored nutrition education: results of a randomized controlled trial. *Health Educ Res.* 2001;16(6):647–660.

32. Marshall AL, Leslie ER, Bauman AE, Marcus BH, Owen N. Print versus website physical activity programs: a randomized trial. *Am J Prev Med.* 2003;25(2):88–94.

33. Hyman DJ, Herd JA, Ho KS, Dunn JK, Gregory KA. Maintenance of cholesterol reduction using automated telephone calls. *Am J Prev Med.* 1996;12(2):129–133.

34. Piette JD, McPhee SJ, Weinberger M, Mah CA, Kraemer FB. Use of automated telephone disease management calls in an ethnically diverse sample of low-income patients with diabetes. *Diabetes Care.* 1999;22(8):1302–1309.

35. Friedman RH, Stollerman JE, Mahoney DM, Rozenblyum L. The virtual visit: using telecommunications technology to take care of patients. *J Am Med Inform Assoc.* 1997;4(6):413–425.

36. Friedman RH, Kazis LE, Jette A, et al. A telecommunications system for monitoring and counseling patients with hypertension. Impact on medication adherence and blood pressure control. *Am J Hypertens.* 1996;9(4 Pt 1):285–292.

37. Delichatsios HK, Friedman RH, Glanz K, et al. Randomized trial of a "talking computer" to improve adults' eating habits. *Am J Health Promotion.* 2001;15(4): 215–224.

38. King A, Friedman R, Marcus B, Napolitano M, Castro C, Forsyth L. *Increasing regular Physical Activity Via Humans or Automated Techonogy: The CHAT Trial.* Salt Lake City, UT: Society of Behavioral Medicine; 2003.

39. Pinto BM, Friedman R, Marcus BH, Kelley H, Tennstedt S, Gillman MW. Effects of a computer-based, telephone-counseling system on physical activity. *Am J Prev Med.* 2002;23(2):113–120.

40. Jarvis KL, Friedman RH, Heeren T, Cullinane PM. Older women and physical activity: using the telephone to walk. *Womens Health Issues.* 1997;7(1):24–29.

41. Ramelson HZ, Friedman RH, Ockene JK. An automated telephone-based smoking cessation education and counseling system. *Patient Educ Counsel.* 1999;36(2): 131–144.

42. Bertakis KD, Franks P, Azari R. Effects of physician gender on patient satisfaction. *J Am Med Womens Assoc.* 2003;58(2):69–75.

43. Delgado DH, Costigan J, Wu R, Ross HJ. An interactive Internet site for the management of patients with congestive heart failure. *Can J Cardiol.* 2003;19(12): 1381–1385.

44. Abel E, Painter L. Factors that influence adherence to HIV medications: perceptions of women and health care providers. *J Assoc Nurses AIDS Care.* 2003;14(4): 61–69.

45. Moyer CA, Stern DT, Dobias KS, Cox DT, Katz SJ. Bridging the electronic divide: patient and provider perspectives on e-mail communication in primary care. *American Journal of Managed Care.* 2002;8(5):427–433.

46. Health SPoICa. *Wired for Health and Well-Being: The Emergence of Interactive Health Communication.* In: Eng T, Gustafson DH, eds. Washington, DC: U.S. Department of Health and Human Services, U.S. Government Printing Office; 1999.

47. Silk KR, Yager J. Suggested guidelines for e-mail communication in psychiatric practice. *J Clin Psychiatry.* 2003;64(7):799–806.

48. Taylor H. Cyberchondriacs update. *The Harris Poll,* no. 21, vol. 2003; 2002.

49. Fox S, Raine L. *How Internet Users Decided What Information to Trust When They or Their Loved Ones Are Sick.* Pew Internet & American Life Project Survey, March 1–31, 2002.

50. Interactive H. Patient–physician online communication: many patients want it, would pay for it, and it would influence their choice of doctors and health plans. *Health Care News.* 2002;2:1–3.

51. Interactive H. New data show Internet, website, and email usage by physicians all increasing. *Health Care News.* 2001;8:1–3.

52. Hobbs J, Wald J, Jagannath YS, et al. Opportunities to enhance patient and physician e-mail contact. *Int J Med Inf.* 2003;70(1):1–9.

53. Patt M, Houston T, Jenckes M, Sands D, Ford D. Doctors who are using e-mail with their patients: a qualitative exploration. *J Med Internet Res.* 2003;5(2):e9.

54. Sittig D. Results of a content analysis of electronic messages (email) sent between patients and their physicians. *BMC Med Inform Decis Mak.* 2003;3(1):11.

55. Stewart M, Brown J, Donner A, et al. The impact of patient-centered care on outcomes. *J Fam Pract.* 2000;49:796–804.

56. Gustafson DH, McTavish FM, Boberg E, et al. Empowering patients using computer based health support systems.[see comment]. *Quality in Health Care.* 1999;8(1):49–56.

57. Brennan PF, Moore SM, Smyth KA. The effects of a special computer network on caregivers of persons with Alzheimer's disease. *Nurs Res.* 1995;44(3):166–72.

58. Kinzie MB, Schorling JB, Siegel M. Prenatal alcohol education for low-income women with interactive multimedia. *Patient Educ Counsel.* 1993;21(1–2):51–60.

59. Scheerhorn D. Creating illness-related communities in cyberspace. In: Street R, Gold W, Manning T, eds. *Health Promotion and Interactive Technology: Theoretical Applications and Future Directions.* Mahwah, NJ: Lawerence Erlbaum Associates; 1997.

60. Smaglik P, Hawkins RP, Pingree S, Gustafson DH, Boberg E, Bricker E. The quality of interactive computer use among HIV-infected individuals. *J Health Commun.* 1998;3(1):53–68.

61. Gustafson DH, Wise M, McTavish FM, et al. Development and pilot evaluation of a computer-based support system for women with breast cancer. *J Psychosoc Oncol.* 1993;11:69–93.

62. Potts HW, Wyatt JC. Survey of doctors' experience of patients using the Internet.[comment]. *J Med Internet Res.* 2002;4(1):e5.

63. Pittenger DJ. Internet research: an opportunity to revisit classic ethical problems in behavioral research. *Ethics & Behavior.* 2003;13(1):45–60.

64. Smith R. Almost no evidence exists that the Internet harms health [see comment]. *BMJ.* 2001;323(7314):651.

65. Sutherland LA, Campbell MK, Haines P, Wildemuth B, Viles C, Symons M. The results of an online tailored nutrition education pilot project for low income women. *JADA.* In press.

66. Purcell GP, Wilson P, Delamothe T. The quality of health information on the internet. *BMJ.* 2002;324(7337):557–558.

67. Winker MA, Flanagin A, Chi-Lum B, et al. Guidelines for medical and health information sites on the internet: principles governing AMA web sites. American Medical Association. *JAMA.* 2000;283(12):1600–1606.

68. Kunst H, Groot D, Latthe PM, Latthe M, Khan KS. Accuracy of information on apparently credible websites: survey of five common health topics. *BMJ.* 2002;324(7337):581–582.

69. Jadad AR, Gagliardi A. Rating health information on the Internet: navigating to knowledge or to Babel? [comment]. *JAMA.* 1998;279(8):611–614.

70. Gagliardi A, Jadad AR. Examination of instruments used to rate quality of health information on the internet: chronicle of a voyage with an unclear destination [comment]. *BMJ.* 2002;324(7337):569–573.

71. Eysenbach G, Kohler C. How do consumers search for and appraise health information on the World Wide Web? Qualitative study using focus groups, usability tests, and in-depth interviews. *BMJ.* 2002;324(7337):573–577.

72. Bader JL, Strickman-Stein N. Evaluation of new multimedia formats for cancer communications. *J Med Internet Res.* 2003;5:e16.

73. Eysenbach G, Powell J, Kuss O, Sa ER. Empirical studies assessing the quality of health information for consumers on the world wide web: a systematic review. *JAMA.* 2002;287:2691–2700.

74. Wilson P. How to find the good and avoid the bad or ugly: a short guide to tools for rating quality of health information on the internet. *BMJ.* 2002;324(7337): 598–602.

75. Dutta-Bergman M. Trusted online sources of health information: differences in demographics, health beliefs, and health-information orientation. *J Med Internet Res.* 2003;5(3):e21.

76. Biermann J, Golladay G, Greenfield M, Baker L. Evaluation of cancer information on the Internet. *Cancer.* 1999;86(3):381–390.

77. Kunst H, Khan KS. Quality of web-based medical information on stable COPD: comparison of non-commercial and commercial websites. *Health Information & Libraries Journal.* 2002;19(1):42–48.

78. Lee CT, Smith CA, Hall JM, Waters WB, Biermann JS. Bladder cancer facts: accuracy of information on the Internet. *J Urol.* 2003;170(5):1756–1760.

79. Bernhardt JM, Lariscy RA, Parrott RL, Silk KJ, Felter EM. Perceived barriers to Internet-based health communication on human genetics. *Journal of Health Communication.* 2002;7(4):325–340.

Chapter 18

Conclusion

Hayden B. Bosworth
Morris Weinberger
Eugene Z. Oddone

LESSONS LEARNED

Adherence to treatments with proven efficacy, including both medications and lifestyle, is a primary determinant of the effectiveness of treatment (1). As reviewed throughout this volume, adherence clearly and directly optimizes clinical benefit and health-related quality of life of patients with disease (secondary and tertiary prevention), as well as prevent onset of disease (primary prevention). In addition, higher rates of adherence confer direct economic benefits by, for example, reducing costs associated with acute exacerbations of disease (e.g., hospitalizations, emergency department visits, expensive treatments). Indirect savings may result by enhancing patients' quality of life and decreasing workdays lost to illness. When adherence programs are combined with regular treatment and disease-specific education, significant improvements in health-promoting behaviors, cognitive symptom management, communication, and disability management have been observed.

Despite these benefits, adherence is often far from optimal; this is especially true for lifestyle behaviors where, for example, poor diet and lack of exercise contribute to the growing obesity epidemic. The evidence is clear that we require large-scale, multidisciplinary studies that rigorously evaluate innovative, behaviorally sound, multicomponent interventions in different service delivery environments. Interventions that promote adherence can help reduce the schism between the clinical efficacy of interventions and their effectiveness.

The authors of this volume have reviewed the considerable amount of empirical, descriptive research that has identified correlates and predictors of treatment adherence. It is clear that there are few consistent demographic characteristics associated with nonadherence. Rather, investigators should focus on factors consistently associated with adherence, including the complexity and duration of treatment, characteristics of the illness, iatrogenic effects of treatment, costs of treatment, and interactions among patients with practitioners and other sociological factors. And, these interventions must overcome patient-related barriers: adherence such as forgetfulness; psychosocial stress; anxieties about possible adverse effects; low motivation; inadequate knowledge and skill in managing the disease symptoms and treatment; lack of self-perceived need for treatment; lack of perceived effect of treatment; negative beliefs regarding the efficacy of the treatment; misunderstanding and nonacceptance of the disease; disbelief in the diagnosis; lack of perception of the health risk related to the disease; misunderstanding of treatment instructions; lack of acceptance of monitoring; low treatment expectations; low attendance at follow-up, or at counseling, motivational, behavioral, or psychotherapy classes; hopelessness and negative feelings; frustration with health care providers; fear of dependence; anxiety over the complexity of the drug regimen; and feeling stigmatized by the disease (2).

Despite evidence to the contrary, there continues to be a tendency to focus on patient-related factors as the causes of problems with adherence, to the relative neglect of the various provider, and health system, community, and policy determinants (see chap. 13, this volume). In terms of providers, clear, accurate communication and involving the patient in the decision-making process is essential. When patients participate in their health care planning, they are more likely to assume responsibility for it and are therefore more likely to adhere to their regimen.

Another clear lesson gleamed from the book is that the health systems must evolve to improve treatment adherence. The health care system, for example, directs appointment length and providers report that their schedules do not allow time to adequately address adherence behaviors (3). Health care systems determine whether telephone communication (4) and/or self-management support (5–8) are reimbursed; both may be pragmatic, cost-effective strategies for improving treatment adherence. The health care system often determines fee structures, as well as whether services such as patient counseling and education are reimbursed. Health care systems determine continuity of care and patients demonstrate better adherence behavior when they receive care from the same provider over time (9).

METHODOLOGICAL ISSUES

Methodological issues related to treatment adherence are provided throughout this book. One lesson is the need to consider the reasons for dropout when estimating treatment adherence. Patients who drop out for reasons related to the treatment need to be distinguished (i.e., experience adverse events) from those who discontinue participation because of the study itself. Anstrom et al. (chap. 15, this volume) provide an excellent and informative example and description of the implications of assumptions associated with the way drop out and nonadherence is addressed in studies. In addition to having implications for estimating the efficacy and effectiveness of adherence interventions, factors involved in dropping out have cost implications for the trial (see chap. 14, this volume).

Much current research depicts adherence as an "all-or-none phenomenon" rather than a continuum of multidimensional behaviors along a normalized spectrum. However, as with many complex human behaviors, treatment adherence may be viewed as a relative term that spans the full spectrum from full adherence to complete nonadherence. It is more reasonable to assume that adherence is normally distributed. Most people adhere to medical regimens to some incomplete extent (the larger area under the curve), and fewer people exhibiting full adherence or complete nonadherence (at either end of the curve). Various factors (e.g., regimen complexity, side effect profile, etc.) may shift the curve to the left or right. For example, inordinately complex regimens would likely shift the curve in such a way that fewer individuals would be likely to fully adhere to the prescribed regimen at any given time; successful adherence strategies would likely shift the curve in the opposite direction.

Another methodological issue concerns the link between adherence and outcomes, which may be conceptualized in multiple ways. Kravitz et al. (10) present four alternative models of the relationship between adherence and outcomes (Fig. 18.1). In the on–off model, which may be applicable to highly active antiretroviral therapy, benefit is negligible unless adherence approaches 100%. In the linear and curvilinear models, benefit increases with increasing adherence, as might be the case with antihypertensive therapy. In the threshold model, benefit is limited below a certain threshold and maximal or near maximal above the threshold. For example, aspirin will not prevent myocardial infarction if taken once a month, but because of the ability of aspirin to inhibit platelet aggregation for a full 7 days—it might be highly effective if taken once a week.

With the realization that full adherence is probably not a realistic expectation for the majority of individuals under most circumstances, some experts suggest that less than complete adherence should be considered acceptable if the desired outcome can still occur (11). However, determining

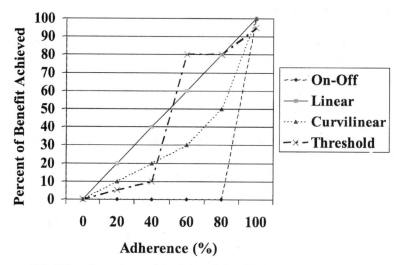

FIG. 18.1.   Alternative models of the relationship between adherence and outcomes. (10)

what constitutes the threshold at which treatment adherence will result in a therapeutic/deleterious effect is not well established for most medical conditions (12). Complicating this problem is that this threshold may change over time. For example, adherence to only 3 days of antibiotic therapy for sinusitis would at one time have been defined as very poor adherence, until a randomized controlled trial demonstrated equivalent outcomes between 3 days and 10 days of antibiotic therapy for sinusitis (13). Lack of adherence to daily antituberculosis medication led to a revised, less frequent, regimen and a new method for delivering it: directly observed therapy. Consistent performance of what was previously defined as "partial" adherence has led to better adherence (14). Nevertheless, closer examination of the growing body of evidence related to medical adherence will bring us one step closer to a fuller understanding of this important and ubiquitous health care problem, and perhaps one step closer to a solution.

INTERVENTIONS

Although there are ample interventions available to improve adherence to medical regimens, the adherence problem continues to persist. One reason involves the implementation of these interventions. There has been a tendency to focus on single strategies (rather than multiple components) that focus on patient-related factors (rather than provider or system interventions). Authors of this volume suggest that no single intervention targeting patient behavior is effective and the most promising methods of improving adherence behavior use a combination of the strategies such as, patient education, behavioral skills, self-rewards, social support, telephone follow-up, self-monitoring, goal setting, behavioral rehearsal, corrective feedback, behavioral contracting, and relapse prevention (15–17). Thus, the field of treatment adherence research is ready for practitioners to tailor scientifically based adherence interventions to the development stage of the patient. For example, in a recent systematic review of the effectiveness of interventions to increase adherence to blood pressure–lowering medication, the authors conclude that it "would seem logical that future studies should try to adopt a tailored approach aimed at patients" and addresses barriers to adherence (18). As interdisciplinary expertise is brought to bear on developing scientifically based policy for addressing the developmental aspects of adherence and managing care, the gaps in the understanding of the nonadherence should begin to close. However, a remaining stumbling block is a lack of understanding what occurs in the "black box." As interventions become more complex, there will be an increasing need to assess not only study outcomes, but the processes involved in changing the particular behavior.

Because providers have such a significant role in initiating and maintaining patient adherence, designing interventions to influence their behavior seems a reasonable strategy. However, few investigations of this subject have been reported in the literature or translated into practice (see chaps. 12 and 16, this volume). As these authors clearly point out, changing providers' behavior and getting them to accept evidence-based practices can be a real challenge, but is required to improve outcomes and adherence to prescribed regimens.

In addition to tools and strategies, providers need further education on patient adherence including graduate/medical education and continuing education for those in the workforce. Such educational training would ideally provide information on patient adherence and tools for optimizing treatment adherence (35). Though new technology and innovative strategies hold out powerful hope for improving patient adherence, several practical suggestions made by the authors offer more immediate help to providers trying to optimize patient adherence. First, providers need to assess the potential for nonadherence with every patient contact. Providers can examine previous refill patterns if available and look at responsiveness to the treatment regimen. Second, providers can elicit feedback from patients about their experience with the treatment regimen. For example, do the patients believe in the value of the prescribed treatment regimen? Are they having difficulty affording their dietary regimen? Are they experiencing side effects? Third, when problems or barriers are found, providers can help the patient problem solve. Fourth, providers can make, whenever possible, the regimen less complex. Use once-a-day rather than twice-a-day dosing regimens; suggest the use of diaries or PDA-based programs for self-monitoring performance (e.g., diet, exercise). Fifth, providers can involve the patient's support system and allow significant others to gain an understanding of the patient's condition and health care needs. Sixth, with certain chronic diseases and/or age-related cognitive declines, providers should remember that nonadherence to a treatment regimen may develop gradually over time. Finally, patients' choice of whether or not to adhere to a particular treatment regimen is the patient's right.

QUESTIONS FOR FUTURE RESEARCH

Useful research into treatment adherence should take into account a wide range of approaches to enquiry, including qualitative and quantitative research methods. Further studies should be designed with the following aims:

- Define the theoretical models that underlie interventions to promote adherence to treatment therapies.
- Describe patterns of adherence (e.g., patients who take their medication sporadically, those who regularly take less than prescribe, and those who discontinue it completely).
- Identify time points in the treatment at which different types of adherence strategy may have increased impact.
- Determine the efficacy and cost-effectiveness of specific interventions to improve adherence, as part of a complex health intervention necessary to achieve a high rate of treatment success.
- Examine how multicomponent strategies may interact to improve treatment adherence.

The concept of adherence is likely to continue to change as proponents of patient-centered care argue that helping patients to become more informed and involved in their care leads to better clinical outcomes and is the right thing to do (19, 20). Under this philosophical change, the goal of the provider is then not to badger the patient into submission, but rather to engage the patient as a partner in a therapeutic alliance. Providers should be sure that patients understand the consequences of nonadherence and, when possible, address any medical, social, and emotional factors that undermine adherence (10). This position means we will need new metrics that indicate not only whether the patient follows providers' recommendations, but also whether the patient performs behaviors that maximize his or her own personal utilities.

REFERENCES

1. The World Health Report. *Reducing Risks, Promoting Healthy Life.* Geneva: World Health Organization; 2002.
2. World Health Organization. *Adherence to Long-Term Therapies: Evidence for Action.* Geneva: World Health Organization; 2003.
3. Ammerman AS, DeVellis RF, Carey TS, et al. Physician-based diet counseling for cholesterol reduction: current practices, determinants, and strategies for improvement. *Prev Med.* 1993;22(1):96–109.
4. Haynes RB, McKibbon KA, Kanani R. Systematic review of randomised trials of interventions to assist patients to follow prescriptions for medications. *Lancet.* 1996;348(9024):383–386.
5. Wheeler JR, Janz NK, Dodge JA. Can a disease self-management program reduce health care costs? The case of older women with heart disease. *Med Care.* 2003;41(6):706–715.
6. Schermer TR, Thoonen BP, van den Boom G, et al. Randomized controlled economic evaluation of asthma self-management in primary health care. *Am J Respir Crit Care Med.* 2002;166(8):1062–1072.
7. Gallefoss F, Bakke PS. Cost-benefit and cost-effectiveness analysis of self-management in patients with COPD—a 1-year follow-up randomized, controlled trial. *Respir Med.* 2002;96(6):424–431.
8. Lorig KR, Ritter P, Stewart AL, et al. Chronic disease self-management program: 2-year health status and health care utilization outcomes. *Med Care.* 2001; 39(11):1217–1223.
9. Meichenbaum D, Turk DC. *Facilitating Treatment Adherence: A Practitioner's Guidebook.* New York: Plenum Press; 1987.
10. Kravitz RL, Melnikow J. Medical adherence research: time for a change in direction? *Med Care.* 2004;42(3):197–199.
11. Matsui D. Drug compliance in pediatrics: clinical and research issues. *Pediatr Clin North Am.* 1997;44(1):1–14.
12. Rapoff M, Barnard MU. Compliance with pediatric medical regimens. In: Cramer JA, Spiker B, eds. *Patient Compliance in Medical Practice and Clinical Trials.* Philadelphia: Lippincott, Williams, & Wilkins; 1991:73.
13. Williams JW Jr., Holleman DR Jr., Samsa GP, Simel DL. Randomized controlled trial of 3 vs 10 days of trimethoprim/sulfamethoxazole for acute maxillary sinusitis. *JAMA.* 1995;273(13):1015–1021.
14. Chaulk CP, Kazandjian VA. Directly observed therapy for treatment completion of pulmonary tuberculosis: Consensus Statement of the Public Health Tuberculosis Guidelines Panel. *JAMA.* 1998;279(12):943–948.

15. Roter D, Hall JA, Merisca R, Nordstrom B, Cretin D, Svarstad B. Effectiveness of interventions to improve patient compliance: a meta-analysis. *Med Care.* 1998; 36(8):1138–1161.

16. Miller N, Hill MN, Kottke T, Ockene IS. The multilevel compliance challenge: recommendations for a call to action. A statement for healthcare professionals. *Circulation.* 1997;95:1085–1090.

17. Haynes RB, McDonald H, Garg AX, Montague P. Interventions for helping patients to follow prescriptions for medications. *Cochrane Database Syst Rev.* 2002(2):CD000011.

18. Schroeder K, Fahey T, Ebrahim S. How can we improve adherence to blood pressure–lowering medication in ambulatory care?: systematic review of randomized controlled trials. *Arch Intern Med.* 2004;164(7):722–732.

19. Greenfield S, Kaplan S, Ware JE Jr. Expanding patient involvement in care. Effects on patient outcomes. *Ann Intern Med.* 1985;102(4):520–528.

20. Stewart M, Brown JB, Donner A, et al. The impact of patient-centered care on outcomes. *J Fam Pract.* 2000;49(9):796–804.

Author Index

Subject Index

Note: Page numbers in *italic* refer to figures; those in **boldface** refer to tables.